FACIAL FRACTURES

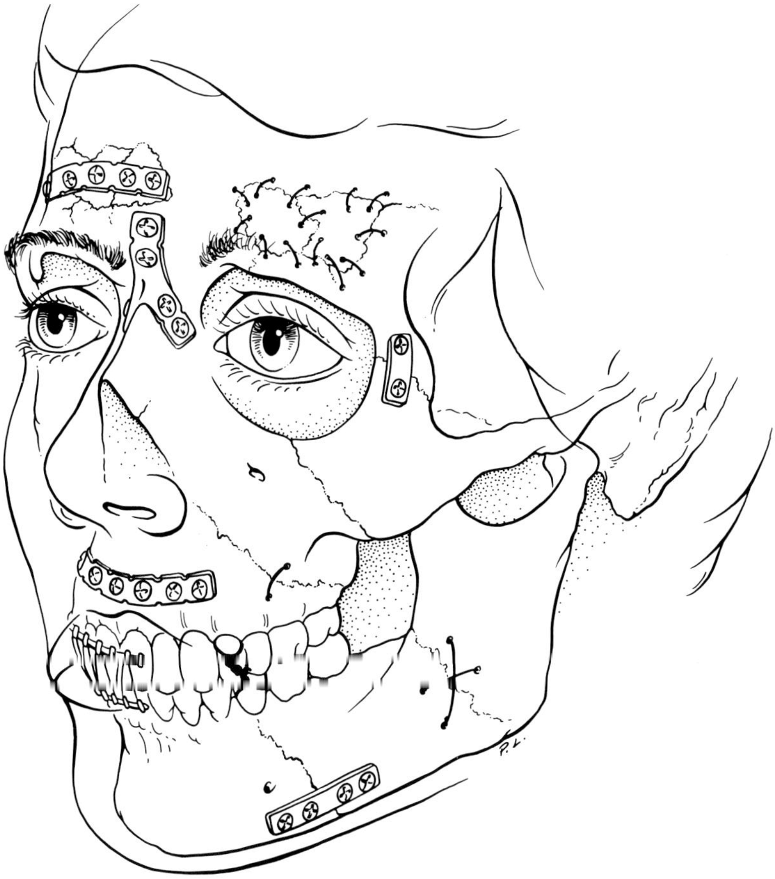

Yesterday and Today

Frontispiece depicts progress in the treatment of facial fractures. Plates and screws (*left*) have replaced the wire loops (*right*) once used for internal fixation.

FACIAL FRACTURES

MUTAZ B. HABAL, M.D., F.R.C.S.C., F.A.C.S.

Director, Tampa Bay Craniofacial Center
Human Resources Institute
University of South Florida
Clinical Professor of Surgery and Adjunct Professor of Material Science
University of Florida
Research Professor, University of South Florida
Tampa, Florida

STEPHAN ARIYAN, M.D., F.A.C.S.

Professor of Surgery and Chief
Division of Plastic Surgery
Yale University School of Medicine
Attending Plastic Surgeon, Yale-New Haven Hospital
New Haven, Connecticut

1989

B.C. Decker Inc • Toronto • Philadelphia

Publisher	**B.C. Decker Inc** 3228 South Service Road Burlington, Ontario L7N 3H8		**B.C. Decker Inc** 320 Walnut Street Suite 400 Philadelphia, Pennsylvania 19106
Sales and Distribution			
United States and Possessions	**The C.V. Mosby Company** 11830 Westline Industrial Drive Saint Louis, Missouri 63146	Asia	**Info-Med Ltd.** 802–3 Ruttonjee House 11 Duddell Street Central Hong Kong
Canada	**The C.V. Mosby Company, Ltd.** 5240 Finch Avenue East, Unit No. 1 Scarborough, Ontario M1S 5P2	South Africa	**Libriger Book Distributors** Warehouse Number 8 "Die Ou Looiery" Tannery Road Hamilton, Bloemfontein 9300
United Kingdom, Europe and the Middle East	**Blackwell Scientific Publications, Ltd.** Osney Mead, Oxford OX2 OEL, England	South America	**Inter-Book Marketing Services** Rua das Palmeriras, 32 Apto. 701 222–70 Rio de Janeiro RJ, Brazil
Australia and New Zealand	**Harcourt Brace Jovanovich Group (Australia) Pty Limited** 30–52 Smidmore Street Marrickville, N.S.W. 2204 Australia		
Japan	**Igaku-Shoin Ltd.** Tokyo International P.O. Box 5063 1–28–36 Hongo, Bunkyo-ku, Tokyo 113, Japan		

NOTICE

The authors and publisher have made every effort to ensure that the patient care recommended herein, including choice of drugs and drug dosages, is in accord with the accepted standards and practice at the time of publication. However, since research and regulation constantly change clinical standards, the reader is urged to check the product information sheet included in the package of each drug, which includes recommended doses, warnings, and contraindications. This is particularly important with new or infrequently used drugs.

Facial Fractures

ISBN 1–55664–084–6

Library of Congress catalog card number: 88–72037

10 9 8 7 6 5 4 3 2 1

To our wives
Randa and Sandy
and to our children

CONTRIBUTORS

STEPHAN ARIYAN, M.D., F.A.C.S.

Professor of Surgery, Yale University School of Medicine; Attending Plastic Surgeon, Yale-New Haven Hospital, New Haven, Connecticut
Airway Management

RONALD M. BARTON, M.D.

Assistant Professor of Surgery, Department of Plastic Surgery, Vanderbilt University School of Medicine; Chief, Section of Plastic Surgery, Veterans Administration Hospital, Nashville, Tennessee
Evaluation of the Patient with Facial Fractures

GREGORY L. BORAH, D.D.S., M.D.

Assistant Professor of Surgery, Division of Plastic Surgery, University of Massachusetts Medical School; Director, Maxillofacial Service, University of Massachusetts Medical Center, Worcester, Massachusetts
Immediate Bone Grafting of Maxillofacial Injuries

GILA BUCKMAN, M.D.

Fellow, Oculoplastic Surgery, Mount Sinai Medical Center, Cleveland, Ohio
Globe Injury

PAUL R. COOPER, M.D.

Associate Professor of Neurosurgery, New York University School of Medicine, New York, New York
Head Injury

MILTON T. EDGERTON, M.D., F.A.C.S.

Professor of Plastic Surgery, University of Virginia Medical Center, Charlottesville, Virginia
Foreword

JOSEPH S. GRUSS, M.B., B.Chir., F.R.C.S.C.

Associate Professor, Department of Surgery, University of Toronto Faculty of Medicine; Head, Division of Plastic Surgery, Sunnybrook Medical Centre, Toronto, Ontario, Canada
Complex and Panfacial Fractures

MUTAZ B. HABAL, M.D., F.R.C.S.C., F.A.C.S.

Director, Tampa Bay Craniofacial Center, Human Resources Institute, University of South Florida; Clinical Professor of Surgery and Adjunct Professor of Material Science, University of Florida; Research Professor, University of South Florida, Tampa, Florida
Team Approach to Management of Trauma Victim

ROBERT A. HARDESTY, M.D.

Assistant Professor, Division of Plastic Surgery, Loma Linda University School of Medicine; Chief, Plastic Surgery, Jerry L. Pettis Memorial Veterans Hospital, Loma Linda, California
Malunion and Nonunion

IVO P. JANECKA, M.D., F.A.C.S.

Associate Professor of Otolaryngology, University of Pittsburgh School of Medicine; Co-Director, Center for Cranial Base Surgery and Chief, Division of Head and Neck Plastic Surgery, Department of Otolaryngology, Eye and Ear Hospital, Pittsburgh, Pennsylvania
Orbital Fractures

DANIEL H. JOHNSON Jr., M.D., F.A.C.R.

Clinical Associate Professor, Departments of Radiology and Otolaryngology—Head and Neck Surgery, Tulane University Medical Center, New Orleans, Louisiana
Diagnostic Imaging

LEONARD B. KABAN, D.M.D., M.D., F.A.C.S.

Professor and Chairman, Department of Oral and Maxillofacial Surgery, University of California School of Dentistry, San Francisco, California
Mandibular Fracture

HENRY K. KAWAMOTO Jr., D.D.S., M.D., F.A.C.S.

Associate Clinical Professor, Division of Plastic Surgery, UCLA School of Medicine, Los Angeles, California
Traumatic Enophthalmos

J. CAMERON KIRCHNER, M.D.

Associate Professor of Surgery (Otolaryngology), Yale University School of Medicine; Attending Physician, Yale-New Haven Hospital, and Consultant, West Haven Veterans Administration Hospital, New Haven, Connecticut
Airway Management

DONALD L. LEAKE, D.M.D., M.D., F.A.C.S.

Professor of Surgery, UCLA Schools of Medicine and Dentistry; Chief of Oral and Maxillofacial Surgery, Harbor-UCLA Medical Center, Torrance, Los Angeles, California
Maxillary Fracture

MARK R. LEVINE, M.D., F.A.C.S.

Associate Clinical Professor of Ophthalmology and Head, Section of Oculoplastic Surgery, Case Western Reserve University School of Medicine; Chief of Ophthalmology, Mount Sinai Medical Center, Cleveland, Ohio
Globe Injury

EDWARD A. LUCE, M.D., F.A.C.S.

Professor of Surgery, Division of Plastic Surgery, University of Kentucky Medical School, Lexington, Kentucky
Frontoethmoidal Fractures

JEFFREY L. MARSH, M.D., F.A.C.S.

Professor of Surgery, Plastic and Reconstructive, Washington University School of Medicine; Medical Director, Cleft Palate and Craniofacial Deformities Institute, and Children's Hospital, St. Louis, Missouri
Malunion and Nonunion

BRUCE M. McCORMACK, M.D., F.A.C.S.

Neurosurgery Resident, New York University Medical Center, New York, New York
Head Injury

J. WAYNE MEREDITH, M.D.

Assistant Professor of Surgery, Section on General Surgery, Bowman Gray School of Medicine of Wake Forest University; Trauma Director, Wake Forest University Medical Center, Winston-Salem, North Carolina
Trauma Victim Management

DOUGLAS K. OUSTERHOUT, D.D.S., M.D., F.A.C.S.

Clinical Professor of Surgery (Plastic), University of California, San Francisco; Consultant, Letterman Army Hospital, and Attending, St. Francis Memorial Hospital, Ralph K. Davies Memorial Center, and Children's Hospital of San Francisco, San Francisco, California
Pediatric Trauma: Resultant Growth Changes

JOHN H. PHILLIPS, M.D., F.R.C.S.C.

Lecturer, University of Toronto Faculty of Medicine; Active Staff, Division of Plastic Surgery, Sunnybrook Medical Centre, Toronto, Ontario, Canada
Complex and Panfacial Fractures

M. ANTHONY POGREL, M.B., Ch.B., B.D.S., F.D.S., R.C.S. (Eng), F.R.C.S. (Edin)

Assistant Professor, University of California School of Dentistry, San Francisco, California
Mandibular Fracture

IRVING M. POLAYES, D.D.S., M.D., F.A.C.S.

Clinical Professor, Plastic and Reconstructive Surgery, Yale University School of Medicine; Attending Staff, Yale-New Haven Hospital and Hospital of St. Raphael, New Haven, Connecticut
Facial Fractures in the Pediatric Patient

JEFFREY I. RESNICK, M.D.

Assistant Clinical Professor, Division of Plastic and Reconstructive Surgery, UCLA School of Medicine, Los Angeles, California
Traumatic Enophthalmos

CLARENCE T. SASAKI, M.D., F.A.C.S.

Professor of Surgery (Otolaryngology), Yale University School of Medicine; Attending Physician, Yale-New Haven Hospital, and Consultant, West Haven Veterans Administration Hospital, New Yaven, Connecticut
Airway Management

EMIL W. STEINHAUSER, M.D., D.D.S.

Full Professor in Oral and Maxillofacial Surgery; Professor and Chairman, Department of Oral and Maxillofacial Surgery, University of Erlangen-Nuremberg, Federal Republic of Germany
Miniplate Fixation

DONALD D. TRUNKEY, M.D., F.A.C.S.

Professor of Surgery, and Chairman, Department of Surgery, Oregon Health Sciences University, Portland, Oregon
Trauma Victim Management

KARIN VARGERVIK, D.D.S.

Professor, Department of Growth and Development, University of California School of Dentistry, and Adjunct Professor, Department of Surgery, University of California School of Medicine, San Francisco, California
Pediatric Trauma: Resultant Growth Changes

HENRY C. VASCONEZ, M.D., F.A.C.S.

Assistant Professor of Surgery, Division of Plastic Surgery, University of Kentucky Medical School, Lexington, Kentucky
Frontoethmoidal Fractures

ROBERT L. WALTON, M.D., F.A.C.S.

Professor of Surgery, Division of Plastic and Reconstructive Surgery, University of Massachusetts Medical School; Chairman, Division of Plastic and Reconstructive Surgery, University of Massachusetts Medical Center, Worcester, Massachusetts
Immediate Bone Grafting of Maxillofacial Injuries

PREFACE

In the immediate post–World War II era, two classic textbooks were widely held to be the "bibles" of both practicing plastic surgeons and students of plastic surgery: the first by Drs. Converse and Kazanjian, the other by Dr. Dingman. Both of these texts dealt with the popularized use of open reduction and internal fixation using wire loops. The old techniques of closed reduction, popping techniques, and simple manipulation were fading; even their most enthusiastic advocates were growing increasingly disenchanted as the results of treated patients were examined over time. Such long-term follow-up documented the findings that most of these fractures did not withstand the effects of time, mechanical stress of growth, and continuous pressure. Patients usually ended up with some type of deformity that required additional corrective surgery.

The same problems were becoming apparent with open reduction with tight wire loop fixation. Even though the tight wires were adequate for immobilization, they produced telescoping of the fragments and improper stabilization of the multiple fractures that did not stand the test of time. Then, for further improvement, two-point and three-point fixation of the fragments became very popular.

However, in the mid-1970s to early 1980s, the success of internal rigid fixation in orthopedic surgery prompted maxillofacial surgeons to develop and refine the use of miniplates and miniscrews. With the assistance of instrument companies, the Champy, Wurzburg, Luhr, Steinhouse, and Synthes systems were developed.

Through his teaching Dr. Paul Tessier single-handedly helped us to understand the fundamental principles of dissection, the basics of bone manipulation, and the steps leading to total repair and reconstruction of multiple facial fractures and post-traumatic deformities.

The extensive use of bone grafts was another major advance. Both of its cardinal principles—in the early phases the limited application of bone grafts in the immediate post-injury phase, to the subsequent total reconstruction with bone grafts in present use—represent a major advance for the trauma victim with facial injury.

These two noteworthy advances in reconstruction, together with the widespread and more precise use of computerized diagnostic imaging, led all practitioners to a more profound understanding of these forms of multiple fractures. Therefore it was inevitable that a new text would be forthcoming. We foresee the day when this book will be available as a soft-cover handbook, such that the surgeon will be able to refer to it conveniently when confronted with a difficult facial-injury patient in the emergency department.

We had hoped that Drs. Converse and Dingman would be able to advise and contribute to this text. However, the project was slow, tedious, and time-consuming and regrettably neither of them is now with us to comment on the book.

We have chosen a group of authors who are authoritative in their approaches to the problems of facial injury, and allowed them to express their opinions freely. We have also selected authors from the three "disciplines" that usually govern the treatment of facial fractures, in order to stress that the best approach is a multidisciplinary one. We believe that working in a collaborative way, surgeons will finally produce the best results in patient care. Working as adversaries often produces an unfavorable outcome and should be avoided at any cost.

Dr. Milton Edgerton has witnessed all of these changes and advances, beginning with early wartime surgery and leading to the recent progress. We therefore believe that he can provide the ideal Foreword to this text.

Mutaz B. Habal, M.D., F.R.C.S.C., F.A.C.S.
Tampa, Florida

Stephan Ariyan, M.D., F.A.C.S.
New Haven, Connecticut

FOREWORD

With this new book on facial fractures, Drs. Habal and Ariyan have made a timely and useful contribution to the literature on plastic surgery.

Rapid strides have been made in recent years in the techniques of craniofacial surgery and in our resultant ability to correct problems of oculo-orbital dysfunction and deformity.

In the 1940s, plastic surgeons learned many lessons while treating the facial fractures and compound wounds of World War II soldiers. In the 1950s, they applied these principles to the correction of congenital craniofacial defects. This wartime experience also improved surgeons' abilities to resect safely massive cancers of the oropharynx and maxillofacial region. To expose the cancer, the cranial cavity was opened deliberately and the brain gently retracted and protected. Tumors encroaching on the base of the skull, the orbits, and the ethmoid regions could then be resected safely with adequate margins. Many patients so treated remained free of disease in the years that followed.

Even more importantly, the wartime experience taught plastic surgeons how to do immediate reconstructions of defects created by the removal of large malignant tumors. That approach to the treatment of advanced head and neck cancer has become almost standard in the years that have followed. Morbidity has gone down while cure rates have improved. We learned that we could safely remove the bone (and at times even the dura and portions of the brain) at the base of the skull, if immediate soft tissue reconstruction were accomplished.

During the 1960s, as surgical confidence grew in the use of craniofacial techniques, surgeons in Europe and in the United States began to find ways to correct the complex congenital deformities of hypertelorism, Crouzon's and Apert's diseases, Treacher-Collins syndrome, craniosynostosis, rare facial clefting, and hemifacial microsomias. Children with these and other challenging problems showed combined growth disturbances of both skeletal and soft tissue components of the craniofacial region.

The results obtained in treating these major deformities have been so promising that we now have a new subspecialty of craniofacial surgery. At least a half dozen centers currently treat a steady stream of patients undergoing corrections of these rare and difficult congenital problems.

Now the wheel has turned full circle. The recent breakthroughs, learned from treating *congenital* deformities, are now being used to add finesse and safety to the care of patients with injuries from auto accidents and other forms of *trauma*.

Drs. Habal and Ariyan and their co-authors have told that story in this new book. Dr. Habal's experience with craniofacial techniques and Dr. Ariyan's extensive background in surgery for head and neck cancer make them synergistic in bringing together many of the most useful new principles in managing facial fractures.

Early chapters give excellent perspective and background. They do not neglect the general evaluation of the total patient. The initial priorities of cardiac function, open upper airway, and fluid and electrolyte resuscitation are correctly stressed.

The modern tertiary medical center must have a well-coordinated team of specialists if it is to handle patients with major trauma properly. The plastic surgeon, neurosurgeon, otolaryngologist, oral surgeon, and ophthalmologist must all know when to call on their fellow specialists for additional help. The orthopedic, thoracic, vascular, or general surgeon may be simultaneously needed to manage injuries that do not involve the head and neck. Dr. Habal outlines an excellent plan for smooth teamwork.

What is the role of computed tomographic scans and magnetic resonance imaging in the diagnosis and treatment of facial fractures? When is three-dimensional computed imaging of value? Are these just expensive methods of providing documentation of the injury? Do these tests serve only to delay treatment? Or do they, in some instances, materially alter the timing and nature of surgical treatment? The authors of several chapters address this issue. Surgery must be of top quality, but it also must be cost effective.

Throughout history, the treatment of fractures in all parts of the body has improved as more exacting diagnosis and repositioning of fracture fragments have been combined with more stable and secure fixation of the bony parts. This progressive improvement in results has also been seen in the treatment of facial fractures.

Membrane facial bone is very thin, and it requires ingenious methods of fixation, but it tolerates loss of soft tissue attachments and it seems to resist absorption when used after a fracture as a free graft. These advantages have spawned a whole generation of mini-bone plates and self-locking screws to help the surgeon "rebuild Humpty-Dumpty again". Drs. Gruss, Luce, Janecka, Leake, Kaban, Pogrel, Marsh, and Ousterhout all describe their favorite methods of bone fixation. The reader will find many of their points persuasive and may wish to choose a little something from each menu. Dr. Emil Steinhauser has provided a particularly useful overview on the total subject of miniplate fixation.

When should a surgeon consider primary bone grafting in reducing a facial fracture? Should the paranasal sinuses be drained routinely (or never)? Will fractures in the facial bones of children be followed by growth arrest of those bones? How can one prevent late telecanthus with a fracture of the nasoethmoid complex? When may arch bars *not* be used in treating mandibular fractures? For the answer to these and other fascinating questions, please stay tuned to the chapters that follow in this book.

Dr. Kawamoto points out methods of late correction of enophthalmos, diplopia, and other orbital dystopias. Plastic surgeons have known for thirty years that residual diplopia after a facial fracture may sometimes be corrected by reconstructions of the bony orbit. Surprisingly, the ophthalmology literature says very little about this possibility. This chapter ideally will encourage ophthalmologists to send more patients with late diplopia to a craniofacial center. Evidence is clear that many of them will gain improved eye function with orbital reconstruction.

I believe *Facial Fractures* to be a thoroughly modern book. The authors of the various chapters do not all agree with one another as to the exact best method for treatment of any particular fracture. The reader will find different priorities, but the authors of each chapter are experienced surgeons with high standards of excellence. The principles advanced are sound, and those who carefully read this book will find that they have learned quite a bit about—facial fractures!

Milton T. Edgerton, M.D., F.A.C.S.
Craniofacial Surgery Center
The University of Virginia
Medical Center
Charlottesville, Virginia

CONTENTS

1

EVALUATION OF THE PATIENT WITH FACIAL FRACTURES

RONALD M. BARTON, M.D.

HISTORICAL PERSPECTIVE

The Smith papyrus, written in the 16th century B.C. and one of the earliest medical documents known, contains descriptions of facial fractures. It accurately details the physical findings of patients with nasal and mandibular fractures and prescribes treatments, many points of which are valid today. The Egyptians recognized the value of splinting, elevation of the head to decrease edema, and the treachery of infected fractures.

The school of Hippocrates during the 5th and 4th centuries B.C. taught the procedure for reducing a displaced fracture of the mandible and provided detailed written instruction on the methods required for splinting using elaborate bandaging techniques. They were also aware of the elements required to produce proper occlusion and that bandages must be applied carefully so as to not displace the fracture.[1]

Our present concept of intermaxillary fixation dates back to the Middle Ages which produced the first description of binding the jaws together.[2] Because metallic arch bars did not exist, the physicians used silk threads to establish occlusion.

The use of internal splints for fractures of the mandible became popular in the early 19th century. The materials designed for intraoral use were often crude and suffered from the fact that they placed too much pressure on the mucosa. The use of gutta percha allowed the early surgeons and dentists to customize the splint to fit the patient more precisely. Gunning, in the mid 1800s, was one of the first to take dental impressions from which vulcanized rubber splints were made.

Periods of armed conflict among nations, as tragically devastating as they have been, stimulated surgical advances in the care of maxillofacial injuries. During World War I facial injuries were of epidemic proportion. Blair[3] states that more than 3,000 of the 8,000 facial wounds incurred by American soldiers were fatal. Among the leading causes of death were aspiration and airway obstruction during transport to medical facilities. This led to the development of airway splints and the abandonment of transporting patients in the supine position. Difficulties in treating maxillofacial injuries were due to the great delay between time of injury and appropriate medical treatment (often days to weeks) and the lack of trained physicians close to the battlefront,[4] which resulted in wound sepsis in nearly all patients. Because open reduction of fractures often resulted in further loss of tissue, surgeons relied on achieving dental occlusion using splints, bandages, and interdental wiring.

Secondary reconstruction of mandibular defects was accomplished by using pedicle bone grafts from the mandible and grafts from the tibia, rib, and ilium. Ivy and Eby[5] reported experience with 103 grafts of which 77 percent were judged successful by the fact that bony continuity was achieved. Hayes[6] described a similar series using tibial and rib grafts with a 65 percent success rate. The basic principles he followed were: (1) elimination of sepsis before grafting, (2) use of aseptic surgical techniques, (3) avoidance of oral communications, (4) firm splinting for segments, and (5) no general anesthesia if intermaxillary fixation was necessary.[4]

The care of maxillofacial injuries during World War II had advanced greatly, owing in part to the introduction of antibiotics, the availability of blood and blood products for resuscitation, and the ability to administer general anesthesia safely. During the preantibiotic era, wounds were routinely left open awaiting delayed primary closure or contraction. In the 1940s wounds could be safely closed up to 24 hours after injury. The use of corticocancellous bone grafts increased the success rate of bony reconstruction.

The common use of open technique and internal fixation in the treatment of facial fractures dates back to the 1940s. Prior to that time maxillofacial surgeons manipulated and held fracture fragments with towel clips, Kirschner wires, or by blind packing of the maxillary sinus. Gillies and others developed techniques whereby the fracture was approached indirectly using incisions in the temporal scalp, but direct visualization of the fracture site was not employed.

Lothrop[7] in 1906 described his use of an incision in the buccal sulcus to approach a fracture of the maxilla. He then opened the sinus through the fracture site or an antrostomy, and by manipulating the fragment with various instruments was able to achieve reduction and good results in six patients. This was the first report of use of the antral approach for reduction of maxillary fractures. For most surgeons during the first half of this century, however, the results were often unpredictable and frequently led to poorly reduced fractures and contour irregularities.

Dingman[8] in 1939 described the use of rubber bands between the mandible and maxilla to reduce displaced fractures of the maxilla and establish occlusal relationships. This was the development of a technique first reported by Tucker in 1852. In a related report Fry and colleagues[9] described the use of intermaxillary fixation and splints to maintain proper occlusion between the mandible and maxilla.

Adams,[10] in a classic publication in 1942, was the first to propose using the open approach and internal wire fixation in the treatment of displaced facial fractures. His technique involved wire fixation of the orbital rims and closed reduction of the lower midface fracture, with position maintained by suspension wires. Although this method simplified the care of patients with these fractures, his method was not widely accepted until after World War II.

Advances in the postwar period have involved improvements in the diagnosis of fractures with the introduction of tomography and computerized tomographic (CT) scans. Surgeons began to take a more active approach to fracture fixation: use of stainless steel and then Vitallium plates has increased the stability, and early bone grafting has appeared to improve the results in extensive midface fractures.[11,12]

INITIAL EVALUATION

The first priority in the evaluation of patients with severe facial trauma is assessment of the airway. Midfacial fractures often result in significant edema extending posteriorly into the nasopharynx, eliminating the nasal airway. Because of the rich vascular supply to this area, bleeding is often severe and may result in limitation of direct vision of the area of injury, pulmonary aspiration, and fatal hypovolemic shock. Mandibular fractures may further compromise the airway. If bilateral anterior fractures have occurred, the tongue loses its support and may prolapse posteriorly, compromising the airway. Teeth and alveolar segments may be fractured and displaced into the pharynx, causing obstruction.

Ideally the examiner, with an assistant providing exposure, examines the oral cavity, removing broken teeth, dentures, or clots that could be causing obstruction. Adequate suction is necessary for clearing the airway of blood and allowing full examination to determine the sources and extent of bleeding. If the tongue prolapses into the pharynx causing obstruction, traction may be exerted by placement of a suture or use of a towel clip. Posteriorly displaced fractures of the mandible may be reduced in the emergency room, which adds a measure of stability to the floor of the mouth and possibly prevents airway compromise. As a temporizing measure, circumdental wires may be used to stabilize this mandibular segment until definitive repair is undertaken. This will also reduce the pain associated with movement at the fracture; however, there is a risk of loosening and displacing teeth with this maneuver.

Tracheostomy or intubation should be an early consideration in the management of patients with severe mid- or lower facial fractures. Associated head, spinal cord, or thoracic trauma with the consequent need for controlled respiration often argues for immediate control of the airway. Patients who will be transferred to another hospital must have their airway assured before leaving the primary facility. Tracheostomy should be performed under the most controlled circumstances possible, usually in the operating room with adequate lighting, instruments, and the invaluable assistance of an anesthesiologist. Many disasters have occurred when this procedure was relegated to the most junior member of the trauma team, to be performed alone in the emergency room.

Patients with either soft-tissue injury or facial fractures may bleed to death. This fact often goes unrecognized until the patient is in shock. The volume of blood lost is difficult to quantitate; there is blood lost at the scene of the accident and en route to the emergency room, some is swallowed, and large amounts can be absorbed in dressings. The scalp laceration is one of the most common sources for exsanguinating hemorrhage (Fig. 1–1). The laceration often transverses the main trunk or a first order branch of the superficial temporal or occipital arteries. There is a tendency to place a "compression" head dressing on the patient in hopes of controlling the bleeding instead of inspecting the wound. Often a well-placed suture or hemostat will save several hundred milliliters of blood before definitive repair is undertaken.

Severe bleeding from the nose occurs infrequently, usually less than 5 percent in reported series. It should be first evaluated by direct inspec-

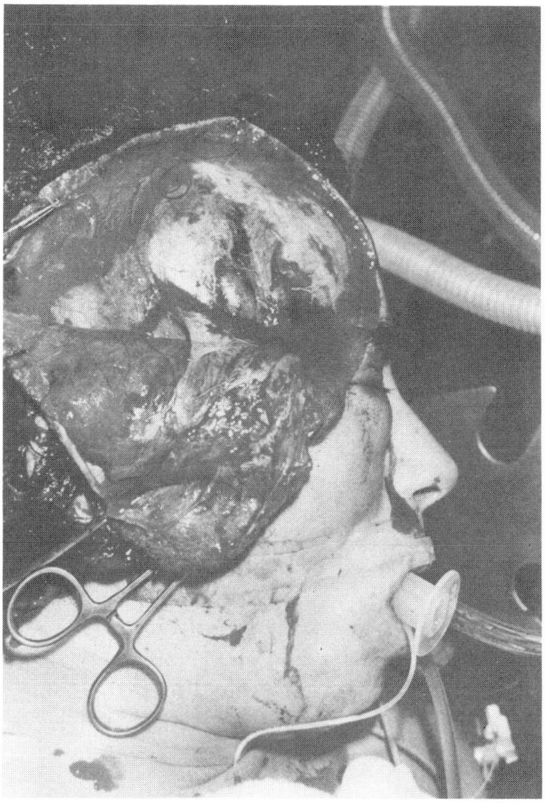

Figure 1–1 Patient with life-threatening hemorrhage from scalp laceration.

tion using a nasal speculum and adequate suction. Discrete bleeding from small vessels can be controlled by suture or cauterization. More severe nasal hemorrhage can be treated by anterior and posterior nasal packs. These are placed by first passing a catheter through the nose into the nasopharynx. The end is retrieved through the mouth and a gauze pack fastened to a withdrawal tape is attached to the catheter and positioned in the posterior nasal cavity by withdrawing the catheter from the nose. The anterior nasal cavity is then packed through the nose, tamponading the bleeding point between the two packs. A closed space is thus created which is prone to infection. These packs should be removed at the first sign of abscess formation or toxicity in the patient.

Massive hemorrhage, usually resulting from severe displacement of midface fractures of the Le Fort type, may require operative reduction and stabilization of the fracture to control the bleeding. Potentially fatal hemorrhage may also result from fractures of the base of the skull with damage to the cavernous sinus or other large vessels. Direct ligation of major vessels has proven effective under certain circumstances. Ligation of the external carotid artery will decrease blood flow to tissues inferior to the turbinates. However, the anterior ethmoid artery, a branch of the internal carotid, supplies bone and soft tissue cephalad to this and may have to be ligated through the medial orbital approach. Ligation of the internal maxillary artery is possible using the transantral approach.

Neurologic evaluation should include all cranial nerves and should be performed as soon as possible in the emergency room before soft-tissue edema makes findings difficult to interpret. The cause of cranial nerve injury (usually limited to the first seven nerves) may either be direct trauma to the periphery or damage to the central nervous system with stretching of the nerve roots.

Patients with fractures involving the naso-ethmoid complex will often suffer anosmia, a fact that is often overlooked until the convalescent phase of injury. The association of facial trauma with loss of the sense of smell was reported as early as 1864 by Jackson.[13] In a series of more than 4,000 patients studied by Zusho and colleagues[14] in 1980, the total incidence of smell disturbances was 3.5 percent, of which 20 percent were transient and 80 percent were permanent. These percentages were reversed by Sumner,[15] who has also noted a correlation between the area of injury and the incidence of anosmia: a 5 percent incidence in patients with frontal trauma, 13 percent with parietal trauma, and 28 percent with injury to the occipital area. In this study, however, there were five times as many patients with frontal as occipital trauma.

Although blindness as a result of facial fractures is uncommon, visual acuity should be carefully documented. Because most facial fractures do not require immediate fixation, there is time to obtain consultation from the ophthalmology service, and injuries involving the optic nerve may require prompt action. I obtain such consultation in all patients with mid- and upper facial fractures who cannot be thoroughly evaluated, who have an obvious injury to the orbital contents, or who have abnormal visual acuity. In addition, because of the risk of injury to the globe and optic nerve during fracture treatment, it is prudent to record any visual loss preoperatively from a legal as well as a medical standpoint. The surgeon should be aware of case reports in which blindness[16] or disk edema[17] was the result of fracture reduction. It is also possible for vision to improve following fracture reduction, and I have seen such a case, although the vision was not completely restored to normal postoperatively.

The oculomotor nerve divides into superior

and inferior branches, the former supplying the superior rectus and levator palpebrae superioris muscles, the latter supplying the medial and inferior rectus and inferior oblique muscles. Each can be tested individually as can the trochlear nerve, which supplies the superior oblique muscle, and the abducens nerve, which supplies the lateral rectus muscle. Differentiation between nerve injury and muscle entrapment will be discussed later.

The facial nerve is rarely injured in fractures without soft-tissue laceration. Muller[18] has reported that 11 percent of displaced mandibular fractures result in damage to the marginal branch of the facial nerve. However, weakness of the muscles of facial expression can result from a neurapraxia. The nerve may also be injured secondary to fractures of the temporal bone and facial canal. Again, it is wise to document any abnormality of facial nerve function, particularly since the marginal mandibular branch is at risk when fractures of the mandible are explored through an external approach.

The infraorbital nerve is frequently damaged in fractures of the orbital floor or at its foramen with zygomatic complex fractures. The resulting decrease or absence of sensation of the cheek, lip, and alveolar mucosa is often one of the most bothersome complaints patients voice. Hypoesthesia in this area is a valuable clinical finding indicating fracture, although contusion resulting in neurapraxia will produce similar findings.

Anesthesia in the distribution of the supraorbital nerve may indicate a fracture of the frontal sinus or supraorbital rim. When associated with cerebrospinal fluid leakage, a fracture of the posterior wall of the frontal sinus, cribriform plate, and ethmoid sinuses should be suspected.

Damage to the inferior alveolar nerve resulting in numbness of the lower lip is a common finding in mandibular fractures. It suggests a fracture occurring between the mandibular foramen on the medial surface of the ramus and the mental foramen. The nerve may either be contused, stretched, or lacerated. If contused, sensation may be expected to return in a few months.

Associated Injuries

Because trauma victims may have multiple injuries of varying severity, the trauma team, composed of members from all surgical specialties, is usually coordinated by a general surgeon. It is his or her responsibility to determine the acuity of all injuries and to establish a logical list of priorities in the treatment plan. Frequently facial injuries are relegated behind neurosurgical, thoracic, and abdominal concerns. Nevertheless, the maxillofacial surgeon should be responsible for ensuring that facial injuries receive prompt and appropriate treatment to prevent long-term functional and cosmetic loss.

The most damaging injuries that occur in association with maxillofacial trauma are to the central nervous system. In an analysis of 6,173 fractures of the facial skeleton, Lentrodt[19] reported a 22 percent incidence of cerebral concussion, the group with the highest incidence being those with midface and combined fractures.

Gwyn and colleagues[20] have reviewed a large series of hospitalized patients with facial fractures and found that 19 percent had a life-threatening injury such as head injury or hemorrhagic shock. Tracheostomy for airway obstruction was required in 2.3 percent, and 1.4 percent sustained a severe pulmonary injury. Other fractures occurred in approximately 20 percent of patients. Eye injuries resulting in blindness occurred in 3.4 percent.

Associated injuries in a group of patients with nasoethmoid fractures have also been described. Sixty-three percent had severe nonfacial injuries, with 51 percent incurring central nervous system trauma and 24 percent chest trauma. This group also had a high incidence of other facial fractures, with 94 percent having orbital floor/rim fractures, 72 percent having a Le Fort fracture, and 27 percent having a mandibular fracture. A motor vehicle was involved in 31 of the 33 cases reported.

The cause of facial fractures varies widely among reported series; however, the leading causes in large urban centers are motor vehicle accidents and interpersonal violence. Both are capable of inflicting damage not isolated to the facial skeleton.

Roentgenographic Examination

After a thorough history and physical examination, roentgenographic evaluation of the patient with suspected facial fracture is usually indicated. This should be done in a timely fashion with thorough consultation of the radiologist, which includes relevant details of the patient's medical condition and the possibility of airway compromise. Often a member of the surgical team should be present to monitor the patient and ensure that the radiographs taken demonstrate or rule out the suspected fracture.

The justifications for complete x-ray evaluation are many:

1. Fractures that may ordinarily be palpated are often obscured by soft-tissue swelling.

2. Some fractures, such as those in the subcondylar and ethmoid areas, may be difficult to palpate even without soft-tissue edema.
3. The degree of displacement is often impossible to judge accurately by physical examination.
4. The design of models and the fabrication of splints is aided by accurate x-ray films.
5. Foreign bodies and fractured tooth roots are better demonstrated by x-ray evaluation.
6. Clinically occult fractures that demand treatment may be missed on physical examination.

Thorough and complete evaluation of the facial skeleton is the standard of care, and failure to do this may have medicolegal consequences. Good documentation of all injuries will serve both the patient and physician well and allow critical evaluation of the progress of the treatment plan. Many patients will have a history of previous injuries that could have resulted in facial fractures. A review of pertinent roentgenograms may disclose old fractures and possibly save the patient an unnecessary operation.

Because of the frequent association of facial fractures with fractures of the skull and cervical spine, evaluation of these areas is usually warranted. Because of the positioning requirements for many of the facial x-ray films, cervical spine films should take precedence. Skull fractures may also warrant neurosurgical evaluation before a full complement of facial x-ray films is taken.

The Waters view is a posteroanterior projection of the facial skeleton with the patient in the prone position with the neck extended. The purpose of this view is to project the orbits, zygomatic arches, and maxillary sinus against the relatively homogeneous area of the posterior skull. Fractures of the orbital rims, lateral maxillary walls, and zygomatic arches are usually identified.

The reverse Waters view is useful if the patient cannot be placed in the prone position, such as after a cervical spine fracture. In this projection the patient is kept supine and the x-ray film placed under his head. The anteroposterior direction of the x-ray beam is tilted in a cephalad direction, again to project the orbital rims and maxillary sinuses against the posterior skull.

The Caldwell view is a posteroanterior projection in which the beam is nearly parallel to the skull base. It is useful in outlining fractures of the frontal sinus and the lateral walls of the maxillary sinuses.

The submentovertex view positions the patient supine with the head elevated and the neck arched. The beam projects an axial representation of the skull with the zygomatic arches outlined.

The Towne's view is an anteroposterior view with the x-ray beam tilted 30 degrees downward. This projects the ascending rami and subcondylar areas of the mandible.

Oblique views of the mandible are useful in demonstrating fractures through the parasymphyseal, body and angle areas. Often the rami are superimposed, which can make fracture definition in these areas more difficult. Other views such as the posteroanterior projection, can define fractures of the rami and the symphysis. Occlusal views with the x-ray film held between the patient's jaws examine the anterior arch of the mandible and can outline the mental symphysis.

The orthopantomograph or pantographic view employs an x-ray tube that pivots around a seated patient to obtain a 180-degree perspective of the mandible from condyle to condyle. It is useful in examination of the entire mandible and allows the surgeon to gain an appreciation of the orientation and placement of multiple fractures (Fig. 1–2). There is representation of cephalocaudal displacement of fracture fragments but little in the mediolateral direction.

Investigation of the mandibular condyles and fossae is often difficult and may be inconclusive by standard methods. Use of tomograms or CT scan may be necessary to define fractures in this area.

ORBITAL FRACTURES

Orbital floor fractures were described in 1844 by MacKenzie.[21] In 1899, Lang[22] described the often cited account of a patient who was struck in the orbit by the shaft of a cart, which eventually resulted in enophthalmos. It was not until 1957 when Smith and Regan[23] coined the term "blowout fracture" that the entity became widely studied. Their hypothesis was that when the orbit was struck with a blunt object, such as a fist, mechanical forces were translated into "hydraulic" forces by the soft tissues of the orbit. These forces then resulted in fracture(s) of the relatively fragile orbital walls or floor, hence the term "blowout." They sought to refute the concept held by Le Fort and others that the fracture was caused by bony transmission of the force through the intact orbital rim. This study based its conclusions, in part, on cadaver dissections in which a ball was propelled toward the globe, similar to the experiments of Le Fort in the late 1800s.

The evaluation of the patient with a suspect-

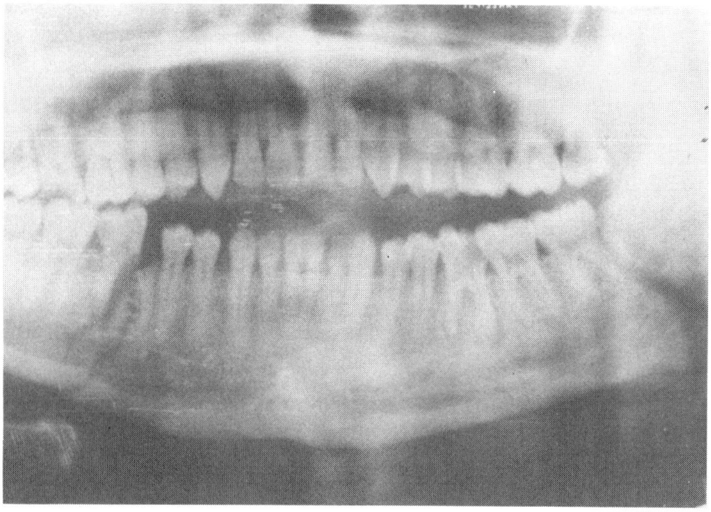

Figure 1–2 Panorex film showing left angle and right body mandibular fractures.

ed blowout fracture of the orbit should include a measure of the function of the extraocular muscles, since entrapment by the fracture fragments may be a cause of diplopia. Restriction of the inferior oblique or inferior rectus muscles will tether the globe and produce diplopia on upward gaze. Testing can be either passive—having the patient focus on an object in a particular field—or active—performing the forced duction test with the patient under local or general anesthesia. The forced duction test entails using an instrument to grasp the muscle and apply gentle traction to determine if muscle entrapment prohibits rotation of the globe in a direction opposite to the muscle's physiologic action (Fig. 1–3). Riley and Mazow[24] have described a four-step test to evaluate extraocular muscle function. It is important to differentiate causes of diplopia not caused by direct muscle entrapment, such as direct trauma to the muscle causing hematoma or edema or damage to the motor nerve. The examiner should document at what point in the field of gaze diplopia occurs. The primary field of gaze is defined as within 20 degrees of the central axis, and diplopia in this range will be much more debilitating.

Enophthalmos is posterior displacement of the globe usually caused by an increase in the orbital volume relative to the orbital contents. This may be the result of a fracture of the bony orbit with displacement of the fragments, loss of ligament (e.g., Lockwood's ligament) support, scar contracture, escape of orbital fat (most often inferiorly or medially), or necrosis of fat. Objective measurements of the degree of enophthalmos can also be made with the Hertel exophthalmometer. This device measures the position of the cornea relative to the lateral orbital rim; a difference of greater than 5 mm when compared with the normal side is significant. However, when the bony landmark is displaced, the measurement becomes unreliable. In this instance CT scan with careful and precise placement of the patient's head will enable the radiologist or surgeon to measure the position of the cornea from a fixed point, which is then compared with the normal side.

In a study by Manson and colleagues[25] the bony and soft-tissue changes occurring after orbital fracture were studied; they concluded that or-

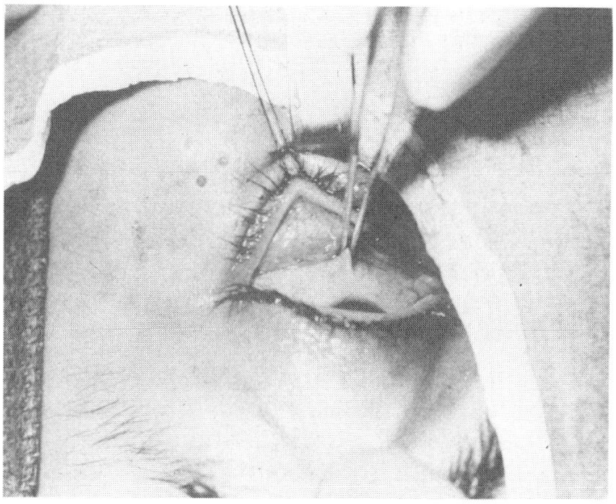

Figure 1–3 Forced duction test showing no muscle entrapment.

bital volumes increased up to 18 percent whereas fat and globe volumes did not differ significantly. Furthermore, they stated that these volume changes could be reversed following reconstruction.

The surgeon should be aware that the superomedial aspect of the orbital roof may also be damaged. If the defect is large and the dura disrupted, the brain may herniate into the orbit resulting in pulsating exophthalmos.

Traditional methods of radiologic investigation have included the standard Waters view and tomography. Converse and associates[26] recommended these techniques to locate the fracture and noted the classic "hanging drop" sign in which the prolapsed orbital contents produced an opacity when viewed against the air-filled maxillary sinus (Fig. 1–4). In a later study, Crikelair and colleagues[27] reviewed their x-ray findings and determined that routine plain films had a 47 percent error rate when compared to tomography. However, tomography had a 14 percent incidence of false positive results when their patients underwent operative exploration.

Hammerschlag and associates[28] have shown that CT scan is superior to conventional radiology in evaluation of the orbit, particularly with regard to soft tissue such as extraocular muscles. Finkle and colleagues[29] have shown the superiority of CT scan compared to clinical examination and linear tomography in fractures of the infraorbital rim, lateral wall, orbital roof, and orbital floor with accuracy approaching 90 percent. The authors cite potential advantages of CT scanning of the trauma patient, particularly when facial edema prevents accurate physical examination. They also present a case in which CT scan correctly identified herniation of the inferior rectus muscle through the orbital floor. The study of Gilbard and colleagues[30] found that those patients in whom the inferior rectus muscle appeared to be trapped on CT examination continued to experience diplopia, while all of those with a free inferior rectus had resolution of "clinically significant" diplopia.

The use of reformatting techniques as an adjunct to CT scanning can provide additional views in the coronal, sagittal, or parasagittal planes without the necessity of further scans. Reformatted images can be oriented in any direction, such as along the long axis of the orbit (Fig. 1–5). Marsh and Gado[31] have used case presentations as well as illustrations to document its utility. Such images can define specific structures such as the optic nerve and can more accurately determine if a fracture of the orbital apex is impinging on the nerve. In addition, direct measurements can be made of the position of the globe to estimate more accurately the degree of enophthalmos.

Two-dimensional CT images can also be reformatted to give three-dimensional projections of the facial skeleton (see the chapter entitled *Diagnostic Imaging*). With the current technology employing 0.5-mm sections, this can determine positional and rotational changes due to fractures. It is less useful, however, for identifying relatively nondisplaced fractures of thin bones such as the orbital floor (Lineaweaver and Barton, unpublished data).

CT scanning is not without drawbacks. It is ex-

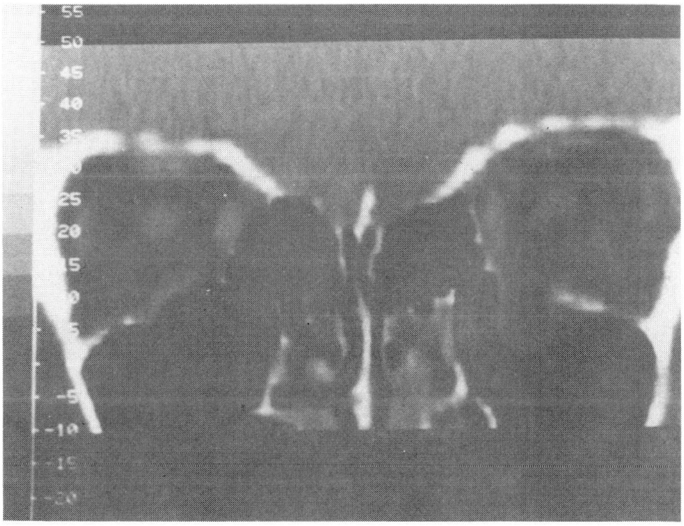

Figure 1–4 CT scan showing prolapse of orbital contents into maxillary sinus ("hanging drop" sign).

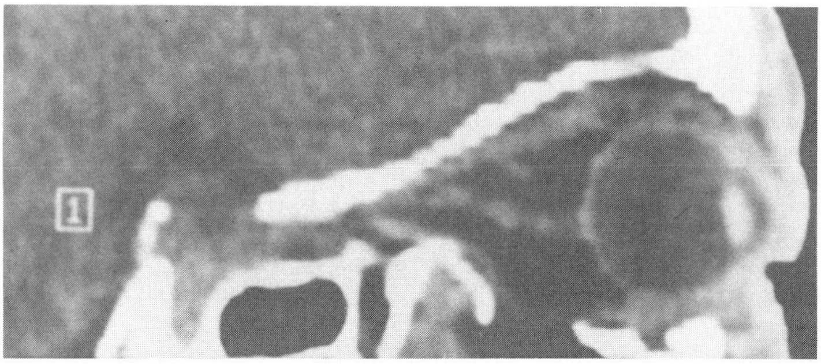

Figure 1–5 Reformatted CT scan along axis of orbit.

pensive and produces a significant radiation dose. One should be aware that cataract formation can result from more than 200 rad delivered to the lens.

Nuclear magnetic resonance has potential advantages in that it does not expose the patient to irradiation and the definition of soft-tissue detail is improved when compared to CT scans. Its use thus far in facial fractures is limited and it has yet to be determined whether it will be a useful technique.

ZYGOMATIC FRACTURES

The precise diagnosis of a zygomatic fracture is essential for its correct treatment. The difficulty encountered in diagnosis by physical examination relates to the often severe swelling of the soft tissues which may obscure the bony landmarks. Other pitfalls are mistaking a normal irregularity in the infraorbital rim or the infraorbital foramen for a displaced fracture. When subconjunctival ecchymosis is present it is indicative of a zygomatic fracture only when it extends past the limits of the observable sclera (Fig. 1–6). This is because the hemorrhage begins laterally and then dissects medially beneath the sclera. Isolated scleral hemorrhages do not indicate zygomatic fractures.

Anesthesia or hypoesthesia in the distribution of the infraorbital nerve (cheek, upper lip, and gingiva) suggests bruising or damage by bony fragments. This occurs because fractures through the inferior orbital rim often pass through the infraorbital foramen. However, similar neurologic findings can be caused by orbital blowout fractures or direct contusion of the nerve without fracture of the zygoma.

Depression of the zygomatic arch may be indicative of a zygomatic complex fracture, but not diagnostic because it can occur as an isolated fracture. Inspection and palpation of the upper buccal sulcus may reveal a bony step-off and submucosal hemorrhage secondary to fracture of the anterior/lateral wall of the maxillary sinus.

When the lines of fracture extend into the posterior orbit and involve the superior orbital fissure, a syndrome of the same name may result. With compression or laceration of the third, fourth, or sixth cranial nerve, the patient may present with ptosis of the upper eyelid, proptosis, a fixed and dilated pupil, loss of corneal reflex, and ophthalmoplegia. If the fracture involves the optic foramen with compromise of the optic nerve, the orbital apex syndrome exists.

Lines of fracture can occur in many orientations and, when combined with different rotational components, can produce an atypical clinical picture. Yanagisawa[32] has modified Rowe and Killey's[34] description of the various types of zygomatic fractures in an attempt to predict the "postreduction stability." He emphasizes that three views (Waters, submentovertical, and Caldwell) are often necessary to make the correct diagnosis.

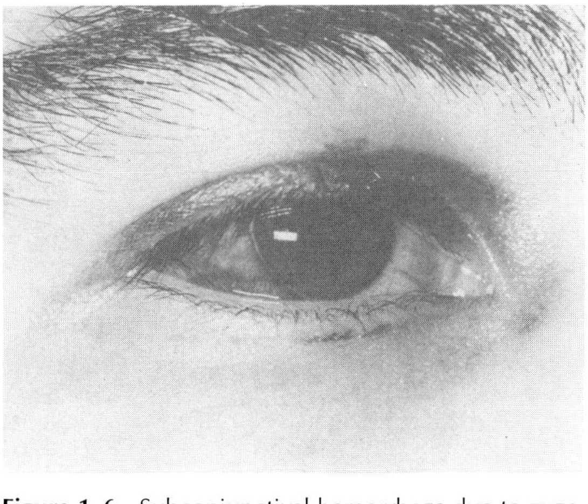

Figure 1–6 Subconjunctival hemorrhage due to zygomatic fracture.

While plain x-ray films are important as a screening test, complete reliance on them has been supplanted by the CT scan.

NASOETHMOID FRACTURES

The nasoethmoid area, consisting of the nasal bones, ethmoid sinuses, and the medial orbital walls (lamina papyracea) is vulnerable to trauma by virtue of its relative fragility and the fact that it is often fractured when the more substantial frontal and maxillary processes are injured. Because of their location adjacent to the orbits, cranium, frontal sinus, and nasal airway, untreated fractures may have serious sequelae.

In an attempt to understand better these often complex fractures, Gruss[34] has proposed a system of classification based on five types ranging from isolated nasoethmoid-orbital injury to more extensive fractures involving maxilla, cranium, orbit, or bony loss.

Fractures extending through the cribriform plate may result in anosmia, cerebrospinal fluid rhinorrhea, or central nervous system injury. Fractures of the lamina papyracea and lacrimal bone may injure the lacrimal duct and sac or may result in telecanthus by disrupting the medial canthal tendons which attach posterior to the lacrimal crest.

Often direct trauma to this area will displace this complex of thin bones posteriorly in a telescoping fashion, resulting in a midface depression which is very difficult to correct secondarily.

Physical findings of patients with nasoethmoid fractures include an acute glabellar angle due to the depressed fracture of the nasal process of the frontal bone; edema and ecchymosis in the glabellar region extending to one or usually both orbital areas; bleeding from the nose which may be significant if the ethmoid artery has been injured; and fracture of the nasal septum with dislocation and submucosal hemorrhage. If fractures have disrupted the vomer, nasal septum, and nasal process it is possible for the examiner to displace the nasal tip into the piriform aperture.

It is important to recognize the possibility of medial canthal tendon disruption early in the patient's course. This can best be accomplished by palpation of the tendon near its insertion while lateral traction is placed on the eyelids. If the tendon cannot readily be identified with a stable relationship to the medial orbit, the examiner can presume a fracture has occurred. Normal intercanthal distance is between 32 and 34 mm, and any increase should alert the examiner to the possibility of canthal disruption.

If the fracture has injured the nasolacrimal duct resulting in obstruction, the patient often complains of epiphora. This can be determined by placing a drop of fluorescein dye (1 percent) into the eye and looking for appearance of the dye at the inferior meatus beneath the inferior turbinate. This can be facilitated by placing a dry cotton swab adjacent to the meatus for several minutes and then examining the end with a Wood's lamp.

Any clear fluid from the nose should be tested immediately using a gauze sponge; samples should be sent for a determination of glucose concentration to rule out cerebrospinal fluid rhinorrhea.

FRONTAL SINUS FRACTURES

Fractures of the frontal sinus are common occurrences, comprising 8 percent of all facial fractures reported by Luce.[35] However, they are often overlooked and may result in disastrous sequelae. They are often comminuted in an eggshell fashion, and unless the fracture is associated with a laceration over the fracture line, palpation of the fracture may be obscured by soft-tissue edema. It is incumbent on the examiner to palpate carefully the underlying bone in all lacerations and to obtain appropriate x-ray films (posteroanterior, lateral, and Waters views) to rule out fractures of the anterior wall of the sinus. The presence of pneumocephalus on a lateral x-ray film is strongly indicative of a fracture of the posterior wall of the sinus.

A CT scan may be necessary to visualize fractures of the posterior table, and in the study by Luce[35] it was helpful in detecting anterior and posterior wall fractures as well as the presence of fluid in the sinus. However, CT scanning was not useful in determining the degree of displacement of the fracture fragments.

Failure to document and treat such fractures may result in a severe cosmetic deformity due to a depressed outer table fracture, mucocele, or chronic sinusitis due to a disruption of the frontonasal duct; or meningitis from a posterior table fracture with cerebrospinal fluid leak. A patient who presents with clear fluid leaking from the nose and nasoethmoid bruising or swelling should be presumed to have a posterior table fracture with laceration of the dura and cerebrospinal fluid rhinorrhea until proven otherwise.

In a review by Newman and Travis,[36] 63 frontal sinus fractures were studied in which 30 involved the anterior wall, supraorbital rims, or anterolateral sinus floor; 16 involved the nasofrontal duct; and 17 involved the posterior wall of the sinus. This study reported instances in which the examiner could palpate a fracture not shown on x-ray film and stated that frontal and lateral scout films rarely adequately defined the extent of the fracture.

Finkle and colleagues[29] have evaluated the diagnostic accuracy of various methods of evaluation in frontal sinus injuries. Clinical examination was accurate in 91 percent of patients, linear tomography in 97 percent, and CT scan in 97 percent.

NASAL FRACTURES

Because of its prominence, the nose is often fractured in facial trauma. Schultz,[37] studying a series of 1,031 consecutive facial fractures, reported that nasal fractures were the most common, comprising 37 percent of all fractures.

Examination of the nose should begin with external inspection. Often the eye is more sensitive than the palpating finger in determining small deviations. Unfortunately, this is possible only very soon after nasal trauma, as edema begins early and lasts for many days to weeks. A single light source placed directly over the patient's head will be reflected from the nasal dorsum and can be used as a guide to judge irregularities or deviation. Very few persons have a perfectly straight and symmetric nose, and careful questioning can often reveal previous facial trauma having occurred in childhood.

Palpation should start in the glabellar region and proceed distally with a gentle side-to-side movement. The finding of crepitance indicating a fracture is often subtle and usually painful. Depression in the area of the nasal root resulting in a "saddle" deformity may also indicate underlying fracture of the ethmoid complex. Often the nasal tip is rotated upward with this fracture. Bruising may extend to one or both orbits and result in subconjunctival ecchymosis beginning near the medial canthus.

Intranasal inspection requires a nasal speculum and a spotlight or headlamp. The presence of a septal hematoma requires early drainage through a small incision. Using two fingers, one can assess the position and integrity of the septum, with particular attention paid to fractures or dislocations. The normal septum rests in a groove in the nasal spine and the examiner can usually determine if a dislocation is recent or remote.

Routine lateral x-ray views of the skull or facial bones are often too penetrated, which obscures the nasal bones. It is important to specifically request nasal views in both the posteroanterior and lateral orientations.

MIDFACE FRACTURES

The diagnosis and treatment of extensive midface fractures has roots in the early 20th century. Le Fort was the first to experimentally reproduce and to categorize fractures in the human facial skeleton. He did this by subjecting the heads of cadavers to a wide variety of trauma using multiple instruments, angles of attack, and methods of support or nonsupport for the head in order to try and reproduce the clinical findings in patients.[38] This work led to a systematic classification of maxillary fractures which is still useful today. Le Fort grouped these fracture lines into three types: I (transverse, also known as the Guérin fracture), II (pyramidal), and III (craniofacial disjunction). Morgan[39] has reviewed 300 cases of midface fracture and reports the relative frequency of Le Fort fractures: I:II:III in a ratio of 7:8:1.

On examination all midfacial fractures demonstrate malocclusion and often have elongation of the midface. The trauma causing these fractures forces the maxillary fragments posteriorly and inferiorly. This forces the upper molars into premature contact with those of the mandible, resulting in an open bite. The patient appears to have a relative retrognathia. The posterior displacement of Le Fort fractures may be so severe as to obstruct the nasal airway completely and compromise the oropharynx.

Le Fort I and II fractures disrupt the periosteum anterior to the orbital septum and cause periorbital ecchymosis, particularly in the lower eyelid. The intraorbital edema resulting from type II and III fractures may cause diplopia which usually resolves spontaneously.

Mobility of the maxilla is identified by grasping the upper dental arch and gently moving it while holding the skull stable. By palpating each region of the midface in sequence, the examiner can determine the lines of fracture. Inspection of the buccal vestibule will reveal ecchymosis in type I and II fractures.

Cerebrospinal fluid leaks result from tears in the dura caused by disruptions most commonly in the cribriform plate or anterior skull base. The fractures are often associated with midface fractures, particularly of types II and III. Occasionally cerebrospinal fluid leaks manifest themselves several days after injury.

Enophthalmos may result from Le Fort II or III

fractures when the orbital volume has increased owing to separation of the fragments. In addition, these types of fractures may cause a decrease in the extraocular muscle function, deformity of the medial canthus, paresthesia of the infraorbital nerve, diplopia, and subconjunctival ecchymosis.

Steidler[40] has reviewed 240 patients with midface fractures with the following findings: loss of consciousness (62 percent); residual cerebral disturbance (15 percent); cerebrospinal rhinorrhea (33 percent of Le Fort II and 47 percent of Le Fort III); infraorbital nerve deficit (37.5 percent); anosmia (5 percent); cranial nerves II, III, VI, VII, and VIII defect (all under 2 percent), and blindness (19 cases, of which 16 were due to penetrating trauma to the globe). The authors concluded that 98 percent of patients had a satisfactory outcome with regard to occlusion following surgery.

The Le Fort classifications are merely guidelines used to identify frequent lines of midface fracture. By definition, Le Fort fractures are bilateral. However, many patients do not have fractures that meet these exact criteria; their fractures may be asymmetric, partial, or more extensive than Le Fort's original illustrations.

X-ray examination using the Waters projection will often confirm the findings on physical examination. CT scan has been extremely valuable in making precise diagnoses in complex fractures of the midface.

MANDIBULAR FRACTURES

Mandibular fractures are extremely common, with an incidence second only to nasal fractures. Reported series usually note a rate of between one-third and one-half of all facial fractures.

Examination of the mandible begins by palpation of the lower border in the midline and moves posteriorly; the examiner compares symmetry and looks for any areas of bony step-off. The condyles are best examined simultaneously with the examiner's finger either in the patient's external auditory canal or just anterior to the tragus. The patient is asked to open and close his jaw slowly while the normal anterior and inferior displacement of the condylar head is palpated. Dislocation of the condylar head will often be felt anterior to the articular eminence while the glenoid fossa is empty.

The most important aspect of the mandibular examination is evaluation of occlusion. Although it is important to ask the patient if he feels his teeth meet normally, this is not foolproof. Nor have all patients had the benefit of orthodontia, so they may not have enjoyed Class I occlusion prior to their injury. Rarely, obtaining records from the patient's dentist will give valuable clues to the patient's preinjury status. Unilateral fracture or dislocation will result in a cross-bite or displacement of the midline. Bilateral dislocations may maintain midline relationships but can result in an anterior open bite or a shift toward Class III occlusion.

Pertinent findings to look for during the intraoral examination are step-offs in the bony alveolar margin. Since most mandibular fractures communicate with the oral cavity either through lacerations or ruptures of the periodontal membrane, blood in the oral cavity without other lesions should lead the examiner to suspect a fracture. A hematoma in the floor of the mouth is almost pathognomonic of a mandibular fracture. Hematomas may also occur in the buccal sulcus and may be palpated intra- or extraorally. The cant of the occlusal plane should be noted; asking the patient to bite on a tongue depressor will provide a point of reference to compare with the maxilla. Gently trying to manipulate suspected areas of fracture will often identify the point of fracture and the interdental space involved. Anesthesia of the mucosa implies damage to the nerve. Cracked or loose teeth should also be noted; it is possible to salvage some loose teeth, while others should be extracted to prevent displacement and possible aspiration. Finally, the presence and position of wear facets will often determine the premorbid occlusion, particularly in patients who may not have had normal occlusion prior to injury.

Because the mandible, despite its articulations with the skull, does not behave like a complete ring explains why not all fractures are multiple. However, there are certain patterns of fracture occurrence which are frequently encountered, such as a body or angle fracture with a contralateral subcondylar fracture, or a (para)symphyseal fracture with bilateral subcondylar fractures.

Radiologic evaluation usually includes lateral and oblique views, Towne's view, and a panoramic radiograph. Occlusal views will define segments of the mandible and teeth in greater detail. Rarely, a clinically suspicious fracture will not be evident on conventional x-ray films. Alternatives in this situation are to repeat the radiographs in a few days (I have seen more than one fracture become apparent, possibly owing to bony absorption at the fracture site) or obtain a CT scan. Tomography has been particularly valuable in the evaluation of fractures of the condyle.

REFERENCES

1. Hoffmann-Axthelm W. The treatment of maxillofacial fractures and dislocations, in historical perspective. In: Kruger E, Schilli W, eds. Oral and max-

illofacial traumatology. Vol 1. Chicago: Quintessence Publishing, 1982:17.
2. Rowe NL. The history of treatment of maxillofacial trauma. Ann R Coll Surg Engl 1971; 49:329.
3. Blair VP. Relation of the early care to the final outcome of major face wounds in war surgery. Milit Surg 1943; 92:12–17.
4. Kelly JF. Management of war injuries to the jaws and related structures. Washington, DC: US Government Printing Office, 1977.
5. Ivy RH, Eby JD. Maxillofacial surgery. Part 2, Vol II. Washington, DC: US Government Printing Office, 1924.
6. Hayes GB, ed. Maxillofacial surgery: histories of 146 selected cases of facial wounds treated at the American Ambulance, Paris, France (1914–1917), 1920 (Unpublished)(As quoted in Kelly JF[4], p.6).
7. Lothrop HA. Fractures of the superior maxillary bone, caused by direct blows over the malar bone. A method for the treatment of such fractures. Boston Med Surg J 1906; 154:8. (As quoted in Converse JM. Reconstr Plast Surg 1977, p.713)
8. Dingman RO. Use of rubber bands in treatment of fractures of bones of face and jaws. J Am Dent Assoc 1939; 26:173–183.
9. Fry WK, Shepherd PR, McLeod AC, Parfitt GJ. The dental treatment of maxillofacial injuries. Oxford: Blackwell Scientific Publications, 1943.
10. Adams WM. Internal wiring fixation of facial fractures. Surgery 1942; 12:523–540.
11. Manson PN, Crawley WA, Yaremchuk MJ, et al. Midface fractures: advantages of immediate extended open reduction and bone grafting. Plast Reconstr Surg 1985; 76:1–10.
12. Gruss JS, Mackinnon SE. Complex maxillary fractures: role of buttress reconstruction and immediate bone grafts. Plast Reconstr Surg 1986; 78:9–22.
13. Jackson JH. Defects of smell. Clin Lect Rep Lond Hosp 1864; 1:388.
14. Zusho H, Takeuchi M, Tokita N, et al. Post-traumatic anosmia. Nippon Jibhnkoka Gakkai Kaiho 1980; 83:402.
15. Sumner D. Post-traumatic anosmia. Brain 1964; 87:107–129.
16. Gordon S, Macrae H. Monocular blindness as a complication of the treatment of a malar fracture. Plast Reconstr Surg 1950; 6:228–232.
17. Kaplan LJ. Unilateral disk edema following tripod fracture repair necessitating optic nerve decompression: case report. Plast Reconstr Surg 1982; 70:375–378.
18. Muller W. Frequency, site and causes of facial skeleton fractures. In: Reichenbach E, ed. Maxillofacial traumatology. Munich: Barth.
19. Lentrodt J. Maxillofacial injuries—statistics and causes of accidents. In: Kruger E, Schilli W, eds. Oral and maxillofacial traumatology. Vol I. Chicago: Quintessence Publishing, 1982.
20. Gwyn PP, Carraway JH, Horton CE, et al. Facial fractures—associated injuries and complications. Plast Reconstr Surg 1971; 47:225–230.
21. MacKenzie W. Traite pratique des maladies des yeux. Traduit de l'anglais avec notes et additions par S Laugier et G Richelot. Paris: B. Dusillon, 1844:vii.
22. Lang W. Traumatic enophthalmos with retention of perfect acuity of vision. Trans Ophthalmol Soc UK 1899; 9:41.
23. Smith B, Regan WF Jr. Blow-out fracture of the orbit; mechanism and correction of internal orbital fracture. Am J Ophthalmol 1957; 44:733–739.
24. Riley WB, Mazow ML. Recognition and avoidance of ocular motility pitfalls in plastic surgery. Plast Reconstr Surg 1980; 66:153–157.
25. Manson PN, Grivas A, Rosenbaum A, et al. Studies on enophthalmos: II. The measurement of orbital injuries and their treatment by quantitative computed tomography. Plast Reconstr Surg 1986; 77:203–214.
26. Converse JM, Smith B, Obear MF, Wood-Smith D. Orbital blowout fractures: a ten-year survey. Plast Reconstr Surg 1967; 39:20–36.
27. Crikelair GF, Rein JM, Potter GD, Cosman B. A critical look at the "blowout" fracture. Plast Reconstr Surg 1972; 49:374–379.
28. Hammerschlag SB, Hughes S, O'Reilly GV, et al. Blow-out fractures of the orbit: a comparison of computed tomography and conventional radiography with anatomical correlation. Radiology 1982; 143:487–492.
29. Finkle DR, Ringler SL, Luttenton CR, et al. Comparison of the diagnostic methods used in maxillofacial trauma. Plast Reconstr Surg 1985; 75:32–38.
30. Gilbard SM, Mafee MF, Lagouros PA, Langer BG. Orbital blowout fractures: the prognostic significance of computed tomography. Ophthalmology 1985; 92:1523–1528.
31. Marsh JL, Gado M. The longitudinal orbital CT projection: a versatile image for orbital assessment. Plast Reconstr Surg 1983; 71:308–317.
32. Yanagisawa E. Pitfalls in the management of zygomatic fractures. Laryngoscope 1973; 83:527–546.
33. Rowe NL, Killey HC. Fractures of the facial skeleton. Baltimore: Williams & Wilkins, 1968:276.
34. Gruss JS. Naso-ethmoid-orbital fractures: classification and role of primary bone grafting. Plast Reconstr Surg 1986; 75:303–315.
35. Luce EA. Frontal sinus fractures: guidelines to management. Plast Reconstr Surg 1987; 80:500–508.
36. Newman MH, Travis LW. Frontal sinus fractures. Laryngoscope 1973; 83:1281–1292.
37. Schultz RC. Facial injuries. Chicago: Year Book Medical Publishers, 1977:217–227.
38. Le Fort R. Etude experimentale sur les fractures de la machoire superieure. Rev Chir (Paris) 1901; 23:208–227.
39. Morgan BDG, Madan DK, Bergerot JPC. Fractures of the middle third of the face—a review of 300 cases. Br J Plast Surg 1972; 25:147–151.
40. Steidler NE, Cook RM, Reade PC. Residual complications in patients with major middle third facial fractures. Int J Oral Surg 1980; 9:259–266.

2

TRAUMA VICTIM MANAGEMENT

J. WAYNE MEREDITH, M.D.
DONALD D. TRUNKEY, M.D., F.A.C.S.

Resuscitation of the severely traumatized patient is a team effort involving surgeons, emergency physicians, anesthesiologists, nurses, and other health professionals. It is critically important that the trauma team approach the patient in an organized, logical manner, since the initial resuscitation and management of such a patient significantly affect the eventual outcome.

The exact approach to the trauma patient cannot be learned by rote but must be determined from each patient's presentation. If the patient's condition is unstable, the assessment and resuscitation must be simultaneous; if his condition remains unstable or deteriorates despite initial resuscitation measures, operation for control of hemorrhage becomes a part of the resuscitation. The trauma surgeon must orchestrate the efforts of the other team members using guidelines based upon a knowledge of the principles of treating shock and a knowledge of the order of priorities in the management of the trauma patient (Table 2–1).

INITIAL ASSESSMENT AND RESUSCITATION

The initial assessment is the same in virtually every trauma patient, regardless of how stable or unstable the patient's condition. It is designed so that one can, within a few minutes, evaluate the patient's overall condition and identify and correct immediately life-threatening conditions. Most early trauma deaths result from inadequate ventilation, shock, or severe head injury; therefore, early evaluation and resuscitation are aimed at ensuring proper ventilation, which includes an open airway and adequate breathing, whether spontaneous or mechanical. Then the trauma surgeon must ensure adequate circulation; when that is achieved, he must do a rapid neurologic examination to identify patients who must undergo early evacuation of intracranial hemorrhage. Since the primary goal of resuscitation is preservation of tissue oxygen delivery, adequate ventilation is the most important and the first order of priority in the management of the trauma patient.[1]

TABLE 2–1 Priorities in Management of the Trauma Patient

Airway and/or breathing
Cardiovascular
Pump
Volume
Hemorrhage
Neurologic
Fracture stabilization
Definitive diagnosis
Definitive treatment of injuries
Recovery
Rehabilitation

Ventilation

Adequate ventilation first requires a patent airway, and the first maneuver in establishing an airway is to clear the oropharynx. In the unconscious patient, the oropharynx is best cleared by inserting a finger in the mouth and sweeping out any clots, debris, bone fragments, teeth, or vomitus that may be present in the upper airway. In the conscious patient, one can clear most of the obvious debris by aspirating the airway with a tonsil sucker. Before deciding to intubate a patient, one should make every effort to restore the airway by lifting the angle of the mandible or pulling the tongue forward.

Insertion of a nasopharyngeal or oropharyngeal tube should be reserved for unconscious patients, since inserting these devices may induce vomiting in patients with an intact gag reflex. Most conscious patients who have respiratory effort can have an adequate airway established without intubation. Occasionally, however, a patient with a head injury or some other cause of depressed mental status (e.g., severe alcohol or drug intoxication) will require intubation and assisted ventilation. The choice between nasotracheal and orotracheal intubation requires judgment and experience. Generally, nasotracheal intubation is preferred in patients who are breathing spontaneously. Patients with extensive facial fractures or gunshot wounds of the face or larynx causing severe soft tissue injury present a particular challenge and are the type of patients in whom a surgically created emergency cricothyrotomy or tracheostomy may be needed.

After an airway has been established, one's attention must turn to ensuring adequate alveolar ventilation. Ineffective respiratory effort due to head injury or altered mental status from intoxicants requires intubation and positive-pressure ventilation. Other important causes of ineffective respiratory effort are abnormalities of the chest wall or lungs, such as open pneumothorax. For this problem, a chest tube should be inserted immediately and an occlusive dressing placed over the open site.

Circulation

The other essential element in providing adequate tissue oxygen delivery is adequate circulation. Problems that cause inadequate circulation can, in general, be categorized as pump failure or inadequate volume (Table 2–2).

Pump Failure. An easily observable indicator of pump failure in the trauma victim is distention of the neck veins. Patients with distended neck veins are likely to have tension pneumothorax, pericardial tamponade, myocardial contusions or infarction, or coronary air embolism.

The most common, easily treated, immediately life-threatening injury causing inadequate circulation due to pump failure is tension pneumothorax, which, in addition to distended neck veins, presents with tracheal shift away from the side of injury, decreased breath sounds, and decreased chest excursion on the side of the pneumothorax. Tension pneumothorax should be decompressed immediately, either by inserting a needle through the second intercostal space anteriorly or by inserting a large caliber chest tube through the fourth or fifth intercostal space in the midaxillary line. If the diagnosis is made clinically, radiographic confirmation is not necessary before insertion of the tube, and, in the unstable patient, waiting for an x-ray film is undesirable.

Pericardial tamponade is also a life-threatening emergency. The hallmark of the diagnosis is Beck's triad, which is shock, elevated central venous pressure (as manifested by distended neck veins), and muffled heart sounds. If the tamponade is secondary to penetrating trauma, there is usually an obvious injury to the chest, although the entrance wound may be in the neck, back, or abdomen. Pericardial tamponade is less common in blunt trauma, although it should be considered when the patient has a steering wheel injury or similar anterior chest trauma.

If pericardial tamponade is diagnosed before the patient is in extremis, pericardiocentesis or pericardial window drainage of the tamponade may temporarily improve the patient's hemodynamic status. Pericardiocentesis is done by inserting a needle in the subxiphoid area (Larrey's point) at a 45-degree angle, aiming it toward the left shoulder. Aspiration of as little as 20 to 30 ml of nonclotting blood can have a dramatic effect on the patient's hemodynamic status. A subxiphoid pericardial window is established by making an incision in the midline beginning over the xiphoid process and extending 8 cm inferiorly. The linea alba is incised and a substernal plane established. The pericardium is identified, grasped, and opened over a distance of 2 to 3 cm. The escape of blood associated with hemodynamic improvement confirms the diagnosis of pericardial tamponade. As a diagnostic maneuver this method provides fewer false-negative and false-positive results than pericardiocentesis,[2] and it also provides better continued drainage when used as a temporizing measure until definitive treatment can begin.[3] If the patient arrives in extremis, has cardiac arrest from tamponade, or exhibits early deterioration, immedi-

TABLE 2–2 Traumatic Shock

Cause	*Treatment*
Pump failure	
Tension pneumothorax	Decompression
Pericardial tamponade	Operation
Myocardial contusion	Inotropic support, afterload reduction
Air embolus	Occlude pulmonary hilum
Hypovolemia	
Mild	Crystalloids
Moderate	Blood
Severe	Blood, blood, blood
"Spinal shock"	Restore effective blood volume

ate emergency thoracotomy is indicated.[4] The chest should be prepared in a sterile manner if possible, but the procedure should not be delayed for that preparation if it cannot be done immediately. With the nipple as a guideline, an incision is made in the fourth intercostal space from the sternal border as far laterally as possible. A chest retractor is inserted and the wound enlarged. The pericardium is opened vertically, parallel and anterior to the phrenic nerve. The clot is removed and bleeding vessels are controlled with digital pressure or suture while the patient is resuscitated and taken to the operating room for definitive management.

Myocardial contusion and myocardial infarction are other causes for pump failure; they are more likely to follow blunt than penetrating injury. Most lethal manifestations occur shortly after injury and are often disturbances in cardiac rhythm. Dysrhythmias are treated by standard pharmacologic means and by avoiding hypoxia, acidosis, hypercarbia, and hypokalemia. The patient should have constant cardiac monitoring for the first few days. If cardiogenic shock is a problem, it is managed by inotropic support (e.g., with dopamine or dobutamine), by afterload reduction (e.g., with nitroglycerin or nitroprusside), or rarely, by intra-aortic balloon pump counterpulsation.

Coronary air embolus, a not infrequent cause of pump failure, occurs in approximately 4 percent of all patients with major thoracic trauma,[5] although it often goes unrecognized, even at autopsy.[6] Air embolism is produced by a fistula between a bronchus and a pulmonary vein following blunt or penetrating trauma, although more commonly it is the result of penetrating thoracic trauma. Diagnosis is usually based on four signs, alone or in combination: sudden cardiovascular collapse or pump failure, especially following recent intubation; direct visualization of air in the coronary circulation; the appearance of focal or lateralizing neurologic signs in a patient without head injury; and the appearance of froth when the initial blood specimen is drawn.

The mechanism for sudden cardiovascular collapse following intubation is based on simple physiologic principles. The injury causes a fistula between a bronchus and a pulmonary vein so that, upon intubation, the increase in airway pressure provides a pressure gradient, which causes air to cross the fistula into the pulmonary vein; through the pulmonary vein the air enters the left atrium and can be ejected into the coronary circulation, thereby producing ischemic cardiomyopathy and pump failure. Any patient with sudden, unexplained cardiovascular collapse, especially immediately following intubation and positive-pressure ventilation, should be assumed to have a coronary air embolus and should undergo immediately thoracotomy with cross-clamping of the pulmonary hilum.[7]

Hypovolemia. Patients who have suffered trauma and who are in shock without distended neck veins are generally suffering from hypovolemia.[1] The variables for assessing the degree of shock and the adequacy of resuscitation are outlined in Table 2–3.

Blood pressure is the time-honored variable used to ascertain the degree of shock. Unfortunately, blood pressure alone does not provide an adequate measure of the patient's volume status. Young, healthy patients can lose 15 to 20 percent of their intravascular blood volume before any change in blood pressure is detected. Elderly patients, on the other hand, who have lost some of their compensatory mechanisms, may show a decline in blood pressure with a loss of only 5 to 10 percent of blood volume. Furthermore, there is no absolute normal value for blood pressure. Some patients have perfectly adequate tissue perfusion with a systolic blood pressure of 90 mm Hg, while others may have inadequate tissue perfusion even at 120 mm Hg.

Pulse rate is a more sensitive indication of hypovolemia than blood pressure, but it too is nonspecific. Pain, anxiety, or drugs may alter the heart rate in a manner independent of the patient's volume status. Heart rate is nonetheless an important variable, and tachycardia should be regarded with some concern.

Evaluation of the patient's peripheral skin perfusion is another very helpful tool in assessing volume status. Warm, pink skin with good capillary refill indicates adequate tissue perfusion, since these signs quickly disappear in the presence of volume loss.

Another indicator of adequate tissue perfusion is maintenance of urinary output. The patient suffering major trauma should always have an indwelling urinary bladder catheter inserted unless a urethral injury is suspected. Urine outputs of

TABLE 2–3 Indices of Successful Resuscitation

Peripheral perfusion	Warm, dry, good capillary refill
Urine output	0.5–1.0 ml/kg/hr
Level of consciousness	Alert
Atrial filling pressures	
Central venous	8–12 mm Hg
Pulmonary capillary wedge	8–10 mm Hg
Cardiac index	>3 L/M²/min

0.5 to 1.0 ml per kilogram of body weight per hour indicate adequate visceral tissue perfusion.

The last indicator for assessment of adequate volume is measurement of the central filling pressures. Exact measurement is usually unavailable early in the patient's management, but a very effective tool for assessing central pressure is observing the filling status of the peripheral veins. Normal distention of peripheral veins of the feet and hands and rapid refill after stripping are good indications of adequate volume replacement. If a more precise measurement of central venous pressure is required, a central venous pressure line can be inserted. This is usually not necessary until a later phase in the management of the trauma patient.

Treatment of hypovolemia requires access to the circulatory system. The most reliable, least risky method is through peripheral intravenous catheters, most commonly large-bore 14- or 16-gauge catheters placed in each antecubital fossa. A minimum of two such catheters is necessary. If these sites are unavailable or if the upper extremity veins cannot be cannulated, we recommend cannulation of the saphenous vein through a cutdown at the ankle. An experienced surgeon can usually, within a minute or so, place an intravenous extension tube directly into the saphenous vein. Large volumes of fluid, blood, or both can then be administered rapidly through this type of access. In general, one should avoid inserting a cannula in an obviously injured extremity, or where there is injury proximal to the cannulation site. As the first intravenous line is being established, blood should be drawn for typing and crossmatching, as well as for measurement of hematocrit. Part of the specimen should be reserved for determinations of electrolytes, blood urea nitrogen, creatinine, amylase, glucose, and toxicology determinations, if indicated later. In general, 2L of balanced salt solution should be infused in the adult hypovolemic patient. The amount of fluid will vary from patient to patient and should be determined by the physiologic response to resuscitation (see Table 2–3).

Neurologic Status

The neurologic examination is an important part of the initial assessment of the trauma patient. Early or rapid deterioration of neurologic status commonly mandates prompt neurosurgical intervention. The most important sign of immediate concern is the patient's level of consciousness, which can be assessed on the basis of whether the patient is awake and alert, and whether he responds to vocal stimuli, only to painful stimuli, or is unresponsive (Table 2–4). The awake state is easily recognized and is the state of those patients who respond appropriately to questioning. The second category is broader and constitutes the group of trauma patients who, though responding sluggishly or in a confused manner, do nonetheless respond to vocal stimuli. The third category consists of those patients who do not respond to verbal stimuli but do respond to painful stimuli, either by purposeful movement to eliminate the source of pain or by abnormal posturing. Finally, there is the group of patients who make no response to verbal command or pain.

Neurologic assessments should be repeated frequently in any patient who has an altered mental status or who has obvious head, face, or neck injuries. Most treatable intracranial lesions produce a deteriorating level of consciousness, and lives may be saved by recognizing this deterioration early and treating it promptly. A more detailed neurologic examination is part of the upcoming secondary survey.

SECONDARY SURVEY

The secondary survey consists of a brief history and physical examination. The history may be obtained from the patient, his family, the paramedics, and witnesses to the traumatic episode. The history taking should be quick but comprehensive. Information should be obtained concerning the mechanisms of injury. For vehicular accidents this includes the speed and angle of the impact, the extent of damage to the vehicles, and the condition of other passengers; with penetrating trauma, this may include the caliber of a gun or the size of a knife blade. A minimal essential past medical history includes any current or past diseases, a list of all medications the patient is taking, prior operations, any allergies, and when the patient last ate.

Following the initial evaluation and institution of resuscitation, if the patient remains stable, a thorough examination of all body systems should be undertaken in an orderly manner, the goal being to search for other injuries and to gather information required to plan definitive therapy.

The secondary survey begins with the head and evaluates the scalp and all facial bones for lacerations or fractures. Pupillary size and extraocular motions should be reevaluated; the external auditory canal must be examined for hemotympanum or otorrhea. Patients with midfacial fractures who may have a fracture of the cribriform plate

TABLE 2–4 Correlation Between Clinical Signs and Level of Central Nervous System Function

Neurologic Sign	*Example*	*Anatomic Region*
Cognitive functions	Follows commands, purposeful movements	Cerebral cortex
Abnormal posturing	Flexion/extension posturing	Brainstem
Level of awareness	Spontaneous eye opening	Reticular activating system
Abnormal eye reflexes	Corneal reflex	Pons, CN V, VII
	oculocephalic or oculo-vestibular	Pons, CN VIII, VI
Vital functions	Breathing	Medulla, CN III

CN = cranial nerve

should not undergo nasogastric or nasotracheal intubation, since the result might be inadvertent intracranial intubation.

While in-line traction is applied, the cervical spine should be examined for tenderness, pain, and deformity.

In the noisy emergency room, examination of the chest is often best performed visually searching for areas of flail and for proper and symmetric chest expansion. One can commonly palpate the crepitation of fractured ribs or subcutaneous emphysema. In the responsive patient, gentle sternal pressure or gentle lateral compressive force applied at both midaxillary lines should indicate the presence or absence of rib fractures. The chest should be auscultated for symmetry and quality of breath sounds, for distant heart sounds, for pericardial friction rub, and for new murmurs, which could indicate valvular or septal disruption. The chest radiograph is an essential part of the evaluation of the chest and is the only radiograph that is absolutely required before the patient is taken to the operating room.

Although examination of the abdomen is fraught with inexactitude in the blunt trauma patient, the abdomen must nonetheless be examined carefully for evidence of intra-abdominal injury. The examiner must remember that the abdominal contents extend as high as the fifth intercostal space above the costal margin. Pelvic stability should be evaluated and a good rectal examination performed: during the latter one should palpate for a high-riding or mobile prostate gland in the male patient and at the same time evaluate sphincter tone.

The extremities are then examined for contusions, deformity, pain, or crepitus.

An in-depth neurologic evaluation, including assessment of the Glasgow Coma score (Table 2–5), cranial nerves, muscle strength, reflexes, and sensory function, should then be performed.

DEFINITIVE DIAGNOSIS

If the patient's condition is stable, those injuries that have been identified or suspected during the primary and secondary surveys should be confirmed by the appropriate diagnostic technique, generally some sort of radiographic study. However, in the unstable patient, the only radiograph required before the patient is taken to the operating room for control of hemorrhage is the chest x-ray film. Evidence of a widened mediastinum requires arteriography to rule out traumatic disruption of the aorta. Persistent pneumothorax unrelieved by chest tube insertion requires bronchoscopy.

TABLE 2–5 Glasgow Coma Scale

A. Eye opening	
Spontaneous	4
To voice	3
To pain	2
None	1
B. Verbal response	
Oriented	5
Confused	4
Inappropriate words	3
Incomprehensible words	2
None	1
C. Motor response	
Obeys commands	6
Localizes pain	5
Withdraws	4
Flexion posturing	3
Extension posturing	2
None	1
Glasgow Coma Score = A + B + C	

After the chest x-ray film, the next films to be obtained in the stable patient with blunt trauma are those needed for evaluation of the cervical spine. In general, an alert, awake, and cooperative patient will have pain or tenderness in the neck if there is a significant cervical spinal injury. In the absence of these findings, a technically adequate lateral x-ray film that evaluates all seven cervical vertebrae down to the top of T-1 and a satisfactory anteroposterior cervical spinal film should suffice. In patients with suspected head injury, computed cranial tomography (CCT) should be performed if the patient later is going to be unavailable for clinical evaluation, for example undergoing general anesthesia for management of fractures or chest or abdominal injuries. Patients with altered or deteriorating mental status should undergo urgent CCT in an attempt to find a surgically correctable lesion.

The abdomen can be evaluated by diagnostic peritoneal lavage or abdominal CT scan. Peritoneal lavage is performed after making an incision 4 to 5 cm long below the umbilicus. The linea alba is divided, the peritoneum is grasped, a small catheter is directed into the pelvis, and the abdomen is lavaged with lactated Ringer's solution (1 L in adults). This fluid is then aspirated and evaluated for red blood cells, white blood cells, and chemical composition[8] (Table 2–6). In the stable patient, one may elect to perform abdominal CT rather than diagnostic peritoneal lavage. This study provides quantitative and qualitative information and also a better evaluation of the retroperitoneum than does lavage.

A patient with gross hematuria, flank injury, or microscopic hematuria associated with hypotension should be evaluated for renal trauma. This may be accomplished by obtaining a "single shot" intravenous pyelogram after injection of 50 ml of Renografin, or by abdominal CT. As many as 10 percent of pelvic fractures are associated with bladder rupture, and as many as 5 percent with urethral injury. Thus, the patient with pelvic fractures should also have anteroposterior and oblique films obtained after instillation of at least 300 ml of Cystografin into the bladder through a Foley catheter.[7] This must be preceded by a urethrogram in any patient with blood at the urethral meatus or in whom the Foley catheter meets any resistance during its insertion.

TABLE 2–6 Criteria for Positive Peritoneal Lavage

Gross blood on initial aspiration
More than 100 RBC/mm^3
More than 500 WBC/mm^3
Presence of bile, bacteria, or vegetable matter
Efflux of irrigant from Foley catheter or chest tube

RBC = red blood cell, WBC = white blood cell

In the stable patient, any long bones believed to be fractured should be evaluated radiographically. Open fractures should be washed, irrigated, and covered with a clean, sterile dressing before the patient is taken to the operating room for definitive therapy.

DEFINITIVE THERAPY

The first priority in managing injuries should be evacuation of epidural and subdural intracranial bleeding causing increased intracranial pressure. If the head injury is associated with hemorrhage or shock, two surgical teams may be necessary, one to address the head injury and the other to address the hemorrhage elsewhere. The decision whether to operate on chest or abdominal injuries first should be based on the most likely site of active hemorrhage. If the patient with abdominal injuries is hemodynamically stable and has a ruptured thoracic aorta, the aorta should be repaired first. If, on the other hand, the patient is hemodynamically unstable and intra-abdominal bleeding is suspected, the abdominal hemorrhage is the higher priority and the chest injuries should be repaired following control of the hemorrhage in the abdomen.

The trauma patient should be placed supine and his chest and abdomen prepared in a sterile manner from just above the suprasternal notch down to the pubis; the preparation should also include the saphenous vein for use in vascular repair and should extend posteriorly down the patient's flanks as far as the surface of the table. This provides the exposure needed by the surgeon to gain access to any body cavity expeditiously and to place drains and chest tubes properly. The abdomen should be explored through a midline incision. One may start with an upper midline incision and extend the incision below the umbilicus if injuries are found. Once entered, if the abdomen is filled with bright red blood, the bowel should be eviscerated and all quadrants of the abdomen quickly inspected and packed with large packs for control of hemorrhage. Minor injuries and minor sources of hemorrhage should not distract the surgeon until all sites of major hemorrhage have been identified and dealt with. After initial control of hemorrhage has been achieved, an attempt should be made to control spillage of gastrointestinal contents. This can be done temporarily by placing a Babcock clamp or a quick running suture.

Then definitive repairs can be performed: first the repair of the bleeding sites and then the repair of the visceral injuries.

Once those repairs have been made, the trauma team must decide whether to proceed immediately with definitive fixation of long bone fractures. We strongly recommend the early stabilization of fractures during the same operation if the patient's clinical status allows it. The only contraindications to immediate stabilization of fractures after abdominal repairs are hemodynamic instability, coagulopathy, and hypothermia. When these problems are present, the patient should be taken to the intensive care unit for further resuscitation, correction of any coagulopathy, and restoration of normothermia. The patient should then be taken back to the operating room for fracture stabilization.

Maxillofacial trauma not associated with airway obstruction should be treated after the patient's condition is completely stabilized and the patient has no untreated major life-threatening injuries.

RECOVERY PHASE

The most common non-neurologic cause of death in patients who survive the first few days following severe trauma is infection (78 percent).[9] Many of these infections are iatrogenic.[10] Therefore, we recommend that catheters and tubes placed in the emergency room for invasive monitoring and treatment be removed and, if their use is still necessary, replaced. It should be assumed that all such devices are contaminated and that they were inserted under less than completely aseptic circumstances. A nasogastric tube contributes to infection by causing continued nasopharyngeal irritation which may then lead to sinusitis. Endotracheal tubes are a common source of respiratory infection, including tracheitis, bronchitis, and bronchial pneumonia. Indwelling urinary catheters left for very long will cause bacteriuria, and some patients will develop urinary tract infections, including prostatitis, cystitis, and pyelonephritis. Surgical drains are notorious for introducing hospital organisms into body cavities; thus it is best to avoid surgical drains unless the advantages of their use outweigh the disadvantages.

Malnutrition is a common problem in prolonged recovery from trauma, and aggressive nutritional support is mandatory in the severely traumatized patient. The enteral route is preferable if it is intact: It not only provides nutrients in proper proportion, but it also helps to maintain the integrity of the gut mucosal barrier.[11,12]

REHABILITATION

Acute rehabilitation includes early procedures for skin protection and passive movement of joints. As soon as the patient is able to cooperate, use of a trapeze bar and active physiotherapy should be routine. Early rehabilitation is an important goal. Long-term rehabilitation programs are often necessary for patients who survive accidents with severe fractures, spinal cord injury, or head injury.

REFERENCES

1. Blaisdell FW. General assessment, resuscitation and exploration of penetrating and blunt abdominal trauma. In: Blaisdell FW, Trunkey DD, eds. Trauma management. Vol 1. Abdominal trauma. New York: Thieme-Stratton, 1982:1.
2. Arom KV, Richardson JD, Webb G, et al. Subxiphoid pericardial window in patients with suspected traumatic pericardial tamponade. Ann Thorac Surg 1977; 23:545–549.
3. Trinkle JK, Toon RS, Franz JL, et al. Affairs of the wounded heart: penetrating cardiac wounds. J Trauma 1979; 19:467–471.
4. Baker CC, Thomas AN, Trunkey DD. The role of emergency room thoracotomy in trauma. J Trauma 1980; 20:848–854.
5. Yee ES, Verrier ED, Thomas AN. Management of air embolism in blunt and penetrating thoracic trauma. J Thorac Cardiovasc Surg 1983; 85:661–668.
6. King MW, Aitchison JM, Nel JA. Fatal air embolism following penetrating lung trauma: an autopsy study. J Trauma 1984; 24:753–755.
7. Trunkey DD, Lewis FR. Current therapy of trauma. 2nd ed. Toronto: BC Decker, 1986:304.
8. Root HD, Keizer PJ, Perry JF Jr. The clinical and experimental aspects of peritoneal response to injury. Arch Surg 1967; 95:531–537.
9. Baker CC, Oppenheimer L, Stephens B, et al. Epidemiology of trauma deaths. Am J Surg 1980; 140:144–150.
10. Schimpff SC, Miller RM, Polakevetz S, Hornick RB. Infection in the severely traumatized patient. Ann Surg 1974; 179:352–357.
11. Seibel R, LaDuca J, Hassett JM, et al. Blunt multiple trauma (ISS 36), femur traction, and the pulmonary failure-septic state. Ann Surg 1985; 202:283–295.
12. Carrico CJ, Meakins JL, Marshall JC, et al. Multiple-organ-failure syndrome. Arch Surg 1986; 121:196–208.

3

TEAM APPROACH TO MANAGEMENT OF TRAUMA VICTIM

MUTAZ B. HABAL, M.D., F.R.C.S.C.

Patients presenting to the emergency department with facial injuries may have no injuries elsewhere or may have a multisystem involvement with trauma in other parts of the body. In this latter circumstance, the surgeon caring for the trauma patient becomes a member of a multidisciplinary team. The team's basic goal is the general care and welfare of the patient; it works for such care and welfare after efforts to save the life of the patient are undertaken by attending to the life-threatening conditions first. With each specialist on the team focusing on his or her own fairly narrow area of expertise, there is a need for a surgeon to oversee all treatment plans and to coordinate "holistic" patient care. In most emergency situations it is the general surgeon, an expert on traumatology, who assumes this larger responsibility and who proceeds with a coordinated plan. Traditionally, general surgeons were already on hand in emergency situations; thus their role as coordinator in such care situations came to seem a natural one and has so remained. However, any surgeon experienced in trauma management and general care can assume such a role if the general surgeon is not available, and if the surgeon is willing to take responsibility.

Surgeons whose primary responsibility and expertise are treatment of facial fractures usually have diverse medical backgrounds. Some may already have had wide experience in the treatment of acutely injured patients and may therefore look at the patient as injured in general, the "body-all" concept. Those with different backgrounds focus more specifically on the head and facial area, in which case overall care must be made the responsibility of another specialist. The coordinator should always bear in mind that associated injuries may well be relevant to the one being treated in the facial region.

The trauma team typically includes specialists whose services are needed immediately for treatment of the patient with a facial injury, such as a general surgeon, a neurosurgeon, and a plastic surgeon. The general surgeon should make sure that other parts of the body are not injured and, if so, a specialist is called to provide specific attention to those areas. Recent reports show that at least 60 to 70 percent of patients with multiple injuries have one of the extremities involved. This makes the orthopedic surgeon an integral part of the trauma team, whose evaluation of the involved extremities is especially important before any treatment plan can be instituted (including functional assessment and diagnostic work-up).[1-3]

We believe that optimal care of facial injuries can be given by a cooperative effort of all those who have expertise in this area of surgical care. However, there are unfortunate occasions in which the personal preferences, and personalities of the surgeons interfere with this coordinated effort, leading to an adversarial discussion of "areas of expertise." We must stress that cooperation of these specialists is clearly in the best interest of the patient. Beyond this principle, the basic goal of every trauma team should be restoration of structure for the preservation of function. Maintenance of this restored function should be achieved by careful and considered long-term monitoring. The goal of the team's efforts should always be long-term, not short-term.

Thus, surgical subspecialists with interest in the head and neck should ideally pool their expertise for the patient's ultimate well-being. Among these specialists, the most experienced practitioner or, in the event of equal expertise, the one with the greatest seniority should assume the role of the "surgeon in charge"; an accepted principle. From the start, care of the patient by the facial-surgical group is presumed to have approximated the treatment plan outlined later in this book. The airway should be under control, and the vascular system should be stable. Then, and only then, facial injury assessment, care, and treatment should be started.

The surgeon in charge should, at the outset, classify the injury as "serious" or "nonserious." Serious facial injuries require prompt attention, whether it be immediate steps to repair the problem or a temporary stopgap until definitive treatment can begin. The most pressing problem calling for immediate treatment is the rupture of the oculus, or any injury as an open area within the central nervous system. Open wounds should be closed immediately, even temporarily, until the patient is ready for definitive surgery. We prefer to use the auto-stapler to change temporarily any open contaminated wounds into closed wounds awaiting definitive treatment. This is considered a useful "tidying" procedure for open wounds. When the patient is ready for definitive treatment, these wounds can be reopened by removal of the staples, a simple maneuver, and further tidying of the areas can take place, followed by débridement and closure of the wounds in layers, with attention paid to the restoration of structures based on anatomic landmarks.

Nonserious injuries are those diagnosed as fractures that remain closed. If the patient's condition is unstable, we typically do not hesitate to wait up to 15 days before we undertake a complete structural repair of the defects. However, if there is need to delay repair further, special attention should be paid to those fibrous bands lying between fractured segments, to ensure the most complete repair and reconstruction.

Specific questions of method then present themselves. What is the best way to repair the fractures? Does one use wire loops, miniplates, or screws for such repair? These questions are ultimately decided by the treating surgeon based on experience, background, and expertise. We all began practicing with wire-loop fixation, for these internal fixations of fractures were originally popularized in wartime trauma repair. Later, it became apparent that the wire loop assured better stability of bony fragments and a better result than no fixation at all for facial fractures. Eventually, there were disadvantages or conditions identified with these new advances. The most important advance has been the utilization of good exposure for miniplate fixation. We attempted to stabilize the fragment, and to avoid any telescoping effect when wire loops are pulled tighter, thus obviating the need to shorten the face after trauma. All of these factors prompted the widespread use of miniplates for internal fixation systems, which provide better stability on a long-term basis and a far superior result. Plating has become the state of the art in fixation of unstable fractures in the face.

After structural repair, maintenance and preservation of function is the most pressing responsibility of the trauma team. Based on widespread experience it appears that normal shifting of the facial structures during healing necessitates close monitoring of the patient's teeth and eyes. For the former, the surgical orthodontist can design whatever program may be necessary to provide an optimal outcome. The eyes may require exophoria surgery or further assessment of the bony platform for addition or subtraction bone surgery in or around the orbits to correct any orbital deformities.

Unfortunately, injuries involving facial fractures, especially the more serious ones, may require extensive use of bone grafting. The maxillofacial surgeon is the team member most likely to do these grafts. If a relatively large area is deficient, bone grafts can be harvested from the cranium, since it is accessible through the same incision, and applied in the deficient sites for the purpose of repair and reconstruction in the "self-sufficiency" principle of craniofacial surgery. However, bone grafts will undergo a course of unpredictable resorption, thereby forcing the treating team to continue evaluations for 12 months after the injury to deal with late sequelae. The need for long-term close follow-up of the post-trauma patient cannot be overstated.

These late sequelae of facial injuries are treated as described in this text, specifically according to the repair needed. On occasion, a major craniofacial procedure will be required, which should be handled by a qualified and recognized craniofacial team. In other patients, only bone grafting may be required. Late sequelae are what tend to make all extensive facial fractures unique in terms of treatment, and the approach needed for the correction of such deformities must be individualized correspondingly.

There are two final and even more specific points upon which to concentrate. One is patient satisfaction, which is of course very important, even though the treating team may find the ultimate results less than optimal. The second point is that children's facial fractures deserve special attention because of ensuing craniofacial growth problems; the nature of that attention, along with a description of late sequelae, is detailed in a later chapter in the book (see chapter 17 entitled *Facial Fractures in the Pediatric Patient*). However, in the initial phase of children's care, a pediatric surgeon should evaluate all treatment of the injured child and a pediatrician should be available to deal with overall concerns.

CLINICAL NOTE

A case history is presented to demonstrate the systematic approach to the care of the victim with multiple injuries and the principles outlined in the care and treatment of such patients.

A 30-year-old patient was involved in a boating accident. He was standing in his highspeed boat, and the rising tide caused it to hit a concrete bridge. He took the major impact on his face and also suffered head, brain, chest, and arm injuries. Because of the severity of his injuries, he was transferred to our unit, where he was provided with airway control and circulatory support (Fig. 3–1).

The initial care was undertaken when the open wounds on his face were tidied, using skin staples to change these open wounds to closed ones. A central venous line was placed for access, and the life-threatening conditions were cared for first. We were unable to save his left eye, which had to be removed because of complete rupture of the interocular structures (Fig. 3–2).

The facial injuries were repaired 10 days later with rigid fixation and extensive use of bone grafting (Fig. 3–3). The bone grafts were removed from the outer table of the skull through the bitemporal coronal approach, which was used to approach and expose all fractures in the facial region. Both bone grafts and the plating for fixation helped to stabilize the patient's facial structures and preserve his identity. The stabilized segments were clearly shown on radiographs (Fig. 3–4).

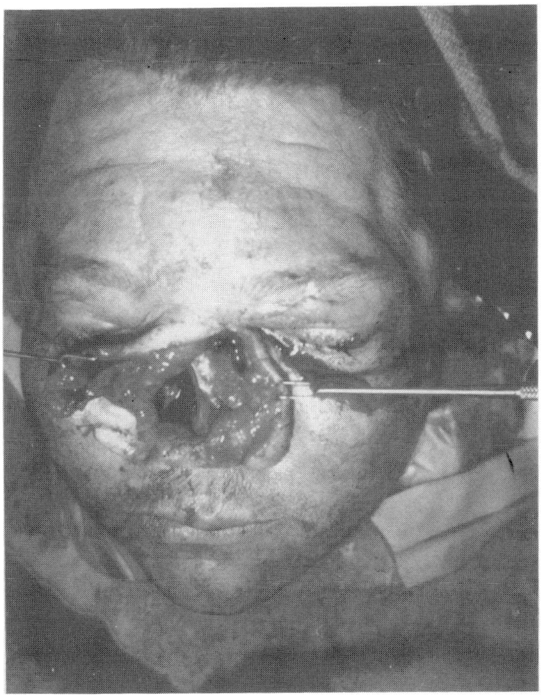

Figure 3–2 Intraoperative view showing the open fractures in the facial region.

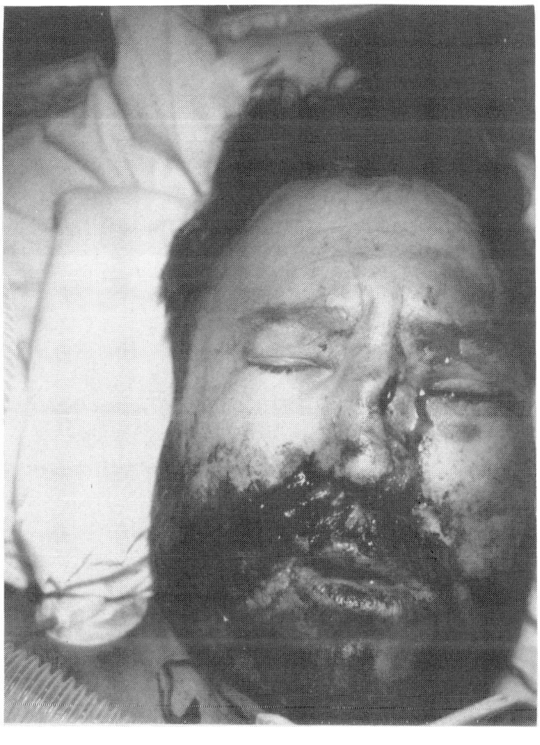

Figure3–1 Patient with extensive panfacial fractures.

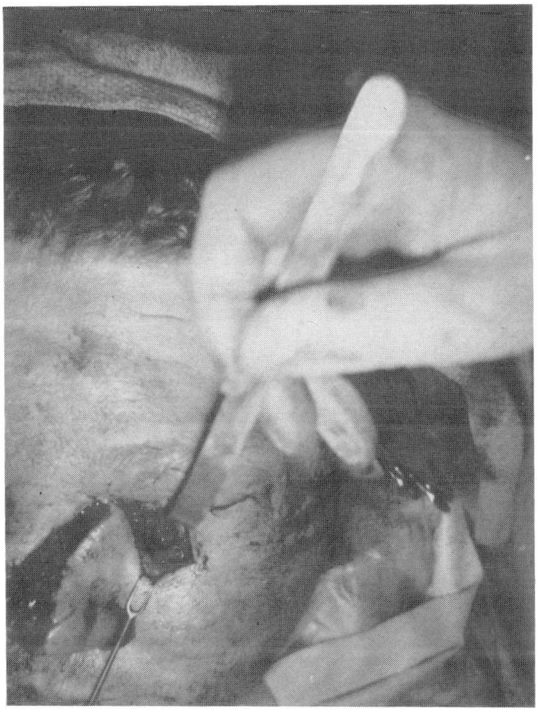

Figure 3–3 Close-up view of the orbit. The patient lost the eye on this side.

An ocular prosthesis was inserted and the patient was able to pursue all normal functions and to resume his preinjury activities (Fig. 3–5).

The two substantive advances in structural repair in the facial region, namely, internal rigid fixation with plating and immediate bone grafting, were primary reasons for the near-normal ultimate

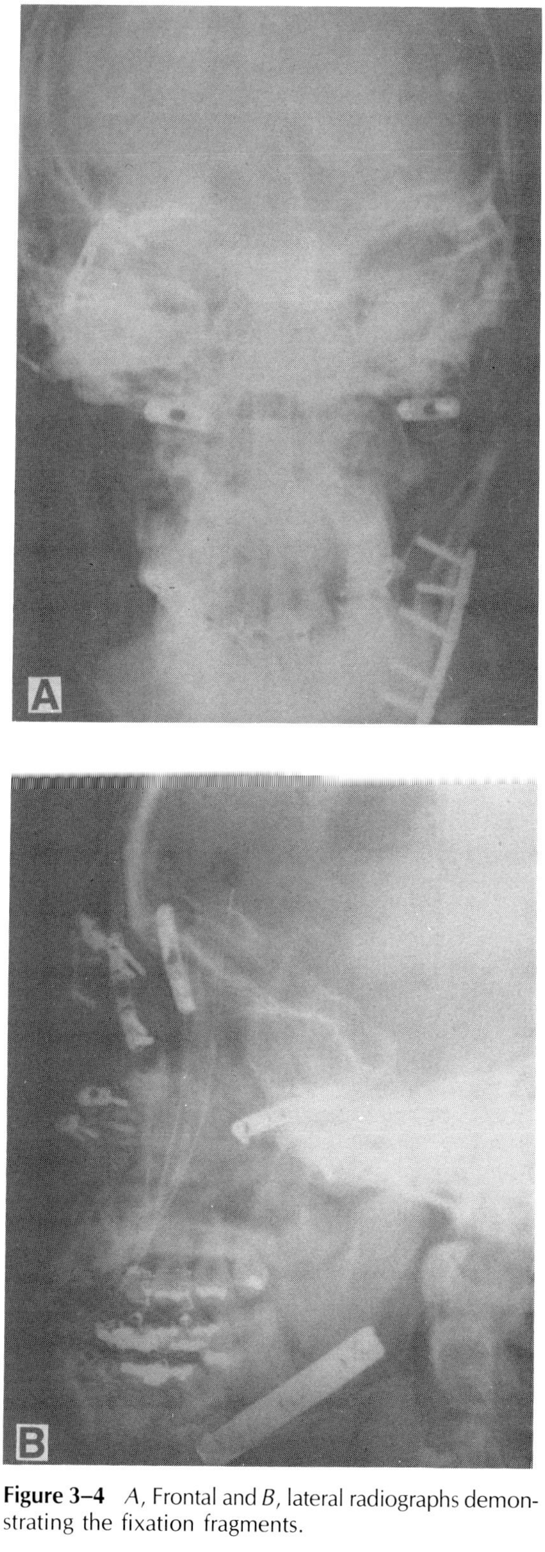

Figure 3–4 *A*, Frontal and *B*, lateral radiographs demonstrating the fixation fragments.

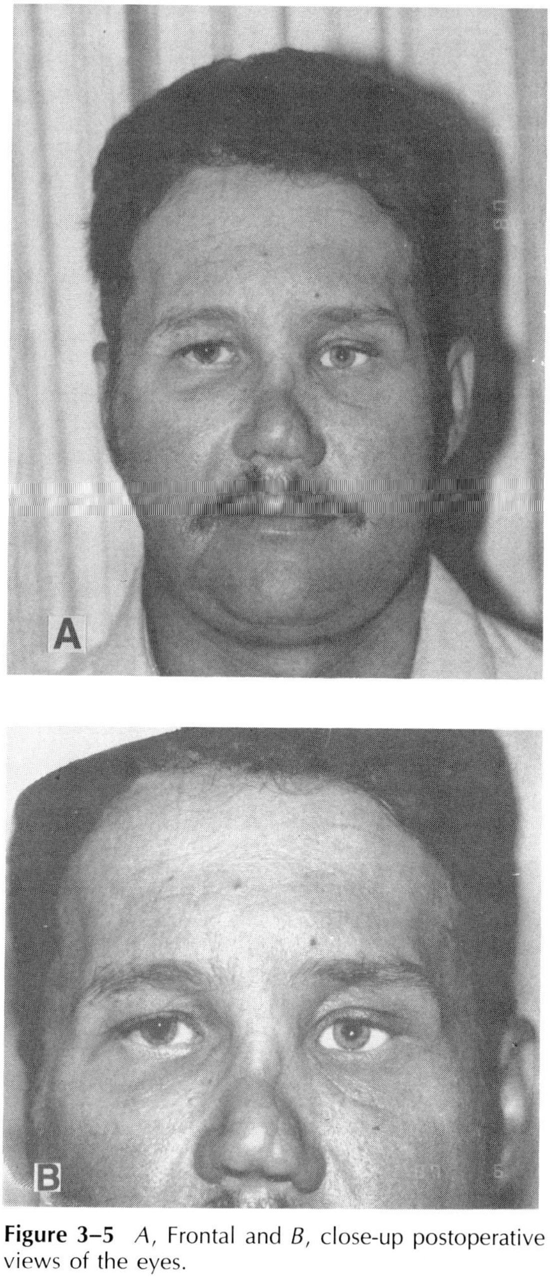

Figure 3–5 *A*, Frontal and *B*, close-up postoperative views of the eyes.

result, maintained 1 year after repair. The outstanding advantage of this new repair technology is the durable stability of all face and body fragments even on long-term follow-up. Figure 3–6 shows the injured patient 1 year after the surgical correction.

Maintenance was achieved partly by orthodontic manipulation, combined with ophthalmic care by an ophthalmologist, as well as neurologic treatment for seizure disorders performed by a neurologist, and otologic care handled by an otolaryngologist. Thus, all necessary maintenance was provided by a coordinated post-trauma care team. It is essential in the care of trauma patients—following immediate resuscitation and recovery of life-threatening situations—that the main functions of normal productive life be restored and maintained as well, and that any further necessary assistance be provided by the trauma team, so that the patient can return to preinjury functions, ideally without any impairment.

A three-dimensional image made 1 year later (Fig. 3–7) demonstrated the stabilization of the fracture fragments and the viability of the bone grafts.

Future repairs as in this patient will include extensive bone grafting and internal fixation (Fig. 3–8). The loop wires continue to be used; how-

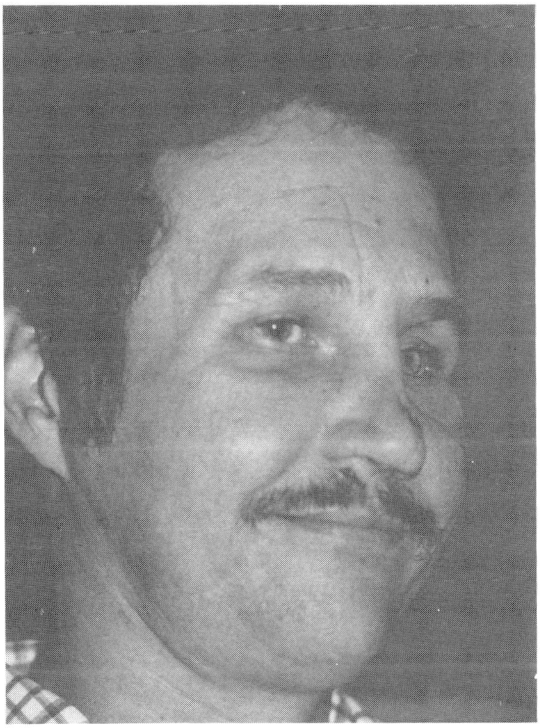

Figure 3–6 One year later, note the normal projection produced by a bone graft.

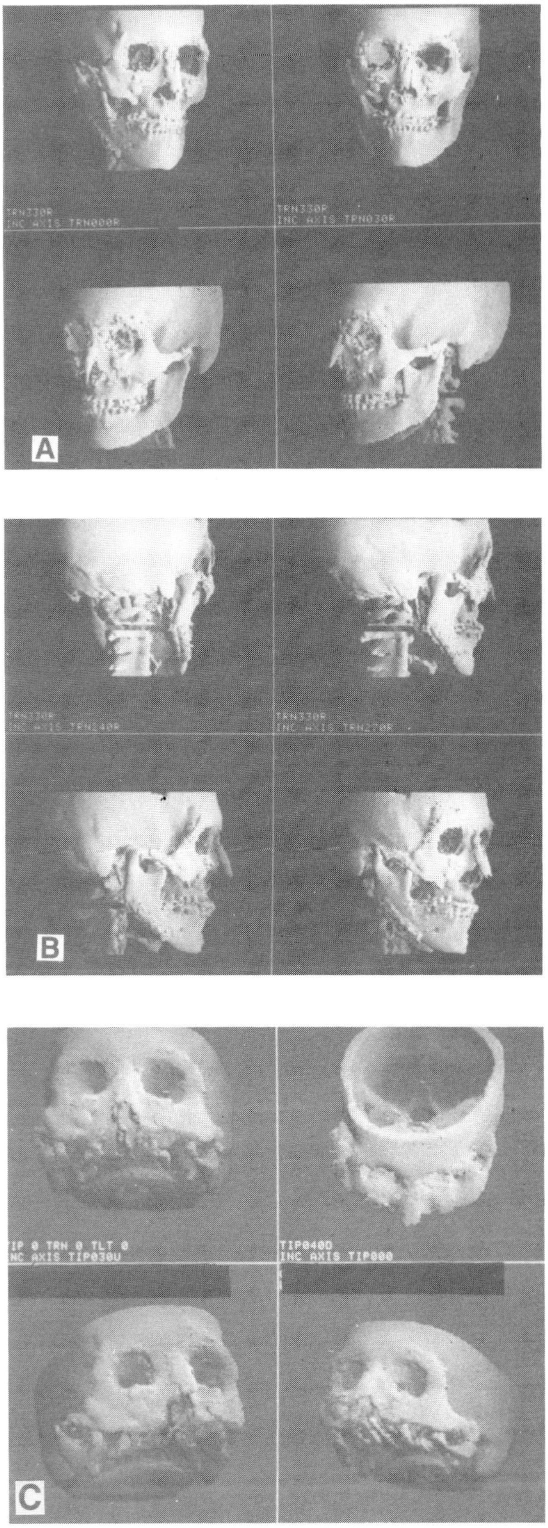

Figure 3–7 Three-dimensional image reformatted from a computed tomographic scan. Note the different bone fragments 1 year after reconstruction.

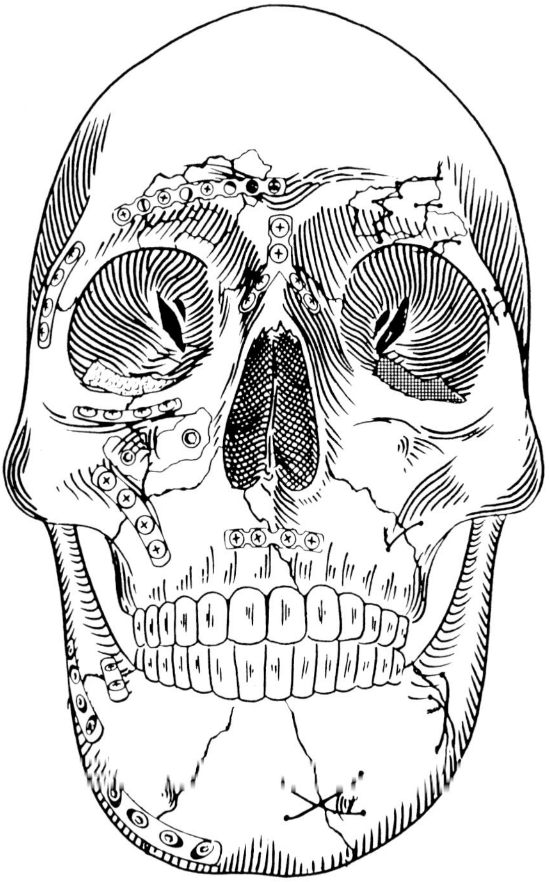

Figure 3–8 A diagram to demonstrate the trauma repair of wire looping of the past in the patient and plating to be undertaken today and in the future.

ever, we have to be careful not to mix metals in the same patient.

To summarize, complex and serious facial fractures deserve special care, since their treatment centers on an important but not life-sustaining part of the individual. We prefer to have the patient seen both individually and collectively by a neurosurgeon, an otolaryngologist, an oral surgeon, and a plastic surgeon as the basic treatment team, with inclusion of other specialized surgeons as indicated. All will do their own diagnostic work-ups on the patient and will then meet to formulate a coordinated definitive treatment plan, with the plastic and maxillofacial surgeon directing the effort. This team of surgeons, each with a different specialty, should work together for the best solution, and all should attempt to avoid the controversies created by specialty boundaries and overlaps. Such an approach, when planned in detail, cooperatively undertaken, and monitored over the long term, provides the patient with his best chance for improvement, care, and recovery (Table 3–1).

TABLE 3–1 Flow Sheet for the Trauma Team

General principles and guidelines
Members of the team
Emergency room physician as triage officer
Who should be in charge? For the face, most experienced
Classify injuries as:
Serious
Nonserious
The head and neck (maxillofacial) team:
Oral surgeon
Surgical orthodontist
Ophthalmologist
Otolaryngologist
Neurosurgeon
The general trauma team:
General surgeon
Thoracic surgeon
Cardiac surgeon
Orthopaedic surgeon
Maintain vital functions—airway, circulation
Diagnostic work-up
Look at restoring structures and function
Follow-up period
Postdischarge care
Maintenance care
Vision
Occlusion
Looking for and treating late sequelae

If patients are satisfied with the ultimate result, they will go back to their original surgeon. If they are not satisfied, they will seek satisfaction by consulting other specialists. This subtle matter of patient acceptance is sometimes unrelated to whether the physician him- or herself is pleased or displeased with the patient's final outcome.

REFERENCES

1. McDermott JE. Rehabilitation of the trauma patient. Bull Am Coll Surg 1985; 70:14–18.
2. Committee on Trauma Report. Multiple trauma: early management in the emergency department. Bull Am Coll Surg 1980; 65:20.
3. Committee on Trauma Report. Evaluation and management of the injured child. Bull Am Coll Surg Report 1987.

4

AIRWAY MANAGEMENT

J. CAMERON KIRCHNER, M.D.
STEPHAN ARIYAN, M.D., F.A.C.S.
CLARENCE T. SASAKI, M.D., F.A.C.S.

Airway obstruction is the most common preventable cause of death following major facial trauma. Prompt assessment of the airway and, if necessary, its re-establishment by artificial means are the first priorities in management of any major trauma victim.

Blunt trauma produces the majority of facial injuries now seen in the United States. Although such injuries may result from sports accidents and assaults with fists or clubs, most severe injuries result from motor vehicle accidents. Motor vehicle accidents account for more than 3,000,000 facial injuries per year in the United States alone.[1] Many of the principles of airway management in victims of blunt trauma also apply to the treatment of penetrating injuries such as stab and gunshot wounds.

PATIENT CARE PRIOR TO HOSPITAL EVALUATION

Following a major motor vehicle accident, victims are assumed to have sustained a spinal injury even if no neurologic deficits are evident. Positioning of a victim for transport to an emergency medical facility is predicated upon this assumption. If the airway appears to be adequate on initial assessment, the patient is placed on a rigid backboard with the head and neck in the neutral position, and the neck is immobilized. The cervical spine is best immobilized by placing a sandbag on each side of the head and neck, and taping the forehead to the sandbags and sides of the backboard and the upper torso to the sides of the backboard (Fig. 4–1). Additional tapes or straps applied across the pelvis and lower extremities will secure the victim to the backboard and thereby further stabilize the neck. (Stiff and soft cervical collars, though used occasionally, do not adequately immobilize the neck.)

After the victim has been secured to the backboard, close observation of the airway is necessary because obstruction may result from the dependent collection of blood, secretions, and even foreign bodies in the pharynx. Additionally, hypopharyngeal obstruction may occur from collapse of the base of the tongue against the posterior wall of the hypopharynx. After arrival in the emergency room, the patient should be maintained in this position without moving the head or neck until the status of the cervical spine has been determined.

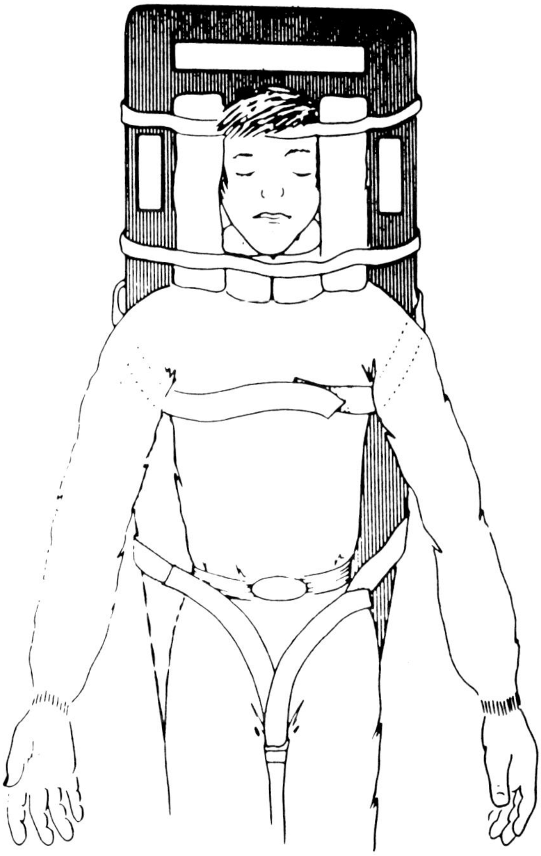

Figure 4–1 Optimal immobilization of the cervical spine. The patient is secured to a backboard, with immobilization both above and below the cervical spine. (Reproduced with permission from McSwain NE Jr., Kerstein MD. Evaluation and management of trauma. Norwalk: Appleton-Century-Crofts, 1987:59.)

INITIAL EVALUATION OF THE AIRWAY

Airway status can be accurately assessed within 15 to 20 seconds. Clothing should be cut away from the neck and chest so that both the upper and lower airways can be examined. Respiratory rate, ease or difficulty of breathing, and the presence or absence of stridor should all be noted. The patient's level of consciousness should be ascertained because it will affect the ability to clear and maintain a patent airway. An unconscious patient may, without warning, stop breathing completely because of an evolving neurologic injury.

Attention should then be directed to brief but vital evaluations of the face, neck, and chest, as injuries to these areas may affect any subsequent decisions regarding the timing and nature of airway support. Fractures of the maxilla and mandible cause airway obstruction at the level of the pharynx and hypopharynx, usually manifested by marked respiratory efforts with minimal movement of air, gurgling respiration, or choking. Significant laryngeal or tracheal trauma may be indicated by hoarseness, subcutaneous emphysema, stridor, odynophagia, dysphagia, pain and tenderness over the laryngeal cartilages, and swelling and ecchymosis of the neck. Chest injuries may be indicated by asymmetric chest movements (e.g., splinting or paradoxic movements), decreased breath sounds over one or both sides of the chest, and sucking chest sounds.

GENERAL CONSIDERATIONS IN AIRWAY MANAGEMENT FOLLOWING MAXILLOFACIAL TRAUMA

Airway obstruction is generally the only sequela of blunt maxillofacial trauma that poses an immediate threat to the life of the patient. Brisk bleeding may follow facial lacerations or lacerations of the oral, nasal, and pharyngeal mucosa, but life-threatening bleeding is unusual because the larger vessels are deeper and relatively well protected. Following penetrating injuries, bleeding may be much more serious and should be controlled as soon as the airway has been secured.

Bleeding following blunt trauma may be controlled by the application of pressure or hemostatic clamps. Use of the latter, however, may be inadvisable unless the bleeding vessels can be clearly visualized because of the risk of possible nerve injury in the anatomically complex head and neck area. Control of nasal bleeding may require the use of nasal packs.

Although maxillofacial injuries may necessitate urgent establishment of an artificial airway, evaluation and definitive repair of the facial fractures can usually wait until long after the patient has been stabilized. Fractures of the mandible which communicate with the oral cavity should be stabilized within 24 hours to minimize the risk of wound infection, but the evaluation and treatment of maxillary fractures, as well as the definitive repair of mandibular fractures, can usually be delayed 5 to 10 days.

Several factors are critical to decisions regarding management of the airway in the early post-trauma period. The first is an understanding of the nature and extent of other injuries, particularly the status of the cervical spine. If an artificial airway must be established before the cervical spine has been evaluated, the options are effectively limited to those that can safely be performed without moving the neck (Fig. 4–2). In the patient at risk for development of airway obstruction, radiologic evaluation should therefore begin with cross table lateral, oblique, anteroposterior, and open mouth views of the cervical spine. A cross table lateral view alone may fail to demonstrate potentially life-threatening fractures (Fig. 4–3).

The importance of evaluating the cervical spine is not diminished by the relative infrequency of fractures in this area. The overall incidence of cervical spine fractures in survivors of serious motor vehicle accidents has been estimated to be 1 to 2 percent,[2,3] but autopsy studies following fatal accidents have demonstrated much higher incidences, up to 24 percent.[4] Lewis and associates[5] suggested that mandibular fractures are more likely to be associated with fractures of the upper cervical spine, and that soft-tissue injuries of the upper face and scalp are more often associated with injuries of the lower cervical spine.

A second factor important to decisions regarding airway management is the patient's neurologic status. Neurologic injuries may affect the patient's ability to maintain a clear airway and may cause vomiting. Decreased levels of consciousness may result not only from head trauma but also from intoxication and the administration of analgesics or tranquilizers.

A third factor should be the assumption that the patient has a full stomach and may therefore vomit and aspirate. This possibility is increased by the presence of certain other injuries, particularly those to the head, spine, and abdomen. In determining whether the stomach is empty, one should determine the time that has elapsed between the

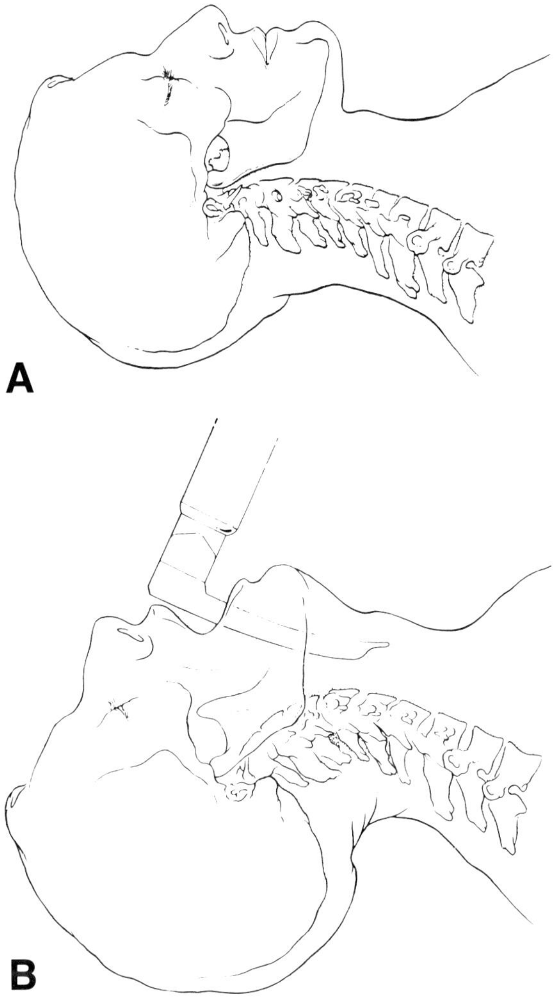

Figure 4–2 Cervical spine in the neutral position (*A*), and when the neck is extended, as for direct laryngoscopy (*B*). Such movement may cause or exacerbate a spinal cord injury in a patient with a cervical spine fracture.

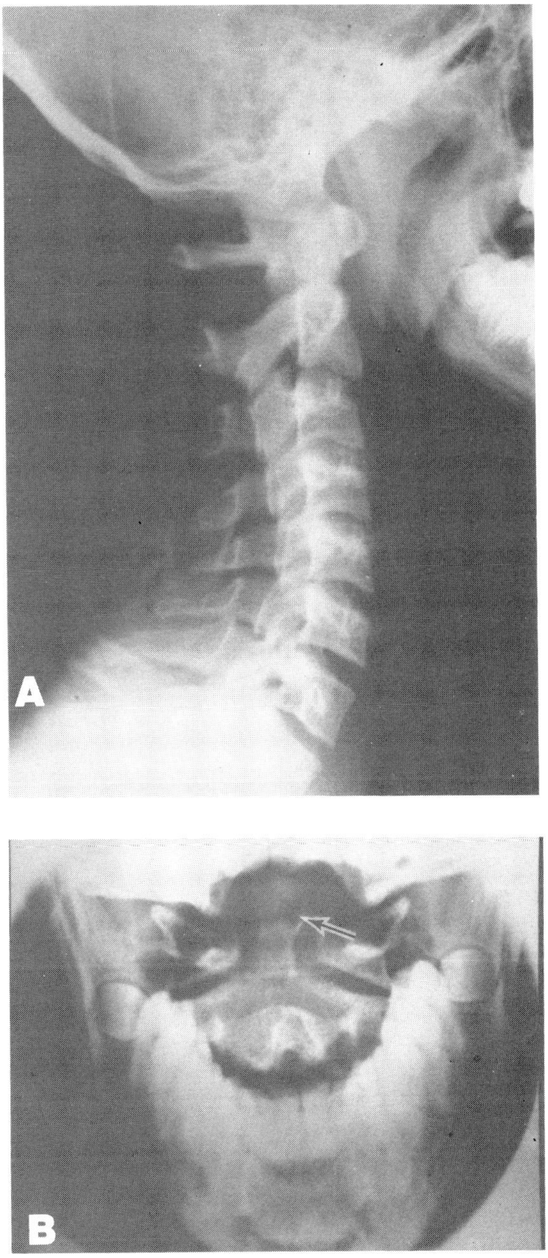

Figure 4–3 Cross table lateral view of the cervical spine (*A*) in a patient who complained of neck pain following a motor vehicle accident. No abnormalities are seen. A subsequent open mouth odontoid view (*B*) demonstrated an odontoid fracture (arrow).

last meal and the accident, rather than the time between the last meal and the evaluation, because gastric emptying effectively ceases for many hours after major trauma.

A fourth factor that affects the options for airway control is the training and experience of the medical personnel in the emergency room when the patient first arrives. Accurate assessment and appropriate management of the airway are best performed by physicians experienced in all aspects of airway control.

If an artificial airway is necessary only after resuscitation has been completed and the patient fully evaluated, securing the airway is generally safer and easier. Even if the stomach has not emptied, the patient's neurologic status may have stabilized. Personnel experienced in airway control will have had time to determine the optimum form of airway management for the patient, and they can establish the artificial airway under more controlled conditions. If the cervical spine has been found to be intact, the neck can be extended for better visualization of the larynx during endotracheal intubation and also for better exposure of the trachea during tracheotomy.

As decisions regarding airway management are so dependent upon the status of the cervical spine and upon the presence or absence of laryngotracheal and thoracic injuries, the following discussion of airway management addresses each of these possibilities. In general, the airway should be secured as soon as possible in patients with progressive or impending airway obstruction so that the particular procedure selected can be performed in a safe and orderly fashion.

MANAGEMENT OF EARLY AIRWAY OBSTRUCTION IN PATIENTS WITH MAXILLOFACIAL INJURIES

Blood, secretions, teeth, bone fragments, dentures, and collapse of the tongue or palate are the most common causes of obstruction soon after injury. Initial management should consist of suctioning the pharynx and hypopharynx with a large Yankauer sucker. Persistent obstruction may be due to the presence of foreign material such as teeth, bone, or denture fragments which can be cleared by sweeping the hypopharynx with the sucker. If obstruction is the result of tongue collapse from loss of consciousness, the mandible may be elevated by placing the index and middle fingers behind the ramus on each side and lifting upward (Fig. 4–4A). Alternatively, if tongue collapse is the result of mandibular fractures, the airway may be re-established either by grasping the symphysis between the thumb and index finger and lifting it forward (Fig. 4–4B), or by pulling the tongue forward with a suture or towel clip. It is essential that the head and neck remain stable during all of these maneuvers.

If the patient cannot clear and maintain a patent airway or is in danger of airway distress because of progressive loss of consciousness or edema of the tongue, pharynx, or floor of mouth, an artificial airway will almost certainly be necessary. Oral airways and nasopharyngeal tubes have been used with some success but are of limited value in these patients for several reasons. First, they do not isolate the airway from the contents of the pharynx and therefore do not prevent aspiration of secretions, blood, or foreign material. Furthermore, as a result of intoxication or head injury, these patients may vomit and aspirate gastric contents. An oral airway will cause a patient who is awake to gag. A nasopharyngeal tube may be used in a patient whose injuries are limited to the mandible but may cause further bleeding and tissue injury in a patient with maxillary fractures.

Of the available airways, the endotracheal tube and tracheotomy tube are the most commonly used and time-tested means of airway support (Table 4–1). In patients whose airway obstruction is the result of maxillofacial trauma, both airways effectively bypass the point of obstruction, limit or eliminate aspiration, provide ready access to the lower airway, and are sufficiently secure that they do not require constant attention. In those patients with significant head trauma, they can be used for mechanical hyperventilation to decrease intracranial pressure.

Orotracheal intubation is frequently employed as a means of both early and late airway management. It is a technique that is familiar to anesthesiologists and many emergency room physicians and can often be performed rapidly. In the patient whose cervical spine status is uncertain, however, intubation may be more difficult because it is most easily performed when the neck is extended, allowing direct visualization of the larynx. Intubation in this setting is facilitated by having an assistant stand alongside the patient, holding both sides of the head between his or her hands and alerting the physician to any head movements noted during direct laryngoscopy. Even if only the epiglottis can be visualized, a physician skilled in intubation may be able to pass the tube into the trachea. The intubation is facilitated by use of an angled stylette (Fig. 4–5A) or a fiberoptic scope passed through the tube (Fig. 4–5B).[6]

Prior to intubation, the patient is placed in the Trendelenburg position and preoxygenated by mask for 30 to 45 seconds. The use of positive pressure ventilation is not advised because it may force blood or secretions into the trachea and air into the stomach. Additionally, it should not be applied if the patient has injuries that could produce a cerebrospinal fluid leak, particularly nasoethmoid complex fractures, as air may be forced intracranially.

If the patient is unconscious, oral intubation may be performed without the use of topical or general anesthesia. If the patient is conscious, the pharynx, hypopharynx, and larynx may be topically anesthetized with 2 percent Pontocaine or 4 percent Xylocaine prior to intubation. Alternatively, rapid induction by administering thiopental sodium and succinylcholine may be employed. If the larynx is intact, the Sellick maneuver[7] may also be

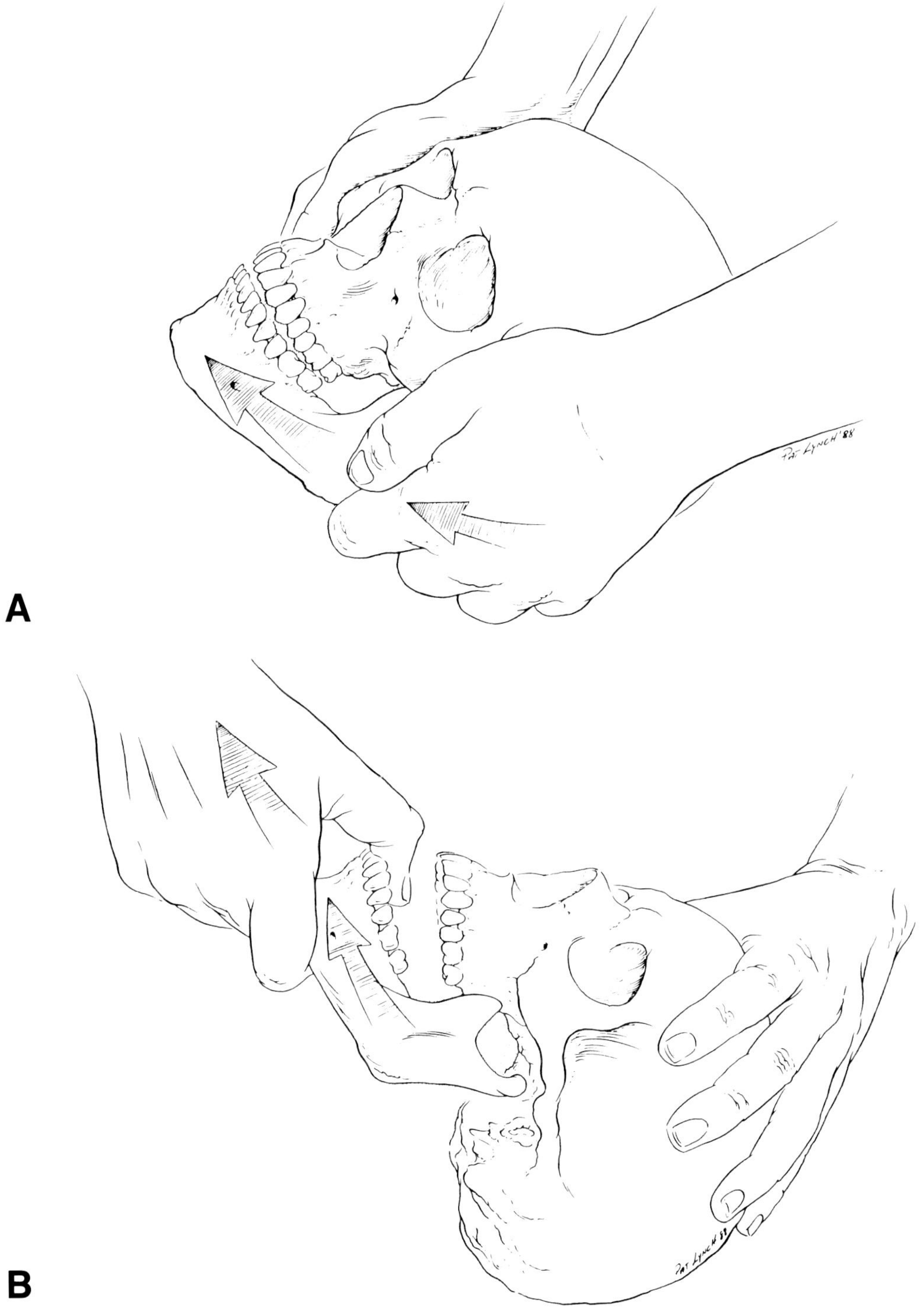

Figure 4–4 Airway obstruction resulting from collapse of the tongue against the posterior pharyngeal wall may be relieved by elevating the mandible. The mandible may be lifted from behind the rami (*A*) or from the symphysis (*B*).

TABLE 4–1 Endotracheal Intubation, Tracheotomy, and Cricothyroidotomy: Indications and Contraindications Following Maxillofacial Trauma

Procedure	*Indications*	*Contraindications*
Orotracheal intubation	Maxillofacial trauma without laryngotracheal trauma	Severe laryngotracheal trauma Inability to visualize larynx Cervical spine fracture (if neck extension is necessary)
Tracheotomy	Inability to intubate Laryngotracheal trauma Long-term airway support	None
Cricothyroidotomy	Inability to intubate	Laryngotracheal trauma

used. It is performed by having an assistant press the cricoid cartilage with the thumb, index, and middle fingers against the cervical spine and is useful immediately before and during intubation to minimize the risk of regurgitation of gastric contents into the pharynx with the attendant risk of aspiration.

If the patient's airway is significantly compromised prior to intubation, use of the rapid induction technique is not advised because mechanical ventilation might not be possible after the patient has been paralyzed. An inhalational technique using oxygen and either enflurane (Ethrane) or isoflurane (Forane) should be employed instead. Both agents cause less elevation of intracranial pressure than halothane, but in patients with significant head trauma, Forane is recommended because it is less epileptogenic than Ethrane.

"Blind" nasotracheal intubation is performed after the nose and pharynx are topically anesthetized by gently advancing the tube through the nose into the hypopharynx while listening to the flow of air through the tube. Successful intubation is signaled by vigorous airflow and frequently a cough through the tube. A cessation of airflow indicates that the tube has been advanced into the pyriform sinus or cervical esophagus. The tube is partially withdrawn and additional attempts made. This technique is of limited value in the early management of patients with maxillofacial trauma. Patients should be conscious, co-operative, and breathing spontaneously.[8,9] In patients with pharyngeal

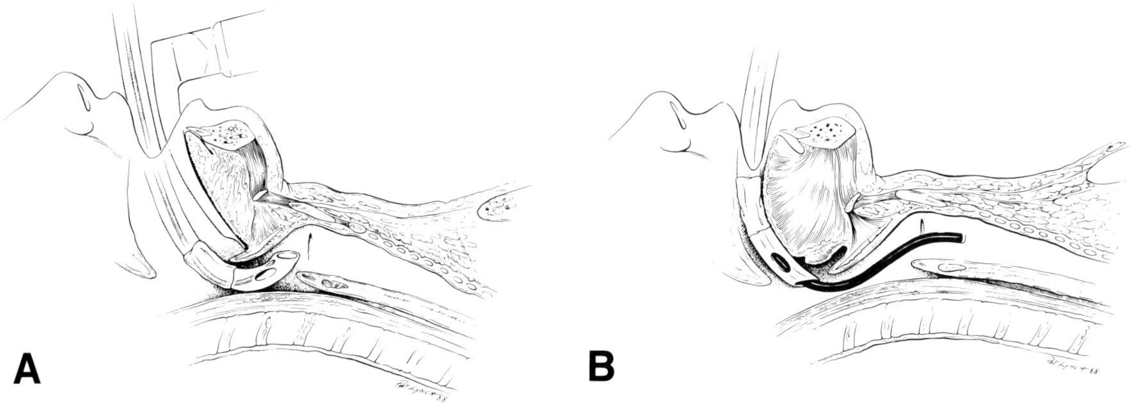

Figure 4–5 In patients with cervical spine injuries, orotracheal intubation must be performed without moving the neck. If the epiglottis can be visualized with a laryngoscope, intubation may be performed by using a stylet to angle the tip of the tube sharply, allowing it to be passed under the epiglottis and through the vocal cords (*A*). Alternatively, a fiberoptic scope passed through the tube into the larynx may be used as a guide over which the tube can then be advanced into the trachea (*B*).

lacerations or nasomaxillary complex fractures, nasotracheal intubation may cause bleeding and further tissue injury. In addition, foreign bodies may be pushed into the trachea.

If orotracheal intubation cannot be accomplished rapidly in a patient whose airway obstruction is progressive, a cricothyroidotomy can safely be performed without extending the neck. The cricoid and thyroid cartilages are generally easily palpable in the anterior midline of the neck. While one stabilizes the larynx between the thumb and forefinger of one hand, a 2-cm transverse incision is made through the skin and anterior one-third of the cricothyroid muscle, with care taken not to cut the cricoid cartilage (Fig. 4–6A). The opening is then widened using a tracheal dilator or hooks placed superiorly and inferiorly around the thyroid and cricoid cartilages, respectively. As the normal distance between the superior edge of the cricoid cartilage and the inferior edge of the thyroid cartilage in an adult is approximately 7 to 8 mm, use of a #4 cuffed tracheotomy tube is recommended, rather than larger tubes which may result in exposure and infection of the cricoid cartilage and the subsequent development of subglottic stenosis (Fig. 4–6B).

Although the long-term risk of developing subglottic stenosis appears to be acceptably low following a well-performed cricothyroidotomy in an uninjured larynx,[10] it is still the practice in many institutions to convert to a formal tracheotomy as soon as the patient's condition permits, preferably within 24 to 48 hours if prolonged ventilatory support is anticipated.

When the larynx has been injured, cricothyroidotomy is contraindicated. The presence of a contaminated opening within the larynx predisposes the injured laryngeal structures to infection, late scarring, and stenosis of the laryngeal airway.

A formal tracheotomy may be performed competently in less than 1 minute by an experienced surgeon, but the complication rate is higher when the procedure is performed by less experienced surgeons in the setting of acute airway obstruction. In addition, it is optimally performed with the neck extended.

As a last resort, percutaneous transtracheal insufflation can be used for the short-term management of acute airway obstruction. A large bore needle or intracath (#12 or #14) is inserted through the cricothyroid membrane or anterior trachea. The needle hub is connected to an oxygen source with a T connector which allows 1-second pulsed insufflations of oxygen every 4 to 5 seconds when the open end of the connector is occluded by the thumb or forefinger (Fig. 4–7). The oxygen flow rate should be set at 15 to 20 L per minute. In this manner, oxygenation can effectively be maintained for 30 to 45 minutes, before the degree of CO_2 retention and respiratory acidosis becomes unacceptable.

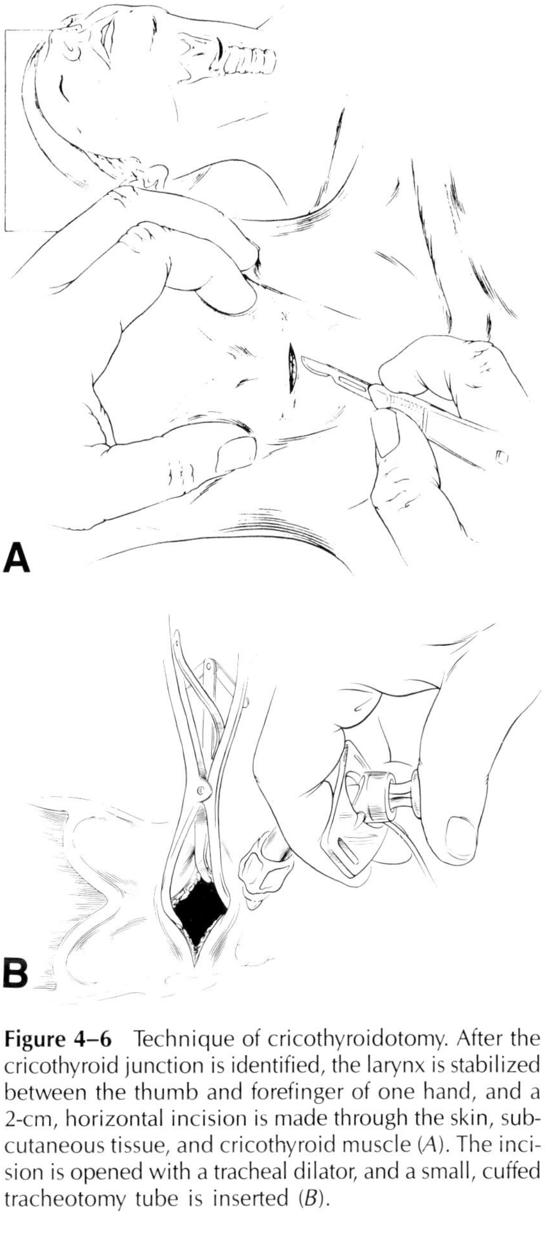

A

B

Figure 4–6 Technique of cricothyroidotomy. After the cricothyroid junction is identified, the larynx is stabilized between the thumb and forefinger of one hand, and a 2-cm, horizontal incision is made through the skin, subcutaneous tissue, and cricothyroid muscle (*A*). The incision is opened with a tracheal dilator, and a small, cuffed tracheotomy tube is inserted (*B*).

MANAGEMENT OF LATE AIRWAY OBSTRUCTION IN PATIENTS WITH MAXILLOFACIAL INJURIES

Establishing an artificial airway after the patient has been fully resuscitated and other major injuries

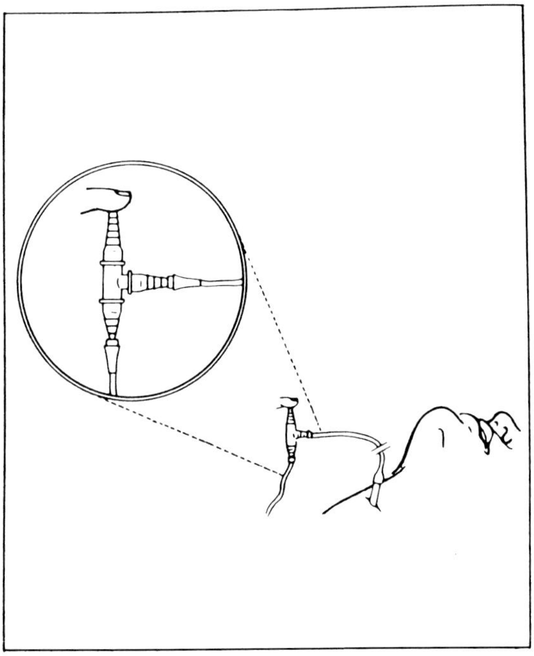

Figure 4–7 Tubing and T connector for percutaneous transtracheal insufflation. (Reproduced with permission from McSwain NE Jr., Kerstein MD. Evaluation and management of trauma. Norwalk: Appleton-Century-Crofts, 1987:66.)

identified is generally easier and safer. If the cervical spine is uninjured and the patient experiences progressive respiratory distress, it may be possible in selected patients, after suctioning the hypopharynx, to turn the patient onto his side in the semiprone position with the head dependent. In this position, the risk of aspiration is reduced because blood and secretions can drain from the mouth rather than pooling in the pharynx, and gravity will reduce the risk of hypopharyngeal obstruction by collapse of the base of the tongue.

Alternatively, if the cervical spine has been determined to be intact, the neck can be safely extended to facilitate orotracheal intubation. If no airway obstruction is present but an artificial airway is necessary for a planned surgical procedure, orotracheal intubation or tracheotomy may be performed. In the patient whose injuries are limited to the mandible, blind nasotracheal intubation can be safely performed under topical anesthesia.

Tracheotomy is a procedure that is often performed electively either under local anesthesia before intubation, or under general anesthesia after intubation. Patients most likely to require a tracheotomy are:

1. Those requiring long-term ventilatory support. Although the risk of laryngotracheal complications following intubation is controversial, it is generally recommended that patients requiring more than 10 days of ventilatory support undergo a tracheotomy. Such patients include those with significant head trauma, multiple mandibular fractures, and extensive injuries of both the maxilla and mandible. Tracheotomy offers several additional advantages in this group of patients. It is more comfortable than an endotracheal tube and may allow the patient to eat and even to talk when the cuff is deflated.

2. Those whose facial injuries are so extensive that reduction and repair are hindered by the presence of an endotracheal tube. These include patients with mandibular, maxillary, and nasal or nasoethmoid complex injuries.

3. Those requiring intermaxillary fixation and at least 1 to 2 days of postoperative respiratory support. Timely reintubation of a patient in intermaxillary fixation whose airway is still compromised after accidental extubation may not be possible. Furthermore, the presence of a nasotracheal tube may predispose the patient to the development of bacterial sinusitis.

Proven techniques for tracheotomy and for avoiding complications have been previously described.[11–13] In brief, with the patient in the supine position and the neck extended, the anterior neck is prepared with antiseptic solution and the skin between the cricoid cartilage and sternal notch infiltrated with 1 percent Xylocaine with 1:100,000 epinephrine. A 3-cm vertical incision is made through the skin strictly in the midline, extending inferiorly from the cricoid cartilage. The vertical incision allows the cannula to move up and down within the surgical field during deglutition, and to find its own tract from the skin to the tracheal lumen during the first 24 to 48 hours after surgery. The risk of trauma to the anterior and posterior walls of the trachea is thereby reduced during deglutition, when movements of the cannula may be restricted by an overhanging skin flap following a horizontal incision (Fig. 4–8).

The incision is carried sharply through the subcutaneous fat, and small blood vessels are electrocoagulated for hemostasis. Vessels 2 mm or larger in diameter are ligated and divided. The strap muscles are separated in the midline. The thyroid isthmus is exposed and isolated by passing a Crile clamp between the isthmus and its attachments to the cricoid cartilage and trachea. The isthmus is

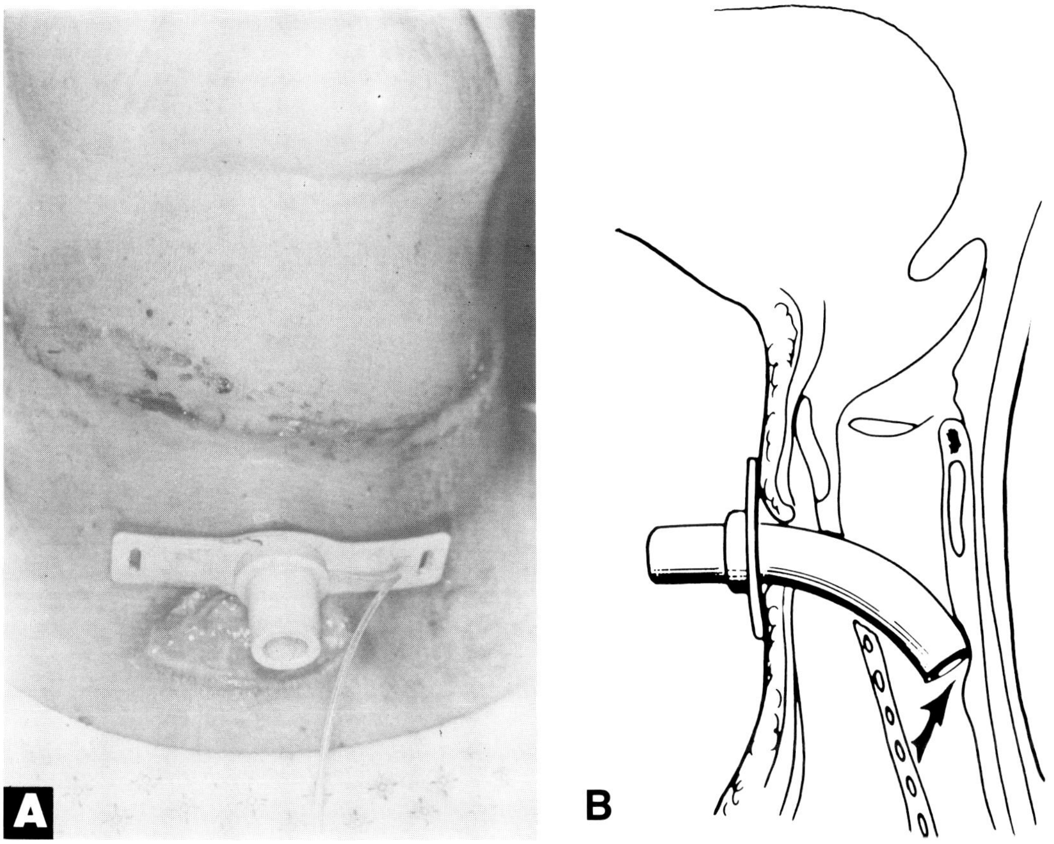

Figure 4–8 A high horizontal incision 24 hours after tracheotomy and laryngeal surgery (*A*). Note redundant tissue overlying the tracheotomy tube. Displacement of the distal end of the tracheal cannula against the posterior tracheal wall by redundant tissue resting on the shaft (*B*). (Reproduced with permission from Kirchner JA. Avoiding problems in tracheotomy. Laryngoscope 1986; 96:55–57.)

doubly clamped and divided and the edges oversewn with 3–0 silk or Vicryl. If the patient is awake, the soft tissue between the second and third tracheal rings, as well as the tracheal lumen, is infiltrated with 2 to 3 ml of local anesthetic. Traction sutures of 2–0 silk may be placed through the anterior tracheal wall above and below the anticipated opening site, or on each side of it, to permit immediate airway access should the tracheotomy tube become dislodged during the early postoperative period, before a tract has formed. Each suture should be knotted approximately 2 cm from the trachea (to facilitate later removal) and taped to the adjacent skin. In the adult, an opening approximately 1 cm wide is made between the second and third rings, and a window of cartilage excised from one of the two rings. (In the child, a vertical incision is made in the anterior midline through the second and third rings.) A cricoid hook is passed under the lower edge of the cricoid cartilage and the larynx pulled superiorly. A cuffed Shiley tracheotomy tube (usually size 6 for women and 8 for men) is then passed under direct vision into the trachea and the cuff inflated. The skin incision is left open to minimize the risk of subcutaneous emphysema from coughing in the early postoperative period. Umbilical tapes are secured snugly around the neck, and dressings consisting of gauze coated with Betadine solution are placed over the tracheotomy site and changed every 8 hours for 7 days to minimize bacterial contamination.

MANAGEMENT OF AIRWAY OBSTRUCTION IN PATIENTS WITH MAXILLOFACIAL AND LARYNGOTRACHEAL INJURIES

Laryngotracheal injuries sufficient to cause airway obstruction may occur in isolation or in association with maxillofacial injuries and may also be associated with injuries of the pharynx, esophagus, and cervical spine. The "clothesline" injury, which occurs when the operator of a motorcycle or snowmobile strikes an unsuspected wire barrier, is typically not associated with maxillofacial injuries. In high-speed automobile accidents, injuries may involve one or both regions.

Airway obstruction may be of gradual or rapid onset and is usually accompanied by signs and symptoms that may include hoarseness, stridor, odynophagia, dysphagia, and subcutaneous emphysema. Ecchymosis and swelling of the neck as well as pain and tenderness over the laryngeal cartilages can be seen. If such an injury is suspected, airway management must be modified appropriately. Even if the cervical spine is known to be intact, direct laryngoscopic visualization of the larynx is not recommended unless one is prepared to perform a tracheotomy immediately, as manipulation of the larynx by the tip of the laryngoscope may result in further injury to the laryngeal soft tissues with increased airway obstruction. The larynx should instead be visualized with a flexible fiberoptic instrument, or even indirectly with a laryngeal mirror. Endotracheal intubation is generally not advised and should be performed only if the subglottic airway can be clearly visualized. If examination demonstrates significant edema of the larynx or mucosal tears and exposed cartilage, a standard tracheotomy performed below the site of injury is the safest procedure and will be necessary in the ultimate management of the patient.

Less serious injuries, with submucosal hematomas and hoarseness but no mucosal disruption or airway compromise, may be treated conservatively with humidification and close observation if the patient's other medical problems do not necessitate an artificial airway.

If the airway is satisfactory or an artificial airway has been inserted, detailed computed tomographic evaluation of the larynx is performed prior to definitive repair of the laryngeal injuries. The integrity of the pharynx and esophagus is also determined by a contrast study using a water-soluble medium such as Gastrografin. Repair should be done as soon as the patient's medical condition permits, preferably within 24 to 48 hours of the injury, to prevent the long-term sequelae of airway compromise and dysphonia from infection and scarring.

Definitive repair of the larynx is preceded not only by a tracheotomy and radiologic studies, but also by direct laryngoscopy, bronchoscopy, and esophagoscopy to assess vocal cord mobility and to look for additional, previously undiagnosed injuries to these structures in the neck or thorax. The larynx is exposed through a U-shaped or horizontal incision and the strap muscles reflected from the thyroid alae (Fig. 4–9). If the vocal cords are mobile and there is no disruption of the laryngeal mucosa, the fractures may be reduced and stabilized with nonabsorbable suture material such as #32 stainless steel wire or 2–0 Prolene, or even with absorbable material such as 2–0 Vicryl. A stent may or may not be necessary, depending on the extent of the injuries.[14–16] Hypopharyngeal and esophageal lacerations are also repaired.

In the presence of lacerated mucosa or exposed cartilage, the larynx should be entered either through one of the fracture lines or through a midline thyrotomy. The latter approach must be performed exactly in the midline to prevent vocal cord injury. Lacerated mucosa is reapproximated using absorbable suture material such as 4–0 chromic catgut. Débridement should be minimal and raw surfaces, if present, covered with mucosa advanced from the pyriform sinus or free grafts of split-thickness skin or cheek mucosa. Exposed cartilage must be covered to prevent subsequent infection and necrosis. A dislocated arytenoid should be reduced, if possible, or removed, depending on the degree of damage. Fractures of the thyroid and cricoid framework are reduced using 2–0 Prolene or Vicryl. If the fractures remain unstable, a stent consisting of molded Silastic or a finger cot filled with sponge rubber may be used. The stent serves to maintain the patency of the laryngeal airway, and free mucosal or split-thickness skin grafts may actually be secured to the larynx by suturing them to the stent. The stent should not extend above the upper edge of the laryngeal inlet. Movement of the stent relative to the larynx during swallowing is prevented by the presence of two stainless steel or nylon sutures passed from one side of the neck to the other through the cartilage and the stent and secured over a button to each side of the neck. Tracking of infection into the larynx along these sutures may be prevented by applying antiseptic dressings around the buttons, burying the buttons in subcutaneous pockets, or burying the wires entirely over the larynx, using no buttons. The wires are later cut and removed under local anesthesia at the time of stent removal.

Tracheotomy dressings moistened with Betadine solution are changed every 8 hours, and systemic antibiotics are administered to reduce the risk of laryngeal soft-tissue infection.

Complete transection of the airway at the cricotracheal junction may necessitate retrieval of the distal trachea from the mediastinum. The edges

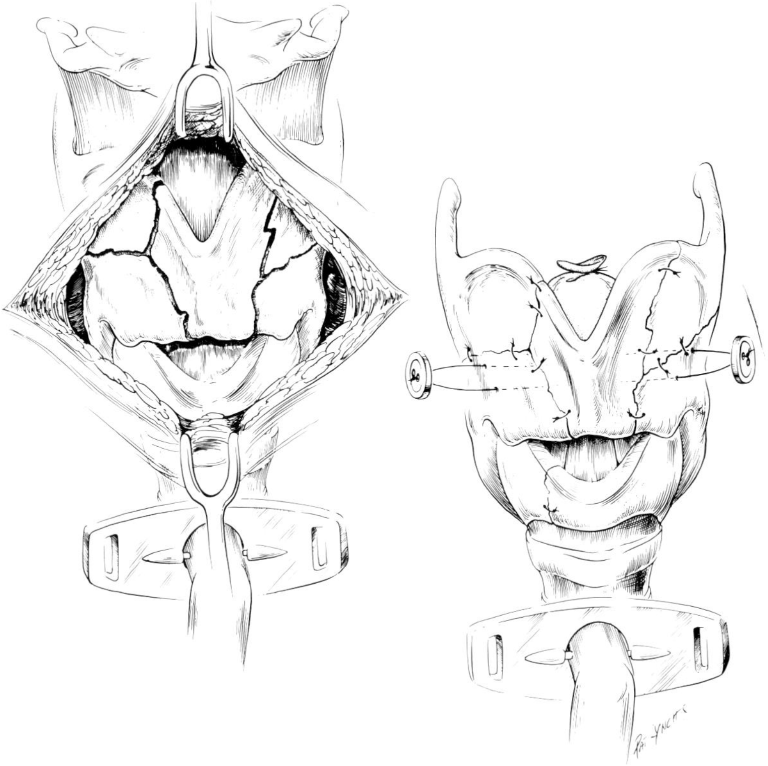

Figure 4–9 Repair of laryngeal fracture. After a tracheotomy has been performed, the larynx is approached through a horizontal skin incision, reflecting the strap muscles (not shown) away from the thyroid and cricoid cartilages. If the intralaryngeal tissues have been disrupted, the endolarynx may be approached and the soft tissues repaired through one of the fracture lines, or through a midline thyrotomy. The fractures are then reduced and sutured. A stent may be used if the reduction remains unstable or if there has been significant disruption of the laryngeal mucosa. A wire or nylon suture passed through the stent, the thyroid alae, and a button on each side of the larynx secures the stent within the larynx. The buttons may be placed on the neck skin or buried in subcutaneous pockets.

should be approximated without tension using 2–0 Vicryl or Prolene sutures. If stenting is necessary, a Montgomery T-tube may be used.[17–19]

MANAGEMENT OF AIRWAY OBSTRUCTION IN PATIENTS WITH MAXILLOFACIAL AND THORACIC INJURIES

Injuries to the thorax, when associated with maxillofacial trauma, often require placement of an endotracheal or tracheotomy tube. Mechanical ventilation and positive end-expiratory pressure are particularly useful in the treatment of flail chest injuries and pulmonary contusions. Tube thoracostomy is performed for the treatment of massive hemothorax, tension pneumothorax, and simple pneumothorax.

SUMMARY

The principles of airway management in patients with maxillofacial trauma may be summarized as follows:

1. Assessment of the airway and, if necessary, establishment of an artificial airway, are the first priorities of management.
2. Airway compromise may result from neurologic, maxillofacial, laryngotracheal, and thoracic injuries.
3. Following major trauma, the patient must be

assumed to have a cervical spine injury until the spine can be evaluated radiographically.

4. The patient must be assumed to have a full stomach during the initial hours after the injury.

5. Secure the airway early in patients who are manifesting signs of obstruction or who are at serious risk for airway obstruction.

6. Endotracheal and tracheotomy tubes offer the best means of airway support because they isolate the airway from the pharynx and allow controlled ventilation.

7. Laryngotracheal injuries are best managed by tracheotomy and primary closure. Stents are useful in maintaining the airway after more serious laryngotracheal injuries but may not be necessary if surgical reduction results in a stable larynx and trachea.

REFERENCES

1. Walton RL, Hagan KF, Parry SH, Deluchi SF. Maxillofacial trauma. Surg Clin North Am 1982; 62:73–96.
2. Huelke DF, O'Day J, Mendelsohn RA. Cervical injuries suffered in automobile crashes. J Neurosurg [illegible]
3. L[illegible] major facial fractures and associated injuries. Plast Reconstr Surg 1979; 63:26–30.
4. Bucholz RW, Burkhead WZ, Graham W, Petty C. Occult cervical spine injuries in fatal traffic accidents. J Trauma 1979; 19(10):768–771.
5. Lewis VL, Manson PN, Morgan RF, et al. Facial injuries associated with cervical fractures: recognition, patterns, and management. J Trauma 1985; 25(1): 90–93.
6. Raj PP, Forestner J, Watson TD, et al. Technics for fiberoptic laryngoscopy in anesthesia. Anesth Analg 1974; 53:708–714.
7. Sellick BA. Cricoid pressure to control regurgitation of stomach contents during induction of anesthesia. Lancet 1961; 2:404–406.
8. Walker WE, Bender HW. Blind nasotracheal intubation. Surg Gynecol Obstet 1981; 152:87–88.
9. Iserson KV. Blind nasotracheal intubation. Ann Emerg Med 1981; 10:468–471.
10. Brantigan CO, Grow JB. Cricothyroidotomy: elective use in respiratory problems requiring tracheotomy. J Thorac Cardiovasc Surg 1976; 71:72–80.
11. Montgomery WW. Surgery of the upper respiratory system. Vol 2. Philadelphia: Lea & Febiger, 1973:324.
12. Kirchner JA. Tracheotomy and its problems. Surg Clin North Am 1980; 60:1093–1104.
13. Kirchner JA. Avoiding problems in tracheotomy. Laryngoscope 1986; 96:55–57.
14. Trone TH, Schaefer SD, Carder HM. Blunt and penetrating laryngeal trauma: a 13-year review. Otolaryngol Head Neck Surg 1980; 88:257–261.
15. Leopold DA. Laryngeal trauma. Arch Otolaryngol 1983; 109:106–111.
16. Olson NR. Surgical treatment of acute blunt laryngeal injuries. Ann Otol Rhinol Laryngol 1978; 87: 716–721.
17. [illegible] ma. Am J Surg 1981; 141:412–417.
18. Huff JS, Magielski JE. Surgical treatment of laryngeal injuries. Otolaryngol Clin North Am 1976; 9: 393–401.
19. Alonso WA. Surgical management and complications of acute laryngotracheal disruption. Otolaryngol Clin North Am 1979; 12:753–760.

5

DIAGNOSTIC IMAGING

DANIEL H. JOHNSON Jr., M.D., F.A.C.R.

In the individual who has sustained trauma to the maxillofacial skeleton, elucidation of the mechanism of injury, determination of the resulting symptoms, and careful physical examination will reveal substantial information about what structures have been damaged. However, imaging has been used for greater insight into what has occurred, at least since the time of Le Fort's work in 1901.[1] Today the field of diagnostic imaging makes the assessment of patients at once more complex and simpler. Complexity stems from the ever growing array of imaging modalities available. Simplicity derives from the facility with which clinically helpful evaluation can be accomplished if the correct modalities are used efficiently.

Of the various forms of imaging currently available, conventional radiographs and computed tomography (CT) are the most important for investigation of the maxillofacial skeleton.[2,3] When the mandible is of interest, panoramic tomography, if available, may be the procedure of choice.[4] If the status of the cartilaginous disc of the temporomandibular joint is of concern, magnetic resonance imaging (MRI) is the procedure of choice for the needed diagnostic information. MRI is not currently used in the typical investigation of injuries to the face for several reasons: It is usually substantially more expensive than CT. Bone gives very little signal with MRI and may be difficult to assess. Where access to MRI is limited, time in the magnet may be a significant drawback. If the patient has difficulty holding still, motion artifact will spoil the study. If the patient is severely injured, he cannot be monitored effectively while in the magnet. Two significant advantages of MRI could, however, make it more desirable if some of the drawbacks can be minimized. First, with state-of-the-art technology, tomographic data can be directly acquired in any plane of a sphere with equal facility. Also, data relative to a volume of tissue can be acquired and then formatted into the desired plane. The other major advantage is the good demonstration of soft tissues. In addition, when some of the technical advances already developed become available, MRI will actually offer the fastest way to acquire data. Thus the concept of using MRI for the investigation of maxillofacial trauma should not be entirely discarded.

This chapter focuses on the use of plain films and CT for an immediate diagnosis of the problem. I will detail a potentially useful method of considering the anatomy for CT purposes; offer an anatomic classification of fractures, correlating bone plane and soft tissue injuries; outline an approach to imaging; and discuss the utility of various planes of imaging. In this analysis of imaging, "conventional tomography" will be left out. I believe that linear and complex motion tomography are virtually obsolete, relying on relatively high amounts of radiation to yield poor information about soft tissues and less than ideal assessment of bone.

ANATOMIC CLASSIFICATION OF FRACTURES OF THE MAXILLOFACIAL SKELETON

The classic work of Le Fort in 1901, in which he produced radiographs of traumatized cadaver heads, resulted in a classification that is used today. In 1968, Valvassori and Hord organized an approach to facial trauma according to its effect on the paranasal sinuses.[5] De Castro and Hanafee, in 1979,[6] divided facial fractures into six groups: the three types of Le Fort fracture and mandibular, orbital, and trimalar fractures. These two approaches address the significant shortcomings of the Le Fort classification. However, none of these methods maximizes the understanding of what CT can demonstrate in the facial skeleton.[2] Recognizing this, Gentry and colleagues, in 1983, published the results of a study in which they repeated Le Fort's concept of imaging traumatized cadaver heads but with CT rather than conventional radiography.[7,8]. The CT observations were confirmed using complex motion tomography and by slicing the anatomic specimens and making contact radiographs of them.

In the Gentry classification, bony structures of the face can be localized to three groups of struts situated at right angles to one another in horizontal, sagittal, and coronal planes.

The horizontal plane consists of superior, middle, and inferior horizontal struts. The roofs of the orbits, the fovea ethmoidalis, and the cribriform plate of the ethmoid bone constitutes the superior horizontal strut. The middle horizontal strut includes the floors of the orbits and the zygomatic arches. The inferior horizontal strut is the hard palate. The alveolus was divided by Gentry into lateral and anterior components as described below, but could instead be considered as a part of the inferior horizontal strut.

The sagittal plane is made up of five parts: a midline partition, two parasagittal struts, and two lateral facial struts. The midline partition is the nasal septum, made up of the vomer, the perpendicular plate of the ethmoid, and the cartilaginous nasal septum. The parasagittal strut on each side is composed of the medial wall of the orbit and the medial wall of the maxillary sinus. The lateral facial strut on each side includes the lateral wall of the orbit, the lateral wall of the maxillary sinus, and the lateral portion of the maxillary alveolar ridge.

There are two coronal struts, anterior and posterior. The anterior coronal strut includes the vertical part of the frontal bone, the zygomaticofrontal buttresses, the nasofrontal complexes, the anterior walls of the maxillary sinuses, and the anterior portion of the maxillary alveolar ridge. The posterior coronal strut is made up of the posterior walls of the maxillary sinuses and the medial and lateral pterygoid plates.

Whereas some of these anatomic structures can be difficult or even impossible to demonstrate with conventional radiographs, they are all readily demonstrated with CT. Often fractures of them occur in combination. Two fairly common such combinations are the zygomaticofrontal fracture and the frontoethmoid complex fracture. I prefer to include these two combinations in a classification of injuries based on Gentry's work (Table 5–1).

TABLE 5–1 More Common Soft Tissue Injuries Accompanying Facial Fractures*

- Horizontal plane injuries
  - Orbital roof fractures
    - Intracranial damage
    - Chance of injury to optic nerve
    - Cribriform plate fracture with CSF leak
    - Extraocular muscle entrapment
  - Orbital floor fractures
    - Muscle entrapment
    - Downward herniation of orbital fat
    - Orbital emphysema
    - Injury to the infraorbital nerve
- Sagittal plane injuries
  - Medial sagittal strut
    - septal hematoma
  - Parasagittal struts
    - Injury to the trochlea, resulting in superior oblique tendon sheath syndrome
    - Herniation of medial rectus muscle and orbital fat into the ethmoid sinus
    - Orbital emphysema
    - Interruption of normal maxillary sinus drainage
  - Lateral struts
    - Disruption of the lateral canthal ligament
    - Damage to the infraorbital nerve
    - Superior orbital fissure syndrome
- Coronal plane injuries
  - Anterior strut
    - Injury to lacrimal gland
    - Injury to nasofrontal duct
  - Posterior strut
    - Injury to neurovascular structures in the pterygomaxillary fissure and pterygopalatine fossa (if this injury is suspected, add a preliminary lateral radiograph for "scout" purposes)
    - Compromise of the eustachian tube
- Combined plane injuries
  - Frontoethmoid complex fractures
    - Disruption of medial canthal ligament, resulting in telecanthus and epiphora
    - Injury of the lacrimal sac
    - Compromise of the nasolacrimal duct
  - Zygomaticofrontal (trimalar) fractures
    - Soft tissue injuries described with fractures of lateral struts and orbital floor
    - Injury to the globe and/or lens

* From Johnson DH Jr. CT of maxillofacial trauma. Radiol Clin North Am 1984; 22:131–144. Reprinted with permission from WB Saunders.

AN APPROACH TO IMAGING OF THE MAXILLOFACIAL SKELETON

In determining how to accomplish optimal imaging of the maxillofacial region, three questions can be posed:(1) when to image, (2) what to image and (3) how to image.

When to image depends primarily on the overall condition of the patient. If some other injury more threatening to the patient coexists with the facial injury, it is perfectly acceptable to delay imaging until the more pressing problem has been successfully managed.[9] If, however, some unexplained phenomenon related to the injury is present such as compromise of the airway or sudden blindness, it may be necessary to image the patient immediately. In cases of massive trauma with evidence of neurologic deficit it is clinically desirable for physical evaluation of the facial damage to closely follow neurological evaluation if interceptive management of the injury is contemplated. Similarly, imaging of the facial injury may be done at the same time as brain imaging. Otherwise, when circumstances permit, it is wise to put off imaging until the opportunity for maximal quality exists. For example, it makes little sense to force CT examination of a facial injury at 3:00 AM using the emergency technologist not accustomed to performing CT, when it would be just as safe for the patient to wait until normal, working hours when optimal staffing will afford a better chance for good demonstration of the anatomic changes that have occurred. The radiologist on call may not be the member of the group with the greatest experience with this type of problem.

Determination of what to image can best be made based on clinical assessment of the patient in consultation with the radiologist. Important clues can be derived from a thorough history and physical examination.[10,11] The mechanism of trauma must be determined: blunt or sharp, focal or massive, isolated or in association with other injuries. Presence of cerebrospinal fluid leakage, abnormality of gaze, abnormal tearing, and anesthesia or unusual pain must be looked for. The presence of fracture can be a predictor of some soft tissue abnormalities. An example would be a fracture of the roof of the orbit, which has the possibility of extending back to injure the optic nerve.[12–14] Conversely, presence of some symptoms and their related soft tissue abnormalities can herald certain fractures. An example of this would be the individual with diplopia following blunt trauma to the eye, suggesting blowout fracture with muscle entrapment.

Combining these clinical findings with a preliminary exaggerated Waters view obtained with the mouth closed and the chin extended a bit more than usual can give important clues about which imaging protocol should be followed. Additional clues may be derived from other images obtained for different purposes, such as skull films and lateral and oblique views of the cervical spine.

The need for good communication between clinician and radiologist becomes greater when determining how to image. In deciding among plain films, panoramic tomography, CT, and other possibilities such as MRI, it is important that the radiologist know what the clinician suspects and what the clinician desires to learn from the imaging procedure, and the degree of diagnostic work-up needed.

Commonly used conventional radiographs include Waters, Caldwell, and lateral facial views. Occasionally, oblique views may be informative, however, I believe that time should not be wasted attempting to obtain extensive plain film examination. The more serious the injury, the more frustrating such attempts are apt to be. Instead, it seems much more productive to focus on the exaggerated Waters projection, as a guide to the need for and advisability of further study. If blowout fracture is suspected, a less exaggerated Waters view might be added for improved visualization of the orbital floor. A lateral radiograph offers a fast way to assess the upper airway in patients suspected of having retropharyngeal hematoma. Ideally, any plain films should be obtained with the patient upright, using a horizontal x-ray beam, in order to capture any air-fluid levels, however, such levels will also be easily seen in axial CT.

CT has several important advantages over other modalities for the diagnostic evaluation of maxillofacial trauma. It offers excellent delineation of bony anatomy and pathology and provides good demonstration of soft tissues. It is fortuitous that axial images are readily obtained with the only requirement of the patient being that he be able to lie supine without moving for the length of the examination. This image plane allows us to visualize both sides at once in a fashion that will permit easy survey of most of the anatomic structures of the face.[15]

Assuming that the condition warrants sophisticated imaging and that CT is to be performed, the several options available with CT need special consideration. If the situation calls for coronal CT images, will the patient's condition permit direct coronal images or will it be necessary to produce reformatted images in another plane? If reformatted three-dimensional (3D) images are needed, it is desirable to obtain thinner sections (1.5 mm or less) for accuracy than might otherwise be employed in a routine diagnostic study.[16] For the "reformatted" images, a series of sequential slices is obtained in the same plane. This "stack" of images can then be "sliced" in the desired alternative plane using computer software designed for that purpose (Fig. 5–1). The patient must be able to hold still while the series is produced or individual slices may be offset and the stack of slices will be distorted, compromising any reformatted images. Some authors suggest using sagittal or oblique sagittal reformations, especially for investigation of the floor of the orbit. [16,17]

The use of 3D reconstruction is becoming more popular in evaluation of the facial skeleton.[18,19] The way 3D images are obtained is quite similar to any other CT examination. A sequential series of slices is obtained in the same plane. For the production of 3D images, the computer manipulation of the data is somewhat more complicated but the result is a two-dimensional display of a model of the anatomic part imaged, which can then be rotated and sliced in an almost infinite variety of ways. Since the beginning of tomographic imaging, one of the advantages of the sectional

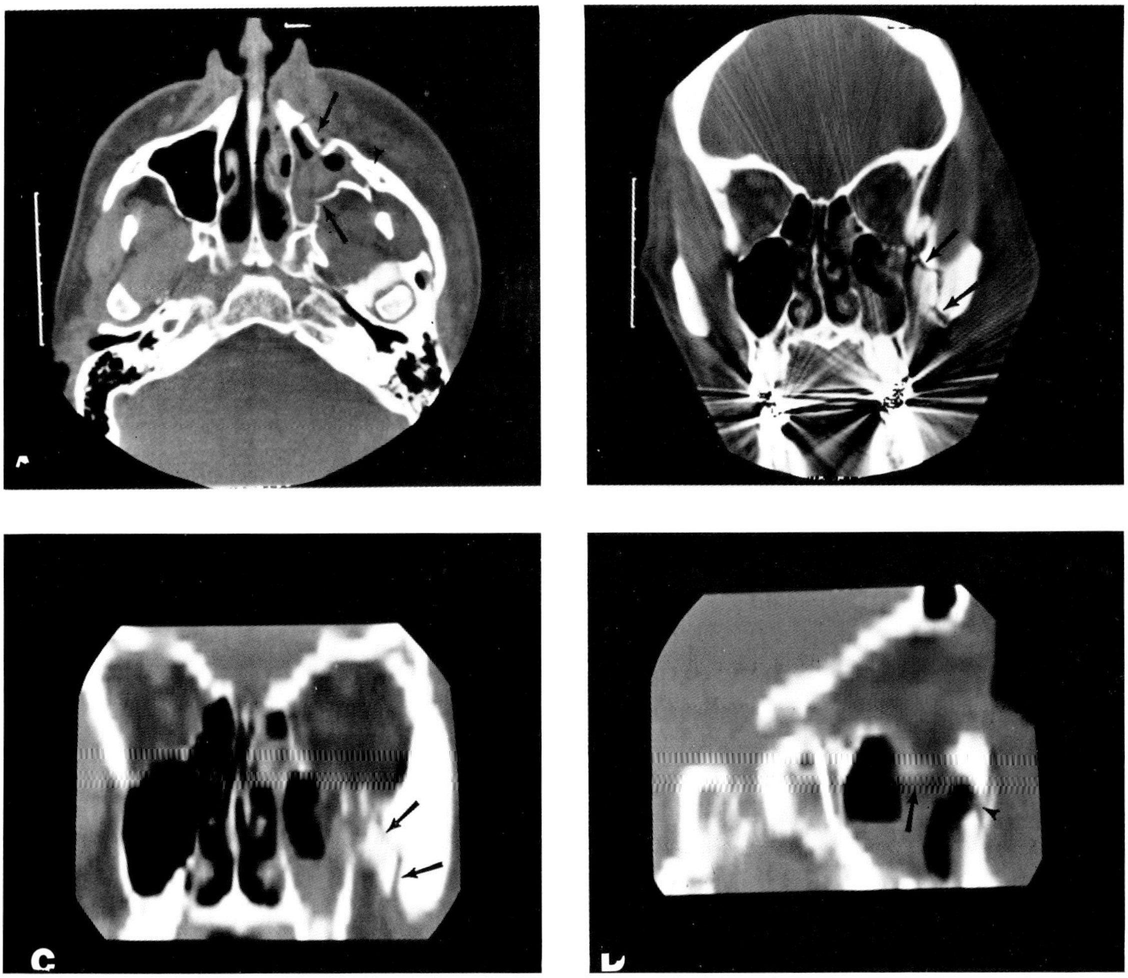

Figure 5–1 Trimalar fracture with reformatted images. *A*, An axial CT image of a patient with a trimalar fracture shows the comminuted fractures of the anterior and posterolateral walls of the maxillary sinus (arrows), with depression of the body of the zygoma (arrowhead). *B*, Coronal CT reveals the irregular fracture line through the medial aspect of the body of the zygoma (arrows). *C*, A coronal reformatted image at a level just anterior to that of B also shows the fracture of the body of the zygoma (arrows) but without the dental artifact. *D*, In this sagittal reformatted image, the fracture of the floor of the orbit (arrow) and that through the anterior wall of the maxillary sinus (arrowhead) are demonstrated. Note the lack of sharpness that results from reformatting 3-mm-thick slices. Images 1.5 mm thick would provide better reformatted images, although the result using 3-mm slices is acceptable. Anything thicker might not yield acceptable reformatting.

concept has been the ability to recreate in the mind's eye a 3D image from a series of two-dimensional sectional images. Thorough knowledge of the relational anatomy of a body part studied with any tomographic procedure will permit an understanding of this procedure. 3D programs can accomplish all of this and display it on a computer monitor and/or on hard copy such as x-ray film, much like the conventional CT images to which we have become accustomed. Marsh and Vannier have described in detail methods for the production of 3D surface images and commented on their potential application.[18,19] Herman and coworkers have described a method for preparing 3D images for stereoscopic viewing.[20]

I believe that such 3D manipulations are of limited value in acute care of trauma patients. The disadvantages are considerable. To obtain good images, the "stack" of original images should consist of thin slices, requiring more images to cover the same area, in turn prolonging the time necessary for the patient to remain motion free. This means that the patient must be totally cooperative, which is not always the case. Once the data have been acquired, considerable additional technologist time and effort are necessary to produce the desired images. This translates into a significant increase in the cost of the study over that of a more conventional CT exam. Availability also still poses a problem. In some newer CT scanners, the program for 3D reconstruction is bundled into the available software for image manipulation. Otherwise, two options exist. Special stand-alone hardware and software systems may be purchased (possibly costing $250,000 or more), or data may be sent to a facility that has the equipment for reprocessing. In either case, the cost per examination is substantial. In the latter situation, it is important to know that the service is commercially available to most institutions, even in very small communities, as long as they have a reasonably modern CT scanner. However, a delay of several days is necessary to ship the data by magnetic tape and allow time for its reprocessing and for return of hard copy images. Figure 5–2 illustrates an application of 3D imaging in a patient with a Le Fort fracture.

The major potential advantage of 3D would appear to lie in the management of the post-traumatic patient with significant residual deformity, for whom reconstructive surgery is planned. In this case the 3D examination permits not only assessment of the deformity, but also the design and production of an accurate prosthetic implant when needed. In at least one instance, the same commercial establishment that processes the 3D images can also produce the appropriate implant. While it will always be difficult to circumvent the potential problems of obtaining 40 or more CT sections without patient motion, computer hardware and software limitations to the widespread availability of 3D surface reconstruction as we know them may be short-lived. Those in the forefront of development of 3D applications to surgical planning have taken advantage of computer-aided design (CAD) employed by major manufacturers of aircraft, automobilies, etc. Similar CAD capabilities have now become quite sophisticated for application with microcomputers available at very reasonable cost, and it seems only a matter of time before software to permit 3D surface reconstructions with microcomputers is commercially available.

Axial images are easily obtained if the patient can lie supine. Coronal images are more difficult for the patient, who must either lie prone with the chin markedly extended or lie supine with the shoulders elevated and the head hanging. However, if neither reformatted images in another plane nor 3D images are desired, slice thickness can be in the 4.5 to 5 mm range, permitting a much more time- and cost-efficient examination.

One concern of many surgeons is the size of the individual images. Modern multiformat cameras, which put the images on x-ray film, are capable of adjusting to create images of variable size depending on how many images are placed on a given size film (typically, 1-on-1, 2-on-1, 4-on-1, 6-on-1, 9-on-1 and 15- or 16-on-1). The scanners themselves can usually produce images in which a segment of the anatomy is enlarged. It is not necessary to have the images depict the anatomy in its actual size. One of the factors in determining the cost of an examination is the cost of film and developing chemicals. Therefore, it is helpful to use an image size that will show the anatomy and pathology clearly but still permit cost-effective use of hard copy image storage. Regardless of what size the images are, it is possible with most CT systems to measure distances very precisely, sometimes to 0.1 mm. Thus, should precise distance measurement be required, the radiologist can provide the surgeon with it on request.

Perhaps the most important option when designing a CT examination for facial trauma is the determination of which plane(s) of imaging to use. To understand and fully explore this dilemma, a review of some of the different injuries using Gentry's classification to organize the survey is in order, with the addition of a category of "combined plane injuries." The examples illustrated are intended to demonstrate the facility with which the anatomy can be visualized and not to show particularly difficult clinical situations. The reader can then extrapolate to the clinical circumstance at hand to decide which plane might work best.

SELECTION OF IMAGE PLANE ACCORDING TO INJURY

Horizontal Plane Injuries

Superior Horizontal Strut Fractures

Fractures of the horizontal plane are usually best imaged in the coronal plane with some important exceptions. Abnormalities of the superior horizontal strut include fracture of the roof of the orbit. This injury is much less common than blowout of the floor and medial wall of the orbit because the roof is relatively stronger (Fig. 5–3). Thus the injury producing the fracture is apt to be more severe, with

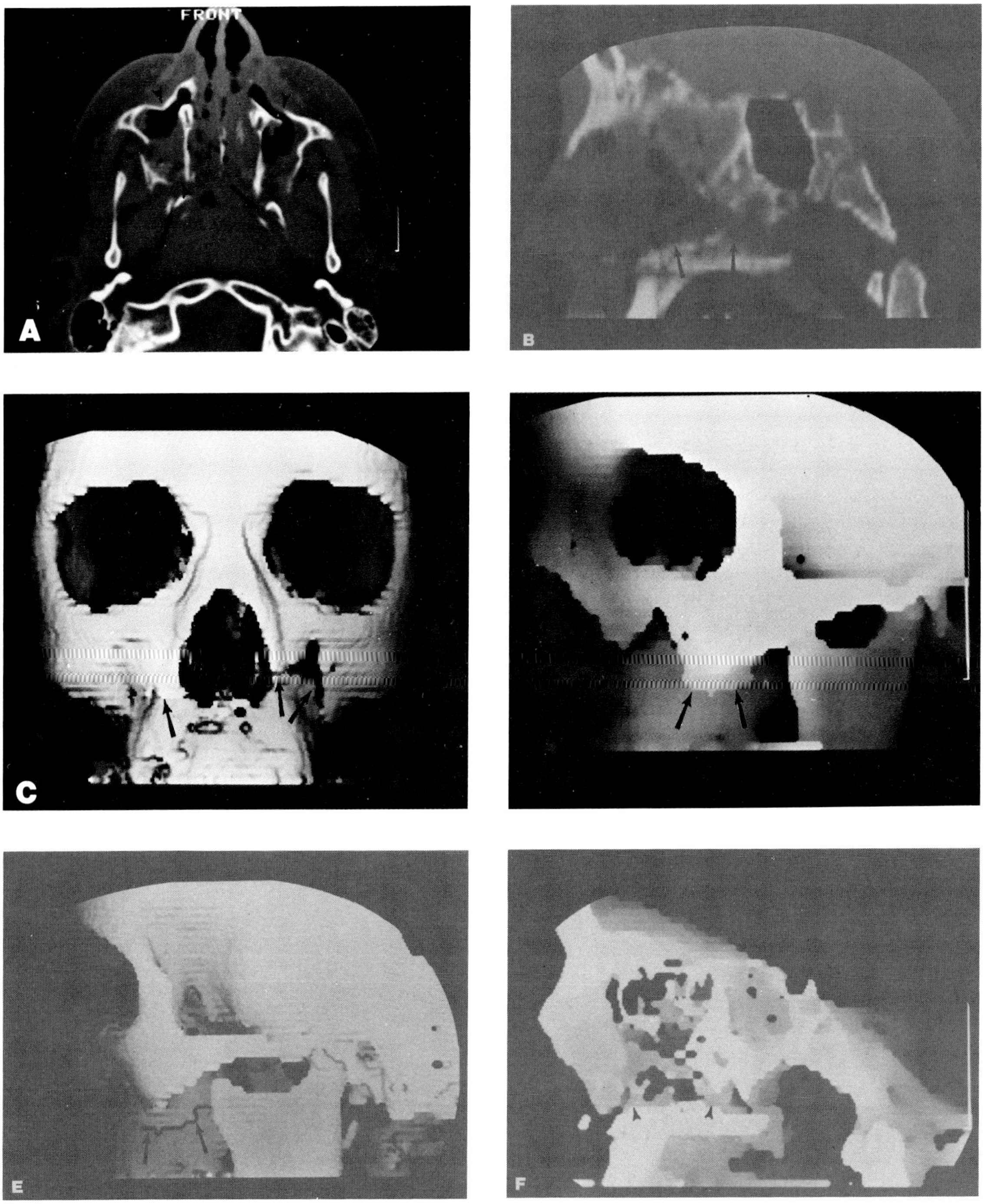

Figure 5–2 Application of 3D to demonstrate a Le Fort I fracture. *A*, A 2-mm-thick axial CT slice of a patient with what is best described as a Le Fort II fracture. Note fractures of anterior, posterolateral, and posterior walls of the maxillary sinuses (arrowheads) and the pterygoid plates (arrows). *B*, A reformatted sagittal slice reveals the mostly horizontal nature of the fracture through the maxilla, just above the alveolar ridge and hard palate. *C*, A 3D anterior surface image reveals the roughly horizontal fractures (arrows). *D*, An oblique 3D surface image again shows the horizontal nature of the fracture nicely (arrows). *E*, A lateral 3D surface image without smoothing actually defines the fracture line above the left alveolar ridge (arrows). *F*, A sagittal slice within the 3D composite yields information (arrowheads) similar to that seen in the sagittal reformatted image in B. (Courtesy of Lindell R. Gentry, M.D., Department of Radiology, University of Wisconsin Clinical Science Center, Madison).

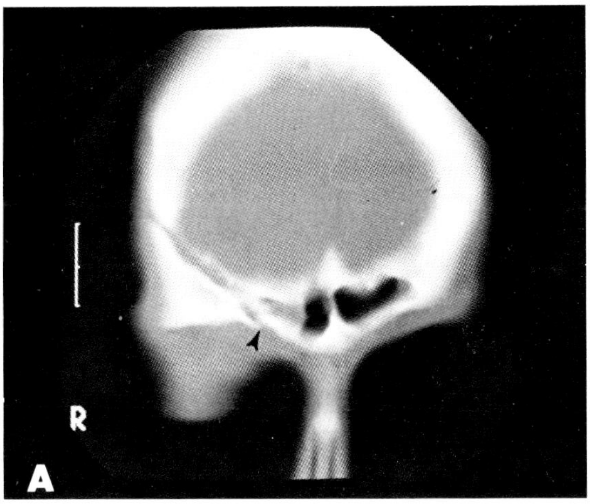

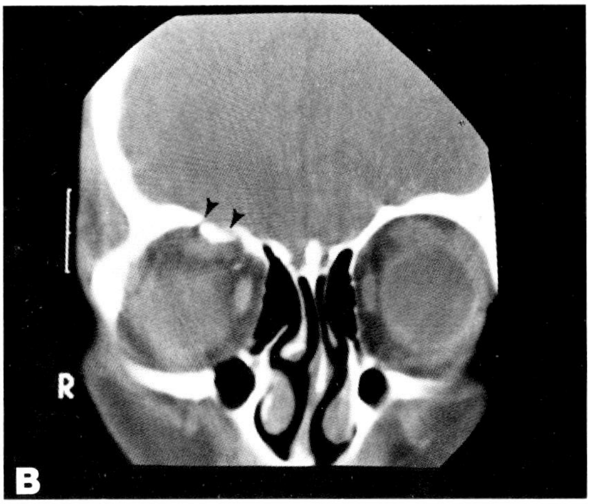

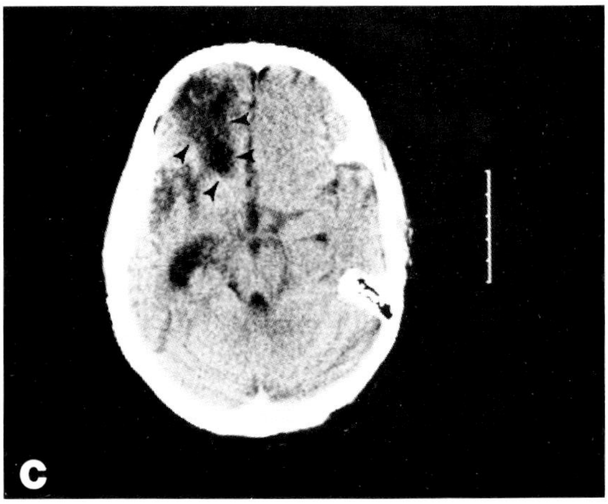

Figure 5–3 Fracture of the roof of the orbit. *A,B*, Coronal CT images reveal fractures of the superior rim of the orbit and orbital roof (arrowheads). *C*, An axial section through the frontal lobes demonstrates a large CSF-containing space at the undersurface of the right frontal lobe, presumably secondary to brain contusion (arrowheads).

a significant risk of intracranial injury and the previously mentioned possibility of posterior extension to the orbital apex with compromise of the optic nerve. In the latter clinical situation, axial images may also become necessary.

A relatively common superior horizontal strut injury is fracture of the cribriform plate, again best seen in the coronal plane if enough distortion of the fracture margins has occurred to result in displacement. This is a common source of cerebrospinal fluid (CSF) leakage.[21,22] It can be a baffling problem to work out, but CT examination after intrathecal administration of water-soluble contrast material can be helpful in determining the precise site of leakage. [16,21,23]

Middle Horizontal Strut Fractures

Blowout fracture of the floor of the orbit, either alone or as a component of the zygomaticofrontal (trimalar) fracture, is a very common clinical problem. The anatomic change of dehiscence of bone with downward herniation of orbital contents may result in diplopia, enophthalmos, and/or hypesthesia in the distribution of the infraorbital nerve.[22,24] The optimal perspective to demonstrate the extent of anatomic alteration is the coronal plane (Fig. 5–4). These injuries can usually be seen in Waters and Caldwell conventional radiographs, but these plain films do not offer a good spatial determination of where the fracture is located along the anterior to posterior axis. Gozum, in a discussion of blowout fractures,[24] has pointed out that the most common site is in the posterior region of the floor, medial to the infraorbital suture and anteromedial to the inferior orbital fissure. Utilizing the tomographic nature of CT, one can accurately determine the location of the fracture (Fig. 5–5).

Assessment of the degree of downward displacement of the floor of the orbit is readily accom-

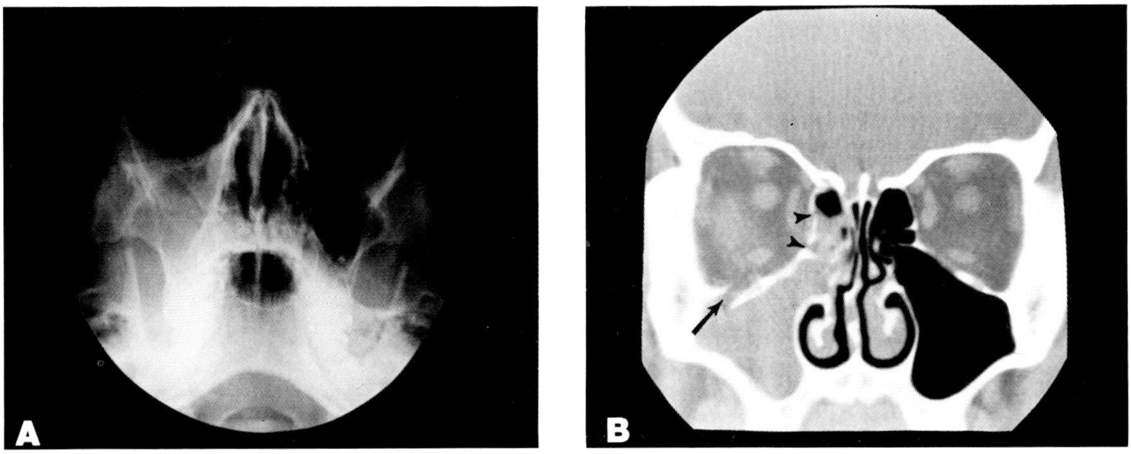

Figure 5–4 Opaque sinus following trauma. *A*, In a Waters view, complete opacification of the right maxillary sinus is a clue to abnormality even though no fracture is identified. *B*, Coronal CT confirms and nicely demonstrates the presence of a blowout fracture of the floor of the orbit but shows that no muscle entrapment has occurred (arrow). Note concurrent fractures of the medial wall of the orbit (arrowheads). Contrast this case with that seen in Figure 5–13.

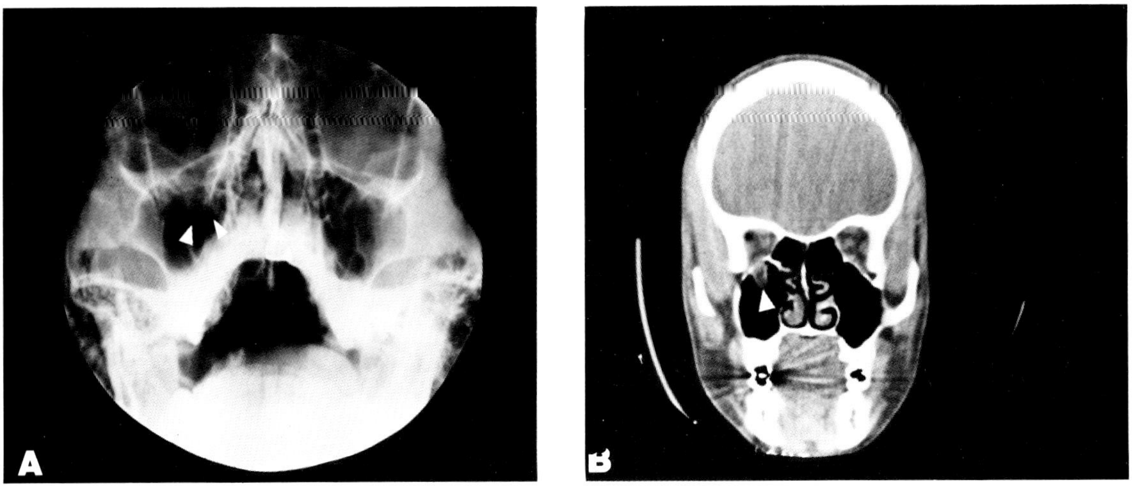

Figure 5–5 Blowout fracture of the floor of the orbit. *A*, Waters view. A "superior polyp sign" consisting of soft tissue extending down from the roof of the right maxillary sinus can be seen (arrowheads) but this is difficult to place from front to back. *B*, The coronal CT section shows the herniating soft tissue in a more posterior section (arrowhead), emphasizing the value of the tomographic nature of the CT study. (From Johnson DH Jr. CT of maxillofacial trauma. Radiol Clin North Am 1984; 22:131–144. Reprinted with permission from WB Saunders.)

plished by coronal images[3] and is potentially important to the patient in terms of preventing posttraumatic enophthalmos.[25] (Axial sections should be obtained if determination of the degree of posterior displacement of the globe is desired.)

One of the exceptions to the use of coronal imaging for horizontal plane fractures is fracture of the zygomatic arch. Although the arch is a component of the middle horizontal strut, it is much more easily evaluated in axial CT images (Fig. 5–6).

Inferior Horizontal Strut Fractures

Inferior horizontal strut fractures are the other exception to the use of coronal plane imaging for the evaluation of horizontal plane fractures. These frac-

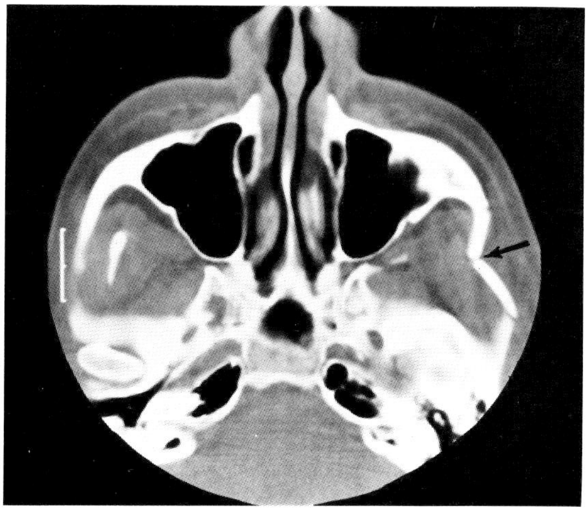

Figure 5–6 In this axial CT image a "bucket handle fracture" of the zygomatic arch is readily seen (arrow). Note that this fracture is well seen in axial images even though it is in the middle horizontal strut.

tures are usually linear in nature and can be easily be seen in axial images (Fig. 5–7).

Sagittal Plane Fractures

Median Strut Fractures

Both recent and old fractures of the bony nasal septum may be readily demonstrated in axial images, although a distinction between recent and old injury may be impossible without previous images for comparison. Septal hematoma is important to recognize[4] and should be easily delineated, although it is difficult to distinguish from localized mucosal thickening.

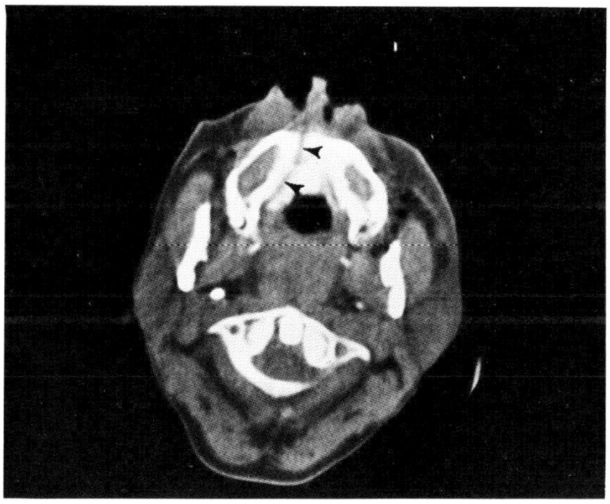

Figure 5–7 Fracture of the hard palate is unusual but readily seen in axial CT (arrowheads) despite the fact that it lies in the inferior horizontal strut. (From Johnson DH Jr. CT of maxillofacial trauma. Radiol Clin North Am 1984; 22:131–144. Reprinted with permission from WB Saunders.)

Parasagittal Strut Fractures

The determination of which plane to use for the investigation of possible fracture of the medial wall of the orbit centers on the question of whether a concurrent fracture of the floor of the orbit has occurred. The medial wall fracture should be visible in both axial and coronal planes (Fig. 5–8). However, the orbital floor fracture will be best demonstrated in the coronal plane.[26] Although there does not seem to be agreement in the literature about the incidence of concurrent medial wall and floor of orbit fractures, several discussions pointed to such concurrence.[5,8,14,26,27] Blowout fracture of the floor of the orbit is the more common injury. Some attribute this difference to the fact that the medial wall is in part supported by the network of septa between ethmoid air cells while the floor of the orbit has no similar support.[5]

Fractures of the medial wall of the maxillary sinus should be visible in the axial plane (Fig. 5–9B) unless they are parallel to the plane of section, in which case coronal images should show them readily.

Lateral Facial Strut Fractures

Fractures of the lateral orbit wall are a component of the trimalar fracture, which will be discussed in the section on complex fractures. They rarely occur as an isolated finding. Thus, while they are best seen in axial images, axial images alone may not suffice for evaluation of the entire injury. Fractures of the lateral wall of the maxillary sinus usually accompany a trimalar fracture (Fig. 5–10) but may occur as an isolated finding (Fig. 5–11). Like fractures of the lateral wall of the orbit, fractures of the lateral portion of the maxillary alveolar ridge are usually clearly seen in the axial perspective.

Fractures in the Coronal Plane

Anterior Coronal Strut Fractures

A particularly vulnerable part of the facial skeleton, the vertical portion of the frontal bone is easily evaluated in axial CT. Fractures of both anterior and posterior tables are readily seen.

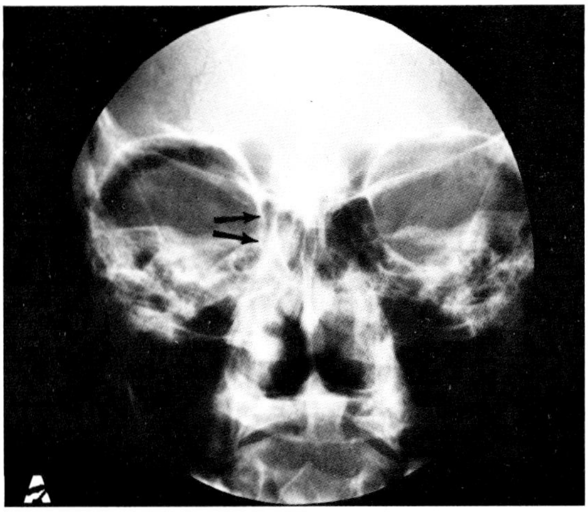

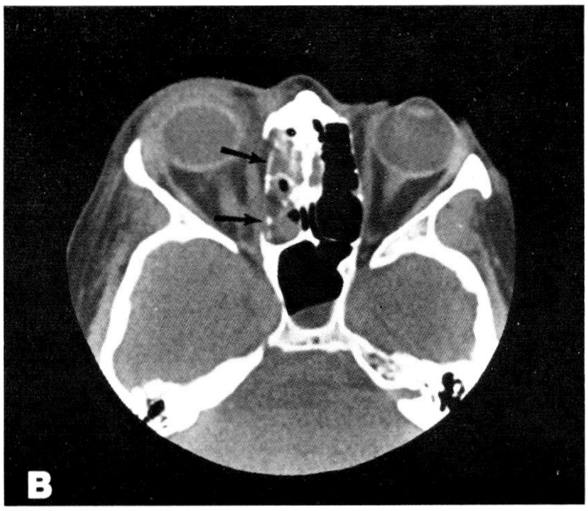

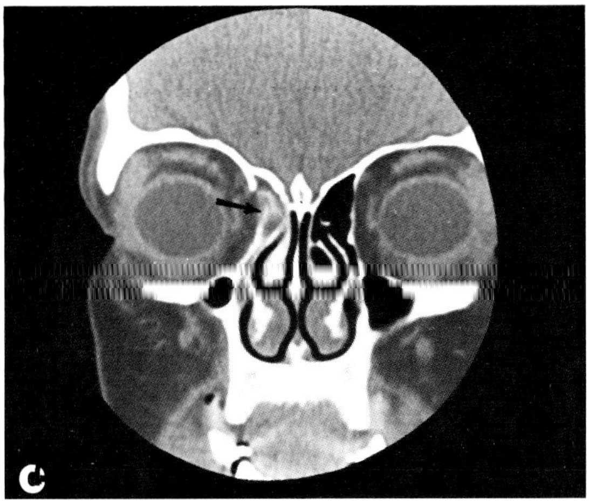

Figure 5–8 Blowout fracture of the medial wall of the orbit. *A*, Caldwell view. The medial wall of the left orbit is intact with aerated ethmoid sinus medial to it, whereas the medial wall of the right orbit is displaced medially with opacification of the right ethmoid sinus (arrows). *B*, Axial CT readily confirms the plain film findings (arrows). *C*, Coronal CT shows the fracture well but adds little to the axial image and plain film demonstration (arrows). Note that the Waters view we usually use for "scout" purposes probably would not have shown the abnormality as well as the Caldwell projection does. (Courtesy of Matthew M. Fluke, M.D., New Orleans Radiology Group).

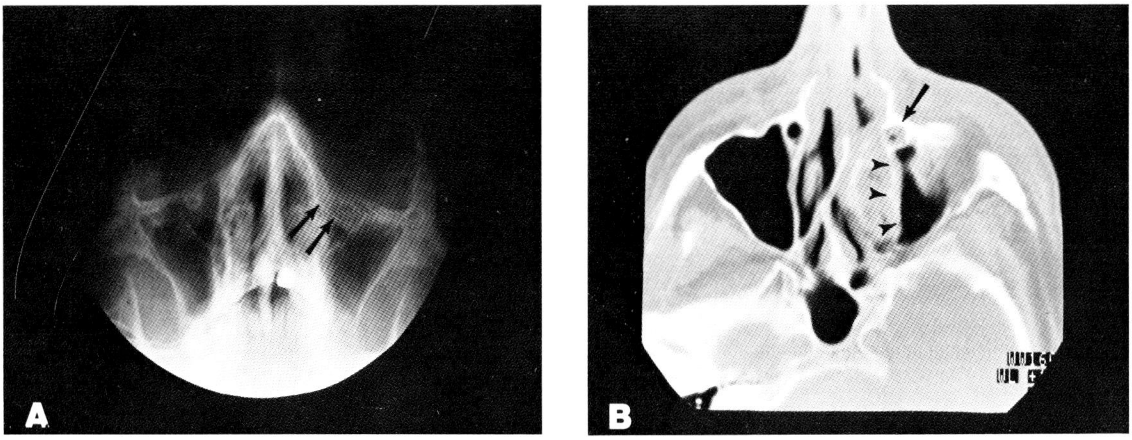

Figure 5–9 Minimal frontoethmoid complex fracture. *A*, In the Waters projection, a thin opaque line at the superomedial aspect of the left maxillary sinus (arrows) should make one suspect an abnormality and is an indication for CT. *B*, Axial CT images confirm the presence of a minimal frontoethmoid complex fracture. The medial wall of the left maxillary sinus is fragmented (arrowheads). Note the slight clockwise rotation of the bony structures forming the lacrimal canal (arrow). Note also fractures of the nasal bones not seen in the Waters projection.

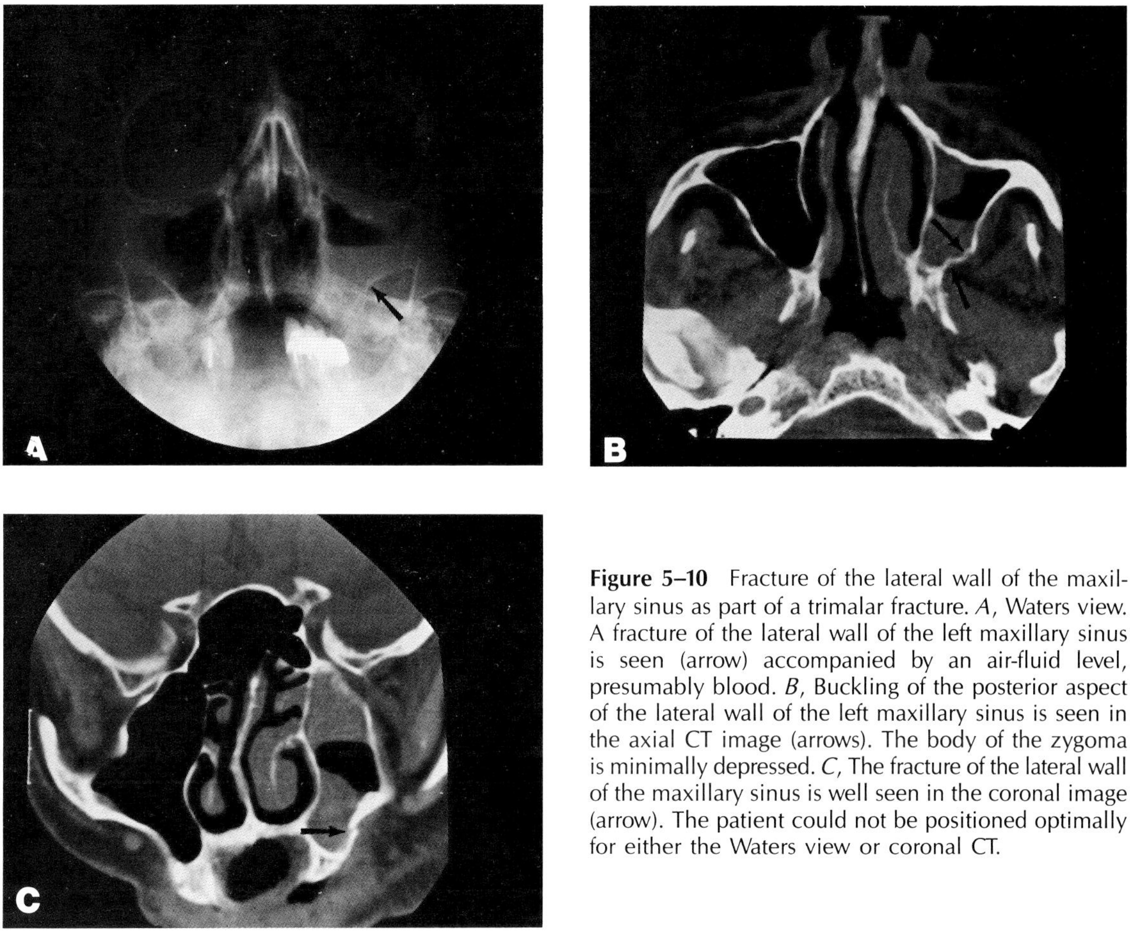

Figure 5–10 Fracture of the lateral wall of the maxillary sinus as part of a trimalar fracture. *A*, Waters view. A fracture of the lateral wall of the left maxillary sinus is seen (arrow) accompanied by an air-fluid level, presumably blood. *B*, Buckling of the posterior aspect of the lateral wall of the left maxillary sinus is seen in the axial CT image (arrows). The body of the zygoma is minimally depressed. *C*, The fracture of the lateral wall of the maxillary sinus is well seen in the coronal image (arrow). The patient could not be positioned optimally for either the Waters view or coronal CT.

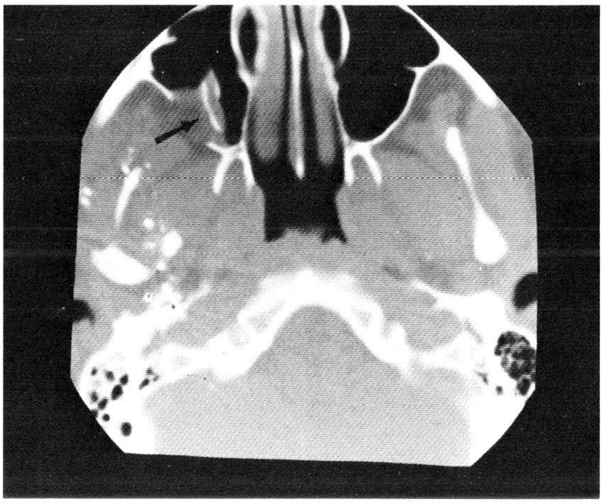

Figure 5–11 Fracture of the posterolateral wall of the maxillary sinus (arrow). This fracture as seen in axial CT, apparently represents a "blow-in" fracture secondary to blast effect of a gunshot wound (note missile fragments around the mandibular condyle).

Figure 5–12 illustrates a fracture of the anterior wall of the frontal sinus. Note the ease with which the axial CT image evaluates the anterior and posterior walls of the sinus. The anterolateral wall of the maxillary sinus is the most common site of isolated maxillary sinus fracture and is best seen in axial sections (Fig. 5–13).

Posterior Coronal Strut Fractures

The components of the posterior coronal strut are complex in their orientation. The pterygoid plates are actually oriented in the anteroposterior or sagittal plane. For convenience, Gentry combines the pterygoid complexes and posterior walls of the maxillary sinuses into one strut. Axial images will usually demonstrate fractures well (see Fig. 5–2A).

Potter's early but still valuable work on sectional anatomy of the head [28] demonstrates in axial sections that portions of the posterior maxilla are separated from the pterygoid plates, forming the

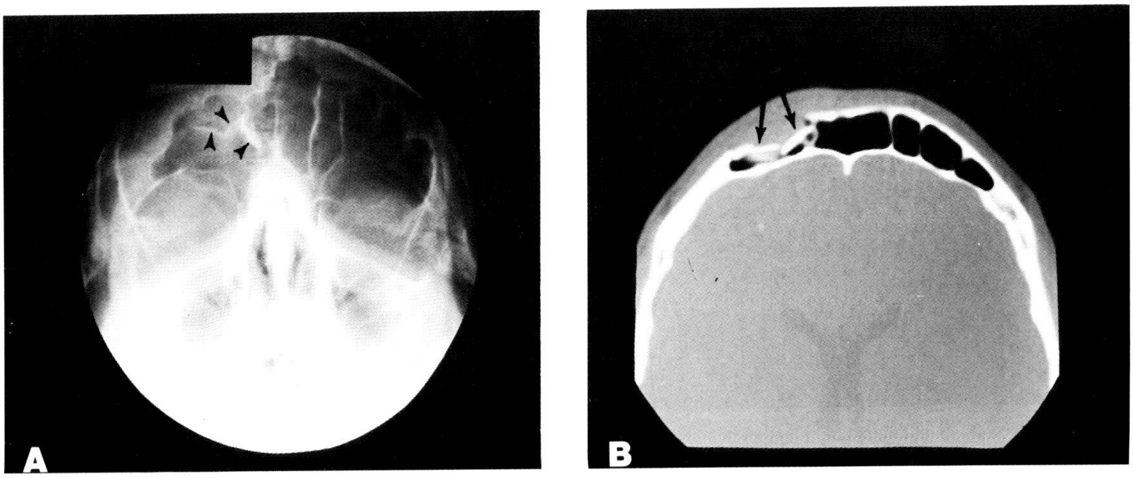

Figure 5–12 Fracture of the anterior coronal strut. *A*, Irregular opaque lines in the right frontal region are strongly suspicious for fracture fragments seen on end (arrowheads). *B*, Axial CT confirms the fracture but shows it to be confined to the anterior wall of the frontal sinus (arrows) and not affecting the posterior wall.

pterygopalatine fossa. In this region it is possible to define a true posterior wall of the maxillary sinus. A fracture of that wall is seen in Figure 5–14.

Combined Plane Fractures

Frontoethmoid Complex Fractures

The frontoethmoid complex fracture, at the junction of the parasagittal, superior, and middle horizontal and anterior coronal struts, is fairly common (see Fig. 5–9). Its special significance lies in the importance of its recognition, so that another associated fracture, such as the trimalar fracture (see Fig. 5–15), does not result in immobilization of an unstable fragment to an unstable fragment. Because all three planes are involved, it is desirable to image in both axial and coronal planes if at all possible. The central landmark is the nasolacrimal canal, readily identified on axial CT and surrounded by relatively thick bone (see Fig. 5–9B). This lies within the medial pillar of support of the face of the anterior aspect of the parasagittal strut. The medial pillar includes the frontal process of the

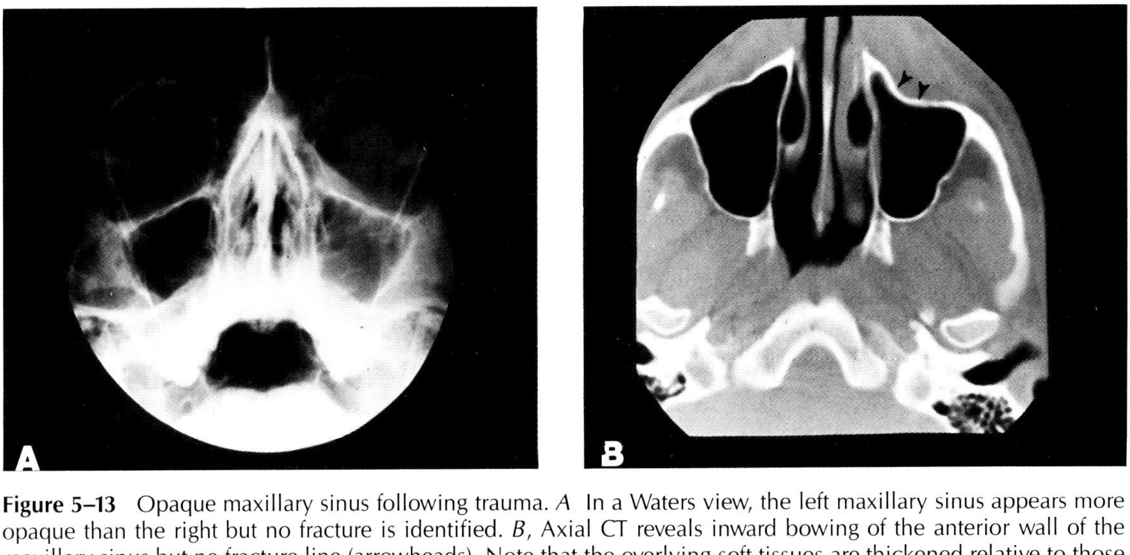

Figure 5–13 Opaque maxillary sinus following trauma. *A* In a Waters view, the left maxillary sinus appears more opaque than the right but no fracture is identified. *B*, Axial CT reveals inward bowing of the anterior wall of the maxillary sinus but no fracture line (arrowheads). Note that the overlying soft tissues are thickened relative to those on the right, which should explain the plain film difference.

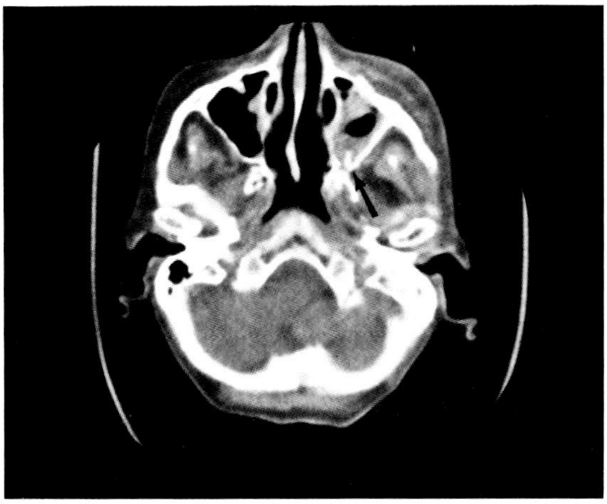

Figure 5–14 Fracture of the true posterior wall of the maxillary sinus (arrow) at the level of the pterygopalatine fossa with the fragment directed anteriorly into the sinus proper. (From Johnson DH Jr. CT of maxillofacial trauma. Radiol Clin North Am 1984; 22:131–144. Reprinted with permission from WB Saunders.)

maxillary bone and the medial portion of the anterior surface of the maxilla extending down to the canine tooth.[29] Fracture across this pillar can disrupt the lacrimal drainage system, causing excess tearing and chronic dacryocystitis.[11] Disruption of the medial canthal ligament may result in traumatic hypertelorism.[8] Other potential complications of this fracture include damage to the trochlea, with impairment of function of the superior oblique muscle, and CSF leakage due to extension into the superior horizontal strut. Figure 5–16 shows a localized variant of this injury in which the upper nose is markedly displaced posteriorly, literally between the orbits.

Zygomaticofrontal (Trimalar) Fractures

The body of the zygoma may be regarded as the cornerstone of the face. Trauma in that region can result in a complex of fractures involving anterior coronal, middle horizontal, and lateral facial struts. Axial CT will demonstrate the rotation and posterior displacement of the body of the zygoma (Fig. 5–17). The preliminary Waters radiograph will usually show the vertical components of the facial skeleton (Fig. 5–18). However, if it is desirable to evaluate the floor of the orbit well, coronal images will be necessary.

Le Fort Fractures

As with the other combined plane fractures, the individual components of the injury can be evaluated with CT. Because of the complex nature of the fractures, images in more than one plane are usually desirable. Because the patient's condition in these more severe images will often preclude direct coronal imaging, reformatted images are apt to become necessary.

The Le Fort I (horizontal) fracture is basically in the axial plane, passing transversely through the maxilla across anterior and posterior struts of the coronal plane and all of the struts in the sagittal plane. While the various components can often be seen in axial images,[3] the use of reformatted images (see Fig. 5–2A, B) and 3D reconstruction

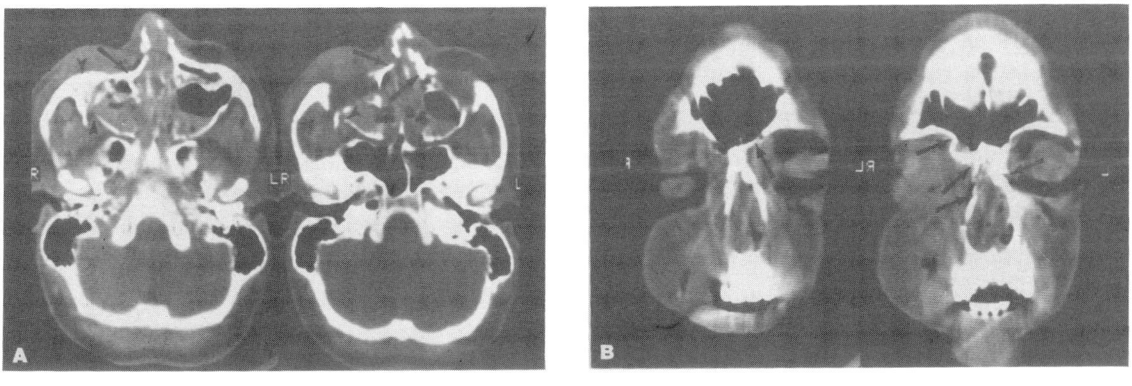

Figure 5–15 Combination of frontoethmoid complex and trimalar fractures. *A*, Axial CT reveals bilateral frontoethmoid complex fractures (arrows) with a right trimalar fracture (arrowheads). *B*, Coronal CT demonstrates the fractures though the frontoethmoid complexes (arrows). This series of fractures could also be classified as a Le Fort II fracture with a right trimalar fracture, illustrating the shortcomings of the Le Fort classification. (Courtesy of Yugi Numaguchi, M.D., Department of Radiology, Tulane Medical Center).

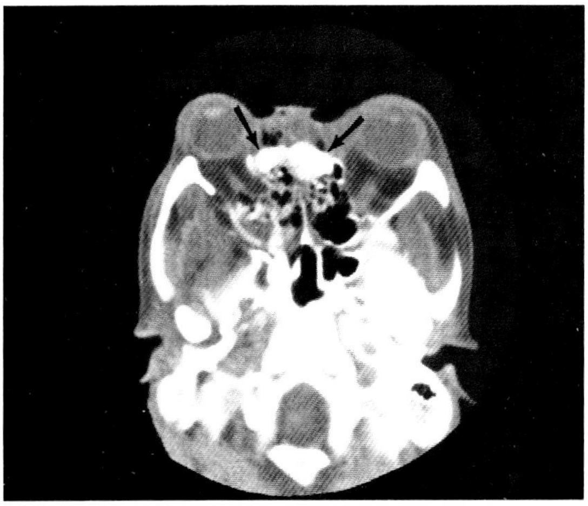

Figure 5–16 This axial CT image reveals marked comminuted depression of the upper nose and anterior ethmoid region (arrows). This particular fracture is difficult to classify, affecting both frontoethmoid complexes and numerous struts. nevertheless, it is nicely shown by axial CT. (Courtesy of Yugi Numaguchi, M.D., Department of Radiology, Tulane Medical Center).

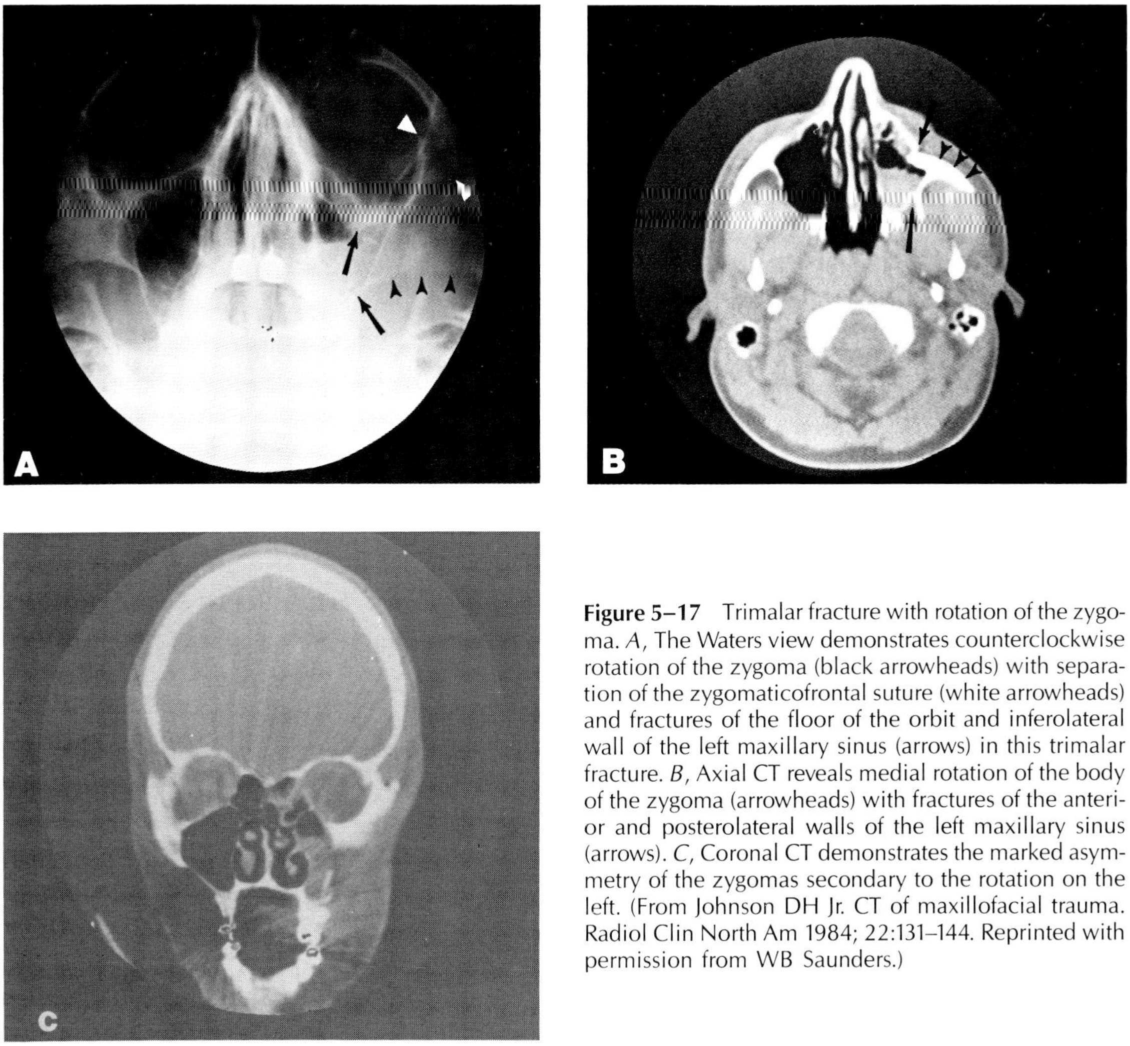

Figure 5–17 Trimalar fracture with rotation of the zygoma. *A*, The Waters view demonstrates counterclockwise rotation of the zygoma (black arrowheads) with separation of the zygomaticofrontal suture (white arrowheads) and fractures of the floor of the orbit and inferolateral wall of the left maxillary sinus (arrows) in this trimalar fracture. *B*, Axial CT reveals medial rotation of the body of the zygoma (arrowheads) with fractures of the anterior and posterolateral walls of the left maxillary sinus (arrows). *C*, Coronal CT demonstrates the marked asymmetry of the zygomas secondary to the rotation on the left. (From Johnson DH Jr. CT of maxillofacial trauma. Radiol Clin North Am 1984; 22:131–144. Reprinted with permission from WB Saunders.)

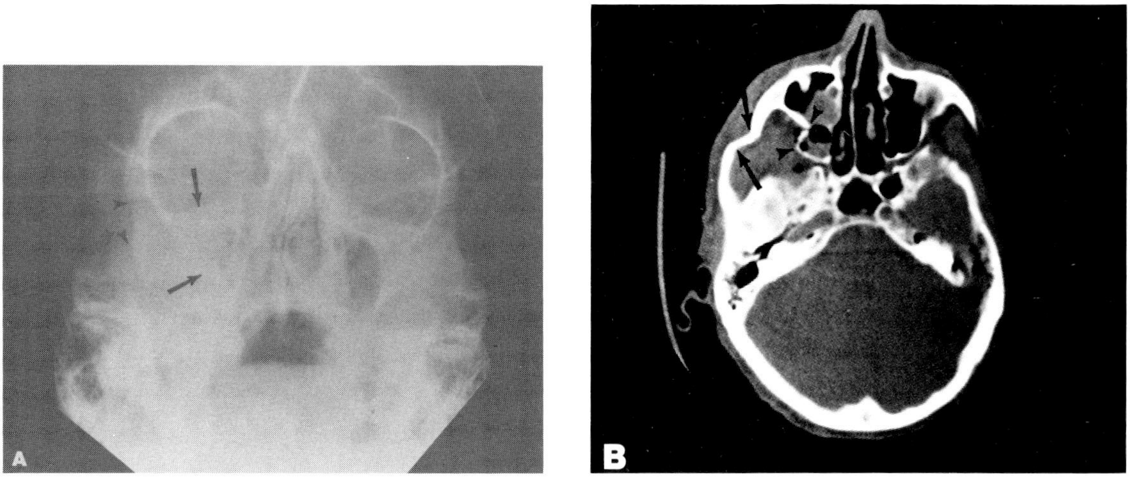

Figure 5–18 Trimalar fracture. *A*, Waters view. Two fractures in the zygomatic arch, a fracture in the frontal process of the zygoma (arrowheads), and counterclockwise rotation of the body of the zygoma with fracture of the inferolateral wall of the maxillary sinus and presumed fracture of the floor of the orbit (arrows) are all demonstrated, nicely complementing the findings in the axial CT study. *B*, Axial CT. Two fractures of the zygomatic arch (arrows), and fractures of the posterolateral wall of the maxillary sinus (arrowheads) are accompanied by lateral rotation of the body of the zygoma.

(see Fig. 5–2C, D, E, F) can be particularly valuable in this complex.

The Le Fort II "pyramidal" fracture extends obliquely across lateral and parasagittal struts of the sagittal plane, anterior and posterior struts of the coronal plane, and the middle horizontal plane. In about 10 percent of cases, there is extension into the ethmoid and frontal sinuses[5] (Fig. 5–19).

The Le Fort III fracture is the most extensive of this type of fracture. This injury results in a complete detachment of the facial skeleton from the base of the skull. These fractures course across all sagittal struts, both coronal struts, and the middle horizontal strut.

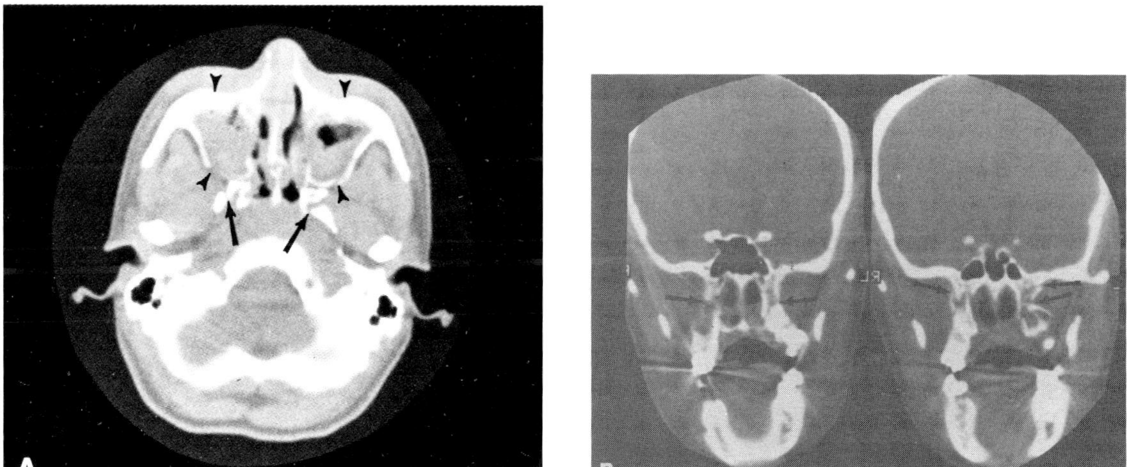

Figure 5–19 Le Fort II fracture. *A*, Axial slice. Note relatively symmetric fractures of the anterior and posterolateral walls of the maxillary sinuses (arrowheads) and of the pterygoid plates (arrows). The bodies of the zygomas are not rotated or otherwise displaced. *B*, A posterior coronal slice shows the fractures of the pterygoid plates (arrows). (Courtesy of Yugi Numaguchi, M.D., Department of Radiology, Tulane Medical Center.)

SUMMARY OF SUGGESTED APPROACHES TO IMAGING OF THE SEQUELAE OF TRAUMA TO THE MAXILLOFACIAL SKELETON

In a patient who has sustained facial trauma, the decision on whether and how to proceed with diagnostic imaging relies on accurate clinical assessment of the entire patient and not simply the facial region. If neurological evaluation is indicated, it should be followed by evaluation of the facial injuries so that a determination can be made whether immediate imaging investigation and treatment of both is indicated. When the nasal bones alone are of interest, plain films will usually suffice. When the mandible has been traumatized, panoramic tomography, if available, is the procedure of choice. Otherwise, plain films should be diagnostic for nasal and mandibular fracture. If CT is performed for investigation of other parts of the facial skeleton, the nose and mandible should be scrutinized.

An exaggerated Waters view with the mouth closed can be used in most patients to indicate whether more sophisticated imaging is indicated. With a clear understanding of the anatomy likely to be affected in a given injury, one can usually establish a satisfactory imaging strategy on the basis of thorough clinical evaluation and the Waters view. So-called conventional tomography is now of limited value, an exception being the situation in which images in two planes at right angles to one another are desired but the patient is too badly injured to assume the position for coronal images and adequate CT image reformatting is not available. Axial CT images and coronal tomography can both be obtained with the patient supine, yielding two image planes at right angles to one another.

Although most authors seem to prefer the coronal plane for imaging of the face, axial sections will show a great majority of the fractures and can be quickly and easily obtained.[11,15] When clinical evaluation, preliminary plain film, and consultation with the radiologist reveal that other imaging will be required, the patient's ability to cooperate must be assessed. If the patient can safely assume the position for any needed coronal images, or if only axial images seem indicated, 4.5- to 5 mm thick images will usually suffice, for a faster, more cost-effective examination. If, for whatever reason, coronal images are desired but the patient cannot assume the position required, indicating that reformatting of axial data into the coronal plane is necessary, and/or if 3D images appear desirable, image slice thickness should be in the range of 1.5 to 3.0 mm; this decision must be made before the examination begins. If the patient is thrashing about and cannot be safely quieted down, a limited preliminary study with thicker sections may suffice until the patient can remain still for the series of thinner slices.

Modern imaging is available in almost all parts of the United States now, but it can be of maximum benefit to the injured patient only when there is meaningful communication between the surgeon managing the patient and the radiologist supervising the diagnostic examination and interpreting the images. The radiologist will be most effective when the surgeon shares with him or her the surgical findings. A simple explanation exists for everything seen on an image; the problem lies in being clever enough to figure it out. Postoperative discussion of findings helps build that cleverness and kindles the interest of the radiologist and, hopefully, the surgeon as well.

REFERENCES

1. Le Fort R. Étude expérimentale sur les fractures de la machoire supérieure. Rev Chir 1901; 23:208–227.
2. Finkle DR, Ringler SL, Luttenton CR, et al. Comparison of the diagnostic methods used in maxillofacial trauma. Plast Reconstr Surg 1985; 75:32–38.
3. Rothaus KO, Rosenthal AM, Kalisman M. Computed tomography—its principles and application to the diagnosis of facial fractures. Clin Plast Surg 1986; 13:433–440.
4. Schultz RC, de Camara DL. Athletic facial injuries. JAMA 1984; 252:3395–3398.
5. Valvassori GE, Hord GE. Traumatic sinus disease. Semin Roentgenol 1968; 3:160–171.
6. De Castro IA, Hanafee WN. Fracturas del esqueleto facial. Rev Interam Radiol 1979; 4:1–9.
7. Gentry LR, Manor WF, Turski PA, Strother CM. High resolution computed tomographic analysis of facial struts in trauma:1. Normal anatomy. AJR 1983; 140:523–532.
8. Gentry LR, Manor WF, Turski PA, Strother CM. High resolution computed tomographic analysis of facial struts in trauma:2. Osseous and soft tissue complications. AJR 1983; 140:533–541.
9. Dolan KD, Jacoby CG, Smoker WRK. The radiology of facial fractures. Radiographics 1984; 4:576–663.
10. Gerlock AJ Jr, Sinn DP, McBride KL. Clinical and radiographic interpretation of facial fractures. Boston: Little, Brown, 1981.
11. Johnson DH Jr. CT of maxillofacial trauma. Radiol Clin North Am 1984; 22:131–144.
12. Potter GD, Trokel SL. Optic canal. In: Newton TH, Potts DG, eds. Radiology of the skull and brain, Vol 1. 1st ed. St. Louis: CV Mosby, 1971: 487.
13. Unger JM. Orbital apex fractures: the contribution of computed tomography. Radiology 1984; 150:713–717.

14. Zizmor J, Noyek AM. Orbital trauma. In: Newton TH, Potts DG, eds. Radiology of the skull and brain, Vol 1. 1st ed. St. Louis: CV Mosby, 1971: 541.
15. Gentry LR, Smoker WRK. Computed tomography of facial trauma. Semin Ultrasound CT MR 1985; 6:129–145.
16. Brant-Zawadzki M, Minagi H, Federle M, Rowe LD. High resolution CT with image reformation in maxillofacial pathology. AJNR 1982; 3:31–37.
17. Hammerschlag SB, Hughes S, O'Reilly GV, et al. Blow-out fractures of the orbit: a comparison of computed tomography and conventional radiography with anatomic correlation. Radiology 1982; 143:487–492.
18. Marsh JL, Vannier MW, Bresina S, Hemmer KM. Applications of computer graphics in craniofacial surgery. Clin Plast Surg 1986; 13:441–448.
19. Vannier MW, Marsh JL, Warren JO. Three dimensional CT reconstruction images for craniofacial surgical planning and evaluation. Radiology 1984; 150:179–184.
20. Herman GT, Vose WF, Gomori JM, Gefter WB. Stereoscopic computed three-dimensional surface displays. Radiographics 1985; 5:825–852.
21. Ghoshhajra K. CT in trauma of the base of the skull and its complications. CT 1980; 4:271–276.
22. Mathog RH, Rosenberg Z. Complications in the treatment of facial fractures. Otolaryngol Clin North Am 1976; 9:533–552.
23. Noyek AM, Kassel EE, Wortzman G, et al. Sophisticated CT in complex maxillofacial trauma. Laryngoscope 1982; 92(Suppl 27):1–17.
24. Gozum E. Blowout fractures of the orbit. Otolaryngol Clin North Am 1976; 9:477–487.
25. Manson PN, Grivas A, Rosenbaum A, et al. Studies on enophthalmos: II. The measurement of orbital injuries and their treatment by quantitative computed tomography. Plast Reconstr Surg 1986; 77:203–214.
26. Zikha A. Computed tomography of blow-out fracture of the medial wall of the orbit. AJNR 1981; 2:427–429.
27. Arger PH. Fractures of the orbit. In: Arger PH, ed. Orbit roentgenology. New York: John Wiley & Sons, 1977: 55.
28. Potter GD. Sectional anatomy and tomography of the head. New York: Grune & Stratton, 1971: 197.
29. Johnson DH Jr, Colman M, Larsson S, et al. Computed tomography in medial maxilla-orbital fractures. J Comput Assist Tomogr 1984; 8:416–419.

6

HEAD INJURY

BRUCE M. McCORMACK, M.D., F.A.C.S.
PAUL R. COOPER, M.D.

In this chapter, the initial evaluation and neurologic examination of head-injured patients is discussed. There is a brief review of intracranial injuries and their management and a more detailed discussion of the treatment of linear, depressed, and basal skull fractures. Traumatic cerebrospinal fluid (CSF) fistulas are also discussed.

THE INITIAL MANAGEMENT OF THE HEAD-INJURED PATIENT

In 1984, there were 470,000 head injuries in the United States.[1] Motor vehicle crashes account for the major proportion of head injuries. However, in urban areas gunshot wounds, assaults, and falls are more frequently encountered. Among 225 patients with severe head injuries, Miller and colleagues[2] found 49 percent with one or more additional systemic injuries, the most common injuries being limb fracture (30 percent) and chest trauma (29 percent). Abdominal injuries occurred in 17 percent of these patients and 6 percent had spinal injuries.[3] Eighty percent of trauma-related deaths occur in patients with injury to more than three body areas.[4,5]

Systemic Assessment and Stabilization

The initial assessment and stabilization of multiply injured patients necessitate the simultaneous activity of several physicians, all under the direction of one physician, usually a general surgeon or trauma surgeon, who assumes the responsibility for total patient care. Close cooperation among the various surgical services is necessary to coordinate the most prudent treatment plan (see chapter 3 entitled *Team Approach to Management of Trauma Victim*). This is particularly important in patients with craniofacial trauma, for whom the expertise of the neurosurgeon, otolaryngologist, plastic surgeon, and oral surgeon is simultaneously needed.

A definitive outline for the care of the multiply injured has been prepared by the American College of Surgeons (Advanced Trauma Life Support). The system is designed to restore rapidly the ABCs—*airway, breathing,* and *circulation*—followed by a more detailed diagnostic examination and adjustment of treatment. Those injuries posing an immediate threat to life, such as cardiac tamponade, tension pneumothorax, impaired airway, or exsanguinating hemorrhage, are assessed and treated. If it is not possible to stabilize these conditions, diagnostic procedures such as computed tomographic (CT) scanning may not be possible, and burr holes are placed if an intracranial hemorrhage is suspected.

Hypoxia

Hypoxia is suspected in all comatose patients and in all patients who are anxious, combative, or apprehensive. Frost and co-workers[6] found a 65 percent incidence of arterial hypoxemia in head-injured patients spontaneously breathing without airway distress. Head-injured patients with hypoxemia have a significantly poorer prognosis than head-injured patients without hypoxemia[7]; it is therefore necessary that an airway be established as soon as possible to provide adequate tidal volume and oxygenation.

Care begins with clearing the upper airway of vomitus, blood, or foreign bodies such as broken teeth, and using the "chin lift" to align the airway anatomically. Once this is done adequate assisted ventilation with a bag and mask will be possible in the majority of patients. If a patent airway cannot be established with these techniques, endotracheal intubation must be performed. Endotracheal intubation can be performed orally or nasally, but in suspected or proven cases of cervical spine injury, nasal intubation is preferred (see chapter 4 entitled *Airway Management*). A surgical alternative to endotracheal intubation is cricothyroidotomy. Extensive craniofacial injuries and tracheal fractures are the most frequent indications for this procedure.

Shock

Shock of varying degrees of severity is present in 13 percent of head-injured patients.[8] The usual cause of low blood pressure is bleeding into the chest or abdominal cavities, or internal hemorrhage in patients with pelvic or long bone fractures. Closed head injuries do not cause hypotension in adult patients. Spinal cord injuries, however, may cause hypotension and associated bradycardia, and this is frequently overlooked in the initial assessment of a patient with multiple injuries. The presence of shock in a patient with a severe closed head injury results in an increase in mortality to 83 percent as opposed to 45 percent when head injury is not associated with shock.[9–11]

The treatment of shock begins with control of external hemorrhage and with fluid resuscitation. Two large-bore 14- to 16-gauge catheters are inserted in the upper extremity and 2 L of crystalloid solution such as Ringer's lactate are infused. Central venous lines are helpful in more severely injured patients. The blood pressure should be maintained above 100 mm Hg for most patients, and fluid administration can be slowed as urine output increases, the central venous pressure rises, and blood pressure is stabilized. Fluid resuscitation should not be withheld in patients with head injuries who have multiple trauma and are hypotensive because of fear of exacerbating cerebral edema. Often raising the blood pressure will improve the patient's level of consciousness and reverse neurologic deficits as cerebral perfusion pressure is raised. Only in patients with isolated head trauma should fluids be used sparingly. If the patient remains hypotensive after receiving 2 L of crystalloid solution, and there is no evidence of cardiogenic or vasogenic shock, blood replacement is indicated. The use of pneumatic antishock garment to sustain blood pressure is not contraindicated in patients with head injury. In a prospective study of 12 patients with severe head injury, there was no abnormal increase in intracranial pressure (ICP) with moderate inflation pressures to 45 mm Hg in each compartment.[12]

Intracranial Hypertension

The single most frequent cause of death in head-injured patients is uncontrolled intracranial hypertension.[13,14] Early recognition of abnormally high ICP and immediate intervention to return it to normal has led to a dramatic reduction of uncontrolled ICP as a cause of death in head-injured patients.

Ideally ICP should be monitored and treated according to values obtained from an ICP monitor. However, a neurosurgeon may not be available immediately for insertion of an ICP monitor. Whether elevated ICP is suspected or confirmed, treatment should begin with hyperventilation. Induced hypocapnea to a range of 25 to 30 mm Hg is the most effective means of rapid reduction of elevated ICP. Mannitol (0.5 to 1 g per kilogram) should be given intravenously if the patient is not hypotensive. These treatments have few risks and may be lifesaving.

Neurologic Assessment

The neurologic assessment is performed simultaneously with cardiopulmonary resuscitation when the patient arrives in the emergency room. The extent of the neurologic evaluation will depend upon the severity of head injury and the extent of the patient's ability to cooperate with the examiner. The poorly cooperative or unconscious patient will have to be examined by observing the response to noxious stimuli and eliciting brainstem reflexes. The complete evaluation should include a history, assessment of state of consciousness, pupillary reactivity, eye movements, and motor abilities.

Information regarding the time, location, and mechanism of injury should be sought from paramedics, police, relatives and witnesses. The mechanism of injury is important; direct blows to the head are likely to cause acute epidural hematomas, whereas acceleration-deceleration injuries commonly cause diffuse cerebral damage and subdural hematomas. The temporal course of the patient's level of consciousness after injury should be elicited. A history of a lucid interval followed by deterioration suggests an expanding intracranial hemorrhage. With diffuse brain injury, the patient will remain comatose and gradually become more alert after the injury. Possible drug or alcohol use should be evaluated with appropriate toxicology screens. If the alcohol level is below 200 mg per deciliter, an alteration in mental status should not be ascribed to the effect of the alcohol.[15] Naloxone should be administered if there is suspicion of narcotic use. Epileptics often present to the emergency room with head injury as a result of seizures. An intracranial hemorrhage should be suspected if there is a postictal neurologic deficit, focal seizures, or status epilepticus in a patient without a prior history of this seizure pattern.[16]

During the neurologic assessment, particular attention should be given to wounds of the head and neck. The entire scalp must be palpated and the wounds debrided while the clinician looks for depressions, fractures, and foreign bodies. Stigmata of a basal skull fracture should be sought; these include otorrhea, rhinorrhea, hemotympanum, periorbital ecchymosis, ecchymosis overlying the petrous bone, and cranial nerve palsies.

Severe head injuries may cause changes in the patient's vital signs. The Cushing reflex of hypertension and bradycardia in response to raised ICP may signify an expanding intracranial hemorrhage but is seen infrequently. As brainstem compression moves caudally, a sequence of respiratory patterns ensues. Cheyne-Stokes breathing characterized by rhythmic waxing and waning of the depth of respiration, with regularly recurring periods of apnea, is followed by hyperventilation, then irregular and ataxic breathing, and finally apnea.

The level of consciousness is the most important clinical sign in the evaluation of the head-injured patient and should be quantified using the Glasgow Coma Scale (GCS) (Table 6–1). This scale records three components: eye opening, motor response, and verbal response. The GCS score is obtained by summing the scores obtained for the individual components. A patient is considered to be in coma when the GCS score is 7 or less. Among the three scores, the motor score has been found to correlate best with the extent of injury and outcome.[17] The GCS has several limitations; it fails to measure pupillary size and reactivity, eye movements, and brainstem reflexes which are also valuable in assessing coma. Difficulties arise if the patient is unable to speak because of facial fractures or intubation, or if the patient cannot open his eyes because of edema or lacerations. These mechanical limitations can skew the assessment because the GCS is heavily weighted toward eye and verbal responses. Infants and small children and an agitated, uncooperative, dysphasic patient cannot be evaluated with the scale. Despite these limitations, the GCS is the most widely used and easiest assessment of the state of consciousness.

If the patient is alert and able to communicate, the mental status examination should be pursued to assess memory and concentration. Memory difficulties are classified as retrograde amnesia (memory loss for events prior to the injury) or anterograde amnesia (loss of memory from the time of injury to the return of continuous memory). Even in severe head injury it is unusual for retrograde amnesia to last more than a few minutes, while anterograde or post-traumatic amnesia may last for months and is a better guide to the severity of the injury.

Eye movements are useful in evaluating head-injured patients. In the cooperative patient, the voluntary eye movements in all fields of vision should be tested. Failure of abduction suggests a sixth nerve palsy and failure of adduction implies a third nerve palsy. Lighter coma is often accompanied by roving horizontal eye movements which indicate that the regions of the brainstem subserving these functions are intact. In deep coma there are no spontaneous eye movements, and the integrity of the brainstem can be assessed by the oculocephalic or doll's eye test, which is performed by rotating the head in a horizontal plane from the resting position. In a normal response, the eyes will maintain their position in space by moving opposite to the position of the head. Failure to elicit this response implies severe depression of brainstem function.

The pupillary light reflex is an important diagnostic test in comatose patients. Metabolic disorders typically spare this reflex, whereas structural lesions such as an intracranial hemorrhage in a head-injured patient will cause unreactive or poorly reactive pupils. Changes in pupillary size and reactivity to light should be carefully noted and may be the earliest sign of incipient neurologic deterioration. A unilateral nonreactive mydriasis or "blown pupil" is an ominous sign in a head-injured patient and is due to an intracranial hemorrhage that pushes the hemisphere across to the other side and then downward. As the medial part of the tem-

TABLE 6–1 The Glasgow Coma Scale (GCS)*

Verbal Response:	
None	1
Incomprehensible sounds	2
Inappropriate words	3
Confused	4
Oriented	5
Eye Opening:	
None	1
To pain	2
To speech	3
Spontaneously	4
Motor Response:	
None	1
Abnormal extensor	2
Abnormal flexion	3
Withdraws	4
Localizes	5
Obeys	6

* The Glasgow Coma Scale (GCS) quantifies the level of consciousness by recording eye movements, verbal response, and motor response. The GCS is obtained by adding the individual scores for each of the three components. Alert and neurologically intact patients have a GCS of 15, while a mute, flaccid patient without eye opening would have a GCS of 3.

poral lobe herniates through the incisura, the third nerve is compressed between the temporal lobe and the brainstem. This leads to pupillary dilation on the same side as the hematoma. If herniation progresses, bilateral mydriasis and ophthalmoplegia will result. Direct trauma to the eye can also cause pupillary abnormalities, and the patient should be examined for periorbital ecchymosis and chemosis which suggest an eye injury before the diagnosis of a catastrophic intracranial event is made. Bilateral miosis or pinpoint pupils may occur with pontine damage, but this is also seen with opiate intoxication.

The motor examination should be tailored to the patient's mental status. In the cooperative patient the strength can be documented on a 0 to 5 scale: 5=normal strength, 4=mild weakness, 3=antigravity movement, 2=unable to overcome gravity, 1 = trace movement, 0 = no movement. Subtle motor weakness can be evaluated by having the patient hold his arms extended in the supine position; a "pronator drift" will appear on the weaker side. In the comatose patient, the response to noxious stimuli should be documented as flexor, extensor, or localizing. The extensor or "decerebrate" posture is characterized by an abnormal extension and pronation of the arm spontaneously or in response to noxious stimuli, while the flexor or "decorticate" posturing is a flexion of the arm and hand to pain. The flexor posture is felt to reflect a more rostral and less severe injury than does the extensor posture. Withdrawal implies purposeful or voluntary behavior.

Hemiparesis may frequently accompany a "blown pupil." The most frequent combination is that of a dilated pupil with contralateral motor deficit. Less frequently, the hemiplegia and dilated pupil are on the same side. The dilated pupil, a manifestation of a third nerve palsy, is the more reliable sign in localizing the mass lesion.

Diagnostic Studies

After the neurologic examination, and prior to any other neuroradiologic procedures, the presence of a fracture or subluxation of the cervical spine must be determined by a lateral radiograph of the neck with visualization caudally to the C7–T1 interspace (Fig. 6–1). Skull films are performed to identify depressed or basal skull fractures, but otherwise have little use. Patients with altered mental status, focal neurologic signs, or penetrating or depressed skull injuries require CT scanning of the head. Angiography is necessary only if a CT scan is unavailable or if a vascular injury is suspected.

BRAIN INJURIES

Trauma to the brain can be classified into focal and diffuse injuries. Focal brain injuries involve destruction of brain tissue related to edema, contusion, laceration, or hemorrhage and can be visualized on a CT scan. These lesions cause neurologic dysfunction both by local brain damage and by causing mass effect within the skull leading to brain shift, herniation, and ultimately brainstem compression. Diffuse brain injuries are associated with global disruption of neurologic function and, in their pure form, are not associated with visible brain lesions. Diffuse brain injuries are the consequence of the shaking effect of the brain within the skull and will range from a mild concussion to diffuse axonal injury with prolonged coma. Once the primary injury has occurred, it may be followed by a series of events which contribute to further injury. These include systemic hypotension, hypoxia, hypercarbia, and intracranial hypertension. This section summarizes the several types of clinically important brain injuries.

Concussion

Concussion is a temporary, reversible neurologic deficiency caused by trauma that lasts less than 6 hours. Mild concussion syndromes are characterized by confusion and disorientation, whereas classic cerebral concussion results in loss of consciousness and is accompanied by post-traumatic amnesia. Because the dysfunction is physiological and not structural, the CT scans in these patients are normal.

Diffuse Axonal Injury

The term "diffuse axonal injury" is used to describe prolonged traumatic coma that is not due to mass lesions or ischemic insults. Violent head motions cause strains and distortions in the brain which result in shearing of nerve fibers with axonal damage. The axonal damage itself cannot be visualized on a CT scan but may be associated with small hemorrhagic lesions in the deep white matter. These patients should be managed with aggressive pulmonary toilet, close monitoring of cerebral oxygenation, and prevention and treatment of cerebral swelling. Although some patients with mild degrees of diffuse axonal injury may recover, most patients with severe manifestations either die or remain in a vegetative state. It has been estimated that diffuse axonal injury causes more than one-third of the deaths in head-injured patients and is most often

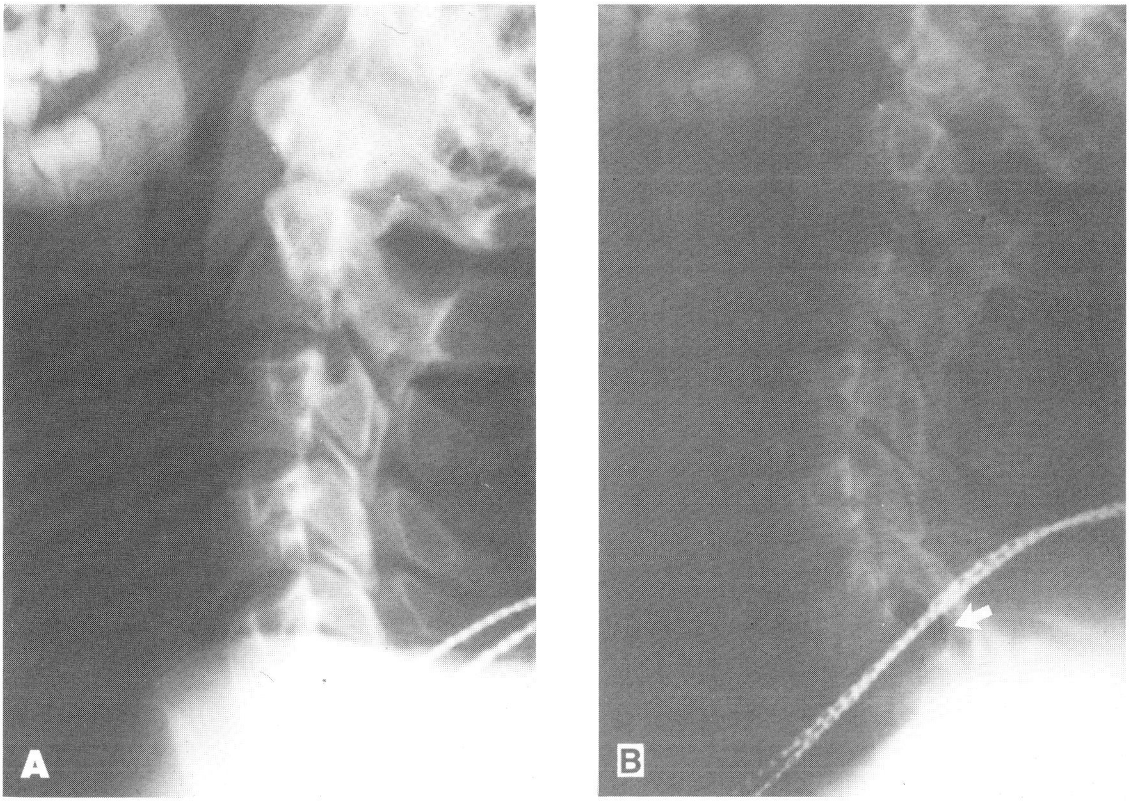

Figure 6–1 These lateral cervical spine films illustrate the importance of visualizing the entire cervical spine. *A*, Initial film fails to visualize the C6–C7 interspace. *B*, Second radiograph with the shoulders pulled down shows a C6–C7 subluxation (arrow).

responsible for the condition of severely disabled and vegetative survivors.[18]

Subdural Hematoma

An impact injury to the head may rupture the veins that bridge the subdural space and cause a collection of blood that compresses the cerebral hemispheres. Acute subdural hematomas are somewhat arbitrarily classified as those hemorrhages that are operated on within 48 hours of injury. The reported incidence of subdural hematoma varies from 1 to 10 percent depending upon the severity of the head injury.[19–21] Diagnosis is established with CT scan and the subdural hematoma appears as a hyperdense lesion that extends diffusely over the cerebral convexity (Fig. 6–2). Medical means to reduce ICP should be used until the patient can be brought urgently to the operating room. The operative treatment should be directed at removing the hematoma, controlling hemorrhage, and resecting associated contusions. Despite optimal treatment, the mortality is 50 percent or more, with a large proportion of the survivors severely disabled.[21–24] Mortality is significantly increased with advanced age,[22] delay in operation,[23] and coma.[21]

The term chronic subdural hematoma refers to those hematomas that present more than 20 days after injury. Elderly patients and alcoholics are particularly likely to develop this complication after apparently minor head injuries. Intermittent headache, slight or severe impairment of the intellectual faculties, and hemiparesis are the most characteristic symptoms. The diagnosis is established with a CT scan; the hematoma appears hypodense compared to brain. However, between the second and third week after injury, most are isodense and may be difficult to visualize on a noncontrast CT scan[25] (Fig. 6–3). Although some patients who are neurologically intact or who have a mild depression of their level of consciousness

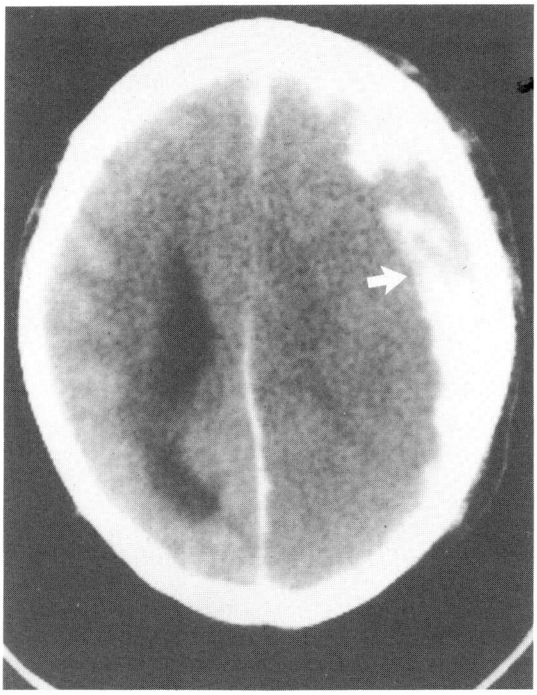

Figure 6–2 Computed tomographic scan showing acute left subdural hematoma (arrow) with effacement of the ipsilateral ventricle.

can be treated medically, the vast majority are best managed with operation. Craniotomy, burr hole, and twist drill evacuation have all been used with success. The reported mortality in most studies is under 10 percent; outcome is most closely related to the patient's neurologic function prior to operation.[22,26,27]

Epidural Hematoma

Epidural hematomas are an infrequent complication of head injuries with a reported incidence of 1.5 percent.[28] An impact to the head, usually but not always associated with a skull fracture, may lacerate the underlying meningeal vessels causing arterial bleeding into the epidural space. As the hematoma accumulates, it progressively strips the dura from the inner table of the skull with compression of the underlying cerebral hemispheres (Fig. 6–4). A history of transient loss of consciousness from a concussion, after which the patient regains consciousness and remains alert until an expanding hematoma results in a second loss of consciousness, is the classic presentation of epidural hematoma. This "lucid interval" is present, however, in less than one-third of the patients.[29,30] Pupillary dilation occurs ipsilateral to

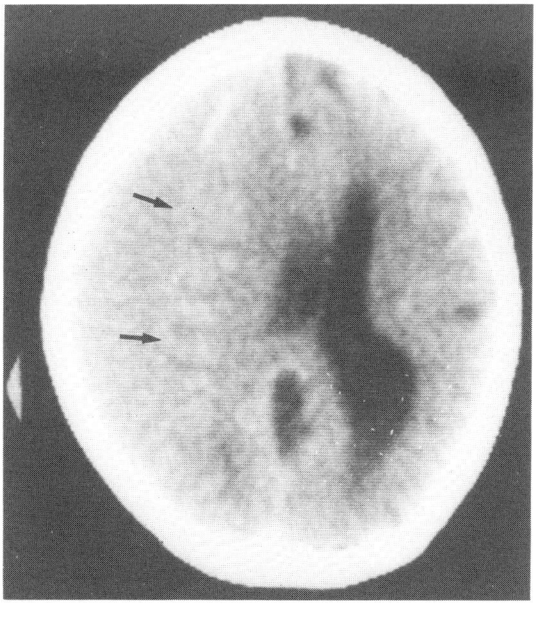

Figure 6–3 Computed tomographic scan of a patient with an isodense chronic subdural hematoma with compression and right to left shift of the lateral ventricles. Arrows delineate the cortical surface pushed away from the inner table.

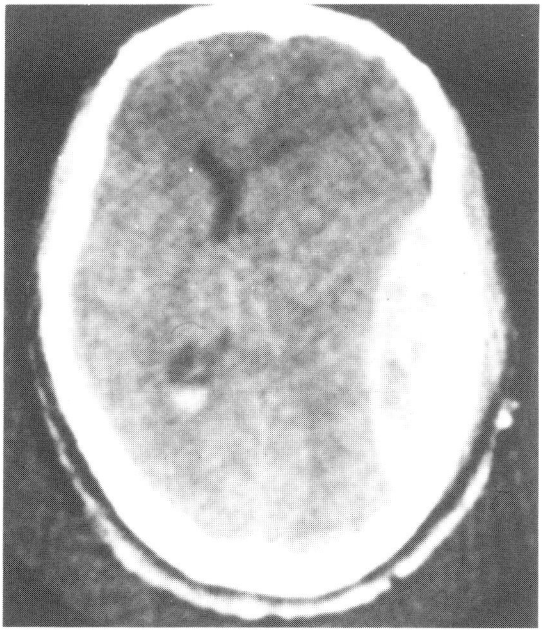

Figure 6–4 Computed tomographic scan showing large left parietal epidural hematoma with hyperdense lenticular appearance beneath the skull. Notice the marked shift of the cerebral ventricles.

the hematoma and motor signs are contralateral to the lesion. Endotracheal intubation, hyperventilation, and diuretics will usually stabilize the patient until a CT scan can be performed. The epidural hematoma appears hyperdense and lenticular beneath the skull. When rapid CT scanning is not possible, or the patient is rapidly deteriorating, the operation should be performed immediately. In this situation, burr holes are placed ipsilateral to the dilated pupil to decompress the hemorrhage until a craniotomy with a bone flap can be performed. The reported mortality varies from 5 to 43 percent and is most closely related to the patient's preoperative neurologic status.[28,30]

Cerebral Contusion

Cerebral contusions are focal areas of pulped brain and hemorrhage which occur at the site of impact (coup), or at points distant from impact (contrecoup) (Fig. 6–5).[31] They are the most frequently encountered parenchymal lesions after head injury and typically occur at the frontal and temporal poles as the brain strikes the irregular bony floor of the frontal and middle fossa. The signs and symptoms of patients with traumatically induced contusions are similar to those that occur as a result of extracerebral collections. Diagnosis is established with CT scan; contusions appear as heterogeneous areas of increased density from multiple small hemorrhages intermixed with edema and necrotic brain. Large contusions (>3 cm) with mass effect are generally treated with operation. Temporal contusions are particularly dangerous because of the proximity of the lesion to the brainstem, and operative removal may be indicated depending on the size of the lesion. Smaller contusions (<2 cm) and deep contusions without superficial extension can be managed medically with close monitoring of ICP and serial CT scanning. Mortality ranges from 25 to 60 percent and is for the most part related to the patient's preoperative condition.[32,33]

Intracerebral Hematoma

Intracerebral hematomas are hemorrhages within the brain parenchyma that range from 1 mm in size to those large enough to involve several lobes of the brain (Fig. 6–6). The reported incidence varies from 4 to 23 percent depending upon the severity of the head injury.[34,35] Intracerebral hemorrhages have a pathogenesis similar to that of cerebral contusions and are found in the same location. These two lesions can be distinguished on CT scan: cerebral hemorrhages appear as homogeneous

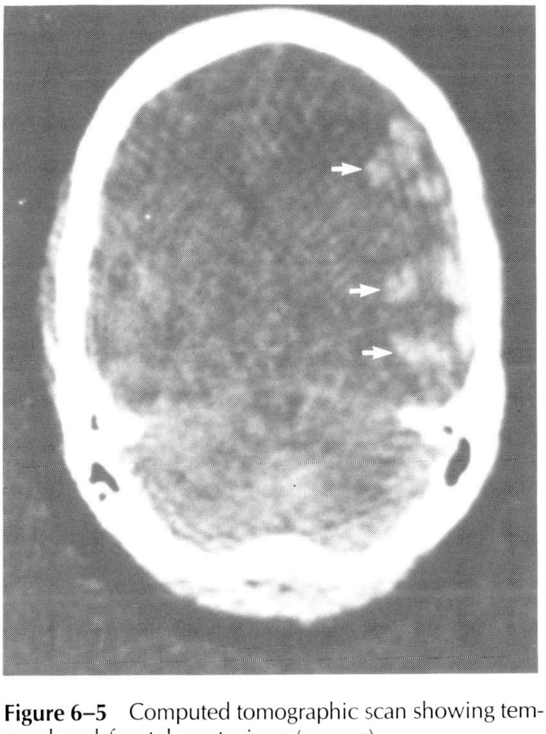

Figure 6–5 Computed tomographic scan showing temporal and frontal contusions (arrows).

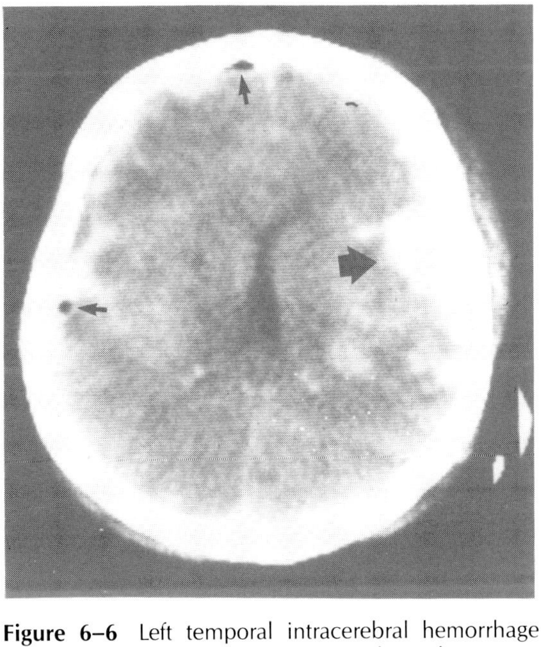

Figure 6–6 Left temporal intracerebral hemorrhage (large arrow) appears as homogeneous hyperdense mass surrounded by multiple contusions which appear as heterogeneous areas of increased density. Notice the intracranial air (small arrows).

hyperdense lesions whereas contusions are heterogeneous. The treatment of cerebral hemorrhages involves the same considerations as that of cerebral contusions. The overall mortality is 25 percent; patients who are unconscious at the time of operation have a mortality of 45 percent, whereas those lucid prior to operation have a mortality of only 6 percent.[36]

IMPACT-ABSORBING FACIAL FRACTURES

Extensive crushing injuries of the facial bones are frequently sustained with little damage to the brain. The compressible, air-filled, energy-absorbing facial bones serve as a cushion to protect intracranial structures located behind them.[37,38] A recent report[39] studied the occurrence of closed head injury and the location of facial fractures in a series of 210 seriously injured patients. The data demonstrated that patients with upper facial fractures were at greatest risk for serious closed head injury, with 50 percent of the patients having moderately severe neurologic findings. Combined fractures to both the mandibular and the midfacial regions with [illegible] a slight neurologic deficit in 50 percent of the patients, while approximately 30 percent were intact. Isolated fractures of the mandible or only in the midfacial region were least likely to be associated with a closed head injury. Approximately one-quarter of these patients had a slight neurologic deficit, while 60 percent were intact. These data are summarized in Figure 6–7.

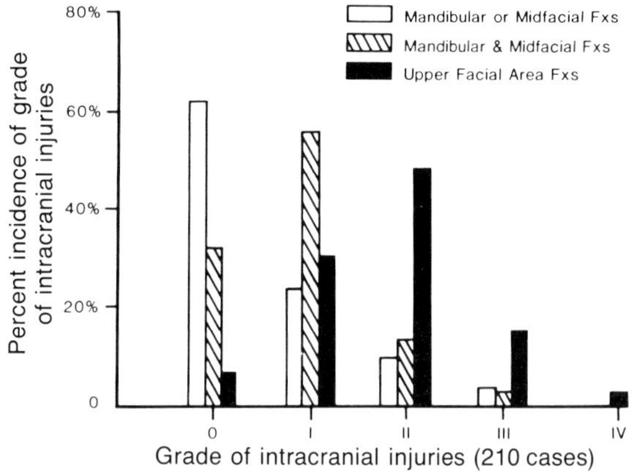

Figure 6–7 Incidence and severity of closed head injuries with facial trauma. The facial fractures were grouped into three regional categories. Head injuries were classified as follows: 0 = normal computed tomographic (CT) scan without significant neurologic deficit; I = minor CT findings with slight neurologic deficit; II = moderately severe CT and neurologic findings; III = severe CT and neurologic findings; IV = grave CT findings with fatal outcome. Severe closed head injuries were more frequently observed in patients with upper facial fractures, whereas the majority of patients with mandibular or midfacial fractures alone demonstrated [illegible] (Reproduced with permission from Lee et al[39].)

LINEAR SKULL FRACTURES

Linear fractures account for approximately 80 percent of skull fractures.[40] Fifty percent of the time these fractures occur in the midportion of the skull and extend toward the skull base. The remainder are divided between the frontal and occipital regions. At the point of impact there is an in-bending of the skull; a simultaneous out-bending occurs at the periphery of the impact. The fracture occurs when the elastic deformation of the skull exceeds the tensile strength of bone. The comminuted or multilinear fracture is the result of a blow transmitting slightly more energy.[41] With increasing energy of impact, a depressed skull fracture may result.

Diagnosis and Significance of Linear Skull Fracture

The most important study in the diagnosis of the linear skull fracture is the skull radiograph. The fracture appears on roentgenography as a lucent line with sharply defined margins. The fracture may be straight, angular, or curvilinear. Linear fractures may frequently be recognized on CT, especially if the window level and window width are adjusted appropriately and the fracture is perpendicular to the scanning plane.

Approximately 2.4 million skull x-ray examinations were requested by emergency room personnel in the United States in 1980 to identify the presence of a skull fracture.[42] In most reports, however, the skull film altered the clinical management of patients less than 2 percent of the time.[43–46] The issues of most concern to the clinician are: (1) relationship between skull fractures and intracranial injuries, (2) diagnosis and significance of the asymptomatic linear skull fracture, and (3) criteria to select patients for skull radiographs.

There is a poor correlation between the presence of a skull fracture and the presence of brain injury. While it is true that among all head-injured patients a skull fracture is associated with a higher risk of intracranial injury than if a fracture were not present, patients with a skull fracture may have no signs or symptoms of brain injury. Conversely, severe brain injury can occur in the absence of a skull fracture. There have been multiple clinical studies of patients with head trauma that have attempted to analyze the relationship between skull fractures and intracranial injuries.[43,44,47–49] Masters and colleagues[50] reviewed the findings in 22,058 patients, of whom 758 (9 percent) had fractures and 138 (0.6 percent) had an intracranial injury. In the patients with skull fractures 91 percent did not have an associated intracranial injury, and 51 percent of patients with intracranial injury did not have a skull fracture.

Treatment of Linear Skull Fracture

Although the value of skull radiographs in head trauma has not been fully defined, the clinician can develop a rational management strategy for dealing with head trauma and skull fractures. For the patient with focal neurologic findings or an abnormal level of consciousness, the presence or absence of a linear skull fracture is less important than the extent of brain injury. These patients should have a CT scan as the initial diagnostic test. Skull radiographs have little place in management.

For the alert and neurologically intact patient, we do not recommend the routine use of skull roentgenograms. Only if the clinician suspects a depressed or basal skull fracture from physical examination or mechanism of injury should skull x-ray films be obtained. This is a controversial policy. Many neurosurgeons will obtain skull radiographs in all patients with a history of loss of consciousness. If a linear skull fracture is diagnosed, the patient is admitted for observation for an intracranial hemorrhage.[51–54] In support of our policy, we cite the work of Cooper and Ho[55] which indicates that more than 90 percent of patients who develop intracranial hematomas have an abnormal level of consciousness at the time of admission and that virtually all of the remainder had other reasons requiring admission not related to the presence of a linear skull fracture. More recently, the United States Food and Drug Administration Skull X-Ray Referral Criteria Panel concluded that a linear skull fracture in asymptomatic patients or those patients with headache, dizziness, scalp hematoma, laceration, or abrasion is rarely, if ever, associated with an intracranial injury and therefore does not have to be diagnosed.[50]

In conclusion, we feel that the linear nondepressed skull fracture in itself requires no specific treatment. The open linear skull fracture requires nothing more than soft-tissue debridement and closure.

DEPRESSED SKULL FRACTURE

A fracture is considered to be depressed when the inner table is depressed more than the thickness of the skull. The term "closed depressed fracture" indicates that the overlying integument is intact, whereas the term "compound depressed fracture" refers to those fractures that occur beneath or immediately adjacent to a scalp laceration. The compound fracture occurs approximately 85 percent of the time.[56,57] The higher incidence of open wounds associated with depressed fractures reflects the amount of energy needed to cause this injury.

The incidence of depressed fracture was estimated to be 20 per million per year in 1970.[56] Most patients with depressed fractures are young—approximately 50 percent are under the age of 16. Among all age groups there are more than twice as many males as females.[56]

Half of depressed skull fractures occur in the frontal area (Fig. 6–8). The remaining injuries are divided between the parietal and posterior regions of the skull. In 25 percent of the cases, more than one convexity bone is affected by the fracture. The more extensive the fracture, the higher the mortality. Occipital depressed fractures are attended by an extremely high mortality because of the frequent association of injury to posterior fossa structures.

Diagnosis of Depressed Skull Fracture

Early diagnosis of a depressed skull fracture can minimize many of the complications. There are many pitfalls, however, that may prevent the examining physician from recognizing the injury. Often the patient may appear to have only a trivial injury. Cabraal and Abeysuriya[58] found that 49 percent of patients with depressed fractures suffered only momentary unconsciousness and 87 percent were alert or mildly drowsy on admission. A penetrating blow to the head absorbs much of the energy of the injury and relatively little force is transmitted to the cerebral hemispheres and brainstem. The level of consciousness is thus not altered and pulped brain may even extrude from the wound while the patient is awake and alert. One

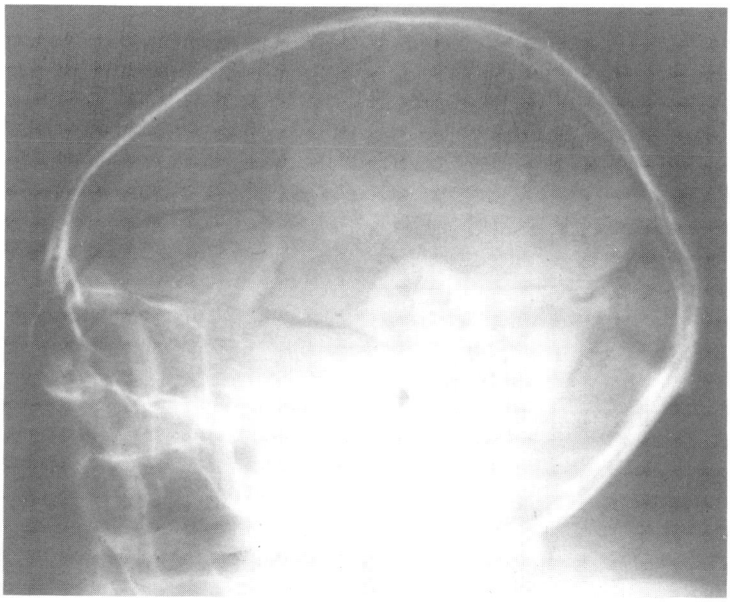

Figure 6–8 Lateral roentgenogram of skull shows stellate skull fracture through the frontal sinus.

study[illegible] found that victims of assault and alcoholics with depressed skull fractures were particularly likely to be disregarded by physicians as having only trivial injuries. The scalp is mobile, and when a laceration is present it may not overlie the depressed fracture. Often the physician will suture the scalp after visually exploring the wound but miss the depressed fracture. A thorough examination of the entire cranial contour and probing of the open wound with a sterile glove are mandatory, especially if there is a history of a blow to the head with an object such as a club or hammer. The presence of leakage of CSF or the presence of brain tissue at the wound edge is prima facie evidence of a dural tear and depressed fracture. Even if the fracture is recognized, the extent of the depression is often underestimated based on visual inspection. This is because the inner table of the skull is always more extensively fractured than the outer table.[59]

The skull radiograph is helpful in accurately identifying and localizing skull depressions and should be obtained when the clinician suspects a penetrating injury. Tangential views may delineate a fracture not appreciated on the standard anteroposterior and lateral views (Fig. 6–9). A CT scan should be performed to identify associated intracranial injuries.

Treatment

Simple Fractures

A depressed fracture without an overlying scalp laceration can be treated conservatively in most cases. The risk of intracranial infection is nil and elevation of the fracture is unnecessary to prevent central nervous system infection.[57] In the past, it was the practice to elevate all depressed fractures to minimize the incidence of post-traumatic epilepsy. However, Jennett and colleagues[60] have shown that "how the fracture is treated has no obvious effect on the incidence of epilepsy." It is unlikely that elevation of depressed bone fragments will facilitate neurologic improvement when deficits exist. This is because the brain injury is due to the force of the blow struck and not to the presence of a depressed area of bone.[60a]

Severe cosmetic deformity is the most common indication to elevate a closed depressed fracture. If the depression is cosmetically unacceptable, particularly when the forehead is involved, elevation of the fragments can be carried out. Jennett and colleagues[60] found that less than 3 percent of closed depressed skull fractures are complicated by intracranial hemorrhage. In those cases in which the neurosurgeon must operate to evacuate a sig-

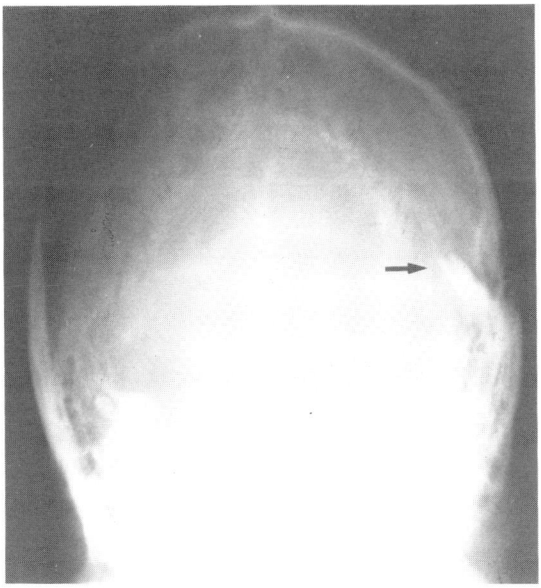

Figure 6–9 Skull radiograph (Townes view) shows a typical depressed skull fracture (arrow).

nificant intracranial hematoma, the depressed fracture is elevated and the dural laceration repaired if present.

Compound Fractures

Compound depressed skull fractures require urgent operation to minimize the potential for infection of the central nervous system. The operation should be performed after a preoperative CT scan is obtained to identify any intracranial hemorrhage that may need simultaneous treatment. Timing is important; Jennett and Miller[61] found that postoperative infectious complications were substantially greater in those patients in whom there was more than a 48-hour delay between the injury and surgical treatment. It is our policy to perform operation within 6 to 12 hours of admission.

The procedure may be performed under local or general anesthesia. The ragged edges of the laceration should be debrided as necessary. The scalp wound can be incorporated into the incision, or the scalp wound can be closed and a classic scalp flap outlined depending upon the size and nature of the laceration. The preoperative CT scan will guide the surgeon as to the size of the flap necessary to gain exposure to any intracranial injury.

An instrument can sometimes be wedged under the fragments to elevate them, or a rongeur used to bite away the depressed fragments. If this is not possible, a burr hole is drilled adjacent to the fracture site and depressed bone is rongeured away and elevated. The bony fragments are saved and placed in antibiotic solution for later replacement. After removal of the bony fragments, the dura is inspected and tears are sutured. If intracranial hemorrhage has been visualized on the preoperative CT scan, the dura should be opened and the hemorrhage evacuated. All foreign bodies, necrotic tissue, and depressed bone fragments are meticulously debrided.[62] The dura is tightly closed; a pericranial graft may be necessary if the dura is extensively torn.

Although some authorities advocate removing all of the bone fragments and performing a subsequent cranioplasty, recent studies[56,57,63,64] have found that replacing bone fragments does not increase the incidence of infection. This strategy has the advantage of avoiding a subsequent cranioplasty. Kriss and associates[63] reported an infection rate of only 2.5 percent in 79 patients in whom the bone fragments were replaced. However, they recommended performing this procedure only if surgery was performed within 24 hours of the injury and the dura was closed. Jennett and Miller[61] have recommended replacing the bony fragments even when surgery is delayed for 24 hours and when the dura is torn. The presence of an established infection was the only absolute contraindication to replacing the bony fragments. In our experience bone fragments can usually be safely replaced except when surgery is delayed for more than 24 hours or the wound is grossly contaminated. If the fragments are not replaced, elective cranioplasty can be performed in 3 or 4 months.

Jennett and Miller[61] advocated the use of prophylactic antibiotics but emphasized that antibiotics in no way replaced surgery and that their use carried an appreciable risk of opportunistic infection. Braakman[56] could not discern any significant difference in infection rates in those patients who received antibiotics compared to those who did not. Mendelow and colleagues[65] have performed the only study on the use of prophylactic antibiotics in compound depressed fractures. Patients treated with ampicillin and a sulfonamide had an infection rate of 1.9 percent, significantly lower than the 10.9 percent incidence in those patients who did not receive antibiotics. In our own experience the infection rate is lower, and it has been our policy not to use prophylactic antibiotics except for established infections or grossly contaminated wounds.

Dural Venous Sinus Injury

The location of a depressed fracture over the midline of the skull or in the occipital region should alert the clinician to a potential injury to the sagittal or transverse sinus. A CT scan using coronal cuts can often be useful in demonstrating the relationship between the depressed fracture and the sagittal sinus. Cerebral angiography or digital intravenous angiography can be used as the definitive study if the relationship of the fracture to the sinus is still in doubt or to identify sinus injury or occlusion.

Because of the potential for severe hemorrhage, Miller and Jennett[57] have stressed that elevation of the portion of the fracture overlying the sinus should not be attempted if the wound is clean. If elevation of the depressed fragment is essential for debridement, this should be performed after blood is available in the operating room and there is adequate bony exposure to obtain proximal and distal control of the sinus. In most cases, active bleeding will begin only when the wound is debrided and the depressed bone fragment tamponading the fracture is removed.

Cooper[66] has advocated a more conservative approach. In patients with a fracture overlying a venous sinus, the scalp over the fracture is debrided but the depressed fragments should be left in place. These patients are observed in the hospital for 7 days for the development of a wound infection or meningitis. Thereafter, they are followed with serial CT scans at 2-week intervals for 6 weeks for the development of a brain abscess. Several CT scans should be obtained for the remainder of the year. Cooper reasons that "although the risk of abscess formation from retained intracerebral bone fragments probably persists for the life of the patient, experience with retained bone fragments after gunshot wounds indicates that risk is greatest in the first months after the injury."[66] He states that late exploration of the sinus "is associated with less risk of hemorrhage than in the acute situation because thrombus is organized and the tear in the sinus wall may have been sealed as a result of the deposition of fibrous tissue."[66]

The surgical principles are the same in both early and late exploration of the sinus. Bleeding can usually be controlled by applying pressure to tamponade the sinus. Minor tears are repaired by suturing the laceration directly, or by suturing a small piece of Gelfoam or a temporalis muscle graft to the rent. Large lacerations of the sinus may require a vein graft. Rarely, the sagittal sinus may have to be ligated to control the hemorrhage. This may be carried out with impunity in the anterior third of the sinus, but posterior to this point, ligation may result in venous congestion, neurologic deficits, and death. Tears of the transverse sinuses can usually be safely ligated, but in cases in which there is a poorly developed transverse sinus on one side, ligation of a dominant transverse sinus may produce dangerous increases in ICP. A preoperative angiogram will clarify the anatomy. In late exploration of sinus wounds where hemorrhage is less likely, Cooper[66] stresses debridement of the infected wound and removal of depressed bone fragments.

Frontal Sinus Fracture

Closed depressed fractures of the anterior wall of the frontal sinus should be elevated when they cause cosmetic deformity or the integrity of the nasofrontal duct is in question.[67] The patient can be observed for a few days to allow resolution of the edema and a better assessment of the cosmetic deformity. Approximately one-fourth of the anterior frontal sinus fractures will involve the nasofrontal duct.[67] Clinical sinusitis and the presence of nasoethmoid complex fractures should alert the physician to a possible disruption of the duct.[68] Treatment consists of a bicoronal scalp flap posterior to the hairline which is reflected anteriorly. The bony fragments are exposed and elevated. The mucosa of the sinus is exenterated, the sinus is obliterated with fat, and the nasofrontal duct is plugged with a piece of temporalis muscle to prevent the formation of a mucocele.[69] The anterior wall is then reconstructed by wiring the bony fragments into place. An alternative to ablating the sinus which has been shown to have excellent results is reconstruction of the nasofrontal duct.[70] Open depressed fractures of the anterior wall should be elevated immediately and the wound debrided. Although open fractures can be repaired through the wound[71] this is not advisable. Mobilization of the fracture generally requires enlarging the wound and this is not cosmetically acceptable in the forehead. Moreover, this approach does not allow sufficient exposure for exenteration of the sinus and the risk of suppurative sinusitis and mucocele persists.

All depressed or comminuted fractures of the posterior wall of the frontal sinus require urgent operation. These fractures are compound by definition and result in a connection between the intracranial structures and a contaminated, or potentially contaminated, sinus cavity. Often the dura is lacerated and a CSF leak is present.

Although some authors have advocated a delay of several days before operation,[67,72] we feel that infectious complications can best be avoided by early surgical debridement. Nondisplaced fractures of the posterior wall, however, are infrequently associated with a dural laceration and do not have to be explored unless there is a persistent CSF leak or involvement of the nasofrontal duct.[67]

For posterior wall fractures, a bicoronal incision is made and any depressed anterior wall fragments are elevated and removed and the dura inspected. A frontal craniotomy is performed if frontal lobe exploration is necessary for thorough debridement of the wound or removal of an intracranial hemorrhage. After dural repair, the frontal sinus is "cranialized."[69,72] This procedure entails excision of the posterior wall, exenteration of the mucosa, packing the nasofrontal duct, and reconstructing the anterior sinus wall so as to allow forward migration of the frontal lobes into the dead space. This technique of immediate bone replacement for depressed frontal sinus fractures is safe and avoids a later reconstructive procedure.[64]

Complications and Outcome

Most patients with a depressed fracture of the skull that has been properly treated will recover quickly and completely. The mortality rate ranges from 3 to 12 percent[56,58] and for the most part is related to the severity of the associated central nervous system injury.[56] The two most important sequelae of depressed fractures are neurologic deficit and epilepsy.

Neurologic Deficit

Long-term follow-up of patients with depressed fracture indicates that less than 10 percent of the patients have persistent neurologic deficit.[6,56,57] Braakman[56] reported that persistent neurologic findings, i.e., hemiparesis, dysphasia, and hemianopia, occurred in 15 percent of temporal bone fractures, 12 percent of parietal fractures, 11 percent of frontobasal fractures, and rarely with occipital or frontal fractures. Infection, intracranial hematoma, and dural venous sinus involvement substantially increased the risk of neurologic sequelae.[56,57]

Epilepsy

Depressed fractures are responsible for 20 percent of all cases of post-traumatic epilepsy.[60] In a series of 1,000 patients with depressed skull fractures 10 percent had early epilepsy (seizures occurring within the first week) and 15 percent had late epilepsy. Early seizures are considered separately because they are less likely to augur lifetime epilepsy than seizures beginning after the first week.

Unfortunately, how a depressed fracture is treated "has no obvious effect on the incidence of epilepsy."[60] The clinician's role is to identify those factors that predispose to epilepsy, treat those patients who have a high risk with prophylactic anticonvulsants, and reassure those patients who do not.

The presence of prolonged post-traumatic amnesia is the most important single factor in determining the future risk of epilepsy.[60,73] When the duration of post-traumatic amnesia is less than 24 hours, the incidence of late epilepsy is 5.4 percent, compared to an incidence of 22 percent in those patients who have an amnestic interval of more than 24 hours.[56]

The presence of local brain damage greatly increases the incidence of late epilepsy and is probably why patients with depressed fracture have a fivefold increase in the incidence of late epilepsy (15 percent) compared to those patients with head injury without depressed fractures (3 percent).[60] The more extensive the local brain damage, the greater the risk of late epilepsy. These risk factors are summarized in Figure 6–10.

It has been our policy to institute prophylactic antiseizure therapy with phenytoin on admission in all patients with depressed skull fractures. If the patient's risk of late epilepsy is calculated to be greater than 20 percent, anticonvulsant prophylaxis is continued; if not, the anticonvulsants are gradually tapered and discontinued.

Infection

Infection rates after depressed skull fracture have been reported to range from 2.5 to 10 percent.[63,64,74,75] Jennett and associates[60] distinguished those patients who presented with infection (6 percent) from patients in whom infection developed after definitive surgery (4.6 percent). Established infections were most often due to missed or delayed diagnosis and developed within the first 2 weeks after injury. More than half of the time the infection was intracranial—i.e., brain abscess—or meningitis and associated with a high mortality. Postoperative infections, on the other hand, were confined to the wound 80 percent of the time, delayed in onset, and not associated with mortality. Delay of surgery of more than 48 hours after injury and cranioplasty with foreign

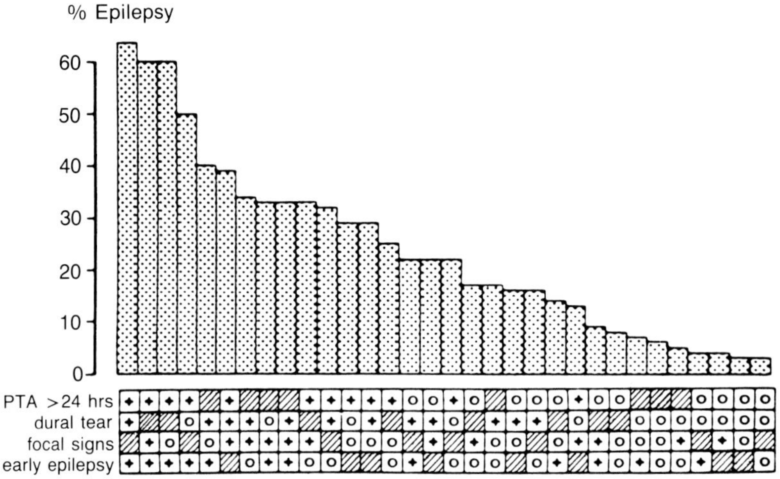

Figure 6–10 The influence of combined risk factors in the development of epilepsy after depressed skull fracture. (Reproduced with permission from Jennett B. Epilepsy after non-missile depressed skull fracture. London: William Heinemann Medical Books, 1975.)

material were associated with a significantly greater risk of postoperative infection.

Wound infections can be diagnosed by inspection and should be treated with debridement of infected bone, evacuation of the abscess, and administration of antibiotics. Osteomyelitis of the adjacent skull is a less frequent complication of head injury and can be diagnosed with plain skull films 50 percent of the time.[76] The combined use of bone and gallium scans is very sensitive in diagnosis if the skull films are negative.[76] The treatment is surgical debridement of infected bone.[77] The craniectomy should extend 5 to 10 mm beyond the area of osteomyelitis. The efficacy of antibiotics after surgical debridement is unclear; it has been our policy to continue them for 7 to 10 days postoperatively.

The intracranial infectious complications of depressed skull fractures include meningitis, subdural empyema, and brain abscess. The treatment of meningitis is discussed at length in the section on CSF fistulas. Subdural empyemas are a rare complication of depressed fractures. Symptoms include headache, fever, neck stiffness, seizures and focal neurologic deficit. We favor an aggressive surgical approach if this complication is suspected because outcome is directly related to the time between the onset of symptoms and surgery.[77,78] Burr holes or craniotomy are used for drainage of the pus and antibiotics are administered.[78]

The most feared infectious complication of depressed fractures is brain abscess (Fig. 6–11). Clinical diagnosis may be difficult; fever is present in only 50 percent of the cases,[79a] and focal neurologic findings are present less than half the time.[79] Headache and an altered mental status are more commonly seen. A high index of suspicion is need

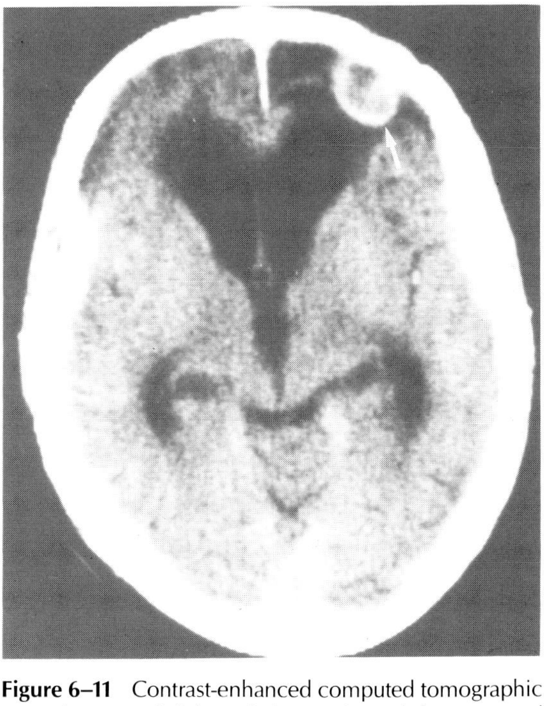

Figure 6–11 Contrast-enhanced computed tomographic scan showing a left frontal abscess (arrow) that occurred at the site of a depressed skull fracture that was inadequately debrided.

ed to make an early diagnosis. Lumbar puncture should not be performed if a brain abscess is suspected because it may result in cerebral herniation and death.[79a] The diagnosis is established with serial contrast CT scans. The abscess appears as a ring pattern of enhancement with a low-density center. Operative drainage is the treatment of choice, although carefully selected patients may be treated with antibiotics alone.[80] We favor an aggressive surgical approach. Although needle aspiration of the abscess has been used with increasing frequency, the presence of a foreign body or bone next to the abscess necessitates a craniotomy and debridement of the fragments. Antibiotics are begun prior to the procedure and continued for 10 to 14 days postoperatively.

BASAL SKULL FRACTURE AND CEREBROSPINAL FLUID FISTULA

Whereas fractures of the vault are often of little significance, basal skull fractures are particularly important because their presence places the patient at risk for meningitis. Adhesions between the dura and bone are more pronounced at the skull base, and even small fractures can tear the dura and place the central nervous system in contact with contaminated or potentially contaminated paranasal sinuses.

Most skull base fractures are extensions of fractures of the vault.[81] Less frequently, blunt trauma to the head may cause a basal skull fracture due to stress concentration at the many foramina at the base. Blows to the lower jaw are particularly likely to cause these fractures because of transmission of force through the condyloid processes. The fracture may occur in any of the five bones that form the base of the skull: the ethmoid, orbital plate of the frontal bone, sphenoid, petrous portion of the temporal bone, and the occipital bone.

Fractures of the petrous bone are classified as longitudinal or transverse depending on the orientation of the fracture line to the long axis of the petrous pyramid.[82] Longitudinal fractures are due to a blow to the side of the head, with the fracture extending into the skull base. This fracture is the most common and accounts for 70 to 90 percent of petrous fractures.[83] Transverse fractures of the petrous bone are due to violent blows to the back of the head and are associated with a high mortality.[84]

Basal Skull Fracture Without Cerebrospinal Fluid Fistula

The reported incidence of basal skull fractures in head trauma varies from 3.5 to 24 percent.[85,86] This difference may be explained by the difficulty in diagnosing these fractures using conventional radiologic techniques. The reported incidence will depend upon the diligence displayed in diagnosing these fractures.

The presence of a basal skull fracture can be inferred from the clinical signs and symptoms. Bilateral periorbital ecchymosis (raccoon's eyes), anosmia, and CSF rhinorrhea are manifestations of fractures involving the sphenoid, frontal, or ethmoid bones. Petrous bone fractures are suggested by ecchymosis of the scalp overlying the mastoid bone (Battle's sign). The clinical syndrome will depend on the type of fracture. Longitudinal fractures of the petrous bone extend through the external and middle ear, and these patients will present with a bloody discharge from the ear, tympanic membrane perforation, and conductive hearing loss due to disruption of the ossicular chain.[84] The seventh and eighth cranial nerves are usually spared in longitudinal fractures because the nerves lie posterior to the fracture line. A transverse petrous fracture typically crosses the internal auditory meatus or the bony labyrinth and will injure the seventh and eighth cranial nerves 50 percent of the time.[87] Patients with this fracture will not have blood in the external auditory canal or a tympanic membrane rupture. They will present with sensorineural hearing loss, tinnitus, vertigo, and facial paresis.[84]

Patients suspected of having a basal skull fracture should be admitted to the hospital. If there is no evidence of a CSF fistula or cranial nerve injury, the radiologic investigation can be limited to plain skull films, with CT scanning if an intracranial injury is suspected. The skull film may rarely visualize fragmented spicules of bone or an extensively comminuted fracture. If the patient's condition permits, Schuller, Towne-Chamberlain, Stenvers, and basal views should be obtained to visualize the fracture. CT scanning is more helpful in identifying intracranial injuries but less helpful than routine tomography in visualizing the base of the skull. Further diagnostic tests are not necessary unless a CSF fistula or cranial nerve injury develops.

Use of nasogastric tubes should be avoided. The tube may be inadvertently inserted into the intracranial fossa with lethal consequences.[88–90] After 3 or 4 days of observation, the patient is discharged with instructions to return at once if otorrhea, rhinorrhea, or symptoms of meningitis develop.

Brawley and Kelly[86] proposed antibiotic coverage for 5 days to suppress organisms in the paranasal sinuses and nasopharynx until there is healing of any potential dural tear to decrease the incidence of meningitis. However, the weight of evidence from clinical trials suggests that antibiotics are not helpful in preventing meningitis. Einhorn and Mizrahi[85] reported that in a series of 46 children with basal skull fractures, there were no infections regardless of whether or not antibiotics were given. Hoff and colleagues[91] prospectively studied 160 patients with basal skull fractures and randomized these patients to no therapy, low-dose penicillin, or high-dose penicillin therapy. None of the groups became infected, and the author abandoned the use of antibiotics in the absence of a CSF fistula. Ignelzi and VanderArk[92] in a prospective analysis of 129 patients with basal skull fractures also concluded that antibiotics were not helpful and possibly harmful. Similar studies in patients with acute traumatic CSF rhinorrhea or otorrhea[93] have not shown any benefit from the use of prophylactic antibiotics in preventing meningitis. Furthermore, the use of antibiotics may suppress the normal pharyngeal flora and result in a predominance of gram-negative organisms.[92] It has been our policy not to use prophylactic antibiotics for patients with basal skull fractures.

Basal Skull Fracture with Associated Cerebrospinal Fluid Fistula

The incidence of post-traumatic fistula has been estimated to be 2 to 3 percent among all head-injured patients and may be as high as 6 percent among patients with severe head injury.[94–96] Post-traumatic CSF fistula is rare in children because the base of the skull is more flexible and the sinuses are not yet fully developed.[97]

In the majority of patients the leak will appear immediately or within 48 hours after the injury, and it will spontaneously cease in more than 85 percent of the patients within a week.[98] In delayed CSF fistulas, the leak may begin weeks to years after the injury, but in 90 percent of these patients the leak will be present within the first 3 months.[98] These delayed fistulas presenting many years after head injury[99] generally require operative therapy.

Cerebrospinal Fluid Rhinorrhea

Patients with CSF rhinorrhea have sustained a dural tear overlying a fracture of the ethmoid, sphenoid, or frontal bone which allows the egress of CSF into the paranasal sinuses. Occasionally, with a fracture of the petrous portion of the temporal bone, CSF may gain entrance to the middle ear, and if the tympanic membrane is intact, CSF will drain into the nose. This phenomenon, otorhinorrhea, should be kept in mind when localization of the site of a CSF fistula is difficult.

The clinical presentation of rhinorrhea is usually straightforward. The patient will have clear, watery drainage from the nose, often from one nostril. Rhinal or allergic discharges tend to be opalescent and drain from both nostrils. If the rhinorrhea is unilateral, the dural tear will be ipsilateral to the leak 95 percent of the time.[100] Bilateral rhinorrhea, however, will be associated with bilateral tears only 50 percent of the time. Anosmia in the presence of rhinorrhea suggests a fracture of the ethmoid bone.

A maneuver that may be helpful in localizing the leak is to have the patient stand or sit erect and flex the neck after awakening. A profuse discharge from the nose is called the "reservoir sign" and is consistent with a fluid collection in any of the larger sinuses.

There are a number of diagnostic tests that utilize the fact that CSF contains more glucose than nasal secretions. If enough secretions not contaminated with blood can be collected, the presence of a glucose concentration greater than 30 mg per deciliter confirms the diagnosis of a CSF fistula.[26] The use of Clinistix, Diastix, or Tes-Tape for bedside determination of glucose when there is scanty drainage is not recommended. In our experience, and that of others,[101] these tests are unreliable.

If there is minimal drainage, an immunofixation test may be useful because it may be performed with a minute drainage sample and is not affected by blood, tears, saliva, or mucous. This method detects the B-2 fraction of transferrin and is specific for CSF.[102]

Plain skull films should be taken on admission, although a skull series will demonstrate the site of the leak only 21 percent of the time.[103] A fracture may be visualized, and the presence of air-fluid levels in the paranasal sinuses or pneumocephalus should alert the clinician to the possibility of a CSF leak. Tomograms have been used in the past to visualize skull defects not appreciated on the skull films. Today, multiplanar high-resolution CT scanning can be used to demonstrate fractures of the skull base. In a recent study, CT scanning could demonstrate 90 percent of petrous bone fractures.[104]

There are a number of more sophisticated techniques that can be used to localize the site of the fistula; each technique has advantages and disadvantages. The use of radioisotopes has been shown to be very sensitive when identifying very small or intermittent leaks. The tracer is injected into the lumbar subarachnoid space and the leak is detected by packing the nasal passages and ear canals with cotton pledgets and then analyzing them for radioactivity. Indium (^{111}In DTPA) is the most frequently used isotope and is able to detect very small or intermittent leaks with a 25 percent success rate.[105] In theory, increased radioactive uptake in the posterior pharyngeal wall pledget indicates that CSF is entering via the eustachian tube, whereas staining of the anterior nasal roof pledget means that the cribriform plate or anterior ethmoid bone may be the site of the leak. Unfortunately, in practice the radioactive tracers have not been helpful in accurately localizing the site of the fistula.

Cisternography, using water-soluble contrast media such as iopamidol, is the best diagnostic test if the patient is actively leaking. Contrast is injected into the lumbar subarachnoid space and the patient is scanned in the coronal plane. The contrast medium can be seen flowing through the fistulous tract into the paranasal sinuses (Fig. 6–12). The major disadvantage of this technique is that the patient must be actively leaking at the time of the study in order to demonstrate the fistula. False-negative studies are common because many leaks are intermittent. Valsalva maneuvers, careful positioning of the patient, and overpressure infusion of artificial CSF have been used to circumvent this problem with some success.[106–108]

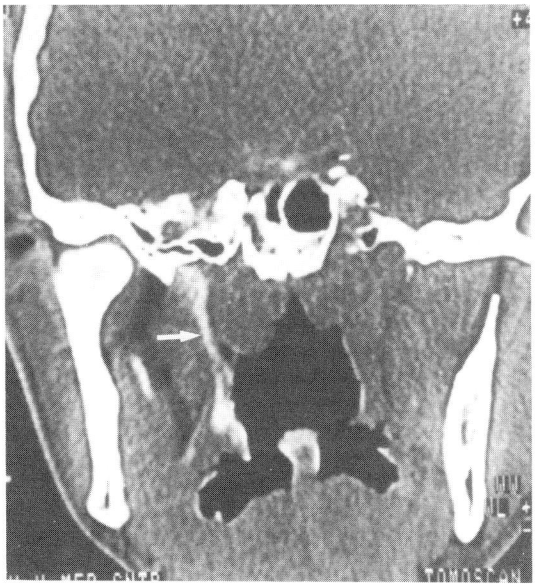

Figure 6–12 Coronal computed tomographic scan performed after subarachnoid administration of water-soluble contrast. Contrast is seen in the eustachian tube (arrow) draining into the nasopharynx.

In the majority of patients with CSF rhinorrhea, a trial of nonoperative management is appropriate. The patient is placed at bed rest with the head of the bed elevated to 30 degrees. The patient is cautioned against sneezing and nose blowing. Laxatives and stool softeners are given to avoid increased ICP associated with Valsalva maneuvers.

After 72 hours, if the leak has not stopped, a trial of continuous spinal drainage employing a lumbar subarachnoid catheter may be instituted. About 150 ml of CSF are removed each day, for 3 to 5 days. The fistula will usually cease in this time, but if it continues to drain or recurs following removal of the drain, operation is indicated.

Surgical repair should be performed in patients whose fistulas persist in spite of medical management, patients with delayed onset fistulas, and in those who have recovered from meningitis. In these cases operation is not an emergency and is performed after appropriate tests are done to localize the fistula. Indications for emergent repair of CSF fistula are: (1) a fistula associated with a significant intracranial hemorrhage, (2) the presence of an open wound that communicates with the dura, (3) radiographic evidence of comminuted bone fractures with extensive dural tearing and brain penetration, and (4) brain herniation into one of the paranasal sinuses (Fig. 6–13). Most neurosurgeons would also argue that the presence of pneumocephalus mandates urgent repair.

The operative repair of CSF rhinorrhea can be performed via an intracranial or extracranial approach. We prefer the trans-sphenoidal or trans-ethmoidal extracranial approach because it is associated with a lower morbidity than the intracranial procedure, does not result in loss of the sense of smell when it existed preoperatively, and it has a greater than 95 percent success rate.[95,109,110] These techniques provide excellent exposure of the sphenoid, parasellar, and posterior ethmoid area and good visualization of the posterior wall of the frontal sinus, the cribriform plate,

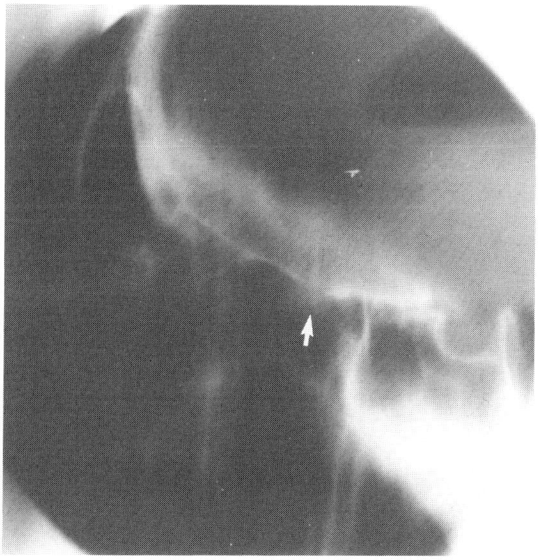

Figure 6–13 Tomogram of the skull showing intraventricular air and an ethmoid fracture with herniation of soft tissue into the ethmoid sinus (arrow). Operation confirmed a skull base fracture with brain herniation into the sinus.

and the fovea ethmoidalis. A nasal septal mucosal flap is created and rotated to cover the cribriform plate and the ethmoid or sphenoid sinus, depending upon where the leak is located. Calcaterra[95] also recommends using a free fascial graft which is then covered by the septal flap. In all postoperative patients, CSF is drained using a lumbar subarachnoid catheter for 3 to 5 days. The extracranial approach is contraindicated if there are coexisting intracranial hemorrhages requiring craniotomy.

An intracranial approach through a unilateral or bilateral bone flap will allow direct visualization of the dural tear and removal of any intracranial hemorrhages. When preoperative studies indicate that the fistula is unilateral, a unilateral bone flap is fashioned on the side of the leak. If there are bilateral fractures or the site of the fracture cannot be determined, a bicoronal incision and a bifrontal bone flap is performed. Mannitol and spinal drainage are used to relax the brain and minimize the retraction necessary for exposure of the leak. The dura is opened and intradural exploration of the floor of the frontal fossa is performed.

Once the tear is located, intradural repair of the laceration is performed. Frequently this is not possible if the laceration is located medially or posteriorly in the frontal fossa. If this occurs, the dura mater is dissected off the floor of the frontal fossa and repaired from an extradural approach. For large dural rents, a graft of pericranium or fascia lata may be necessary. Should the site of the fistula remain unclear, the craniotomy can be extended into the temporal region to expose the middle fossa. Suspicious bony defects can be obliterated, and, if necessary, the tuberculum sella can be opened and the sphenoid sinus packed with fat, muscle, or fascia lata. The cribriform plate should then be covered with fascia lata. These techniques will occlude the majority of unidentified leaks.[111] Spinal drainage is used postoperatively for 3 or 4 days to decrease the chance of recurrent fistula formation.

Cerebrospinal Fluid Otorrhea

CSF otorrhea will occur when the petrous bone is fractured, a dural tear is present, and the tympanic membrane is ruptured, allowing the egress of CSF into the external ear. Diagnosis may be obscured by the presence of blood in the ear, but attempts to probe or irrigate the ear should be avoided because this may increase the risk of meningitis. A sterile nontamponading bag should be placed over the ear to decrease the chance of infection and collect the fluid for diagnostic studies. The management of these patients and the techniques of fistula localization are the same as those discussed for patients with rhinorrhea. In virtually every case, the leak will spontaneously stop without operation.

If an operation is indicated, the procedure may be undertaken by a neurosurgeon or an otolaryngologist. Otolaryngologists have preferred a mastoidectomy approach for repair of the dural defect; a variety of different foreign and autogenous materials can be used.[82] In the absence of useful hearing, a tympanotomy may be performed.[82,112] This procedure entails obliterating the middle ear with free temporalis muscle and fascia and thus eliminating the potential pathway of infection from the nasopharynx to the subarachnoid space. If the tympanic membrane is perforated, a myringoplasty is performed at the same time.

Neurosurgeons have repaired these fistulas by fashioning a bone flap in either the middle or posterior fossa depending on the location of the petrous fracture. An intradural exploration is performed and the dural tear is repaired primarily or a graft of pericranium or fascia lata is used. In experienced hands this technique is 98 percent successful in stopping the leak.[113]

Pneumocephalus

Pneumocephalus, or intracranial air, has been reported to occur in 0.5 to 9.7 percent of head injuries and is a frequent accompaniment of basal skull fractures.[114,115] Pneumocephalus has the same implication as a CSF fistula; they are both associated with a dural tear (Fig. 6–14).

Intracranial hypotension due to loss of CSF may permit air to enter the cranial cavity in an "inverted bottle effect," or the patient may force air up into the intracranial cavity with straining, coughing, or sneezing. The air may be present as single air bubbles, small pockets, or as a large collection called a pneumatocele. The air is usually distributed in the subarachnoid space of the frontal and temporal regions and is occasionally intracerebral and rarely intraventricular. It is often difficult on the basis of CT scanning to determine whether the air is extradural, subdural, or subarachnoid.[115]

The treatment of patients with pneumocephalus is controversial. Park and colleagues[115a] have argued that the presence of pneumocephalus implies a large dural tear that will not heal spontaneously and that will place the patient at great risk for meningitis. They advocate aggressive medical management with antibiotics, or immediate operation. Steudel and Hacker[115] recommended that patients with large collections of air acting as a space-occupying lesion should be operated on as soon as possible. If the pneumocephalus is associated with persistent rhinorrhea, the CSF fistula should be repaired. Ommaya[116] considered the presence of intraventricular air an indication for immediate operation.

Complications

The major complication of CSF fistula is infection. The fracture will allow contamination of the intracranial space by the bacterial flora of the nasopharynx or external environment. Meningitis is the most frequent complication. Brain abscess may occur rarely. The reported incidence of meningitis with CSF fistulas varies from 3 to 50 percent.[92,93,98,117] The longer the CSF fistula is present, the greater the chance of infection.

The interval between the trauma and the onset of meningitis is important in predicting the causative organism. In patients with a skull fracture and CSF fistula who develop meningitis within 3 days of injury, the organism is almost always *pneumococcus*[99,118] and penicillin is the treatment of choice. In children between the ages of 6 months and 6 years, post-traumatic meningitis may be due to *Hemophilus influenzae* and therefore ampicillin and chloramphenicol are appropriate

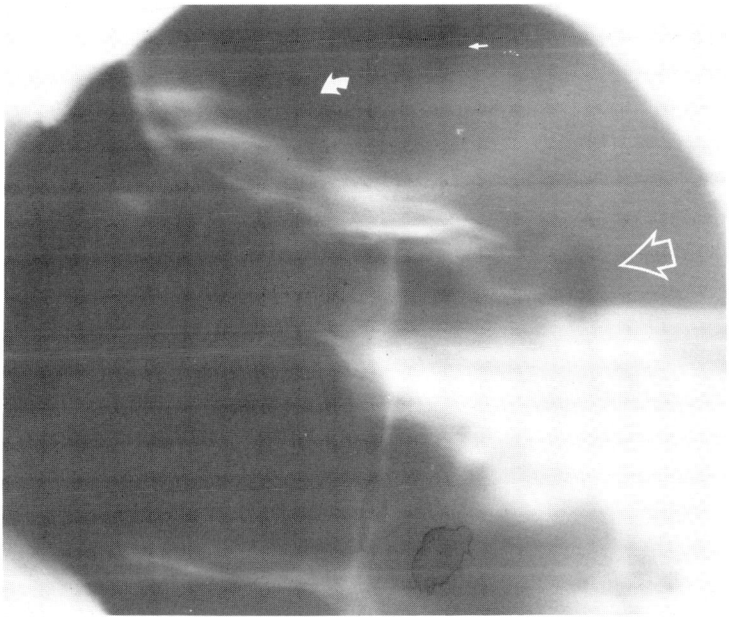

Figure 6–14 Tomogram of skull demonstrating intraventricular, (small arrow), intracerebral (curved arrow), and subarachnoid air (open arrow).

treatment. In patients hospitalized more than 3 days and those patients treated with prophylactic antibiotics who develop meningitis, gram-negative organisms and *Staphylococcus aureus* are the most likely organisms. A third-generation cephalosporin and nafcillin will provide adequate treatment for these patients. These are general guidelines; the ultimate antibiotic coverage is determined by the Gram's stain of the CSF and CSF cultures. A lumbar puncture should be performed immediately if a mass lesion—i.e., brain abscess—is not a consideration.

REFERENCES

1. Draus JF. Epidemiology of head injury. In: Cooper PR, ed. Head injury. 2nd ed. Baltimore: Williams & Wilkins, 1987:8.
2. Miller JD, Butterworth JF, Guderman SK, et al. Further experience in the management of severe head injury. J Neurosurg 1981; 54:289–299.
3. Miller JD. Physiology of trauma. Clin Neurosurg 1982; 29:103–130.
4. Baker CC, Oppenheimer L, Stephens B, et al. Epidemiology of trauma deaths. Am J Surg 1980; 140:144–150.
5. Hoffman E. Mortality and morbidity following road accidents. Ann R Coll Surg Engl 1976; 58:233–240.
6. Frost EAM, Arancibia CU, Shulman K. Pulmonary shunt as a prognostic indicator in head injury. J Neurosurg 1969; 50:768–772.
7. Eisenberg HM, Cayard C, Papanicolaou AC, et al. The effects of three potentially preventable complications on outcome after severe closed head injury. In: Ishii S, Nagai H, Brock M, eds. Intracranial pressure. V. Tokyo: Springer-Verlag, 1983:549.
8. Youmans JR. Causes of shock with head injury. J Trauma 1964; 4:204–209.
9. Clarke R, Fisher MR, Topley E, Davies JWL. Extent and time of blood-loss after civilian head injury. Lancet 1961; 2:381–386.
10. Newfield P, Pitts L, Kaktis J, Hoff J. The influence of shock on mortality after head trauma. Crit Care Med 1980; 8:254 (Abstract).
11. Olsen WR. Shock and the accident and trauma victim. In: Frey CF, ed. Initial management of the trauma patient. Philadelphia: Lea & Febiger, 1976:71.
12. Gardner SR, Maull JD, Swenson EE, Ward JD. The effects of the pneumatic anti-shock garment on intracranial pressure in man: a prospective study of 12 patients with severe head injury. J Trauma 1984; 24:896–900.
13. Youmans JR. Causes of shock with head injury. J Trauma 1964; 4:204–209.
14. Marshall LF, Smith RW, Shapiro HM. The outcome with aggressive treatment in severe head injuries. I. The significance of intracranial pressure monitoring. J Neurosurg 1979; 50:20–25.
15. Galbraith S. Misdiagnosis and delayed diagnosis in traumatic intracranial hematoma. Br Med J 1976; 1:1438–1439.
16. Tabaddor K, Balagura S. Acute epidural hematoma following epileptic seizures. Arch Neurol 1981; 38:198–199.
17. Overgaard J, Hvid-Hansen O, Land AM, et al. Prognosis after head injury based on early clinical examination. Lancet 1973; 2:631–635.
18. Graham DI, McLellan D, Adams JH, et al. Neuropathology of the vegetative state and severe disability after non-missile head injury. Acta Neurochir (Suppl) 1983; 32:67.
19. Echlin FA, Sordillo SVR, Garvey TQ Jr. Acute, subacute and chronic subdural hematoma. JAMA 1956; 161:1345–1350.
20. Kennedy F, Wortis H. "Acute" subdural hematoma and acute epidural hemorrhage. A study of seventy-two cases of hematoma and seventeen cases of hemorrhage. Surg Gynecol Obstet 1936; 63:732–734.
21. Jamieson KG, Yelland JDN. Surgically treated traumatic subdural hematomas. J Neurosurg 1972; 37:137–149.
22. Mckissock W, Richardson A, Bloom WH. Subdural haematoma. A review of 389 cases. Lancet 1960; 1:1365–1369.
23. Seelig JM, Becker DP, Miller JD, et al. Traumatic acute subdural hematoma. Major mortality reduction in comatose patients treated within four hours. N Engl J Med 1981; 304:1511–1518.
24. Ransohoff J, Benjamin MV, Gage EL Jr, Epstein F. Hemicraniectomy in the management of acute subdural hematoma. J Neurosurg 1971; 34:70–76.
25. Scotti G, Terbrugge K, Melancon D, Gelanger G. Evaluation of the age of subdural hematomas by computerized tomography. J Neurosurg 1977; 47:311–315.
26. Cameron MM. Chronic subdural haematoma: report of 167 cases. J Neurol Neurosurg Psychiatry 1978; 41:834–839.
27. Luxon LM, Harrison MJG. Chronic subdural haematoma. Quart J Med 1979; 189:43–53.
28. Jamieson KG, Yelland JDN. Extradural hematoma. Report of 167 cases. J Neurosurg 1968; 29:13–23.
29. Bricolo AP, Pasut LM. Extradural hematoma: towards zero mortality. A prospective study. Neurosurgery 1984; 14:8–12.
30. Reale F, Delfin R, Mencattini G. Epidural hematomas. J Neurosurg Sci 1984; 28:9–16.
31. Courvill CB. Coup coutre-coup mechanism of craniocerebral injuries. Arch Surg 1942; 45:19–43.
32. Schonauer M, Schisano G, Cimino R, Viola L. Space occupying contusions of cerebral lobes after closed brain injury. Considerations about 51 cases. J Neurosurg Sci 1979; 23:279–288.
33. Heiskanen O, Valpalahti M. Temporal lobe contusion and haematoma. Acta Neurochir 1972; 27:29–35.
34. Mckenzie KG. Extradural haemorrhage. Br J Surg 1938; 26:346–365.

35. Zimmerman RA, Bilaniuk LT, Gennarelli T, et al. Cranial computer tomography in diagnosis and management of acute head trauma. Am J Roentgenol 1978; 131:27–34.
36. Jamieson KG, Yelland JDN. Traumatic intracerebral hematoma. Report of 63 surgically treated cases. J Neurosurg 1972; 37:528–532.
37. Halazonetis JA. The "weak" regions of the mandible. Br J Oral Surg 1968; 6:37–48.
38. Murray JF, Hall HC. Fractures of the mandible in motor vehicle accidents. Clin Plast Surg 1975; 2:131–142.
39. Lee FK, Wagner LK, Lee EY, et al. The impact-absorbing effect of facial fractures in closed-head injuries. An analysis of 210 patients. J Neurosurg 1987; 66:542–547.
40. Gurdjian ES, Webster JE. Head injuries. Boston: Little, Brown, 1958:211.
41. Gurdjian ES, Webster JE. Head injuries. Boston: Little, Brown, 1958:65.
42. Bunge RE, Heiman CL. Radiation experience data (RED): documentation and results of the 1980 survey of U.S. hospitals. Rockville, MD: Dept of Health and Human Services, 1986 (DHHS publication no. (FDA) 86–8253).
43. Masters SJ. Evaluation of head trauma: efficacy of skull films. AJR 1980; 135:539–547.
44. Roberts F, Shopfner CE. Plain skull roentgenograms in children with head trauma. Am J Roentgenol Radium Ther Nucl Med 1972; 114:230–240.
45. Eyes B, Evans AF. Post-traumatic skull radiographs: time for a reappraisal. Lancet 1978; 2:85–86.
46. McClean PM, Joseph LP, Rudolph H. Plain skull film radiography in the management of head trauma: an overview. Ann Emerg Med 1984; 13:607–611.
47. Royal College of Radiologists. A study of the utilization of skull radiography in 9 accident-and-emergency units in the U.K.: a national study by the Royal College of Radiologists. Lancet 1980; 2:1234-1237.
48. Jones JJ, Jeffreys RV. Relative risk of alternative admissions policies for patients with head injuries. Lancet 1981; 2:850–853.
49. Thornbury JR, Campbell JA, Masters SJ, et al. Skull fracture and the low risk of intracranial sequelae in minor head trauma. AJR 1984; 143:661–664.
50. Masters SJ, McClean PM, Ararese JS, et al. Skull x-ray examinations after head trauma. N Engl J Med 1987; 316:84–91.
51. Mendelow AD, Campbell DA, Jeffrey RR, et al. Admission after mild head injury: benefits and costs. Br Med J 1982; 285:1530–1532.
52. Dacey RG. Neurosurgical complications after apparently minor head injury. J Neurosurg 1986; 65:203–210.
53. Jennett B. Some medicolegal aspects of the management of acute head injury. Br Med J 1976; 1:1383–1385.
54. Jennett B. Skull x-ray after recent head injury. Clin Radiol 1980; 31:463.
55. Cooper PR, Ho V. Role of emergency skull x-ray films in the evaluation of the head-injured patient: a retrospective study. Neurosurgery 1983; 13:136–140.
56. Braakman R. Depressed skull fracture: data, treatment, and follow-up in 225 consecutive cases. J Neurol Neurosurg Psychiatry 1972; 35:395–402.
57. Miller JD, Jennett WB. Complications of depressed skull fracture. Lancet 1968; 2:991–995.
58. Cabraal SA, Abeysuriya SC. The management of compound depressed fractures of the skull. Ceylon Med J 1969; 14:105–115.
59. OH S. Clinical and experimental morphological study of depressed skull fracture. Acta Neurochir 1983; 68:111–121.
60. Jennett B, Miller JD, Braakman R. Epilepsy after non-missile depressed skull fracture. J Neurosurg 1974; 41:208–216.
60a. Glaser MA, Shufer FP. Depressed fractures of the skull. Their surgery sequelae and disability. J Neurosurg 1945; 2:1403153.
61. Jennett B, Miller JD. Infection after depressed fracture of the skull. Implications for management of non-missile injuries. J Neurosurg 1972; 36:333–339.
62. Cushing H. A study of a series of wounds involving the brain and its enveloping structures. Br J Surg 1918; 5:558–684.
63. Kriss FC, Raren JA, Kahn EA. Primary repair of compound skull fractures by replacement of bone fragments. J Neurosurg 1969; 30:698–702.
64. Nadell J, Kline DG. Primary reconstruction of depressed frontal skull fractures including those involving the sinus, orbit, and cribriform plate. J Neurosurg 1974; 41:200–207.
65. Mendelow AD, Campbell D, Tsementzis SA, et al. Prophylactic antimicrobial management of compound depressed skull fracture. J Roy Coll Surg Edin 1983; 28:80–83.
66. Cooper PR. Skull fracture and traumatic cerebrospinal fluid fistulas. In: Cooper PR, ed. Head injury. 2nd ed. Baltimore: Williams & Wilkins, 1987:97.
67. Newman MH, Travis LW. Frontal fractures. Laryngoscope 1973; 83:1281–1290.
68. Levine B, Towe L, Keane W, Atkins J. Evaluation and treatment of frontal sinus fractures. Otolaryngol Head Neck Surg 1986; 95:19–22.
69. Donald PJ, Bernstein L. Compound frontal sinus injuries with intracranial penetration. Laryngoscope 1978; 88:225–232.
70. Baron SH, Dedo HH, Henry CR. The mucoperiosteal flap in frontal sinus surgery (the Sewall-Boyden-McKnaught operation). Laryngoscope 1973; 83:1266–1280.
71. Luce E. Frontal sinus fractures: guidelines to management. Plast Reconstr Surg 1987; 80:500–508.
72. Peri G, Chabannes J, Nenes R, et al. Fractures of the frontal sinus. J Maxillofac Surg 1981; 9:73–80.
73. Russell WR, Smith A. Post-traumatic amnesia in closed head injury. Arch Neurol 1961; 5:4–17.

74. Jamieson KG, Yelland JDN. Depressed skull fractures in Australia. J Neurosurg 1972; 37:150–155.
75. Sande GM, Galbraith SL, McLatchie G. Infection after depressed fracture in the west of Scotland. Scottish Med J 1980; 25:227–229.
76. Gamache FW, Drucker TB. Alterations in neurological function in head injured patients experiencing minor episodes of sepsis. Neurosurgery 1982; 10:468–472.
77. Bullitt E, Lehman RAW. Osteomyelitis of the skull. Surg Neurol 1979; 11:163–166.
78. Bhondari YS, Sarkuri NB. Subdural empyema—a review of 37 cases. Neurosurgery 1970; 32:35–39.
79. Sameson D, Clark K. A current review of brain abscess. Am J Med 1974; 54:201–210.
79a. Carey ME, Chou SN, French LA. Experience with brain abscess. J Neurosurg 1972; 36:1–9.
80. Rosenblum M, Hoff JT, Norman D, et al. Nonoperative treatment of brain abscesses in high-risk patients. J Neurosurg 1980; 52:217–225.
81. Gurdjian ES, Webster JE. Head injuries. Boston: Little, Brown 1958:76.
82. Henry RC, Taylor PH. Cerebrospinal fluid otorrhea and otorhinorrhea following closed head injury. J Neurosurg 1978; 92:743–756.
83. Hough JVD, Stuart WD. Middle ear injuries in skull trauma. Laryngoscope 1968; 78:899–937.
84. Hicks GW, Wright JW Jr, Wright JW III. Cerebrospinal fluid otorrhea. Laryngoscope 1980; 90 (Suppl 25):1–25.
85. Einhorn A, Mizrahi EM. Basilar skull fractures in children. The incidence of CNS infection and the use of antibiotics. Am J Dis Child 1978; 132:1121–1124.
86. Brawley BW, Kelly WA. Treatment of basal skull fractures with and without cerebrospinal fluid fistulae. J Neurosurg 1967; 26:57–61.
87. Tos M. Fractures of the temporal bone. The course and sequelae of 248 fractures of the petrous temporal bone. Ugeskr Laeger 1971; 133:1149–1456.
88. Freemstad JD, Martin SH. Lethal complications from insertion of nasogastric tube after severe basilar skull fracture. J Trauma 1978; 18:820–824.
89. Galloway DC, Grudis. Inadvertent intracranial placement of a nasogastric tube through a basal skull fracture. South Med J 1979; 72:240–241.
90. Wyler AR, Reynolds AF. An intracranial complication of nasogastric intubation. Case Report. J Neurosurg 1977; 47:297–298.
91. Hoff JT, Brewin A, U HS. Antibiotics for basilar skull fracture. J Neurosurg 1976; 44:649.
92. Ignelzi RJ, VanderArk GD. Analysis of the treatment of basilar skull fractures with and without antibiotics. J Neurosurg 1975; 43:721–726.
93. MacGee EE, Cauthen JC, Brackett CE. Meningitis following acute traumatic cerebrospinal fluid fistula. J Neurosurg 1970; 33:312–316.
94. Braakman R. Survey and follow-up of 225 consecutive patients with depressed skull fracture. J Neurol Neurosurg Psychiatry 1971; 34:106.
95. Calcaterra TC. Extracranial surgical repair of cerebrospinal rhinorrhea. Ann Otol 1980; 89:108–116.
96. Lewin W. Cerebrospinal fluid rhinorrhea in closed head injuries. Br J Surg 1954; 42:1–18.
97. Harris P. Head injuries in childhood. Arch Dis Child 1957; 32:448–491.
98. Brisman R, Hughes JE, Mount LA. Cerebrospinal fluid rhinorrhea. Arch Neurol 1970; 22:245–252.
99. Hand WL, Sanford JP. Post-traumatic bacterial meningitis. Ann Intern Med 1970; 72:869–874.
100. Leonidas JC, Ting W, Binkiewicz A, et al. Mild head trauma in children. When is a roentgenogram necessary? Pediatrics 1982; 69:139–143.
101. Katz RT, Kaplan PE. Glucose oxidase sticks and cerebrospinal fluid rhinorrhea. Arch Phys Med Rehab 1985; 66:391–393.
102. Irjala K, Sunopaa J, Laurent B. Identification of CSF leakage by immunofixation. Arch Otolaryngol 1979; 105:447–448.
103. Lantz EJ, Forbes GS, Brown ML, Laws ER Jr. Radiology of cerebrospinal fluid rhinorrhea. AJNR 1980; 1133:391–398.
104. Yamaki T, Yoshino E, Higuchi T, et al. Value of high-resolution computed tomography in diagnosis of petrous bone fracture. Surg Neurol 1986; 26:551–556.
105. Schaefer SK, Diehl JT, Griggs WH. The diagnosis of CSF rhinorrhea by metrizamide CT scanning. Laryngoscope 1980; 90:871–875.
106. Naidich TP, Moran CJ. Precise anatomic localization of traumatic sphenoethmoidal cerebrospinal fluid rhinorrhea by metrizamide CT cisternography. J Neurosurg 1980; 53:222–228.
107. Magnaes B, Solheim D. Controlled overpressure cisternography to localize cerebrospinal fluid rhinorrhea. J Nucl Med 1977; 18:109–111.
108. Ahmadi J, Weiss M, Segall H, et al. Evaluation of cerebrospinal fluid rhinorrhea by metrizamide computed tomographic cisternography. Neurosurgery 1985; 16:54–60.
109. Cooper PR. Skull fracture and traumatic cerebrospinal fluid fistulas. In: Cooper PR, ed. Head injury. 2nd ed. Baltimore: Williams & Wilkins, 1987:103.
110. Spetzler RF, Wilson CB. Dural fistulae and their repair. In: Youmans J, ed. Neurological surgery. Philadelphia: WB Saunders, 1982:2209–2227.
111. Selman W, Spetzler R. Cerebral spinal fluid fistulae. In: Tindall G, ed. Contemporary neurosurgery. Vol 6. Baltimore: Williams & Wilkins, 1984:4.
112. Calcaterra TC, Rand RW. Tympanic cavity obliteration for cerebrospinal otorhinorrhea. Arch Otolaryngol 1973; 97:388–390.
113. Bousquet C, Vaneecloo FM, Julliot JP, et al. Les otoliquorrhes traumatique. A propos de 50 malades opérés. Neurochir 1980; 26:369–375.
114. Markham JW. Pneumocephalus. In: Vinken PJ, Bruyn SW, eds. Injuries of the brain and skull. Vol 24. New York: Elsevier, 1976:201–213.
115. Steudel WI, Hacker H. Prognosis, incidence and

management of acute traumatic intracranial pneumocephalus: a retrospective analysis of 49 cases. Acta Neurochir 1986; 80:93–99.
115a. Park JI, Strelzow VV, Friedman WH. Current management of cerebrospinal fluid rhinorrhea. Laryngoscope 1983; 93:1294–1300.
116. Ommaya AK. Spinal fluid fistula. Clin Neurosurg 1976; 23:363–392.
117. Leech PJ, Paterson A. Conservative and operative management for cerebrospinal fluid leakage after closed head injury. Lancet 1973; 1:1013–1016.
118. Raaf J. Post-traumatic cerebrospinal fluid leaks. Arch Surg 1967; 95:648–651.

7

COMPLEX AND PANFACIAL FRACTURES

JOSEPH S. GRUSS, M.B., B.Chir., F.R.C.S.C.
JOHN H. PHILLIPS, M.D., F.R.C.S.C.

With the advent of regional trauma centers and rapid air transport systems, more patients with extremely complex craniomaxillofacial trauma are now being seen. The major problem of high-velocity facial injuries with multiple facial fractures, particularly in the multiply injured patient, concerns the severity of the bony injury. The majority of these fractures, particularly in the midface, are unstable and often have multiple comminuted segments. Segments of bone are often markedly displaced or actually dislocated, and, in addition, segments and areas of bone may be so severely damaged as to preclude any form of fixation, or they may actually be missing, having been lost through large skin or mucosal lacerations. Attempts at closed reduction or internal wire suspension of these comminuted areas result in eventual bony collapse and soft-tissue shrinkage. The traditional treatment of a bony gap is some form of external fixation to try and maintain the bone segments in their position and allow soft-tissue healing in anticipation of secondary bone grafting. External fixation techniques will maintain the position of mandibular segments but cannot maintain the position of comminuted midfacial bony segments. The inability to stabilize these midfacial segments results in rapid soft-tissue shrinkage and makes secondary bony correction very difficult, or impossible.

The solution to the problem of midfacial bony collapse and soft-tissue shrinkage and scarring lies in the early exposure of all fracture segments and their repair, using internal fixation techniques. This will result in the re-establishment of normal craniofacial skeletal anatomy and maintain soft-tissue expansion during the healing phase. Comminuted, or missing, bone is replaced by immediate bone grafting.[1–5] The use of these techniques will allow the repair of even the most severe injury in one stage with an insignificant increase in the rate of infection and prevent the development of secondary deformity which may be very difficult, or impossible, to correct adequately.

PRINCIPLES OF REPAIR

Whenever possible, the facial injuries are repaired immediately—or within the first few days—depending on the magnitude of coexisting multisystem trauma. Careful coordination and planning among involved surgical disciplines facilitate early repair. Definitive repair can be delayed for up to 2 weeks, but this makes adequate reduction and fixation more difficult. The decrease in facial edema and discomfort is striking following early and rigid internal fixation and repair. Once the diagnosis of a complex injury has been made, a coordinated approach, based on principles derived from reconstructive craniofacial surgery, is employed.

Direct Exposure of Fractures

All fractures are exposed directly (Fig. 7–1) and the degree of comminution and displacement and the pattern of the fractures are accurately assessed by direct inspection. It is essential to expose all fractures, as only this allows the exact fracture pattern to be assessed and the position of each bony fragment or bone segment to be assessed directly, in relation to its neighboring segment. A logical plan for repair can then be formulated.

Failure to expose all fractures and bone segments adequately will not infrequently result in bone segments being stabilized in their unreduced, or displaced, position because the surgeon can only assess each fracture site individually. This is particularly true in the orbital region where supposed reduction of fracture segments through small incisions can be easily accomplished without the surgeon becoming aware of other fractures and displacements elsewhere in this region. This will result in the development of severe secondary deformities, particularly in the orbital and nasoethmoid region.

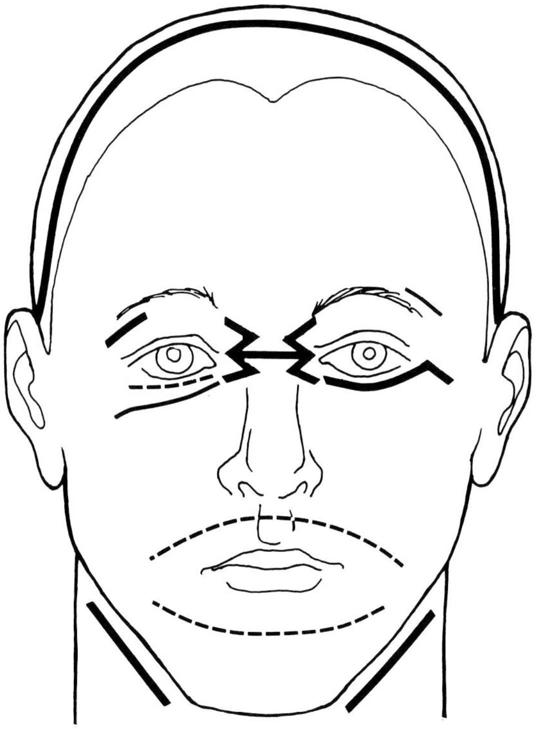

Figure 7–1 Incisions for exposure of craniofacial skeleton. The usual incision combines a full coronal incision, subciliary muscle–splitting incision, and upper buccal sulcus incision with intraoral or extraoral incisions to expose mandibular fractures. It is essential that all incisions communicate subperiosteally so that the entire craniofacial skeleton can be visualized.

Reduction and Internal Fixation

All fractures are reduced and internally fixed with meticulous interosseous fixation, with fragments and bone segments linked to adjacent fragments and to areas of the intact craniofacial skeleton until mechanical stability is obtained. This may involve fixation with interosseous wiring or metal plates and screws, where necessary.

Primary Bone Grafting

All severely damaged or absent bone is replaced, whenever possible, by means of immediate bone grafting (Fig. 7–2). Deficits in bony contour can be similarly augmented at the time of initial repair.

The use of these techniques will allow the repair of even the most severe injuries in one stage and minimize the occurrence of secondary deformities. External fixation techniques are rarely needed and internal craniofacial suspension wires are never used.

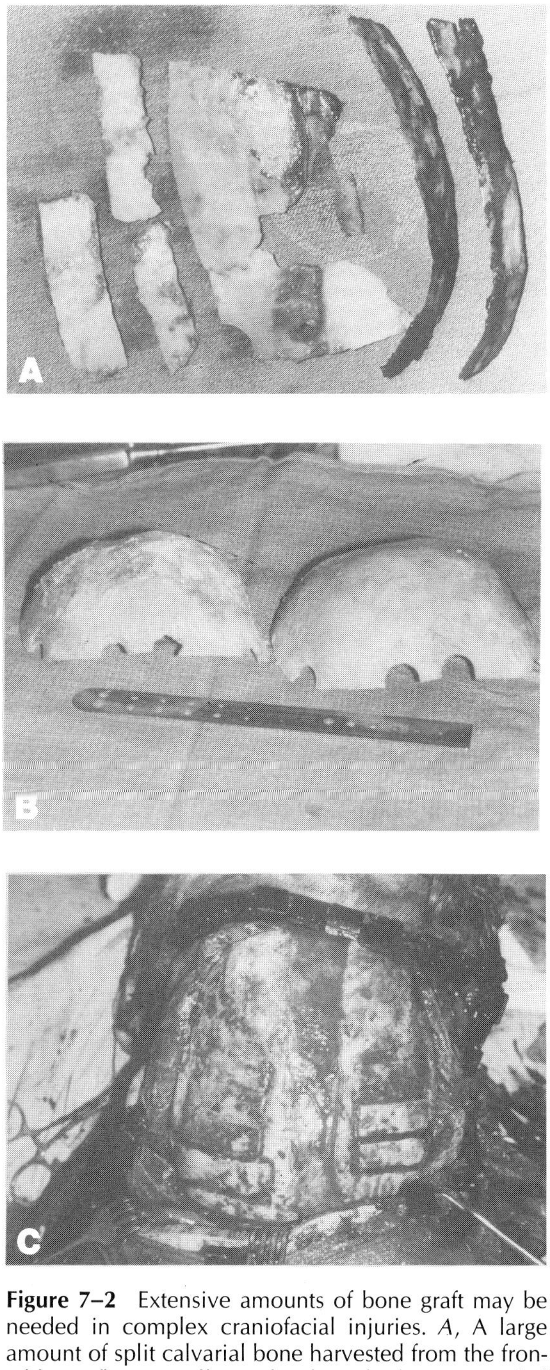

Figure 7–2 Extensive amounts of bone graft may be needed in complex craniofacial injuries. *A*, A large amount of split calvarial bone harvested from the frontal bone flap as well as split rib grafts that are needed in one patient with extensive craniofacial bone loss. *B*, Perfect splitting of the inner and outer table into two large pieces using oscillating reciprocating saws and chisels. This produces a large amount of bone for craniofacial repair. *C*, Extensive harvesting of split calvarial grafts from the intact skull, taking multiple strips of calvarial graft from both sides of the midline. Care must be taken not to take bone overlying the sagittal sinus in the midline of the skull.

INCISIONS AND APPROACHES

Whenever present, preexisting lacerations are taken advantage of in combination with planned incisions (see Fig. 7–1). All incisions are linked to each other subperiosteally to provide direct visualization of the entire involved facial skeleton. No attempt is made to preserve periosteal attachment to small segments of bone, as this compromises the adequacy of exposure. Only this approach will allow direct access to all fractures and facilitate adequate reduction and fixation.

The coronal incision is used for access to the upper craniofacial skeleton and zygomatic arch. When it is used in combination with local eyelid incisions and an upper buccal sulcus degloving incision, direct access to the entire craniofacial skeleton can be obtained.

METHODS OF INTERNAL FIXATION

Interosseous Wiring

Interosseous wiring is the most common traditional form of internal bony fixation (Figs. 7–3 to 7–5). In our experience, it is adequate in the relatively stable and undisplaced fractures, usually localized to one area of the craniofacial skeleton. Unfortunately, in severely unstable, displaced, and comminuted fractures of multiple areas of the facial skeleton, interosseous wires have been found to be less useful. An interosseous wire will provide only two-dimensional stability and will not prevent rotation around the wire. Even with the use of multiple wires, there is still movement of bony segments. In many of our earlier patients treated with extensive interosseous wiring and bone grafting, the early correction obtained on the operating table was not maintained consistently when soft-tissue and bony healing progressed. At the present time, interosseous wire fixation is primarily used for comminuted segments of the cranium and in repair of the infraorbital rim in selected patients in whom adjacent segments have been rigidly fixed with miniplates.

Lag Screws

Lag screw fixation of bone is the most sophisticated form of bony fixation available. The lag fixation principle involves drilling a hole in the outer, or more proximal, bone to a diameter that approximates the outer diameter of the screw threads. The inner, or more distal, hole is drilled with a drill diameter that approximates the inner, or core,

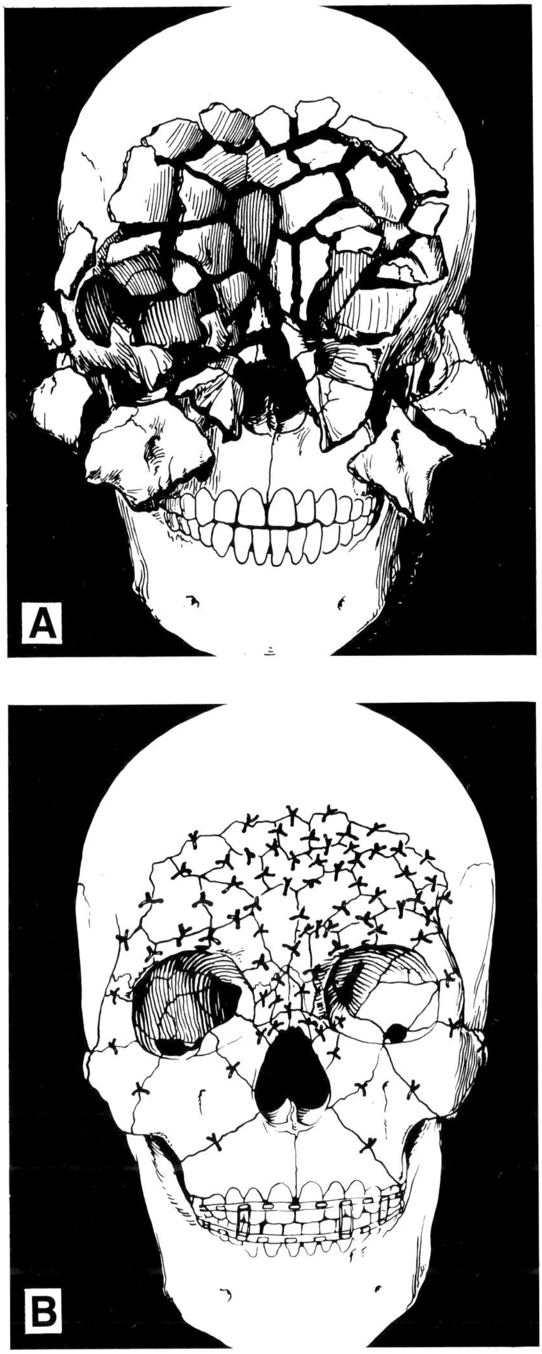

Figure 7–3 *A, B,* Massive panfacial injuries that involve both the cranium and face and result in massive comminution of the craniofacial skeleton including the cranial vault require that the cranial vault first be stabilized with either interosseous wiring or plate and screw fixation. Once the cranial vault has been repaired, the remainder of the craniofacial skeleton can be fixed to this now intact cranial vault using interosseous wires or, preferably, miniplates and screws.

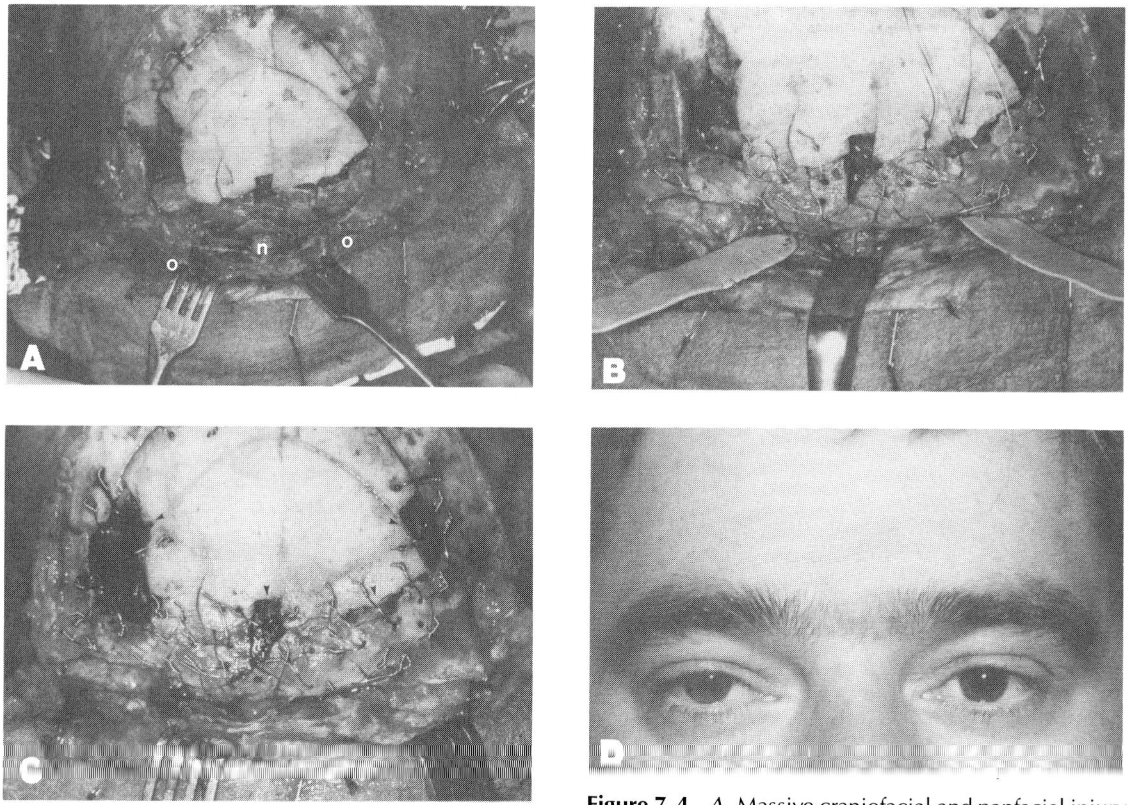

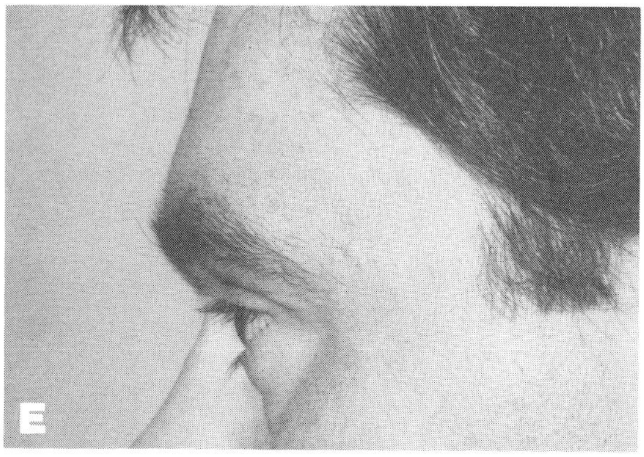

Figure 7–4 *A*, Massive craniofacial and panfacial injury following dural repair and replacement of the frontal bone flap. Extensive comminution can be seen extending right across the cranio-orbital region (O=orbit, N=nose). *B*, Cranio-orbital repair is now completed with extensive interosseous wiring using chain-link wiring where necessary. The residual defect in the cranial skeleton can be seen. *C*, These residual defects (black and marked with arrows) are filled in with carefully contoured calvarial grafts split from the inner table of the frontal bone flap. Comminuted cranial injuries such as this can be repaired quite adequately in most cases with interosseous wiring, as there are minimal muscle forces acting on this craniofacial bone. *D*, Final result at 3 years shows perfect restoration of craniofacial contour. *E*, Lateral view shows restoration of craniofacial projection.

diameter of the screw. This principle can be used with both self-tapping and tapped screws. Thus, when the screw passes through the outer, or gliding, hole, it slides through without any form of fixation and as it engages in the distal bone segment, the screw threads will engage this bone, either by cutting threads in a self-tapping system, or by engaging along precut threads in a tapped system of fixation. As the head of the screw engages in the proximal segment and the screw threads engage in the distal segment and the screw is tightened, the outer and inner bone segments are lagged together, producing direct interfragmentary compression of the bone. Rotation of bone is still possible around a single lag screw and thus more than one lag screw usually is needed for adequate bony fixation. This form of fixation is the most sophisticated and rigid of all forms of bony fixation, as it provides direct interfragmentary compression at each screw site. Lag screw fixation is ideally applied to oblique fractures in various areas of the midface and mandible and can be used in combination with miniplates in the midface and compression and reconstruction plates in the mandible. In addition, lag screws are the ideal form of fixation for bone grafts.

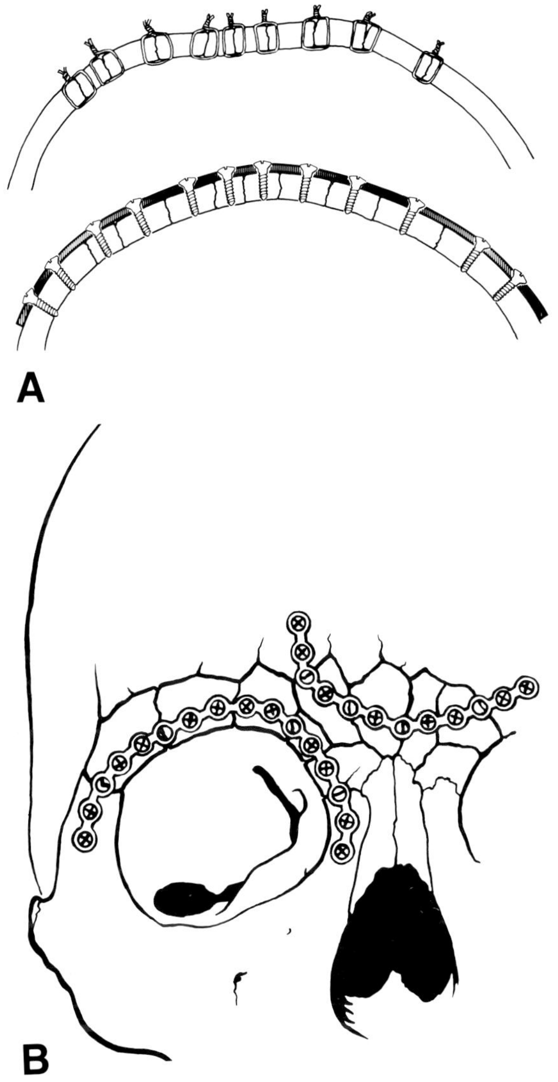

Figure 7–5 *A*, When extensive comminuted fractures of the frontal bone are repaired with interosseous wires, there is a tendency for collapse of the contour of the cranial vault due to rotation around the wire fixation and inability to provide three-dimensional reconstruction. Use of long, carefully contoured adaptive miniplates with separate screws placed in each fragment will prevent this deformity and restore perfect contour to the frontal and cranio-orbital region. *B*, Long adapted miniplates can be ideally used to restore contour and continuity to the supraorbital and nasoglabellar regions. They can be combined with interosseous wire fixation where necessary.

Miniplates and Screws

Specially designed miniplates and screws[6] (Figs. 7–6 to 7–11) have revolutionized the care of upper and midfacial injuries. These provide accurate, three-dimensional stability to the repaired bone

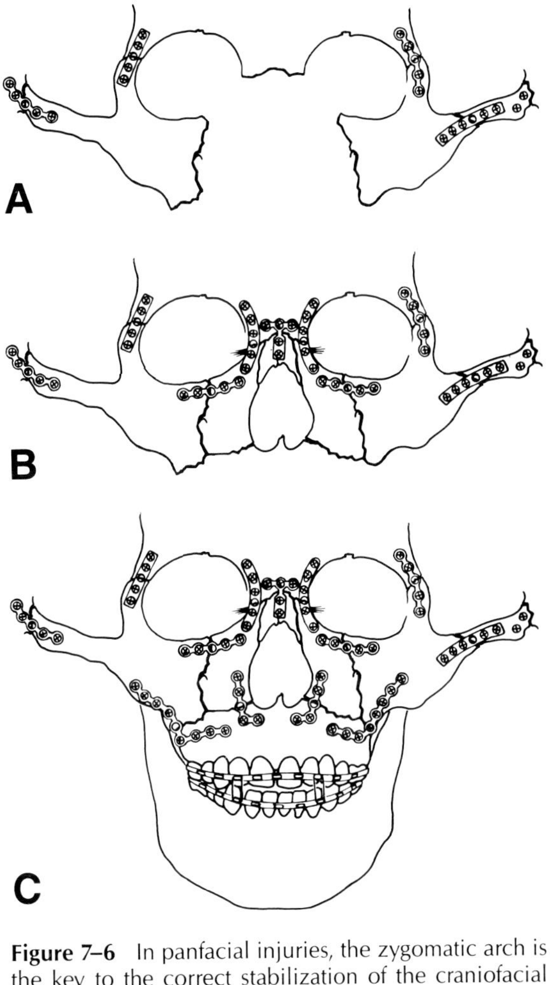

Figure 7–6 In panfacial injuries, the zygomatic arch is the key to the correct stabilization of the craniofacial skeleton. Exact repositioning of the zygomatic arch will re-establish an outer frame with the correct anteroposterior facial projection and transverse facial width. *A*, *B*, *C*, Stabilization of both zygomatic arches and zygomatic bodies in the correct position. This establishes an outer facial frame with the correct facial projection and width. The inferior orbit and nasoethmoid reconstruction can now be completed within this outer facial frame, establishing a perfect upper facial skeleton. The lower facial skeleton can now be placed into the correct intermaxillary fixation and the anterior maxillary buttress is repaired with miniplates completing the lower facial repair. Additional plate and screw fixation can be used on the mandible, if necessary, resulting in a three-dimensional reconstruction of the craniofacial skeleton and ensuring the correct projection and facial width.

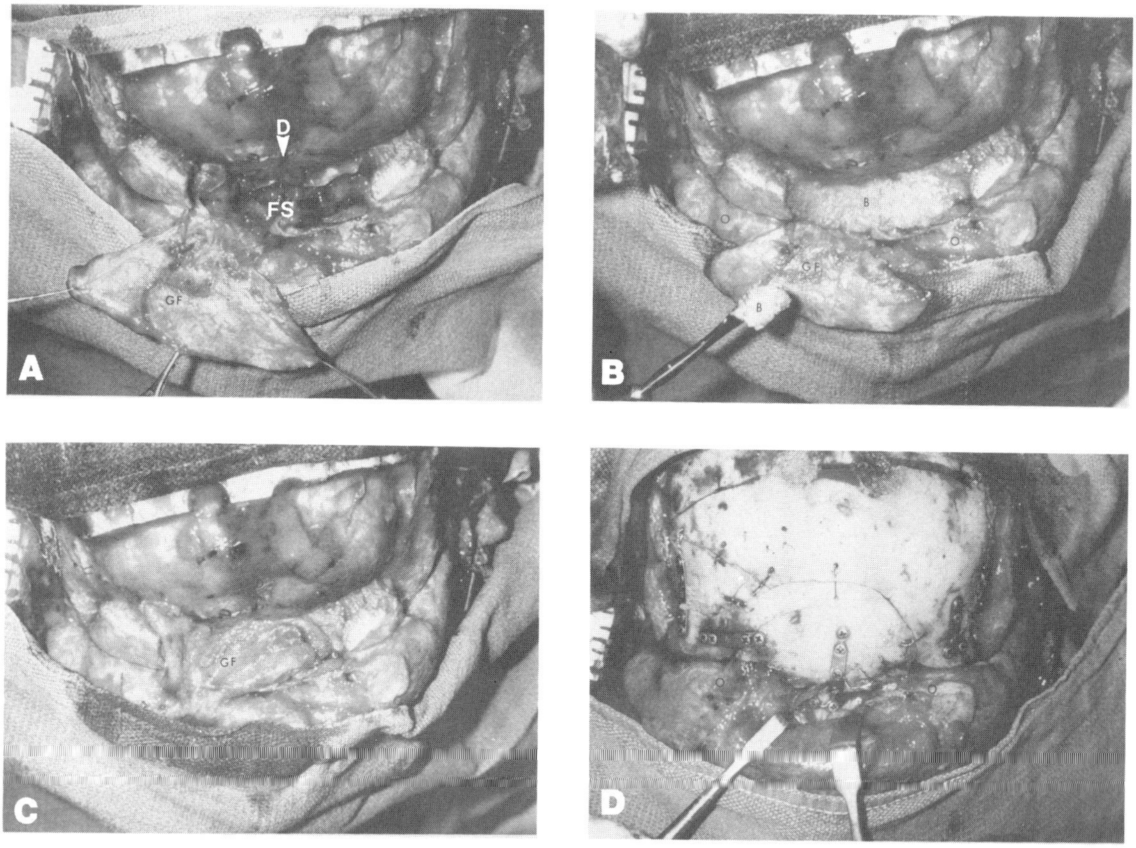

Figure 7–7 Massive craniofacial injury following industrial accident. Injury involves the frontal sinus with marked comminution of the floor of the frontal sinus, resulting in direct communication between the cranial cavity and the nasopharynx. *A*, Repair of the dura (D) by neurosurgeons. The floor of the frontal sinus (FS) can be seen in direct communication with the nasal cavity. Galeal frontalis flap (GF) has been raised from the frontal region on the undersurface of the coronal flap and is ready for transfer into the cranial cavity. *B*, Bone paste (B) has been harvested from the frontal bone flap and packed down into the base of the frontal sinus to seal it off from the nasopharynx. *C*, The galeal frontalis flap is now sutured across into the base of the frontal sinus and anchored along its posterior margin to the dura to seal off the cranial cavity totally from the nasopharynx with a well-vascularized flap. *D*, Completed repair of the complex craniofacial injuries using multiple miniplates combined with interosseous wires. An L-shaped miniplate in the center can be seen extending from the nasoglabellar region onto the bridge of the nose.

Figure continues on opposite page

and bone segments and allow for their exact repositioning without the risk of secondary relapse. Self-tapping screws should always be used in the thin midfacial bone. The use of long miniplates with multiple screws is the ideal method of fixation for long comminuted segments, as the miniplate can be fixed at each end to the relatively stable bone segments and then each comminuted segment can be anchored to the plate by means of multiple miniscrews. Miniplates have proven to be the ideal method of fixation at the frontozygomatic suture line, the zygomatic arch, the nasoethmoid orbital region, and the anterior maxillary buttresses. In addition, they are the ideal method of fixation of various bone grafts, in particular, bone grafts to the lateral orbit and cantilever grafts to the nose.

Compression Plates

Dynamic compression plates producing compression at the fracture site are the ideal method of fixation for mandibular fractures. These compression plates are much stronger than miniplates to counteract the deforming forces acting on the mandible. They aim to produce primary bone healing at the fracture site. As in all plate and screw fixation, at least two screws are needed on either side of the fracture site to prevent any rotation around a single screw.

Reconstruction Plate

The reconstruction plate is a specially designed plate that is three-dimensionally bendable to mimic

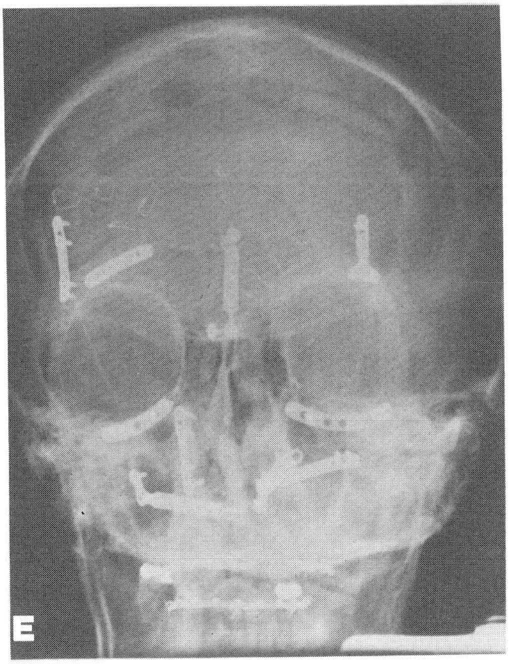

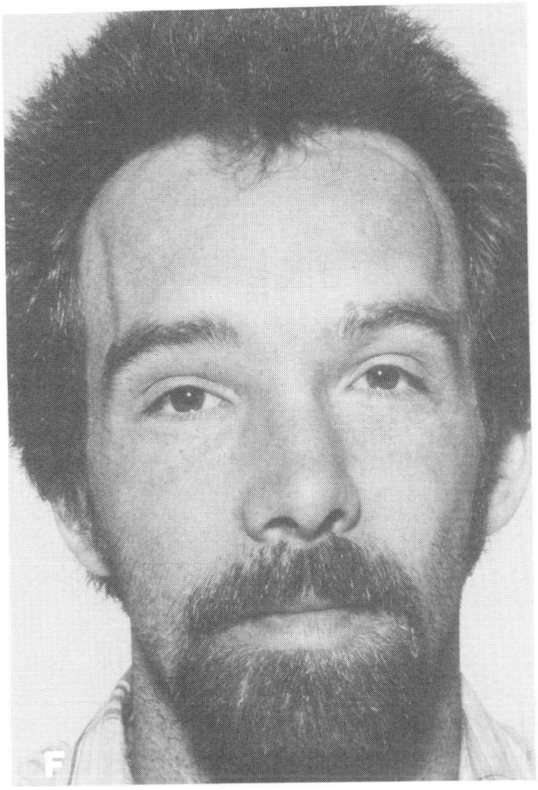

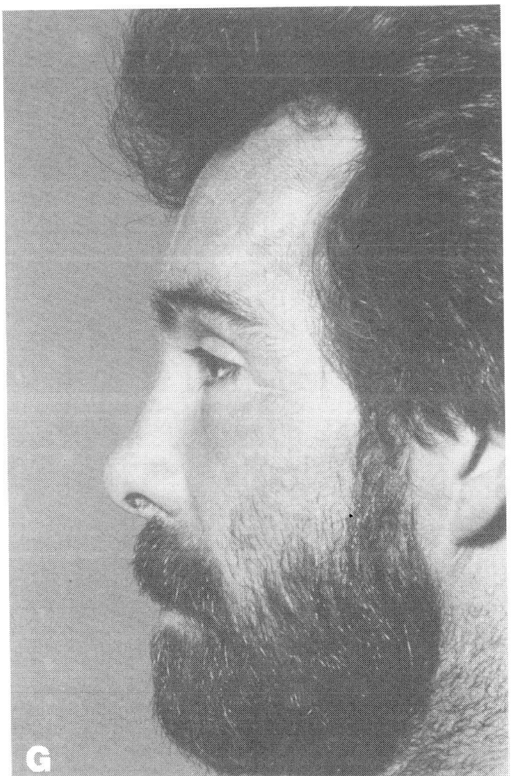

Figure 7–7 Continued. *E*, Roentgenogram demonstrates extensive fixation of multiple complex craniofacial injuries. *F*, Final result at 2½ years showing restoration of preinjury status. *G*, Lateral view shows restoration of craniofacial contour and projection.

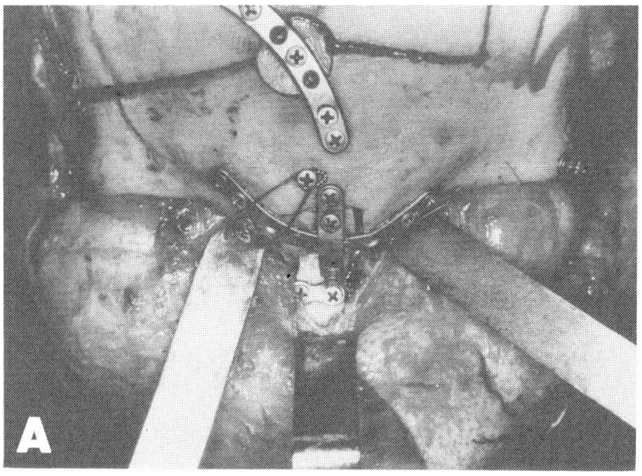

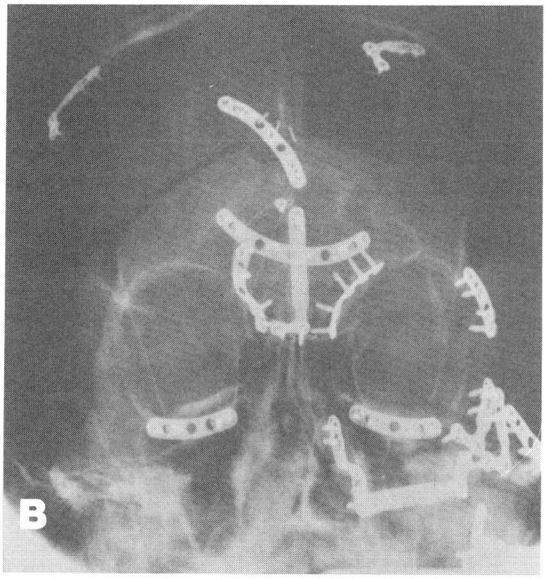

Figure 7–8 *A*, Complex craniofacial injuries showing application of miniplate and screw fixation to stabilize frontal bone flap, burr hole, and complex nasoglabellar fractures. *B*, Roentgenogram showing extensive miniplate and screw fixation of complex craniofacial injuries and nasoethmoid injuries.

exactly the intricate anatomy and shape of the mandible. Reconstruction plates are ideally suited to stabilize long segments of comminuted or segmental fractures of the mandible, or to bridge bony gaps in the mandible such as those caused by gunshot wounds. Their use is not infrequently combined with the use of miniplates, lag screws, and compression plates, all in the same patient.

Principles of Fixation

The status of the zygomatic arch is the key to the repair of complex orbitozygomatic and midfacial injuries (see Fig. 7–6). The position of the zygomatic arch between its temporal attachment posteriorly and the zygomatic body and lateral orbit anteriorly predetermines the position of the lateral and midfacial bones. A careful review of our early patients treated with extensive midfacial fixation and immediate bone grafting without zygomatic arch fixation has shown late flatness of the zygomatic bodies and midface and an obvious shortening of the zygomatic arch, both clinically and on x-ray films, in a significant number. In all complex orbitozygomatic and midfacial fractures that show a shortening or loss of projection of the zygomatic

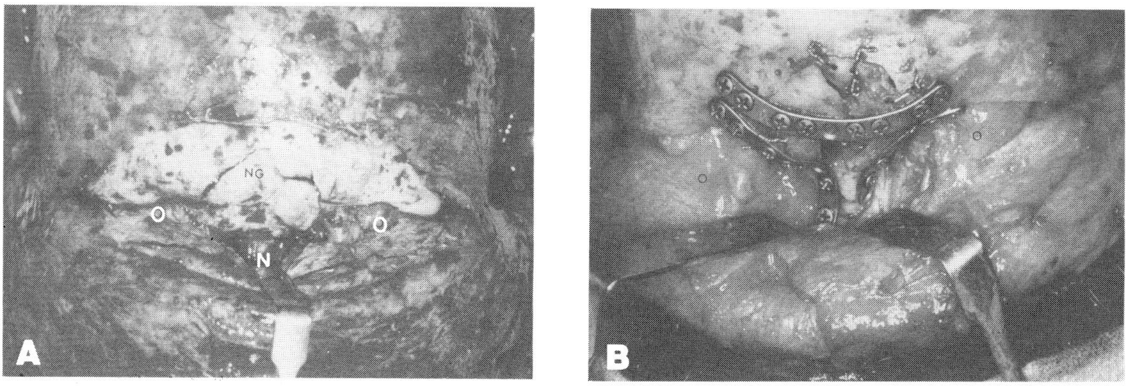

Figure 7–9 *A*, *B*, Severe craniofacial injuries involving the nasoglabellar (NG), nasoethmoid (N), and orbital (O) region. Carefully molded miniplates are used to effect reconstruction in the glabellar region combined with interosseous wiring of the anterior wall of the frontal sinus and carefully molded miniplates extending down the nasoethmoid region.

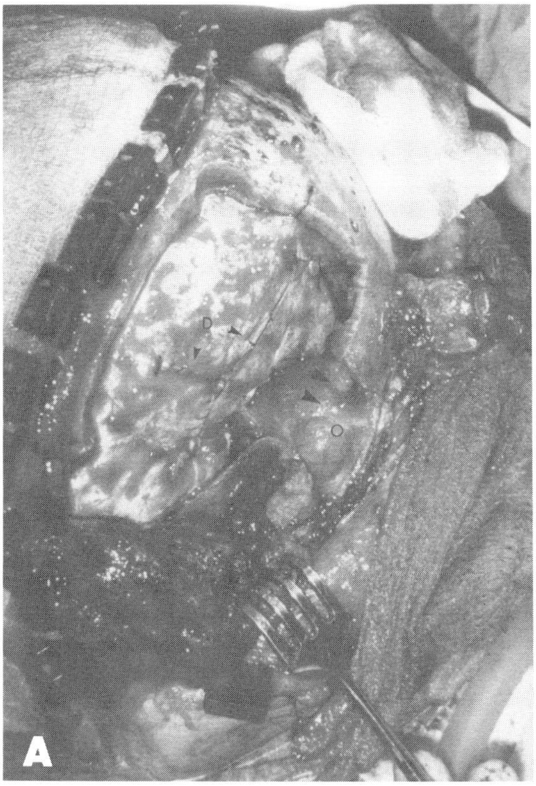

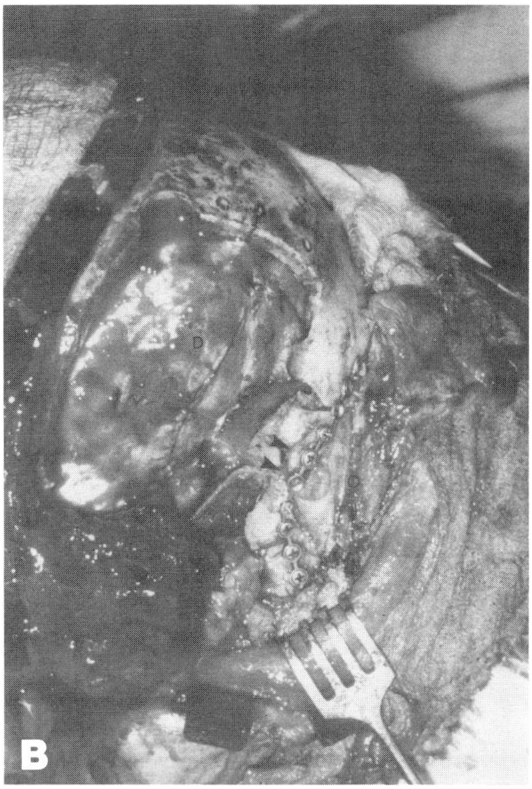

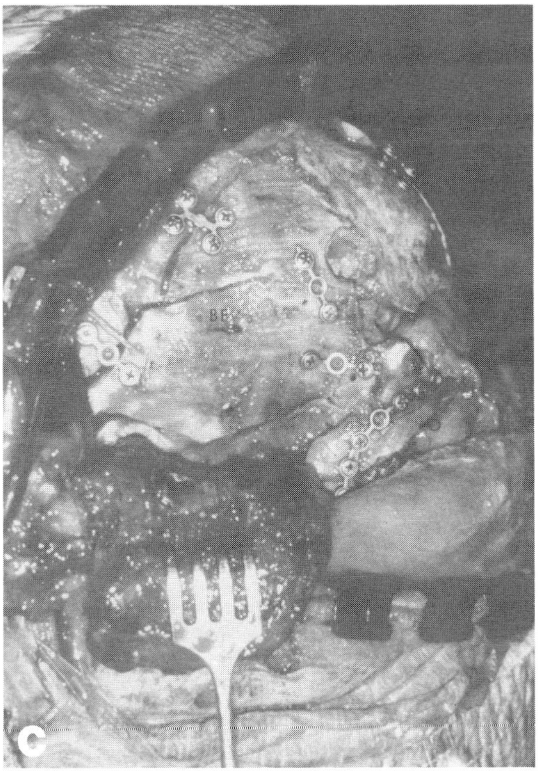

Figure 7–10 *A*, Complex cranio-orbital and facial injury following neurosurgical repair of the dural laceration (small arrows) (D). Extensive injury to the roof of the orbit can be seen with multiple comminuted fractures of the orbit. The comminuted pieces of the orbital roof have been removed to allow access to the dural repair (large arrows). Orbital contents can be seen (O). *B*, Reconstruction of the orbital rim and orbital roof is now performed using a long contoured miniplate. The orbital roof is repaired with a bone graft (large arrows) to separate the cranial cavity from the periorbital contents. *C*, The bone flap (BF) is now replaced and stabilized very rapidly with multiple miniplates.

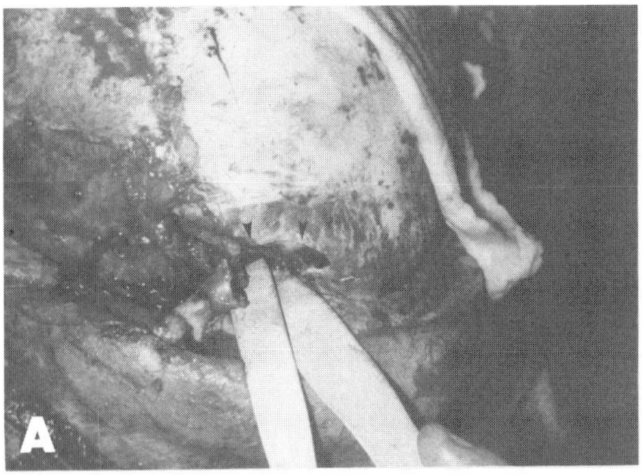

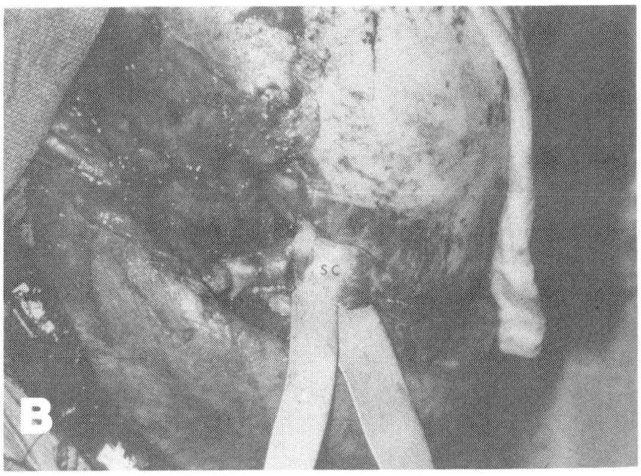

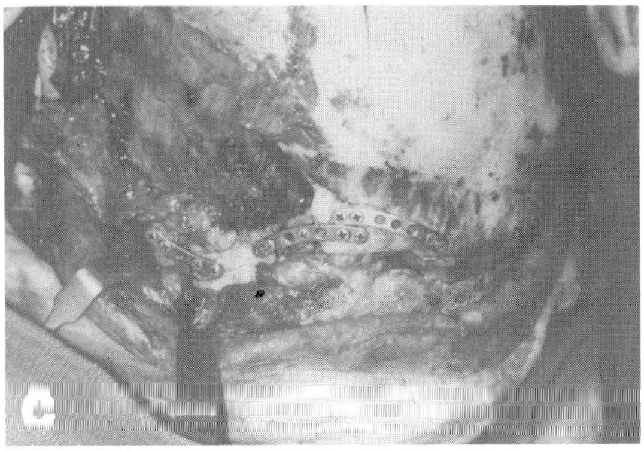

Figure 7–11 *A*, Severe cranio-orbital injury with loss of entire anterior frontal sinus and superior orbital rim and roof (arrows). *B*, Split calvarial bone graft is harvested and carefully contoured to fill in the defect in the orbital roof and anterior wall of the frontal sinus (SC). *C*, Multiple miniplates are now used to stabilize this bone graft rigidly in place, and an additional miniplate can be seen stabilizing the right zygomatic arch.

arch on axial computed tomographic (CT) scanning, it is essential first to stabilize the zygomatic arch. Careful stabilization of the zygomatic arch itself, using miniplates and lag screws in combination with miniplate fixation at the frontozygomatic suture line, will produce exact restoration of correct zygomatic body and lateral orbital wall projection in relation to the cranial base. This produces an intact outer facial frame. The inner facial frame, composed of the orbital rims, naso-orbital ethmoid, and maxillary buttresses, can now be exactly repositioned within this outer facial frame, producing an exact three-dimensional anatomic reconstruction with normal midfacial projection.

All fractures are exposed and reduced, with each fragment linked to its adjacent fragment, until all links in the chain are restored. With an intact mandibular arch, correct maxillary/mandibular occlusion is re-established first. Reduction and repair are commenced with the zygomatic arch and lateral orbit. This results in reconstruction of an outer facial frame with restoration of vertical and transverse facial height. Anterior, posterior, or horizontal facial height and projection are re-established by reduction and fixation of the inferior and medial orbits, nasoethmoid, nose, and central maxillary fractures within this previously established facial frame.

When fractures of the mandibular symphysis, or body, are present, continuity of the mandibular arch is re-established by rigid internal fixation using lag screws, compression, or reconstruction plates. It is essential in the repair of all facial fractures that involve the upper or lower dental arch to re-establish the correct occlusion prior to the application of plate or screw fixations. Failure to do this will maintain stabilized segments in their wrong position, and it is impossible to move these stabilized segments secondarily by any orthodontic means.

PRIMARY BONE GRAFTING

All severely damaged or missing bone is replaced and contour deficits are augmented, whenever feasible, by immediate bone grafting (see Fig. 7–2). Only in the presence of a heavily contaminated or infected wound, or in the absence of adequate soft-tissue cover, may the bone grafting be delayed. In certain cases, such as gunshot wounds with extensive bone and soft-tissue loss, simultaneous primary replacement of the missing soft tissue and bone can be performed with safety. In our experience, bone grafting performed at the time of the original repair always gives superior results compared with secondary bone grafting, the result of which is usually compromised by soft-tissue shrinkage and scarring.

In the majority of patients with craniofacial trauma, split calvarial bone grafts have become our primary source of graft material. However, these are difficult to use and contour in extensive orbital wall defects or if there is extensive bone loss, such as in gunshot wounds. In these situations, we combine the use of split calvarial grafts with split rib grafts, which are easier to bend and shape to large contour deficits of the orbital cavity and very large defects in the maxilla and zygomatic regions and skull.

Split skull and split rib grafts have yielded a readily available source of bone grafting material and have been associated with minimum morbidity and complications. These grafts have an exceptional ability to survive, even if portions of the graft are exposed to the air or through the mucosal lining of the nose or oral cavity, and the risk of possible graft exposure in patients with severe soft-tissue and bony injuries should not preclude their use. Bone grafts, especially in the midface and nasal area, will maintain soft-tissue expansion and projection, even if the segments become exposed. In this situation, they act as an internal splinting mechanism, maintaining the normal stretch and position of the soft tissue during soft-tissue healing and scar maturation. Bone grafts used to reconstruct the anterior wall of the frontal sinus, medial wall, and floor of the orbit and anterior wall of the maxilla survive adequately even though they are placed over an open cavity with healthy soft-tissue coverage on one side only. The failure to use bone grafts will result in rapid shrinkage of soft tissue and make subsequent reconstructive efforts difficult and often inadequate.

Adequate fixation of bone grafts is essential because inadequate fixation predisposes to infection or resorption. Bone grafts are stabilized, whenever possible, using lag screws or miniplates. The addition of lag screw fixation to bone grafts has contributed greatly to the stability of midfacial reconstruction. Bone grafts, either calvarial or rib, that are stabilized with lag screws undergo minimal resorption. Bone grafts used to reconstruct the orbital cavity require no form of fixation and are merely wedged into place and held there by the orbital contents.

SPECIFIC ASPECTS OF INTERNAL FIXATION

Orbitozygomatic Fractures

Injuries to the midface may result in fractures of the orbitozygomatic complex. These fractures may be isolated or may be combined with other midfacial injuries. Orbitozygomatic fractures are wrongly termed tripod fractures and should always be considered as quadrapod fractures, since the fourth site of fracture—or the zygomaticomaxillary buttresses—is one of the keys to the understanding and management of unstable zygomatic fractures. This lateral buttress acts as a direct antagonist to the pull of the masseter muscle and forms the structural support to the zygoma itself. Fractures of this buttress will allow the zygomatic body to tilt downward and inward, resulting in late depression of the zygomatic prominence. Two-point fixation of the frontozygomatic suture line and inferior orbital rim will not prevent downward rotation of the zygomatic body. Direct exposure by means of an upper buccal sulcus incision of this buttress and direct anatomic reconstruction with miniplates or bone grafts will prevent this complication. When fracturing involves the zygomatic arch and results in loss of anteroposterior projection of the zygoma, it is essential to stabilize the zygomatic arch as well. Miniplates are used to stabilize the frontozygomatic suture line, zygomatic arch, and zygomaticomaxillary buttress. The final point of fixation to the inferior orbital rim can be stabilized using a miniplate or interosseous wire. In many cases, an interosseous wire is preferable, since a miniplate may be felt through the thin eyelid skin. Inadequate treatment of orbitozygomatic fractures is the most common cause of secondary deformity following facial fractures. Coexisting orbital wall fractures should always be suspected, particularly in the medial, inferomedial, and lateral walls. These deficits should be carefully outlined and totally reconstructed with immediate bone grafting to prevent the late occurrence of enophthalmos and oculo-orbital displacement.

Nasoethmoid Orbital Fractures

A direct blow to the midface may result in fractures of the bony nasoethmoid orbital complex and injury to the adjacent soft tissues.[3] These injuries may be confined to the nasoethmoid orbital complex but, more frequently, are associated with other facial fractures and are often complicated by multisystem trauma. The injuries result in severe cosmetic and functional deformity due to collapse of the nose, ethmoids, and medial orbits and are accentuated by coexisting injury to the medial canthal ligaments and nasolacrimal apparatus. Extension into the anterior cranial fossa with concomitant dural tear, cerebrospinal fluid rhinorrhea, and cerebral injury may be life threatening.

Nasoethmoid orbital fractures are the most challenging of all craniofacial fractures to treat because of the intricate anatomy of this region and the difficulty in fracture fixation. Inadequate initial treatment will often result in severe deformity which may be extremely difficult, or impossible, to correct adequately. Optimal management involves early surgical exploration and meticulous bony and soft-tissue repair using the principles learned from reconstructive craniofacial surgery. It is essential to understand that the nasal bones, vomerine bone, perpendicular plate of the ethmoid, and ethmoid labyrinth are thin and predisposed to comminuted fractures. Conversely, the nasal process of the frontal bone and frontal process of the maxilla are strong and comminution is rare. The medial wall of the orbit, however, is extremely thin and invariably comminutes. Telecanthus is nearly always produced by the splaying apart of the nasomaxillary buttress which is displaced laterally and downward, taking the medial canthal ligament with it. It is extremely rare for the ligament to be actually lacerated or avulsed from the bone. Correct anatomic repair of the nasomaxillary buttress will allow restoration of a correct intercanthal distance. Attempts at holding this segment in place using multiple interosseous wires have rarely been successful in our experience. The stabilization of this segment using miniplates, both above—attaching the miniplate to the region of the frontal bone and frontal sinus—and below—attaching it to the infraorbital rim, results in a three-dimensionally stable reconstruction and restoration of a correct intercanthal distance. The miniplate can be placed adjacent to the canthal ligament itself, which should be isolated in all cases during medial rim and orbital wall dissection. It is essential not to strip the ligament off the bone during this dissection as it will then have to be rewired to the nasal bone. A transnasal canthopexy, in our experience, rarely gives a perfectly natural appearing medial canthal region. When there is loss of distal nasal support, a cantilever bone graft should be used to restore nasal projection and prevent soft-tissue shrinkage. A split calvarial bone graft is preferred and this is cantilevered by means of a miniplate and fixed to the anterior portion of the frontal bone. By adjusting the angle of the bend in the miniplate, the degree of cantilevering can be varied. Split calvarial grafts, rigidly fixed and cantilevered in this fashion, rarely undergo resorption and produce an excellent long-term nasal reconstruction.

Maxillary Fractures

The paired nasomaxillary, zygomaticomaxillary, and pterygomaxillary buttresses maintain the position of the maxilla in relation to the cranial base above and the mandible below.[4] Exact anatomic reconstruction of the four anterior buttresses, namely the nasomaxillary and zygomaticomaxillary buttresses, will allow exact repositioning of the maxilla in its correct anteroposterior position in relation to the cranial base and allow reconstruction of the exact vertical height and horizontal projection of the maxilla. No reconstruction is needed of the posterior buttress, as the four anterior buttresses will maintain correct position of the maxilla. The intact mandible provides an additional buttress in relation to the cranial base, and the re-establishment of normal maxillary/mandibular occlusion will provide additional support to the reconstructed maxilla.

The anterior maxillary buttresses are exposed through an upper gingival buccal sulcus degloving incision. All unstable buttresses are repaired using miniplates, and missing buttresses are replaced with bone grafts fixed in place with lag screws. When the fractures crossing the buttresses are low and situated close to the tooth-bearing bone, care must be taken not to place screws through the tooth apices. In this situation, it may be necessary to use small bone grafts to reinforce the buttress repair, as the lag screws can be placed exactly between the tooth apices.

Complex Mandibular Fractures

Internal fixation of mandibular fractures using compression plating, lag screws, and reconstruction plates has revolutionized the care of the complex mandibular injury.[7] These techniques are particularly useful in the care of the polytraumatized patient with associated head injuries, cervical spine fracture, and when there are other facial fractures present as well. In addition, they facilitate stabilization in the comminuted or segmental fracture or the mandibular fracture with bone loss.

Airway management is facilitated by the use of rigid internal fixation techniques using plates and screws. In midfacial or mandibular injuries in the multiple trauma patient, or combined injuries of the midface and mandible, the orotracheal tube can be pushed to the side, allowing temporary intermaxillary fixation to establish the correct occlusion. Following rigid internal fixation of the mandible and midface with plates and screws in combination with immediate bone grafting where necessary, the intermaxillary fixation can often be released. This allows endotracheal intubation to be maintained postoperatively until a patent airway is assured. Tracheostomy is needed only in the patient with bilateral condylar neck fractures in whom the position of the mandible has to be maintained in relation to the maxilla. The ability to repair multiple facial fractures without the need for intermaxillary fixation has revolutionized the care of the multiple trauma patient. This allows early fixation of the facial fractures and facilitates airway management in the early postoperative phase without the need for tracheostomy in the majority of patients.

Gunshot Wounds

Gunshot wounds of the face are often formidable wounds that offer a great challenge to the reconstructive surgeon. Frequently there is both bony and soft-tissue loss and the bony loss is usually more severe. This may be further complicated by concomitant injuries to the oral cavity, nasal passages, orbits, cranial cavity, and their contents. Lessons and techniques learned in the management of complex facial trauma using craniofacial surgical techniques, immediate bone grafting, and rigid internal fixation using plates and screws in the midface and mandible can be successfully applied to the management of severe gunshot wounds of the face. Extensive bone loss is replaced using rib and cranial grafts stabilized with lag screws and miniplates. The use of extensive miniplate and lag screw fixation in the midface and large reconstruction plates in the mandible to bridge bone gaps facilitates stabilization and reconstruction in these areas in combination with the bone grafts. Soft-tissue repair can be by means of various local or regional flaps or, in massive soft-tissue loss, by means of a free vascularized omental flap that can be wrapped around the bone grafts. Total nasal reconstruction, using tissue-expanded forehead skin, is an ideal method for nasal reconstruction once initial midfacial reconstruction projection has been obtained.

Combined Injuries of the Cranium and Face: Panfacial Fractures

High-velocity accidents may cause profound injury to the bones of the skull and face. These injuries, craniofacial in the true sense of the word, are a challenge to even the most energetic and well-trained reconstructive surgeon (see Figs. 7–3, 7–4, 7–5, 7–7, 7–10, 7–11 and Fig. 7–12).

The number of patients surviving the initial insult of complex trauma has increased.[8] As a result, surgeons are now often called upon to treat a patient with combined injuries of the cranium and face.[9–25] This requires a synthesis of neurosurgical techniques and techniques derived from reconstructive craniofacial surgery that have been successfully applied to the treatment of complex facial injuries. The management of a concomitant frontal sinus injury is still controversial but remains a key element in the treatment of these injuries.

PATHOGENESIS AND CLASSIFICATION OF FRACTURES

The frontal, ethmoid, and sphenoid bones form a major complex at the junction of the midfacial skeleton and the cranial base. The involvement of this complex and the adjacent buttresses of the facial skeleton establishes the pattern of craniofacial injury.[14,15,17,24] Combined injuries of the cranium and face may be isolated to the cranio-orbital and ethmoid region or extend to involve the midface and mandible.

Central Craniofacial Fractures

Force directed over the frontonasal region creates a central fracture (see Figs. 7–3, 7–4, 7–7, 7–8). The fracture lines involve the frontonasomaxillary and, perhaps, the frontoethmoidal vomerine buttresses, then extend to enter the frontal sinus and ethmoid complex. These fractures involve nasal, vomer, maxillary, ethmoid, and frontal bones. The infraorbital rim is often interrupted and the medial wall of the orbit may be severely comminuted. If the frontal sinus is large, it may absorb a large proportion of the force and the posterior wall may remain intact without exposure of the dura, even when there is severe comminution of the anterior wall. If the sinus is small, fractures may occur in the posterior table. The dura may be intact with

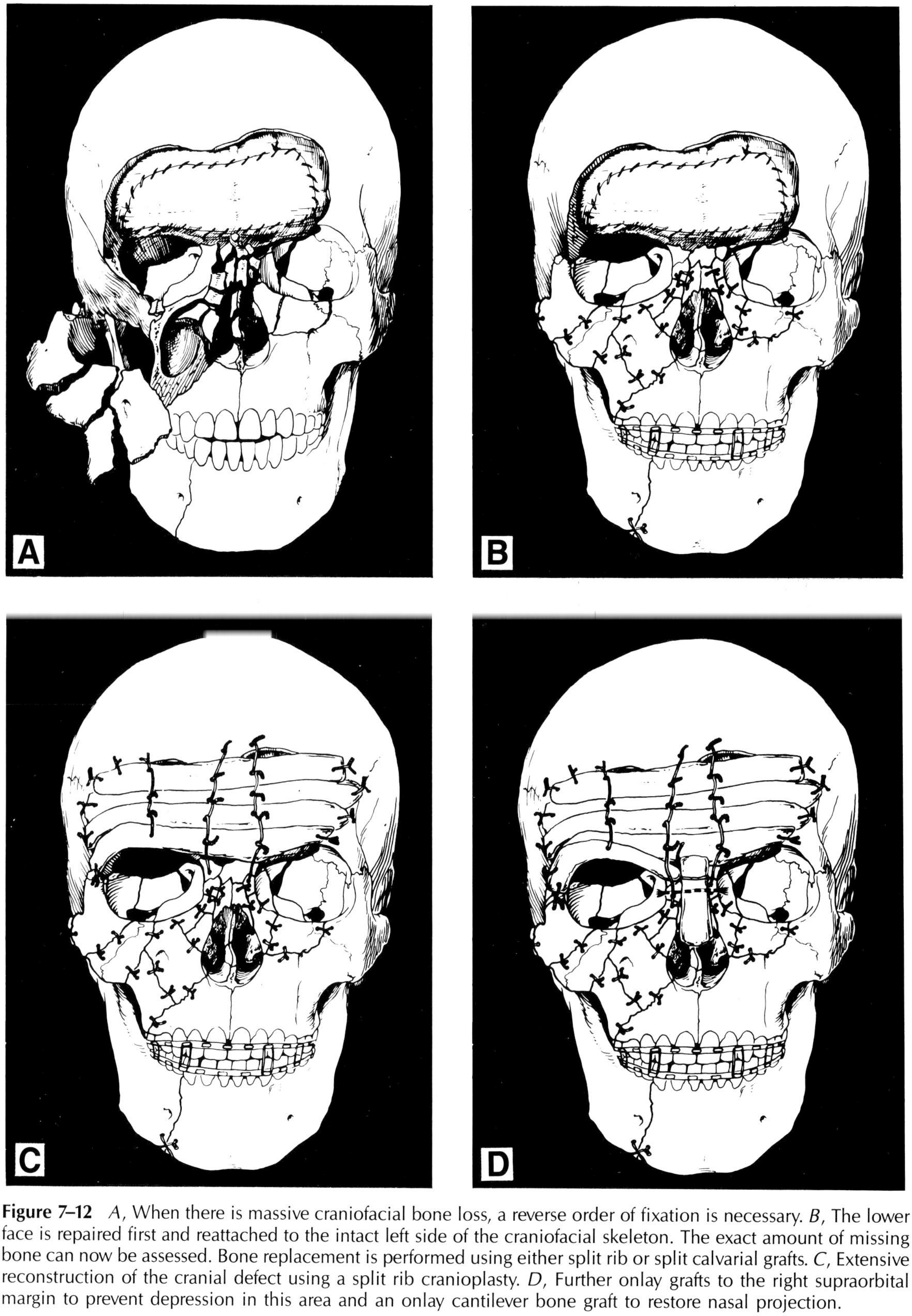

Figure 7–12 *A*, When there is massive craniofacial bone loss, a reverse order of fixation is necessary. *B*, The lower face is repaired first and reattached to the intact left side of the craniofacial skeleton. The exact amount of missing bone can now be assessed. Bone replacement is performed using either split rib or split calvarial grafts. *C*, Extensive reconstruction of the cranial defect using a split rib cranioplasty. *D*, Further onlay grafts to the right supraorbital margin to prevent depression in this area and an onlay cantilever bone graft to restore nasal projection.

small linear cracks in the posterior wall, but with more significant disruption, the dura is commonly injured, resulting in a cerebrospinal fluid leak. If the sinus is rudimentary or the fractures occur outside the sinus, large linear or segmental fractures occur with involvement of the superior orbital rim and orbital roof. These fractures are often impacted and difficult to reduce, even with extended open reduction techniques.

Lateral Craniofacial Fractures

Force applied to the frontozygomatic area initiates fractures in the lateral face and cranium (Figs. 7–10, 7–12). The fracture lines cross the frontozygomaticomaxillary buttress[22] and extend to involve the greater wing of the sphenoid. Fractures of this type commonly involve maxillary, zygomatic, frontal, and sphenoid bones. An ipsilateral Le Fort III pattern is often present in association with a contralateral Le Fort II fracture. In some cases, the adjacent parietal and temporal bones are also involved.

The supraorbital margin is frequently damaged and there may be extension into the lateral aspect of the frontal sinus. The lateral orbital wall and the orbital floor are outwardly displaced, causing orbital dystopia and enophthalmos. In some cases, the lateral orbital wall is severely comminuted. Orbital fat is then displaced into the temporal fossa.

Combined Central and Lateral Fractures

With marked force, fractures involving both the central and lateral skull and face may be produced. Profound instability and dislocation are present. These injuries have a high probability of extension into the anterior, middle, or, rarely, posterior fossa.

EARLY APPROACHES TO REPAIR

Following World War II, combined injuries of the cranium and face were treated differently than they are today. The surgical repair was primarily (and sometimes singularly) directed toward the management of the central nervous system. Clotted peridural blood was evacuated, brain and dura were débrided, and depressed cranial bone was elevated.

The repair of the facial fractures was deferred to a second operation, particularly when the patient was comatose. A limited amount of periosteum was elevated for fear of interrupting the blood supply to the craniofacial bones. Comminuted segments, particularly those of frontal bone, were discarded. Great pains were taken to remove the mucosal lining of the frontal sinus and methods were developed to obliterate the sinus and nasofrontal duct.

Bone grafting was seldom considered and defects in forehead contour were repaired at secondary and tertiary procedures. Foreign substances, such as methylmethacrylate, were often used in the reconstruction of the frontal bone.

CURRENT PRINCIPLES OF MANAGEMENT

Once life support systems have been established and the initial general examination has been completed, attention is directed to the identification and management of the craniofacial injury.

Clinical Examination

The hallmarks of craniofacial fractures are instability and deformation. Marked mobility of the fracture sites is thus a major clue to the presence of a craniofacial injury. The severity of the bony injury in the cranio-orbital region may be underestimated in the presence of marked soft-tissue swelling and ecchymosis and this may lead to inadequate or incorrect treatment and result in secondary deformity. Lacerations, particularly over the frontonasal ethmoid, may communicate directly with the intracranial cavity (Fig. 7–13).

The characteristic instability and deformation reflect the severe dislocation of the fractured segments over a broad area. Centrally, the naso-orbital-ethmoid infrastructure is comminuted. Nasal projection is lost and traumatic telecanthus is present. A similar loss of contour is often palpable in the frontal region. The orbital and zygomatic regions are flattened, accompanied by protrusion of the globe of the eye, due to migration of the greater wing of the sphenoid and blow-in fracture of the orbital roof. More laterally, a step-off along the supraorbital ridge may be noted.

Radiographic Studies

High-resolution CT became available in approximately 1980 (Fig. 7–14). The higher resolution offers greater detail than conventional CT scanning techniques. By choosing a wide or narrow "window," the computer may be programmed for bone or soft tissue, respectively.[26] The higher mode of imaging is able to disclose what would otherwise be occult fractures. Recently, three-dimensional tomography has been used to facilitate diagnosis and treatment planning.

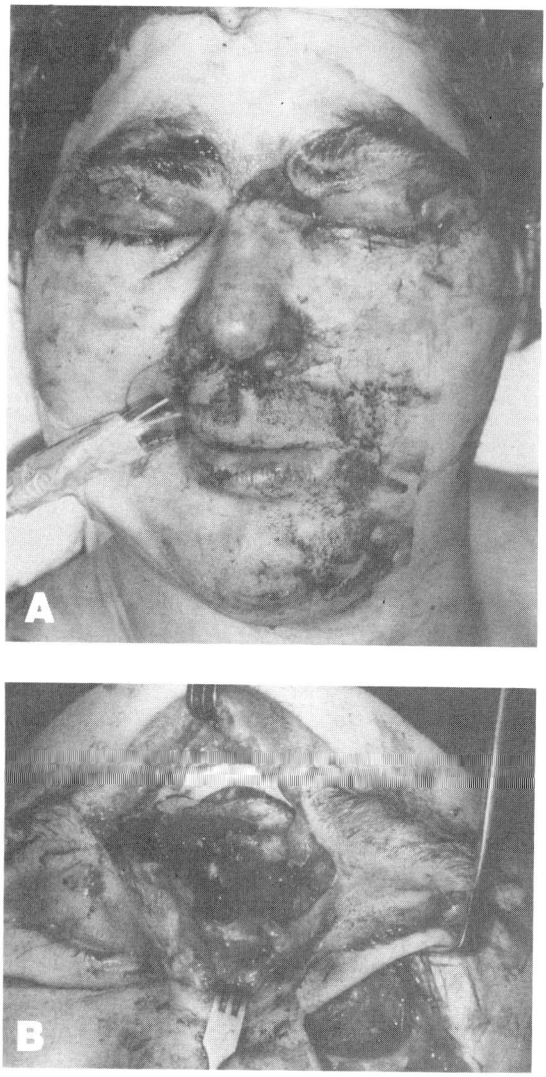

Figure 7–13 *A*, Young man with severe craniofacial injuries that may be underestimated on initial examination owing to marked panfacial edema. *B*, Same patient but with lacerations explored; notice the massive penetrating fractures through the anterior wall of the frontal sinus and cranium directly into the cranial cavity. It is essential to examine these patients very carefully, as small skin lacerations may communicate directly with the cranial cavity.

Surgical Techniques

In our current approach, the patient with craniofacial injuries ideally undergoes treatment within 12 to 48 hours. When possible, the maxillofacial and craniofacial repairs are accomplished at the time of neurosurgical exploration.

General health statistics (trauma scores), age, and the absence of neurologic deficits are used to select patients able to tolerate surgical intervention, even in the presence of coma. Steroid, barbiturate, hyperventilation, and the use of intracranial pressure monitors provide controls.

The neurosurgical procedures are accomplished. Then the fractures of the skull and facial skeleton are reduced. Using sharp instruments, the periosteum is elevated widely.[11] Broad expanses of bone are exposed and the actual fracture pattern assessed by direct inspection. Only then is the final surgical plan formulated. The fragments of bone are wired together[1,27] or stabilized using plates and screws.[5,6,28] Bone, including the anterior table of the frontal sinus, is preserved for use in this subsequent repair.

Primary bone grafting offers the means to repair comminuted areas or osseous deficits in the face or cranium, based on techniques learned from experience in congenital craniofacial surgery.[2,3,4,5,29] Split skull and, occasionally, split rib grafts are used to accomplish the reconstruction in most patients. Splitting the intact skull provides bone for small to medium-sized defects. Splitting the neurosurgical bone flap provides a larger source of cranial bone. Split rib grafts, in combination with split skull, may be needed for reconstruction of extensive and multiple craniofacial defects.

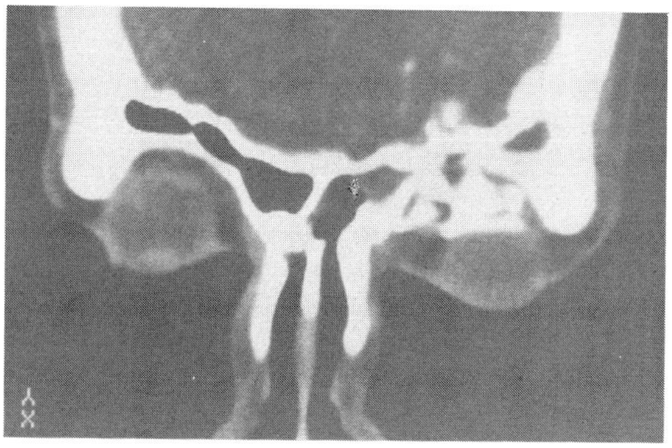

Figure 7–14 Coronal computed tomographic scan of panfacial injury with severe blow-in fracture of orbit showing orbital roof markedly displaced into orbit causing downward shift of ocular globe.

Repair of Frontal Sinus

The management of frontal sinus fractures (see Fig. 7–7) depends on the type of fracture (site and displacement), whether the fracture is open or closed, and the presence or absence of a cerebrospinal fluid leak. Closed, undisplaced fractures of the anterior wall are observed. Open or depressed fractures are explored through a bicoronal incision. Foreign bodies and mucosal shreds are meticulously removed. Copious irrigation is used. The anterior wall is reconstructed. No attempt is made to occlude or drain the nasofrontal duct. Coexisting linear undisplaced fractures of the posterior wall without cerebrospinal fluid leak are left and only the anterior wall is reconstructed. Displaced and comminuted fractures of the posterior wall are usually associated with dural injury. The posterior wall is removed to facilitate access for neurosurgical dural repair. Only the anterior wall is subsequently reconstructed.

With concomitant injury to the floor, the potential for blockage of the nasofrontal duct and subsequent mucocele formation is accentuated. In addition, severe injuries to the floor with comminution and bone loss result in direct communication between the nasal cavity and frontal sinus and with the intracranial cavity when the posterior wall is injured. It is essential to separate the nasal cavity from the frontal sinus and intracranial cavity to minimize the risk of ascending infection. Separation can be accomplished by bone grafting, vascularized soft-tissue flaps, or, preferably, a combination of both.

Our current technique is to place split calvarial grafts, calvarial bone paste and chips, or iliac cancellous bone along the injured floor. Separate plugs of bone can be inserted into the nasofrontal ducts. The posterior wall is removed to "cranialize" the sinus. A vascularized soft-tissue flap of pericranium or, preferably, a galeal frontalis flap is tunnelled into the sinus and sutured to the dura posteriorly to provide a vascularized curtain between the nasal and intracranial cavities.

Sequence of Repair

A sequential approach is often necessary in the presence of craniofacial trauma. The extent of injury, suggested by clinical examination and x-ray studies, is confirmed by wide periosteal elevation and the exposure of all fractured segments. The repair is completed using the following sequence.[2, 24]

1. If there is no loss of cranial bone, first stabilize the cranial vault with rigid interosseous and miniplate fixation. The facial complex is now reattached to the reconstituted cranial vault (see Fig. 7–6).
2. When portions of cranial bone are missing or when massive cranial comminution is present, a reverse order of fixation is employed. First, the midface and mandible are repaired. The reconstituted facial complex is then reattached to the residual cranial vault. The amount of missing frontal, ethmoid, and sphenoid bone can then be assessed. Split rib or split cranial grafts are used to reconstruct the cranial vault (see Fig. 7–12).
3. With associated maxillary, mandibular, or combined maxillary and mandibular fractures, the normal occlusion is first established. Maxillary and mandibular fractures are repaired whenever possible with rigid internal fixation using plates and screws.[4–6] Following completion of craniofacial repair the intermaxillary fixation can be released, thus facilitating airway management with endotracheal intubation in the patient with a head injury, cervical spine fracture, or multiple trauma. Tracheostomy is needed only following prolonged intubation, coma, or other injuries and with associated bilateral condylar neck fractures not amenable to open reduction where the intermaxillary fixation has to be retained. External fixation devices are almost never needed.

DISCUSSION

The techniques used in the repair of combined fractures of the cranium and face should follow, in our opinion, the basic principles of craniofacial surgery used in the repair of congenital deformities.[11,29,30] The repair is a combined procedure involving the neurosurgeon and the reconstructive surgeon. First, the dura is repaired, isolating the cranial contents.[15,31] Then the craniofacial fractures are repaired. The periosteum is widely elevated, despite initial fears by some authors that extensive elevation of the periosteum might cause facial bone necrosis.[14,32] Rigid fixation and the grafting of missing segments are accomplished. Interfragment wiring or plating avoids the use of craniofacial suspension wiring in midfacial fractures which, in our experience, is prone to initiate midfacial compression and shortening of the face.

The mucosa of the frontal sinus is cuboidal, unlike the respiratory epithelium in the nasal cavity.

When the frontonasal duct is obstructed and mucosa is entrapped by fractures of the frontal sinus, chronic infection, or other causes, sinus mucosa tends to develop cysts or true mucoceles. By an unknown mechanism, perhaps by pressure or by the elaboration of an osteolytic enzyme, the mucocele erodes adjacent bone to enter the orbit or the intracranial cavity. If the mucoid contents of the cyst become infected, a mucopyocele results. The mucopyocele, in some instances, leads to orbital or cranial abscess formation, osteomyelitis of the craniofacial bones, or meningitis.

To avoid the implicit hazards of mucocele formation, a number of authors have recommended nasofrontal duct and frontal sinus ablation, or obliteration, in patients with fractures of the frontal sinus.[33–37] This is surprising (in our view), since the indications for obliteration of the sinus using abdominal fat have been rather clearly defined in patients with recurrent infection but not established in those with acute craniofacial trauma.

The studies to date have described experience in a small number of trauma patients, without the benefit of double-blind controls. The most often quoted report is that of Newman and Travis,[13] who described their experience with 63 patients between [illegible] and [illegible]. Operative intervention ([illegible] patients) was delayed for more than 48 hours during a period of observation and antibiotic administration. Newman and Travis favor fat obliteration in patients with fractures of the floor or anterior table. In patients with fractures of the posterior table, they prefer to avoid filling the sinus with fat, citing the risk of placing devascularized fat adjacent to a potentially unsealed cranial vault. In patients with posterior table fractures, the sinus was ablated by removing the anterior table. The overlying soft tissue was allowed to adhere to dura. Reconstruction of the collapsed forehead was deferred to a second operation. The danger of using fat in the frontal sinus in the presence of comminuted or missing sinus walls has recently been emphasized in an animal experiment. In two large series of mucocele,[38,39] trauma played a causative role in only 4 percent and 6 percent of the patients, and primary exploration of the injured sinus was not performed in any patient. May and associates[40] reported four cases of late infection following trauma, but none had been explored primarily. Donald and Bernstein,[41] following the lead of Nadell and Kline[15] and citing two cases, recommend plugging the nasofrontal ducts with temporalis muscle, removal of the posterior wall (cranialization), and repair of the anterior wall.

Dingman and Dickinson in unpublished series, and Schultz[42] chose not to obliterate the sinus nor the nasofrontal ducts in acute trauma cases. The anterior and posterior plates are preserved. The sinus cavity is maintained with the expectation that the nasofrontal duct will continue to function. Reconstruction of the nasofrontal duct and/or obliterative surgery are confined to patients who, at a later date, demonstrate obstruction of the nasofrontal duct. Beziat and colleagues[43] appear to have comparable recommendations.

Our experience is similar to that of the latter group. When bone is securely reduced and grafts are rigidly applied, when dura is repaired and the cranial contents are isolated, and when nondelayed débridement is accomplished, the chance of mucopyocele is minimal. Our long-term follow-up does not exceed 10 years and our study is not highlighted by double-blind controls. Nevertheless, the premise that the nasofrontal duct will resume function in a majority of patients appears to be legitimate. Early intervention and reconstruction are hallmarks of our approach. The presence of improperly reduced bone segments, comminuted sequestra, foreign bodies, and torn mucosal shreds leaves the patient susceptible to the development of mucopyocele, infection, and other complications. Diagnosis and treatment of injury to the floor of the frontal sinus by separating the frontal sinus from the nasal cavity with bone grafts and vascularized soft-tissue flaps, sealing off the frontal nasal duct with bone grafts, and "cranializing" the sinus seem to be the keys to the prevention of long-term complications.

Technical Problems and Pitfalls

In our experience in treating these complex cases, certain technical problems and potential pitfalls have surfaced.

1. Inadequate reconstruction of the supraorbital ridge commonly leads to flatness in this region. The use of a full-thickness rib graft or stacking of bone grafts in layers will prevent this (see Fig. 7–12D).[2, 27]
2. Injury to the orbital roof may result in isolated fractures, comminuted fractures, or areas of bony destruction or loss. Concomitant loss of the posterior wall of the frontal sinus results in direct communication between the anterior cranial fossa and orbit. The orbital roof should always be reconstructed in this situation to separate the two cavities. When the posterior

wall of the frontal sinus is intact, it is not necessary to reconstruct small defects of the orbital roof; however, failure to reconstruct larger defects may lead to herniation and entrapment of orbital contents and possible enophthalmos and diplopia (see Fig. 7–10 and Fig. 7–15).

3. When a total loss of the supraorbital rim is reconstituted with bone grafts, it is difficult to obtain perfect symmetry with the uninvolved orbit. Exophthalmos and downward displacement of the ocular globe may occur if excess bone is inadvertently used, especially when concomitant reconstruction of the orbital roof has been performed. Care must be taken to contour the supraorbital rim and roof correctly and prevent overcorrection of the deformity (see Fig. 7–15).
4. True orbital dystopia[11] may be difficult to recognize clinically when associated with combined injuries of the cranio-orbital region, midface, and orbitozygomatic complex, particularly when there is severe soft-tissue and bony injury. Failure to recognize this and correct it adequately at the time of the initial reconstruction will result in an established orbital dystopia that may be extremely difficult to correct with secondary surgery (see Fig. 7–17). The key to the re-establishment of the orbital position is the adequate exposure and reconstruction of the zygomatic arch and lateral orbital rim and wall. This produces an intact outer facial frame with the correct facial projection and width. The inner facial frame composed of orbital rims and nasoethmoid region can be reconstructed within this outer frame, resulting in exact repositioning of the displaced orbit (Fig. 7–16).
5. Severe injuries in the nasoglabellar region may result in significant bony destruction or loss of the glabellar and/or nasal bones. Glabellar loss is reconstructed with bone grafts and the nasal

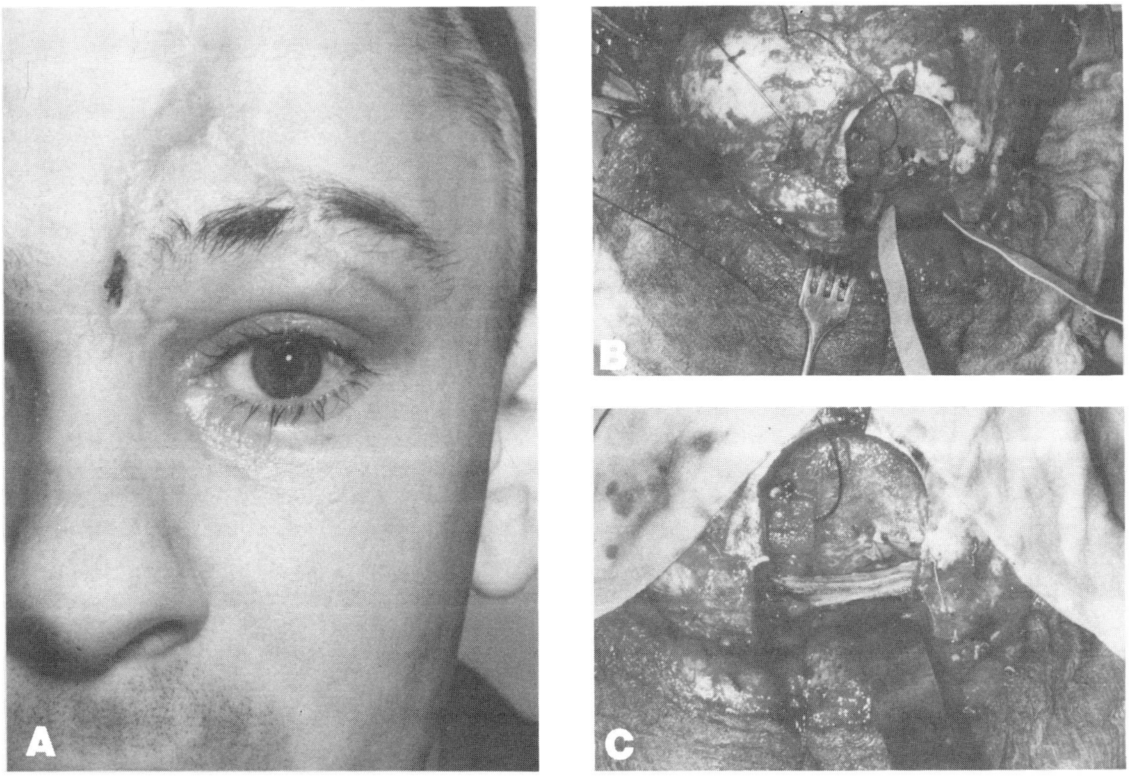

Figure 7–15 *A*, Complex contaminated cranio-orbital injury 8 days following initial débridement of this heavily contaminated penetrating wound into the anterior cranial fossa. *B*, Extensive cranio-orbital deformity with exposure of the orbital contents (O). Direct communication between the cranial cavity and the orbit can be seen through the disrupted orbital roof (arrow). In this situation, it is essential to reconstruct the orbital roof to prevent downward herniation of the dura and direct communication with the periorbita, which may result in a pulsatile exophthalmos. *C*, Reconstruction of the orbital roof with split rib grafts. Inadequate contouring of the split rib grafts can be seen.

Figure continues on the following page

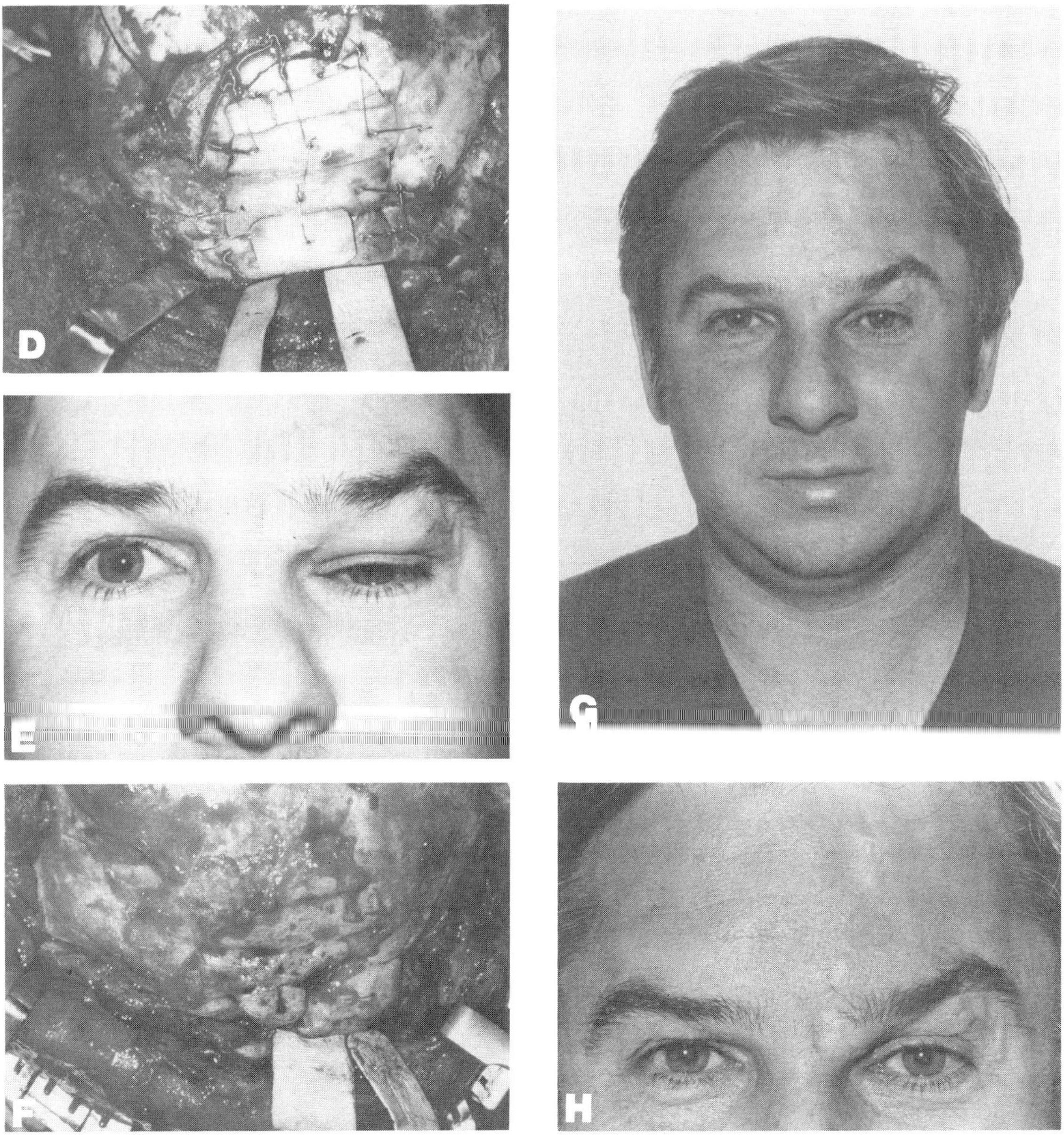

Figure 7–15 Continued. *D*, Completion of the cranial repair using a split rib cranioplasty. *E*, Failure to contour the orbital roof adequately has resulted in a downward displacement of the ocular globe and periorbital contents, producing a vertical ocular dystopia and proptosis. *F*, Secondary exploration of the orbit reveals a perfectly healed cranioplasty but with too much bone in the orbital roof as well as the superior orbital rim. *G*, Following careful contouring of the superior orbital margin and orbit roof, better position of the globe is attained. *H*, Close-up of final orbital reconstruction stresses the importance of the contouring of the orbital roof reconstruction.

bone is then reattached to this rebuilt bony base. When glabellar loss is combined with loss of the nasal bones, glabellar reconstruction is combined with immediate bone graft reconstruction of the nose. The nasal bone graft is attached to the glabellar graft and cantilevered as necessary (see Fig. 7–12).

6. The frontocranial region is under the influence of minimal muscular forces, and thus meticulous interosseous wire fixation can

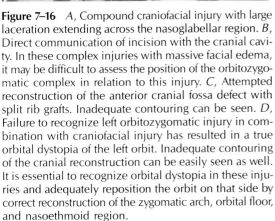

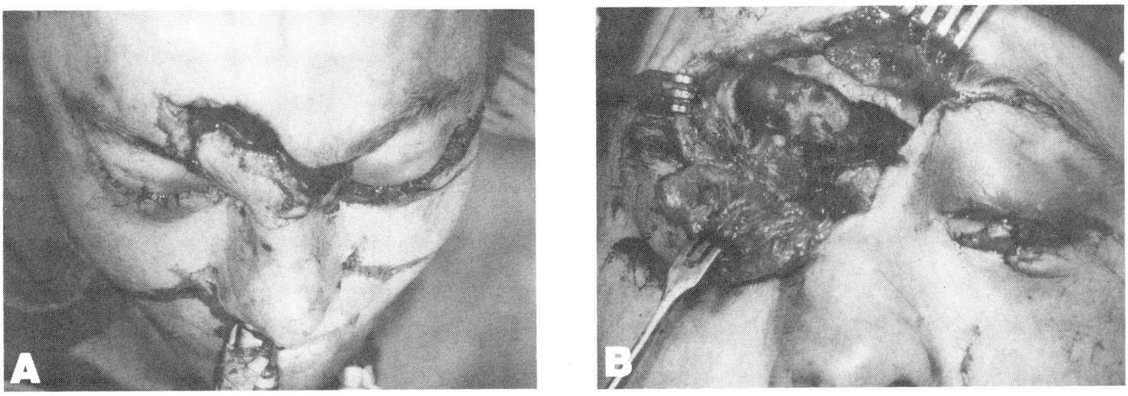

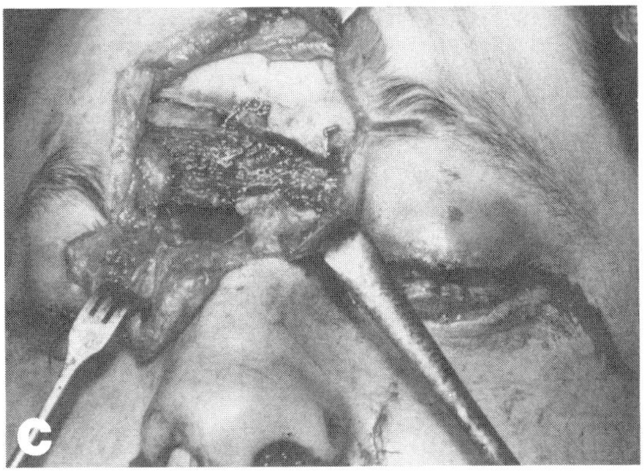

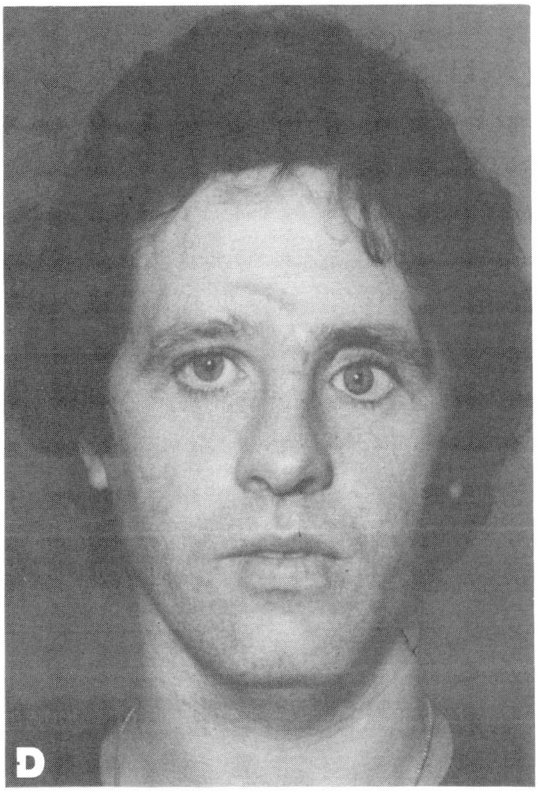

Figure 7–16 *A*, Compound craniofacial injury with large laceration extending across the nasoglabellar region. *B*, Direct communication of incision with the cranial cavity. In these complex injuries with massive facial edema, it may be difficult to assess the position of the orbitozygomatic complex in relation to this injury. *C*, Attempted reconstruction of the anterior cranial fossa defect with split rib grafts. Inadequate contouring can be seen. *D*, Failure to recognize left orbitozygomatic injury in combination with craniofacial injury has resulted in a true orbital dystopia of the left orbit. Inadequate contouring of the cranial reconstruction can be easily seen as well. It is essential to recognize orbital dystopia in these injuries and adequately reposition the orbit on that side by correct reconstruction of the zygomatic arch, orbital floor, and nasoethmoid region.

produce a stable reconstruction in many cases. Maintenance of the correct convex contour is difficult with interosseous wiring alone when extensive comminution is present in the frontal and fronto-orbital regions. Long miniplates can be exactly contoured to the shape of the skull to maintain contour and minimize late collapse. Individual fragments can be fixed to the plate, using specially designed miniscrews that are 3 or 4 mm in length to prevent them from entering the cranial cavity and damaging the dura (see Fig. 7–5).

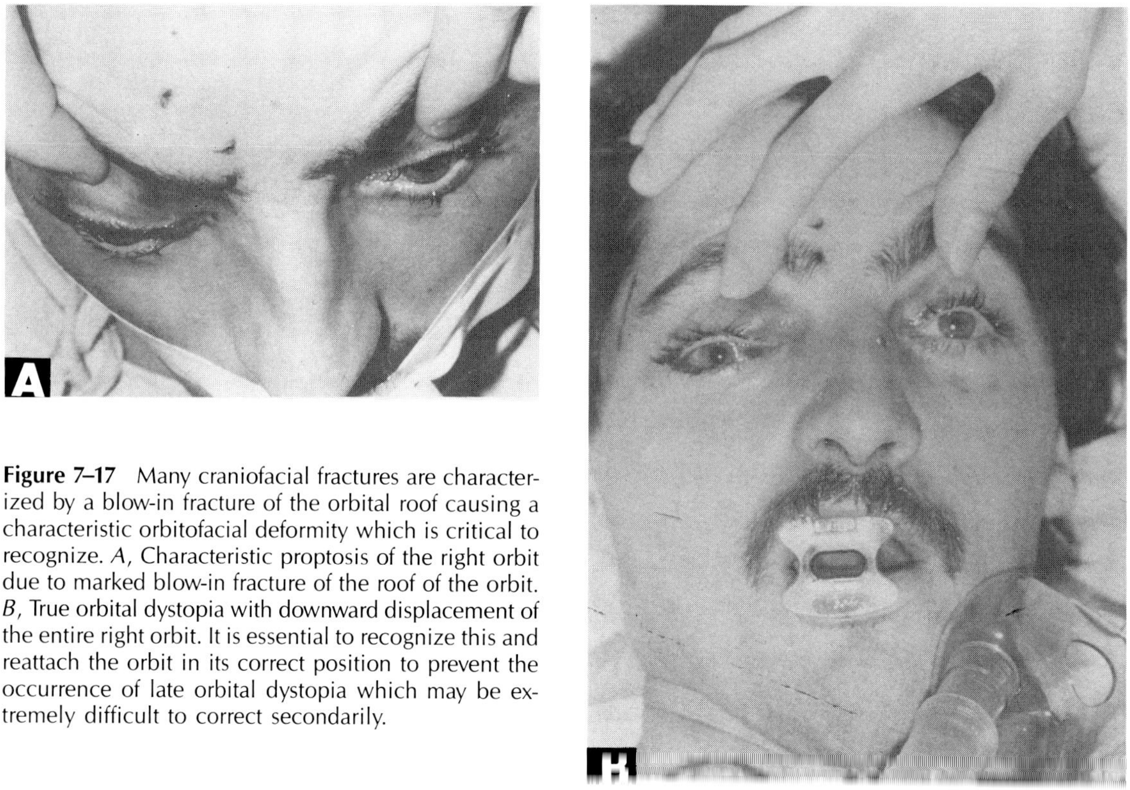

Figure 7–17 Many craniofacial fractures are characterized by a blow-in fracture of the orbital roof causing a characteristic orbitofacial deformity which is critical to recognize. *A*, Characteristic proptosis of the right orbit due to marked blow-in fracture of the roof of the orbit. *B*, True orbital dystopia with downward displacement of the entire right orbit. It is essential to recognize this and reattach the orbit in its correct position to prevent the occurrence of late orbital dystopia which may be extremely difficult to correct secondarily.

REFERENCES

1. Gruss JS. Fronto-naso-orbital trauma. Clin Plast Surg 1982; 9:577.
2. Gruss JS, Mackinnon SE, Kassel EE, et al. The role of primary bone grafting in complex craniomaxillofacial trauma. Plast Reconstr Surg 1985; 75:17.
3. Gruss JS. Naso-ethmoid orbital fractures: classification and role of primary bone grafting. Plast Reconstr Surg 1985; 75:303.
4. Gruss JS, MacKinnon SE. Complex maxillary fractures: role of buttress reconstruction and immediate bone grafts. Plast Reconstr Surg 1986; 78:9.
5. Antonyshyn O, Gruss JS. Complex orbital trauma: the role of rigid fixation and primary bone grafting.
6. Schilli W, Ewers R, Niederdellman H. Bone fixation with screws and plates in the maxillofacial region. Int J Oral Surg 1981; 10:329.
7. Spiess LB. New concepts in maxillofacial bone surgery. Berlin: Springer-Verlag, 1976.
8. Fischer RP, Flynn TC, Miller TW, Duke KH. Urban helicopter response to the scene of injury. J Trauma 1984; 24:946.
9. Finney LA, Reynolds DM, Yates BK. Comminuted subfrontal fractures. J Trauma 1964; 4:711.
10. Dingman RO, Grabb WC, O'Neill RM. Management of injuries of the naso-orbital complex. Arch Surg 1969; 98:566.
11. Tessier P. Total osteotomy of the middle third of the face for faciostenosis or for sequelae of LeFort III fractures. Plast Reconstr Surg 1971; 48:533.
12. Jefferson A, Reilly G. Fractures of the floor of the anterior cranial fossa. Br J Surg 1972; 59:585.
13. Newman MH, Travis LW. Frontal sinus fractures. Laryngoscope 1973; 83:1281.
14. Merville L. Multiple dislocations of the facial skeleton. J Maxillofac Surg 1974; 2:187.
15. Nadell J, Kline DG. Primary reconstruction of depressed frontal skull fractures including those involving the sinus, orbit, and cribriform plate. J Neurosurg 1974; 41:200.
16. Jones WD, Whitaker LA, Mutagh F. Applications of reconstructive craniofacial techniques to acute craniofacial trauma. J Trauma 1977; 17:339.
17. Hybels RL. Posterior table fractures of the frontal sinus. II. Clinical aspects. Laryngoscope 1977; 87:1740.
18. Stranc MF, Harrison DH. Primary treatment of craniofacial injuries. Rev Stomatol (Paris) 1978; 79:363.
19. Cantore GP, Delfini R, Gambacorta D, Consorti P. Cranio-orbito-facial injuries: technical suggestions. J Trauma 1979; 19:370.
20. Psillakis JM, Nocchi VL. Zanini SA. Repair of large defects of frontal bone with free graft of outer table of parietal bone. Plast Reconstr Surg 1979; 64:287.
21. Tajima S, Nakajima H. The treatment of fractures involving the frontobasal region. Clin Plast Surg 1980; 7:525.
22. Sturla F, Absi D, Buquet J. Anatomical and mechanical considerations of craniofacial fractures: an experimental study. Plast Reconstr Surg 1980; 66:815.
23. Whitaker LA. Traumatic craniofacial deformity. Scand J Plast Reconstr Surg 1981; 15:307.

24. Jackson I, Munro I, Salyer K, Whitaker LA. Traumatic deformity. Atlas of cranio-maxillofacial surgery. St. Louis: CV Mosby, 1982.
25. Pollock RA, Gruss JS. Complex facial fractures. In: Foster CA, Sherman JE, eds. Surgery of facial bone fractures. New York: Churchill Livingstone, 1985.
26. Kassel EE, Noyek AM, Cooper PW. CT in facial trauma. J Otolaryngol 1983; 12:2.
27. Munro IR, Chen YR. Radical treatment for fronto-orbital fibrous dysplasia: the chain link fence. Plast Reconstr Surg 1981; 67:719.
28. Ewers R, Harley F. Experimental and clinical results of new advances in the treatment of facial trauma. Plast Reconstr Surg 1985; 75:25.
29. Tessier P. Aesthetic aspects of bone grafting to the face. Clin Plast Surg 1981; 8:279.
30. Munro IR. Craniofacial surgical techniques for aesthetic results in congenital and acute traumatic deformities. Clin Plast Surg 1981; 8:303.
31. Merville LC, Derome P, deSaint-Jorre G. Fronto-orbito-nasal dislocations: secondary treatment of sequelae. J Maxillofac Surg 1983; 11:71.
32. Schultz RC. Facial injuries. Chicago: Year Book, 1977.
33. Failla A. Operative management of injuries involving the frontal sinuses. Laryngoscope 1968; 78:1833.
34. May M, Ogura JH, Schramm V. Nasofrontal duct in frontal sinus fractures. Arch Otolaryngol 1970; 92:534.
35. Bosley WR. Osteoplastic obliteration of the frontal sinuses: a review of 100 patients. Laryngoscope 1972; 82:1463.
36. Merville LC, Real JP. Fronto-orbito-nasal dislocations. Scand J Plast Reconstr Surg 1981; 15:287.
37. Luce EA. Maxillofacial trauma. Curr Probl Surg 1984; 11:1.
38. Chandler JR. Mucoceles: their diagnosis and treatment. J Fla Med Assoc 1960; 46:825.
39. Evans C. Aetiology in treatment of fronto-ethmoidal mucocele. J Laryngol Otol 1981; 95:361.
40. May M, Ogura JH, Schramm V. Nasofrontal duct in frontal sinus fractures. Arch Otolaryngol 1970; 92:534.
41. Donald PJ, Bernstein L. Compound frontal sinus injuries with intracranial penetration. Laryngoscope 1978; 88:225.
42. Schultz RC. Supraorbital and glabellar fractures. Plast Reconstr Surg 1970; 45:227.
43. Beziat JL, Freidel M, Dumas P. Repair of the contour of the frontal bone in injury. Ann Chir Plast 1980; 25:329.

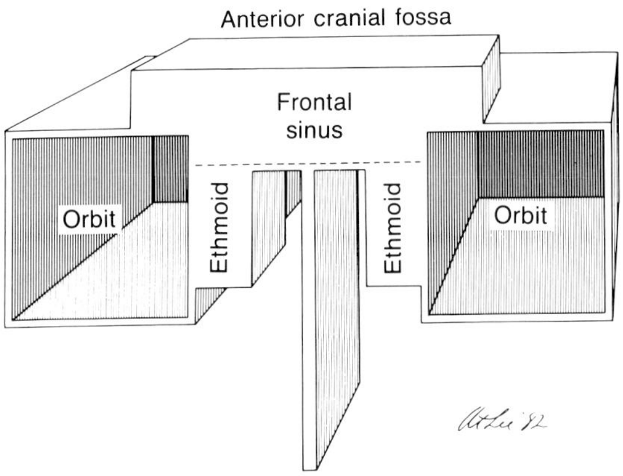

Figure 8–2 Schematic representation of the interorbital space showing the relationship between the anterior cranial fossa, frontal sinus and nasoethmoid orbital areas.

Ethmoid and Frontal Sinuses

The greatest variability in this region depends on the aeration and development of the sinus cavities. The ethmoid sinuses begin development in the second trimester of pregnancy and by the second year of life a true labyrinth of pneumatized cells ranging from 4 to 17 cells can encroach on the bony confines of the frontal, maxillary, sphenoid, and ethmoid structures.[3] Similarly, the frontal sinuses can also extend widely between the anterior and posterior lamellae of the frontal bone; they may actually be absent or rudimentary in about 10 percent of the population. Drainage of these two sinus complexes occurs into the nose and is mediated by their ciliated mucosa. The ethmoid sinuses are divided anatomically by the middle turbinate into smaller, more numerous anterior cells that empty into the middle meatus and larger, less numerous posterior cells that empty into the superior meatus. The frontal sinuses are derived from the frontal recess cells or from air cells of the ethmoid infundibulum and drain into the middle meatus by means of a well-defined nasofrontal duct or an ostium in the anterosuperior portion of the middle meatus.[4]

Proper Nasal Bones

The bones of the nose are paired quadrilateral structures that articulate with the nasal spine of the frontal bone superiorly and the frontal processes of the maxillae laterally. They are also supported on their undersurface by the nasal septum composed of bone and cartilage. The perpendicular plate of the ethmoid and the vomer form the bony portion of the septum and articulate posteriorly with each other and with the sphenoid bone. The cartilaginous septum projects forward from the bone and articulates with the lower third of the nasal bones and the upper lateral cartilages (Fig. 8–3). They give the characteristic profile to the individual and because of their prominent status in the face and their low resistance to G-forces, they are the most commonly fractured bones of the facial skeleton. Deviation and depression of the nasal bones and the septum are common features after moderate to severe injuries and their treatment has been enhanced by early correction and the institution in certain situations of immediate bone grafting.

Blood and Nerve Supply

The blood supply to this region is dual, as it receives contributions from the external and internal carotid arteries. The ophthalmic artery gives rise to the anterior and posterior ethmoidal arteries which nourish the ethmoid complex and medial orbit. They course intracranially and extracranially and serve as a surgical guide to this boundary. The terminal branches, supratrochlear and supraorbital, nourish the skin of this region. They anastomose freely with the terminal branches of the facial artery including the angular and the dorsal nasal vessels. The internal maxillary artery gives rise to

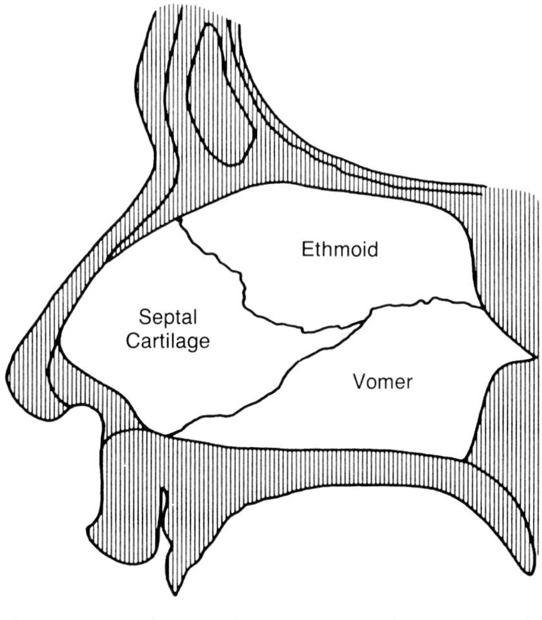

Figure 8–3 The nasal septum. Cartilage anteriorly articulates with bone posteriorly.

nasal and septal branches which also nourish the lateral wall turbinates.

The nerve supply includes sensory, motor, sympathetic, and parasympathetic branches of the fifth and seventh cranial nerves. The olfactory bulb and nerve endings are in intimate contact with these structures and are often injured when these delicate bones are fractured, although partial or complete recovery of smell is the rule. The second, third, fourth, and sixth cranial nerves are also in close proximity and can suffer varying degrees of injury.

DIAGNOSIS

The acute care and management of the facially injured patient is well noted elsewhere in this book. Motor vehicle accidents represent the most common mechanism of injury in the patients seen with maxillofacial trauma. This can be explained by the rapid growth and congestion of our urban centers, although definite geographic differences do exist. It is therefore important to note that the majority of frontal and nasoethmoid-orbital fractures occur concomitantly with other soft- and hard-tissue facial injuries. The experience at the University of Kentucky shows that more than 60 percent of these patients present with significant associated nonfacial injuries that can be life-threatening and demand priority in treatment.[5]

The initial clinical examination including the history and mechanism of injury provides very important information. After the patient has been treated for any life-threatening injuries, the examining physician inspects the soft tissue for skin integrity and looks for nerve deficits and ocular injuries that can vary in degree and may require the urgent consultation of an ophthalmologist to initiate early therapy. Fractures can often be easily documented by the presence of displacement and deformity and by the localized pain elicited on palpation. A crunching or crepitant sensation is noticed in more severe and comminuted fractures.

Specific diagnostic features depending on the zone of injury will now be discussed, although we emphasize that some or all may be present in the same patient depending on the severity of the trauma.

Traumatic Telecanthus

The intercanthal distance is measured routinely in nasoethmoid-orbital fractures. The normal intercanthal distance should roughly equal the palpebral fissure distance or half the interpupillary distance—between 30 and 35 mm in the adult. Traumatic telecanthus or widening of the intercanthal distance due to injury represents a tear of the medial canthus from its insertion on the lacrimal crest, or more commonly its lateral migration due to fracture of the bone-insertion segment. Not only is the intercanthal distance increased but the medial canthal region is rounded instead of elliptical. Marked swelling may make an accurate measurement difficult. It is extremely important, however, to document the presence of telecanthus so that it can be treated primarily. Adequate delayed treatment after the bones and soft tissue have healed can be difficult or impossible.

Nasolacrimal Tract Injury

The nasolacrimal apparatus may also be injured in about one-fifth of patients with nasoethmoid-orbital fractures.[5,6,7] It is especially susceptible when telecanthus is present because the lacrimal tract loses the protective influence of the anterior medial canthal ligament.[6] Primary probing or repair is discouraged except in those cases of obvious injury or laceration, as more damage may be incurred. Open reduction and anatomic fixation of the fractures will usually result in regained lacrimal function.[7] Delayed assessment with irrigation of specific markers, instrument probing, dacryocystography, or radioactive isotope studies can be done if necessary. A dacryocystorhinostomy or other lacrimal bypass procedure can then be performed electively.[8]

Frontal Sinus Fractures

Fractures of the anterior wall of the frontal sinus can produce a visible depression or concavity and are often open because of overlying lacerations. Indeed, deep lacerations or contusions of the supraorbital ridge, glabella, or lower forehead should lead one to suspect frontal sinus fractures, and often palpation with an examining finger through the laceration will establish the diagnosis. Fractures of the posterior wall can lacerate the dura and result in CSF leak or even cause significant brain damage. A careful check for the presence of CSF rhinorrhea should be done.

Cloudiness or an air-fluid level in the sinus due to fracture can easily be seen on a plain posteroanterior or lateral skull film. Pneumocephalus, or the presence of air in the cranial vault, indicates a posterior wall fracture and can also be seen on plain x-ray films but is better evaluated with a computed tomographic (CT) scan. This diagnosis is important in the successful management of this injury (Fig. 8–4).

A variety of classifications of frontal sinus fractures have been proposed.[9,10] We favor a classification that will permit one to establish a treatment plan.[11] The anatomic type of fracture (anterior table, posterior table, anterobasilar, or frontal skull fracture extension), the type of wound (open or closed), and the absence or presence of CSF leak are all considered (Fig. 8–5).

Orbital Roof Fractures

Fractures of the orbital roof are frequently associated with frontal sinus or supraorbital ridge fractures (Fig. 8–6). If the fragments are depressed, the globe may be pushed inferiorly and may even be proptotic. On the other hand, orbital soft tissue can be entrapped into the frontal sinus causing enophthalmos.

A loss of upward gaze with vertical diplopia indicates involvement of the superior rectus and possibly the superior oblique muscles. Exploration and repair of an orbital roof fracture requires a craniofacial approach usually in conjunction with neurosurgical exploration. Major defects are repaired with bone grafts but caution should be used so as not to compress the globe excessively. Treatment is not always necessary. On rare occasions, however, pulsating exophthalmos has been described as a troublesome complication of unrepaired post-traumatic defects of the orbital roof, presumably from transmitted intracranial pressure.

Supraorbital Ridge Fractures

The supraorbital ridge has the highest impact tolerance of the facial skeleton. In a series of 1,000 major facial fractures at our institution, a fracture at this site was associated with a high incidence of life-threatening injuries elsewhere.[12] Supraorbital ridge fractures lateral to the frontal sinus and without significant involvement of the orbital roof are uncommon (about 2 percent of cases) and do not require treatment unless they are depressed. Depressed supraorbital ridge fractures can produce an aesthetic deficit and should be openly reduced, together with neighboring involved structures.

Radiologic and Other Diagnostic Tests

The clinical examination of the patient with facial injuries can at times be limited by the patient's general condition. More severe associated injuries may need to be managed or ruled out. Yet when the patient is stable, a thorough radiologic evaluation should be carried out. Conventional radiography is still useful and gives valuable information regarding fractures and sinus clouding. The Caldwell, Waters, lateral, and basal views are most helpful.[13] There is no doubt, however, that CT scanning with coronal and sagittal sectioning, when possible, is essential for the complete management of complex fractures of this region.

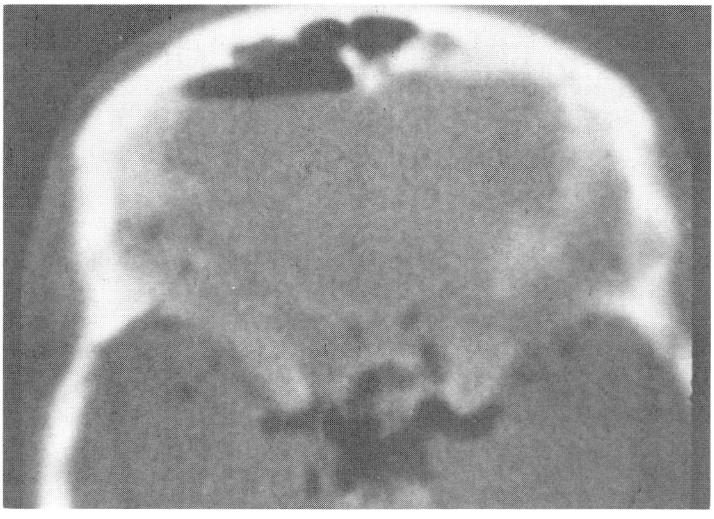

Figure 8–4 Computed tomographic scan showing pneumocephalus due to disruption of the posterior wall of the frontal sinus.

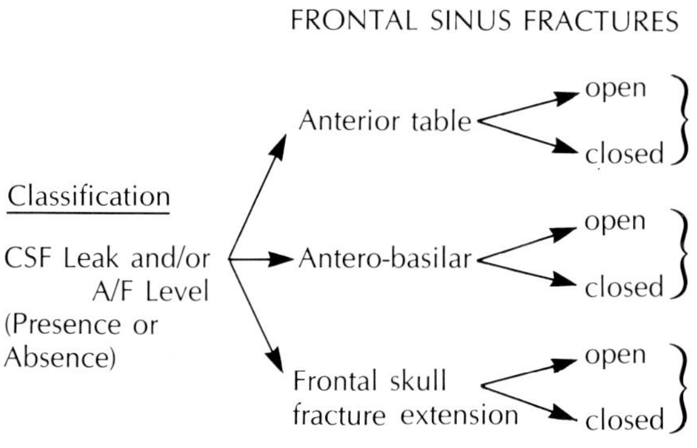

Figure 8–5 Classification of frontal sinus fractures based on the presence or absence of cerebrospinal fluid (CSF) leak and/or air fluid (A/F) level, anatomic type of fracture, and type of wound (open or closed).

Many times these patients are receiving a CT scan of the head to rule out intracranial pathology and it does not take that much more time or increased radiation exposure to continue the scan down to the nasoethmoid-orbital region or lower if necessary. These views give greater detail about the sinus walls and the medial orbit which helps determine a treatment plan. The treatment of frontal sinus fractures depends in great part on the extent of intracranial involvement. The management of enophthalmos due to medial orbital blowout is similar in concept to that of enophthalmos due to inferior orbital blowout and therefore the diagnosis becomes critical.

The use of three-dimensional CT reconstruction is becoming more and more popular in many aspects of surgery, in particular craniofacial surgery.[14,15] Its application in craniomaxillofacial trauma is just beginning to be exploited. It has obvious potential as a diagnostic and planning tool (Fig. 8–7).

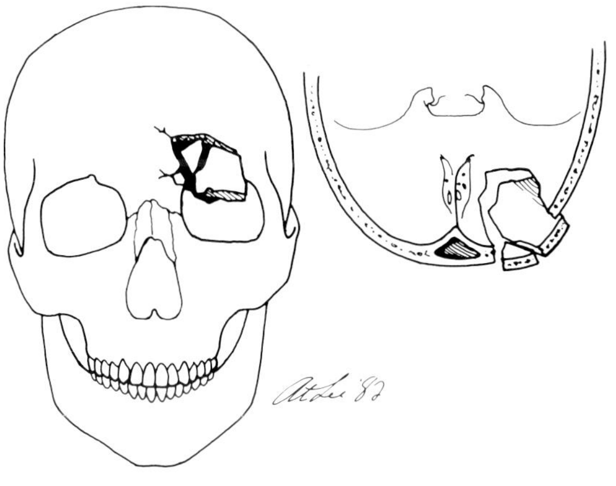

Figure 8–6 Orbital roof fracture. Such a fracture is often associated with supraorbital ridge fractures caused by high G impact trauma.

TREATMENT

In general terms, the state of the art in the treatment of facial fractures requires the discussion of three important concepts that have particular relevance in the management of frontal and nasoethmoid-orbital fractures. They are: the surgical approach, bone grafting, and rigid fixation.

Surgical Approach

The operative approach to upper midline facial fractures has been the subject of some controversy, with earlier authors advocating closed reduction techniques[16] or limited local incisions over the fracture sites. The concept of open reduction and internal fixation has the obvious merit of direct exposure and identification of displaced bony fragments and soft tissue. When the trauma is minor and the fracture isolated, local exploration or even closed reduction techniques can be entertained. When the injury is major and complex, however, the bicoronal anterior scalp flap has proved to be very useful, providing ample exposure of the involved elements while at the same time usually leaving an aesthetic, hidden scar. With experience, the flap can be raised quickly and with minimal blood loss. This approach has the added advantage, in combined procedures, of providing the neurosurgeon ready access to perform any necessary intracranial repairs before the facial injuries are addressed.

Bone Grafting

Various sources of autogenous bone have been used with success for bone grafting purposes including rib and iliac bone. Recent studies have shown some benefits with the use of membranous bone in the facial skeleton, especially with regard to the degree of reabsorption.[17] With the increasing popularity of split cranial bone for grafting purposes, the use of a bicoronal incision in moderate to severe cases of upper third facial trauma has definite advantages. As indicated above, this incision provides unsurpassed exposure of the fracture sites and permits ready access for cranial bone harvesting. The cranial bone can be split in situ with the use of a power-driven burr and a set of straight and curved osteotomes. It can also be harvested full thickness when more volume of bone is re-

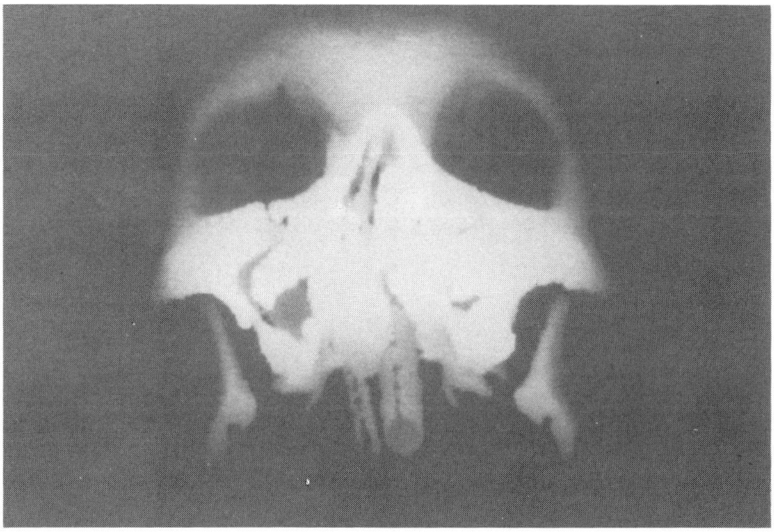

Figure 8–7 Three-dimensional computed tomographic image of infraorbital zygoma fracture with minimal displacement.

quired and then split on the bench. The main drawback with cranial bone is its rigidity and the difficulty in obtaining smooth rounded edges. Rib [illegible] able materials and can initially give better contour in certain areas. Often, nonusable bone or cartilage from certain fracture sites can be used effectively in other areas. For example, in associated maxillary fractures, antral bone can be used for grafting, as it does not contribute significantly to the contour or structural support of this region. This bone is thin and can fill a medial orbital or infraorbital defect or bridge a gap in the anterior frontal sinus.

Work is being done with grafting materials other than autogenous bone, including homografts of bone or cartilage that have been lyophilized or irradiated. Synthetic materials such as hydroxyapatite and Proplast are also being used in elective facial reconstruction.[18–20] Experience in acute, contaminated traumatic wounds, however, is very limited. Infection is a serious complication and must be taken into account when considering these bone substitutes.

Rigid Fixation

Various means of bony fixation have been used since prehistoric times, both external and internal. The application of internal wire fixation for facial fractures by Adams was truly a great advance in the field.[21] However, limitations in wire fixation have been described,[22] the most important being that they do not provide stable rigid fixation in three dimensions. The use of miniplates and screws obviates many of these limitations and has been [illegible] facial fractures.

The popularity of miniplates and screws is evident throughout this book; however, the concept is not new. What is new are the better materials and construction of these fixation devices. The plates are much smaller, thinner, and more custom built for each region of the facial skeleton. They are made of more inert metals such as titanium which can more easily integrate into the bony framework. Wires are still used to fix more delicate bony fragments that will not endure much tension.

Refinements in technology are rapidly being made. Plates and screws are being manufactured that are measured in tenths of a millimeter. Work is also being done on absorbable plates and screws that will provide stability during the healing stage and then disappear.

As with the diagnosis, we will artificially divide the treatment plan so as to deal with each specific problem separately. Quite commonly, however, a particular patient will require that various problems be addressed concurrently.

Nasoethmoid-Orbital Fractures

Three main factors determine the management of nasoethmoid-orbital fractures: (1) the type of fracture—isolated or extended; (2) associated bone and soft-tissue injury; and (3) bone loss or presence of nonfunctional bone. Evaluation of these three factors is needed to prepare a surgical plan. Knowledge of the type of fracture helps establish the method of surgical approach. The approach will also be influenced by the need to expose other injured sites, as in the presence of associated Le Fort-type fractures. Significant bone loss, or more commonly the presence of severely comminuted bone fragments, will require primary bone grafting to restore structural integrity and prevent soft-tissue contracture.[22,23] Gruss' classification of nasoethmoid-orbital fractures[24] uses these criteria and is helpful in understanding their management. The categories proposed are numerous and detailed, reflecting the many combinations of injuries that can occur. Even with our present technology, we cannot always be certain of the diagnosis and neatly fit the patient's injuries into a specific category until the time of surgical exploration. Therefore it behooves the surgeon always to be prepared to extend the exploration and to be ready to perform primary bone grafting if the situation calls for it.

Traumatic Telecanthus

Traumatic telecanthus is caused by a forceful displacement of one or both of the medial canthal ligaments with or without disinsertion. Outfracturing of the canthal-insertion segment is the much more common finding. Therefore, the anatomic reduction and fixation of these fractured segments will often restore the premorbid intercanthal relationship. When a bicoronal dissection is employed, or a direct local approach, isolation of the canthal ligaments is important to avoid their disinsertion from the lacrimal crest. This is easily accomplished by making external medial canthal incisions (Mustardé or Del Campo) and dissecting down to the canthal ligament. This may then be encircled with a fine wire suture until the bone segments are reduced or until the ligaments need to be approximated transnasally. The use of wire permits the ligaments to be approximated to the appropriate distance by simply twisting the sutures. If the canthal ligaments are already disinserted from the bone, they can be transfixed with wire after their dissection and brought closer together transnasally. The use of nasal splints made of lead or plastic is optional after the medial canthi are adequately reduced. Overcorrection of medial canthal approximation medially and posteriorly is the rule, since quite often the results are deficient.

Depressed Nasal Dorsum

Trauma to the proper nasal bones with fracture or collapse of the cartilaginous and/or bony septum can cause posterior telescoping of these anterior structures. The result is a depressed nasal dorsum or saddle deformity. Sometimes this complex can be reduced to restore the proper nasal profile and projection. In severe or comminuted fractures this is not possible and the use of a cantilever bone graft is needed. This should be done during the primary procedure to avoid future contraction of the soft tissue. The bone graft can be fixed in many different ways. We have found the use of a central screw or a plate and screws quite versatile and effective (Fig. 8–8). Dissection along the dorsum down to the tip of the nose is often necessary to obtain the desired projection.

Nasolacrimal Tract Injury

Serious injury to the nasolacrimal apparatus resulting in obstruction or other malfunction occurs in about 20 percent of patients with nasoethmoid-orbital fractures.[5,6,7] The great majority of cases will be corrected or maintain patency if open reduction and meticulous internal fixation of the specific fracture sites are performed.[7] Attempts at assessment in the face of soft-tissue swelling or bony displacement may cause damage to an otherwise intact system. Those patients who will end up with long-term problems can be treated successfully with a lacrimal bypass procedure. However, obvious transection of the superior and inferior canaliculi or lacrimal sac can occur. The latter is reasonably protected by the medial canthal ligament anteriorly, as described above, as it lies within a recess in the lacrimal bone. Unrepaired lacerations of the inferior canaliculus or lacrimal sac will result in obstruction of proper drainage of tears, recurrent episodes of infection (dacrocystitis), and excessive tearing (epiphora). Diagnosis of a transected canaliculus or sac can be made by passing a probe from the punctum near the medial canthus into the wound. Repair of an isolated laceration of the superior canaliculus is usually not necessary, since 80 percent of tears drain through the inferior punctum and canaliculus. Repair of the inferior canaliculus is achieved by the passage of a silk suture or fine Silastic catheter through the superior canaliculus, the sac, and out the inferior punctum. Repair of the sac may be more complex, requiring fine absorbable sutures over a fine Silastic catheter (Quickert tube) passed from the inferior punctum into the nose (Fig. 8–9).

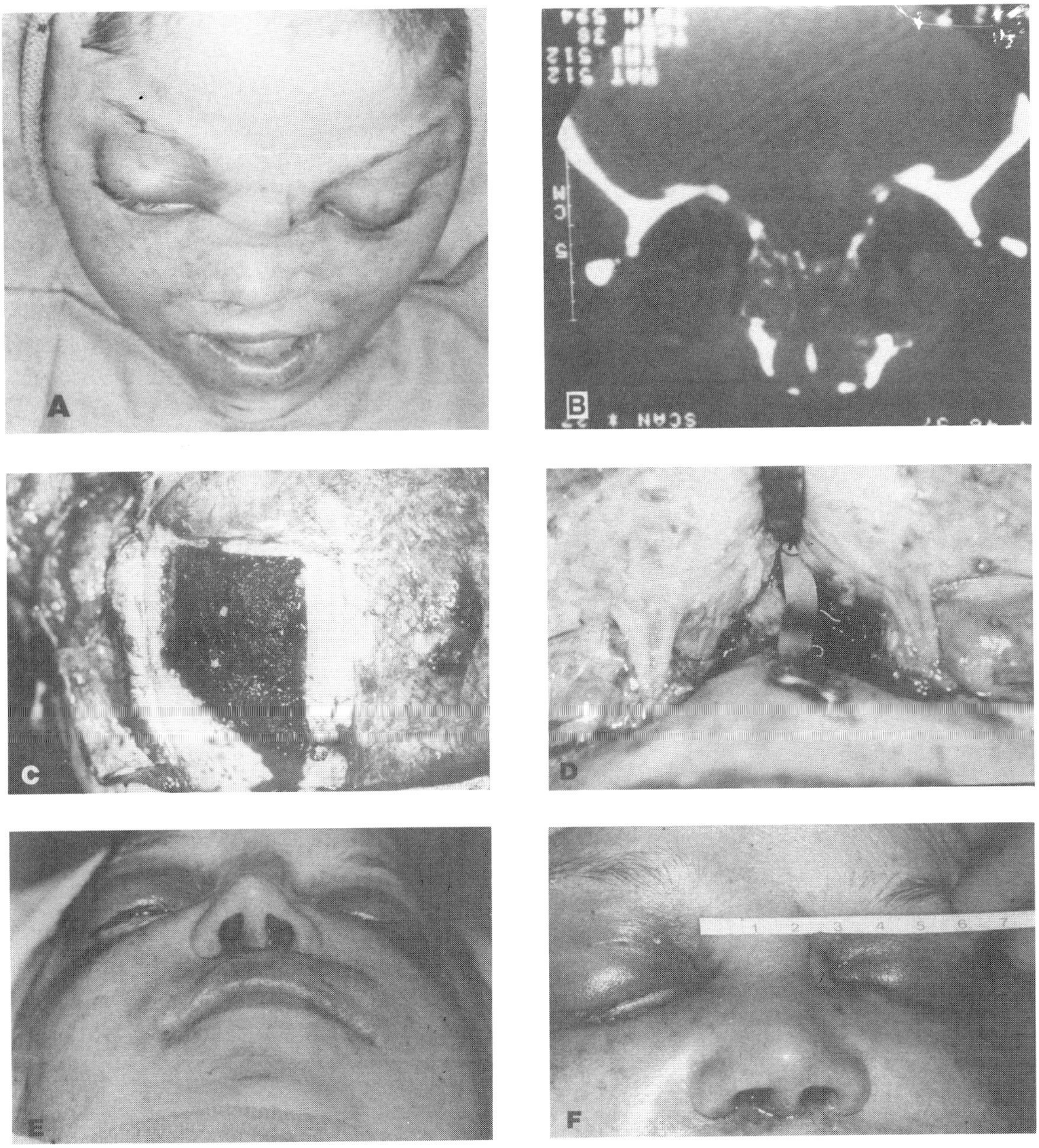

Figure 8–8 *A*, Thirty-nine-year-old female suffered severe facial trauma, including Le Fort III, nasoethmoid orbital, and mandibular fractures. Note telecanthus (over 50 mm) and depressed nasal dorsum. *B*, Computed tomographic scan shows nasal bone and septal collapse as well as medial orbital fractures. *C*, Exposure with a bicoronal incision was used and split cranial bone was harvested for grafting of orbits, maxillae, and nose. *D*, A special L plate was used to fix cantilever bone graft to nose. *E*, Good nasal dorsum and tip projection is obtained. *F*, Final intraoperative result after reduction and fixation of fractures and correction of telecanthus (intercanthal distance is 31 mm).

Frontal Sinus Fractures

The appropriate treatment of frontal sinus fractures is controversial. Some advocate very strongly the ablation or obliteration of the injured frontal sinus to avoid infectious complications.[25,26] Mucopyocele is a late complication of frontal sinus disease and frontal sinus surgery. Localized osteomyelitis and intracranial septic complications are well described.[25,27] A principal thrust of frontal sinus surgery, especially in the otolaryngologic literature, has been to avoid the complication of muco-

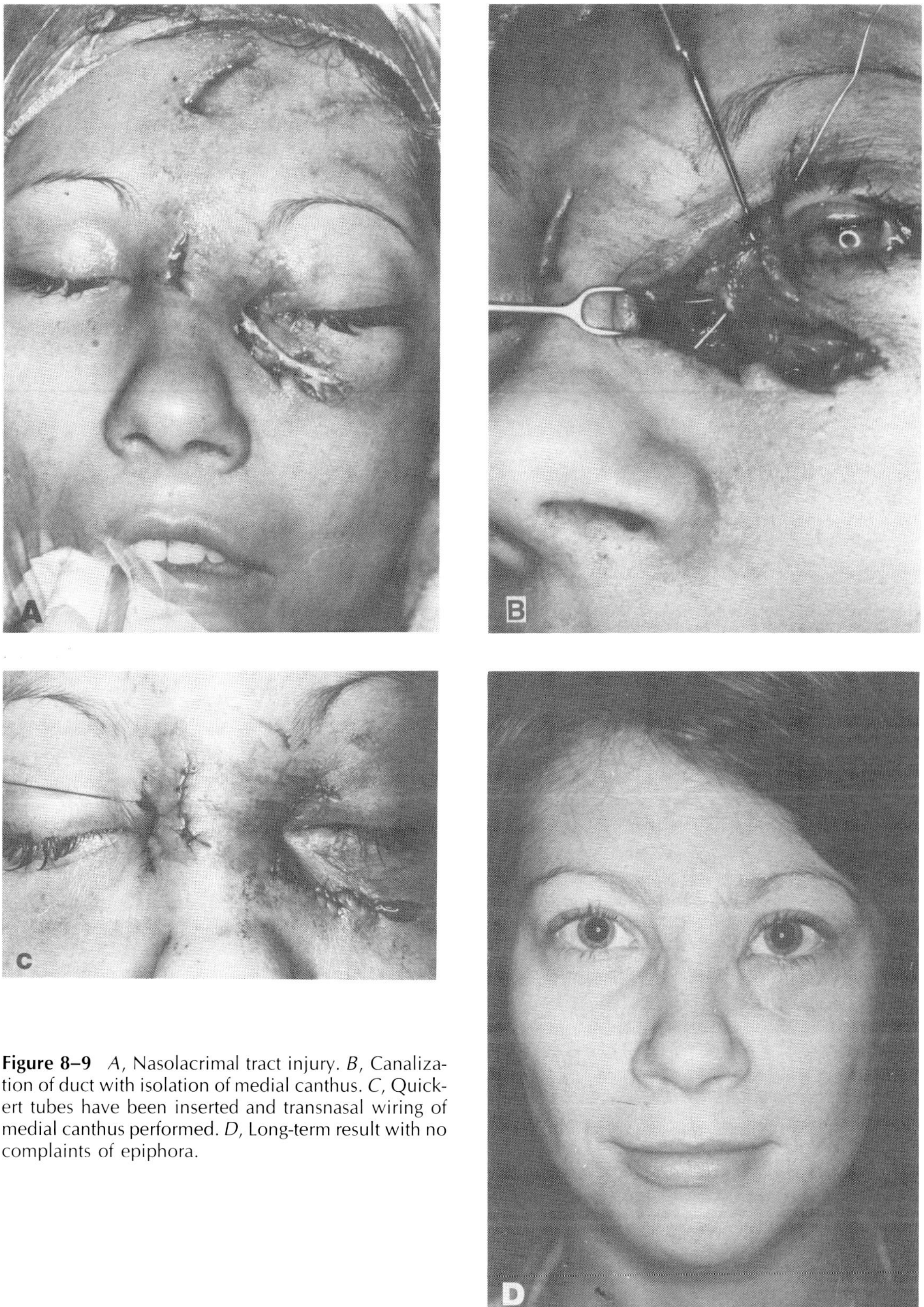

Figure 8–9 *A*, Nasolacrimal tract injury. *B*, Canalization of duct with isolation of medial canthus. *C*, Quickert tubes have been inserted and transnasal wiring of medial canthus performed. *D*, Long-term result with no complaints of epiphora.

pyocele.[28,29] A correlation between the chronically infected sinus and the acutely injured sinus has been proposed.[30] Actually, there is little evidence to suggest that mucopyocele is a common complication of the reconstructed and properly drained frontal sinus. In two large series dealing with the subject of frontal mucocele,[27,31] only 4 and 6 percent were caused by trauma, in sinuses not explored primarily. The large experience of the senior author indicates that surgical treatment is best for the majority of frontal sinus fractures.[11]

A treatment algorithm should be established based on the presence or absence of CSF rhinorrhea, the anatomic type of fracture, and whether it is open or closed (Fig. 8–10). CSF rhinorrhea is highly suggestive of posterior wall involvement and merits exploration to assess fully its configuration, the integrity of the dura and underlying brain, and the patency of the nasofrontal duct.

Open fractures of the sinus region should be explored to clean and débride the area and to reconstruct if necessary with reduction of the fragments and possible bone grafting. Closed anterior wall fractures may have significant bony depression or residual aesthetic deficit that requires repair. These deficits may not be entirely evident until the swelling resolves. Closed anterobasilar fractures without evidence of CSF leak can be managed without surgery, but such patients should have follow-up x-ray films because the fractures may involve the nasofrontal duct(s).

The topic of surgical approach has already been discussed. We favor the bicoronal approach especially when posterior wall or dural involvement is suspected. More extensive dural or brain disruption is best approached through a frontal craniotomy and fascial grafting may be required. Obvious areas of devitalized mucosa are excised, but no attempt is made to remove intact sinus mucosa. The patency of the nasofrontal duct is key. The principal causative factor in the formation of a mucocele, experimentally[32,33] or clinically, is the obstruction of the nasofrontal duct in a diseased or injured sinus. Major damage of the frontal sinus or direct injury to the duct requires placement of a small catheter through the duct into the nose which is left for at least two weeks (Fig. 8–11). Less complex injuries do not need catheter drainage. Patency of the duct is ensured by the instillation of methylene blue or fluorescein irrigation.

Reconstruction of the bony sinus should be accomplished by means of the techniques described above, namely rigid fixation and primary bone grafting.

In frontal skull fractures with extensive injury of the sinus, the technique of "cranialization" is advocated. This procedure is accomplished by excision of the remaining posterior wall, excision of any residual mucosa, plugging of the nasofrontal duct with temporalis muscle or fascia or preferably by using a vascularized galeal or pericranial flap, and allowing the brain to expand to fill the space (Fig. 8–12). The anterior wall is properly reconstructed by reducing the fragments or by primary bone grafting.

Orbital Roof and Supraorbital Ridge Fractures

The orbital roof and the supraorbital ridge are uncommon sites for fractures; such fractures are usually associated with severe or multi-region facial trauma. The supraorbital ridge is very tolerant of G-forces but can suffer direct injury causing depression and fracture extension into the orbital roof. The orbital roof fragments can in turn cause injury or displacement of the globe and the over-

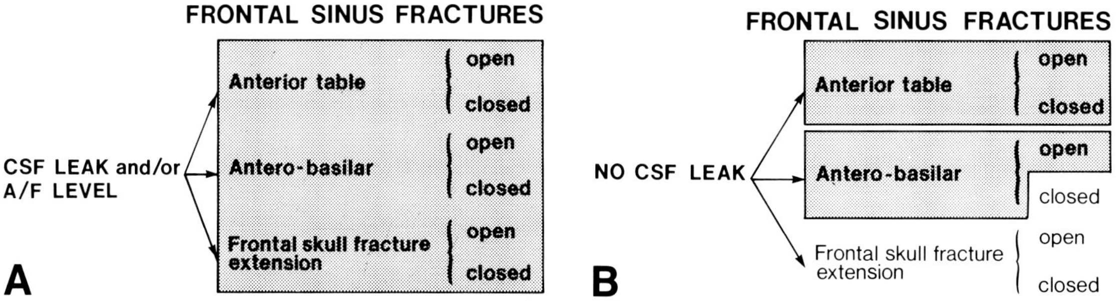

Figure 8–10 *A*, Treatment protocol for frontal sinus fractures with associated cerebrospinal fluid (CSF) leak and/or air fluid (A/F) level. Exploration is the rule. *B*, In absence of CSF leak, the next criterion is that of fracture type. Anterior table fractures are repaired regardless of whether they are open or closed, as are open anterobasilar fractures. Closed anterobasilar frontal sinus fractures or extension of frontal skull fractures involving the frontal sinus can be managed conservatively.

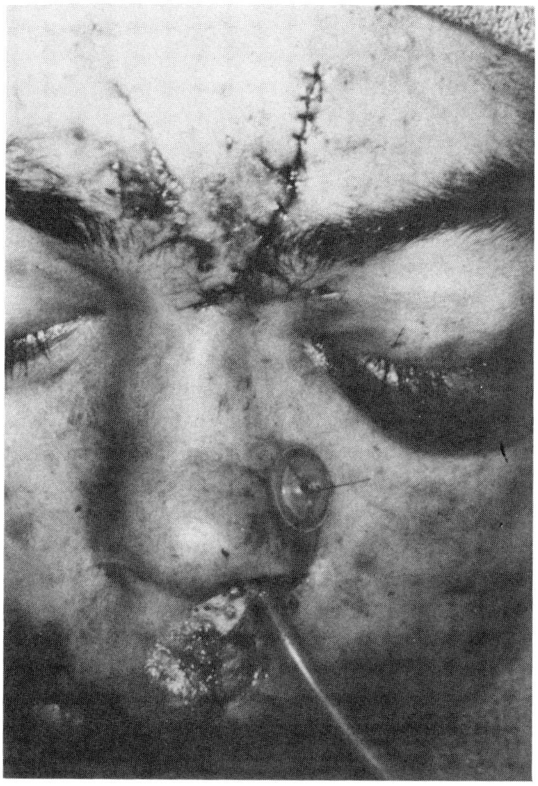

Figure 8–11 Repair of anterior and posterior wall frontal sinus fracture with catheter drainage through nasofrontal duct out of the nose.

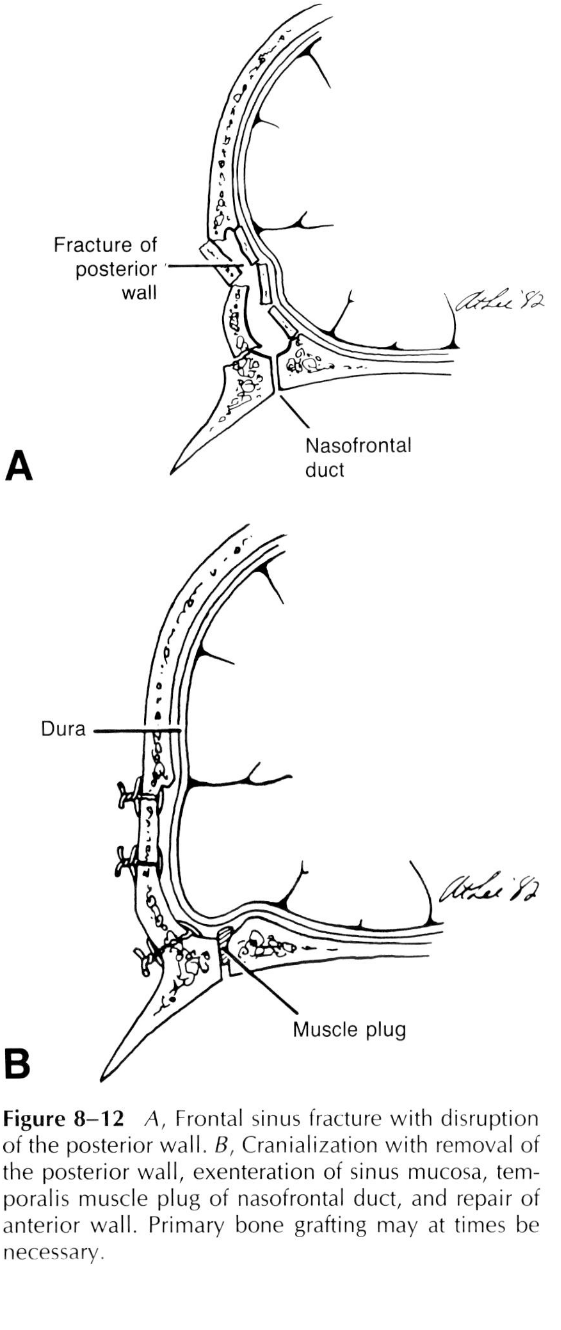

Figure 8–12 *A*, Frontal sinus fracture with disruption of the posterior wall. *B*, Cranialization with removal of the posterior wall, exenteration of sinus mucosa, temporalis muscle plug of nasofrontal duct, and repair of anterior wall. Primary bone grafting may at times be necessary.

lying brain tissue. Repair of the roof becomes important when large gaps exist that may cause problems with orbital volume or pulsating globes. Our choice is for cranial bone which is contoured very nicely for this area. If possible we prefer to fix the bone to avoid later displacement or problems with reabsorption. Repair of supraorbital ridge fractures usually requires reduction and possible bone grafting to restore the very obvious aesthetic contour.

REFERENCES

1. Le Fort R. Experimental study of fractures of the upper jaw. Rev Chir (Paris) 1901; 23(Part I):207–227; 23(Part II):360–379; 23(Part III):479–507.
2. Swearingen JJ. Tolerances of the human face to crash impact. Reprint No. AM-65-20 of Federal Aviation Agency, Oklahoma City, OK, 1965.
3. Ritter FN. The paranasal sinuses—anatomy and surgical technique. Ed. 2. St. Louis: CV Mosby, 1978.
4. Mattox DE, Delaney RG. Anatomy of the ethmoid sinus. Otolaryngol Clin North Am 1985; 18:3–14.
5. Cruse CW, Blevins PK, Luce EA. Naso-ethmoid-orbital fractures. J Trauma 1980; 20:551–556.
6. Stranc MF. The pattern of lacrimal injuries in naso-ethmoid fractures. Br J Plast Surg 1970; 23:339–346.
7. Gruss JS, Hurwitz JJ, Nik NA, Kassel EE. The pattern and incidence of nasolacrimal injury in naso-orbital-ethmoid fractures: the role of delayed assess-

ment and dacryocystorhinostomy. Br J Plast Surg 1985; 38:116–121.
8. Blitzer A, Lawson W, Friedman WH. Surgery of the paranasal sinuses. Philadelphia: WB Saunders, 1985.
9. Peri GJ, Chabannes J, Menes R, et al. Fractures of the frontal sinus. J Maxillofac Surg 1981; 9:73–80.
10. Newman MH, Travis LW. Frontal sinus fractures. Laryngoscope 1973; 83:1281–1292.
11. Luce EA. Frontal sinus fractures: guidelines to management. Plast Reconstr Surg 1987; 80:500–510.
12. Luce EA, Tubb TD, Moore AM. Review of 1000 major facial fractures and associated injuries. Plast Reconstr Surg 1979; 63:26–30.
13. Dolan KD. The ethmoid sinus: plain film and tomographic radiology. Otolaryngol Clin North Am 1985; 18:15–28.
14. Marsh JL, Vannier MW. The "third" dimension in craniofacial surgery. Plast Reconstr Surg 1983; 71:759–767.
15. Vannier MW, Marsh JL, Warren JO. Three-dimensional CT reconstruction images for craniofacial surgical planning and evaluation. Radiology 1984; 150:179–184.
16. Converse JM, Smith B. Naso-orbital fractures and traumatic deformities of the medial canthus. Plast Reconstr Surg 1966; 38:147–162.
17. Zins JE, Whitaker LA. Membranous versus endochondral bone: implications for craniofacial reconstruction. Plast Reconstr Surg 1983; 72:778–784.
18. Salyer KE, Ubinas EE, Snively SL. Porous hydroxyapatite as an onlay graft in maxillofacial surgery. Plast Surg Forum 1985; 8:61.
19. Holmes RE, Hagler HK. Porous hydroxyapatite as a bone graft substitute in cranial reconstruction: a histometric study. Plast Reconstr Surg 1988; 81:662–671.
20. Whitaker LA. Aesthetic augmentation of the malar-midface structures. Plast Reconstr Surg 1987; 80:337–346.
21. Adams WM. Internal wire fixation of facial fractures. Surgery 1942; 12:523–540.
22. Manson PN, Crawley WA, Yaremchuk MJ, et al. Midface fractures: advantages of immediate extended open reduction and bone grafting. Plast Reconstr Surg 1985; 76:1–10.
23. Gruss JS, Mackinnon SE, Kassel EE, et al. The role of primary bone grafting in complex craniomaxillofacial trauma. Plast Reconstr Surg 1985; 75:17–24.
24. Gruss JS. Naso-ethmoid-orbital fractures: classification and the role of primary bone grafting. Plast Reconstr Surg 1985; 75:303–315.
25. Remmer D, Boles R. Intracranial complications of frontal sinusitis. Laryngoscope 1980; 90:1814–1824.
26. Goodale RL. Rationale of frontal sinus surgery. Laryngoscope 1965; 75:981–987.
27. Bordley JE, Bosley WR. Mucoceles of the frontal sinus: causes and treatment. Ann Otol Rhinol Laryngol 1973; 82:696–702.
28. Schenck NL. Frontal sinus disease. I. An historical perspective on research. Laryngoscope 1974; 84:1031–1044.
29. Larrabee WF, Travis LW, Tabb HG. Frontal sinus fractures—their suppurative complications in surgical management. Laryngoscope 1980; 90:1810–1813.
30. Sessions RB, Alford BR, Stratton C, et al. Current concepts of frontal sinus surgery: an appraisal of the osteoplastic flap-fat obliteration operation. Laryngoscope 1972; 82:918–930.
31. Evans C. Aetiology in the treatment of fronto-ethmoidal mucocele. J Laryngol Otol 1981; 95:361–375.
32. Schenck NL, Rauchbach E, Ogura H. Frontal sinus disease. II. Development of the frontal sinus model: occlusion of the nasofrontal duct. Laryngoscope 1974; 84:1233–1247.
33. Schenck NL. Frontal sinus disease. III. Experimental and clinical factors in failure of the frontal osteoplastic operation. Laryngoscope 1975; 85:76–92.

9

ORBITAL FRACTURES

IVO P. JANECKA, M.D., F.A.C.S.

Fractures in and around the orbit involve an anatomical area representing a junction between the cranial and facial skeleton. The presence of significant structures and the proximity of vital organs create special conditions for a potential serious impact of these fractures. A complete understanding of orbital and nasoethmoid anatomy in conjunction with craniofacial surgical technique is fundamental to the diagnosis and repair of such fractures, as well as prevention or treatment of established complications. Reestablishment of normal architecture of the craniofacial skeleton and three-dimensional rigid fixation with supplementary usage of autogenous bone grafts are the principles underlying successful treatment of orbital and nasoethmoid fractures.[1]

CLINICAL ANATOMY

The bony orbits are pyramidal in shape and relatively symmetric. These midfacial structures are separated by interorbital space and surrounded, for the most part, by the periorbital sinuses. They are formed by seven bones: maxilla, zygoma, ethmoid, sphenoid, palatine, frontal, and lacrimal (Fig. 9–1). The orbits have each base directed forward, downward, and outward. The widest diameter is about 1 cm inward from the orbital rims. The angle between the lateral orbital walls is 90 degrees, but between the medial and lateral walls it is only 45 degrees. The medial walls are almost parallel. The orbital region is traversed by several bony support beams permitting suspension of the facial skeleton from the cranium. Vertically, it is the zygomatico-frontal process of the zygoma, jointly with the zygomatic process of the frontal bone, which forms the lateral buttress in conjunction with the pterygoid plates. Medially, this buttress is formed by the nasal process of the maxilla with the nasal process of the frontal bone. Horizontally, the support buttresses run through the superior and inferior orbital rims (Fig. 9–2). The support beams are considered high-resistance bones because it takes between 80 and 200 g (a unit expressing force in excess of gravity) of impact to produce a fracture. The conglomerate of bones forming the orbital space permits entrance of soft-tissue structures through several fissures and foramina which are clinically significant (Fig. 9–3).

Foramina

The *optic foramen* is formed by the sphenoid bone and is located in the apex of the orbit. It permits

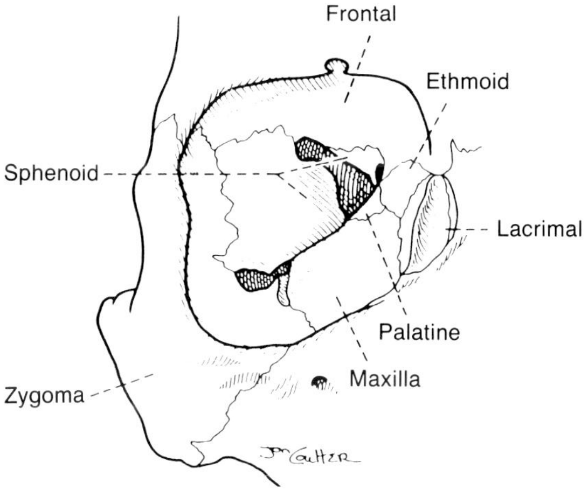

Figure 9–1 Osseous structures of the orbit.

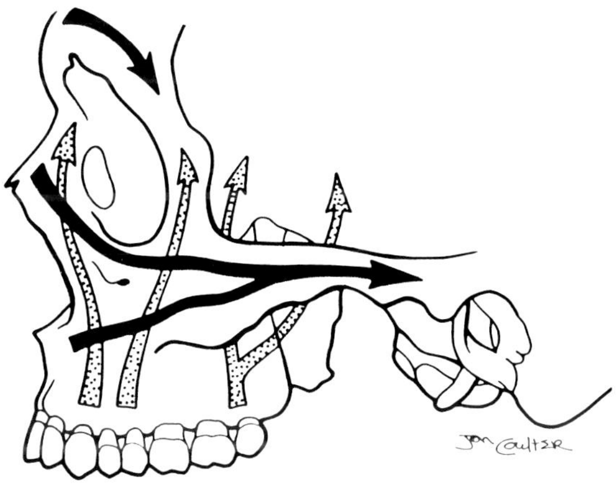

Figure 9–2 Support struts of the orbital region. (Adapted from Foster CA, Sherman JG, eds. Surgery of facial bone fractures. New York: Churchill Livingstone, 1987.)

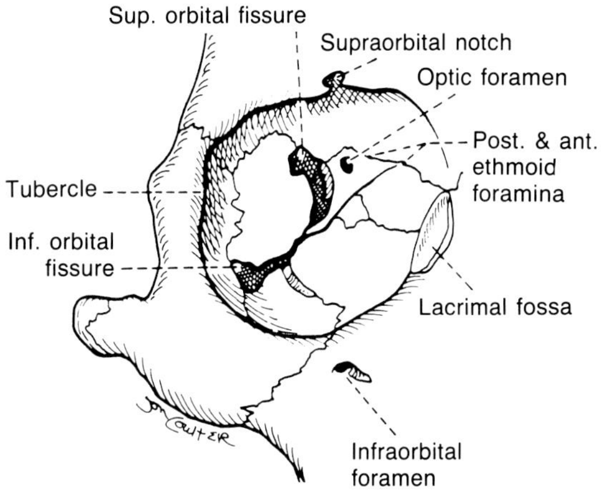

Figure 9–3 Fissures and foramina of the orbit.

passage of the optic nerve and ophthalmic artery to the orbit.

If the optic nerve is injured or severed, the patient will develop the Marcus Gunn pupil (an afferent pupillary defect can be observed). The pupil of the involved optic nerve has minimal or no reaction to light but does react consensually. It is a pupillary contraction to light entering the opposite normal eye which also produces narrowing of the pupil on the involved side. The mechanism is an intact efferent pupillary reflex on the affected side. Without treatment, recovery of sight after optic nerve injury is expected in less than 16 percent of patients. Initially steroids are used following injury, but when no improvement ensues or sight worsens, decompression of the optic nerve can be considered; the frontosphenoid approach with removal of 50 percent of the circumference of the optic canal is used. Other approaches have been described either through the ethmoid and maxillary sinus or through the transorbital route. Scattered data support this concept of surgical intervention.

Ethmoid foramina (anterior and posterior) are formed within the frontoethmoid suture and contain corresponding arteries; the anterior ethmoidal branch and the sphenoethmoidal branch of the nasociliary nerve (from the ophthalmic division of the trigeminal nerve) enter the anterior and posterior ethmoid foramina, respectively.

The *infraorbital canal* ends as a foramen on the anterior aspect of the maxilla and guides the infraorbital nerve (from the second division of the trigeminal nerve) and artery (a branch of the internal maxillary artery).

Infraorbital anesthesia is present in more than 50 percent of patients with zygomatico-orbital fractures.

Fissures

Superior orbital fissure (Fig. 9–4) is also in the apex of the orbit and is formed by the lesser and greater wings of the sphenoid as well as the sphenoid sinus. It contains oculomotor (III), trochlear (IV), trigeminal (lacrimal, frontal, and nasociliary branches of V_1), and abducens (VI) nerves as well as sympathetic fibers from the cavernous sinus plexus entering the globe. The recurrent branch of the lacrimal artery, superior and inferior ophthalmic veins, as well as the orbital branch of the middle meningeal artery also enter the orbit through this fissure.

Superior orbital fissure syndrome includes a dilated pupil, eyelid ptosis, and extraocular muscle dysfunction due to injury to cranial nerves III and IV.

Orbital apex syndrome results from the combination of superior orbital fissure syndrome and optic nerve injury.

The *inferior orbital fissure* is between the floor of the orbit (roof of the maxilla) and lateral orbital wall (formed by the zygoma and the greater wing of the sphenoid). It communicates with the infratemporal fossa. It is traversed by the trigeminal nerve (V_2–maxillary division) which terminates as the infraorbital, anterior, and middle superior alveolar and zygomatic nerves. Also, the infraorbital artery, branches of the inferior ophthalmic vein, and branches of sphenopalatine ganglion are found in this fissure.

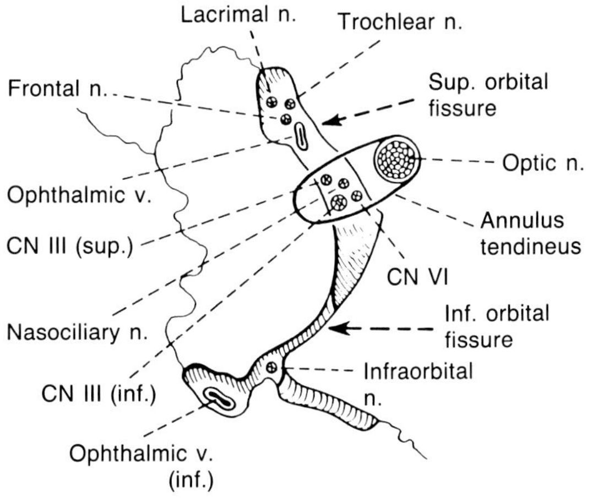

Figure 9–4 Orbital apex.

Orbital Boundaries

The *floor of the orbit* begins with the orbital rim anteriorly which ends medially as the anterior lacrimal crest. The floor receives contributions from three bones—maxilla, zygoma, and the palatine; it is the second thinnest wall of the orbital vault in its posterior portion, where it is continuous with the lamina papyracea of the ethmoid bone. The inferior oblique muscle originates from the medial aspect of the floor just lateral to the nasolacrimal canal.

The orbital floor may or may not be fractured in its entirety (including the rim). In the case of an intact orbital rim, it has been termed "blowout" fracture because of the theoretical concept of sudden posterior displacement of the noncompressible globe which would then cause fractures in the weakest wall of the orbit. The more plausible theory is one emphasizing buckling of the orbital framework causing fractures of the thin, nonelastic components of the orbital framework, e.g., the orbital floor, but not the rim. The bony fragments are displaced inferiorly. If the fracture is comminuted, they remain as free fragments in the maxillary antrum; if they retain some attachment to the orbital floor, they may trap orbital soft tissue (fat, inferior rectus or inferior oblique muscles) and cause limitation in upward gaze. Infraorbital nerve anesthesia is frequent (50 percent of cases). Diplopia is present in 25 percent of cases secondary to fixation of the soft tissue at the site of fracture or entrapment of the inferior rectus muscle by the fracture margin. Injuries to the globe are present in about 4 percent of blowout fractures and in more than 6 percent of orbital rim fractures.

The *lateral orbital wall* is formed primarily by the zygoma and the greater wing of the sphenoid. It contains the tuberculum of Whitnall where the lateral canthal tendon attaches as well as the lateral retinaculum of Hesser (the check ligaments of the lateral rectus muscle, the suspensory ligament of Lockwood, and the lateral extension of the levator muscle aponeurosis). It is located about 1 cm below the zygomaticofrontal suture and 2 mm into the orbit. The outside (lateral) structure of the orbit is the infratemporal fossa, containing the temporalis muscle, and posterolaterally it is the middle cranial fossa (Fig. 9–5).

Separation of the attachment from the tubercle results in shortening and rounding of the palpebral fissure. If the orbital floor is comminuted and cannot provide solid support to the globe, the lateral retinaculum provides the only additional horizontal support to orbital soft tissue. If both structures are dislodged a significant lid and globe malposition results.

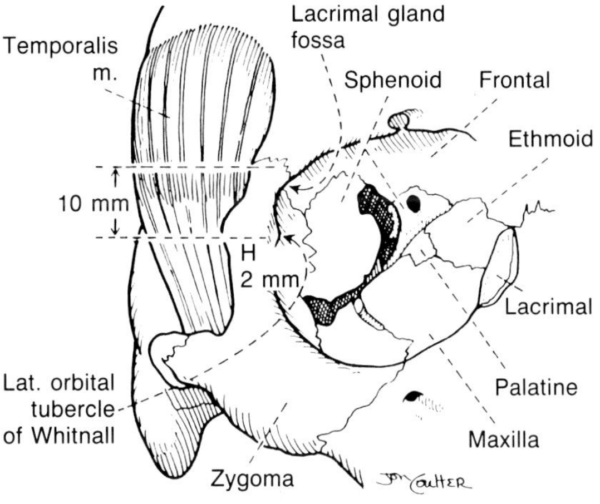

Figure 9–5 Lateral orbital wall.

The *superior orbital wall* is formed mainly by the frontal bone; a small contribution comes from the lesser wing of the sphenoid. The superior orbital notch (in 25 percent of patients it is a true canal and foramen) is located about 2.5 cm lateral to the midline. It guides the supraorbital nerve and artery. The supratrochlear artery and nerve pass medially to this notch. About 5 mm posteriorly is the trochlea, where a cartilaginous pulley of the superior oblique muscle is attached. The orbital roof can be pneumatized by frontal or ethmoid sinuses (which have a common embryologic origin) and therefore may be as thin as 1 mm (Fig. 9–6). Superior to the orbit is the anterior cranial cavity.

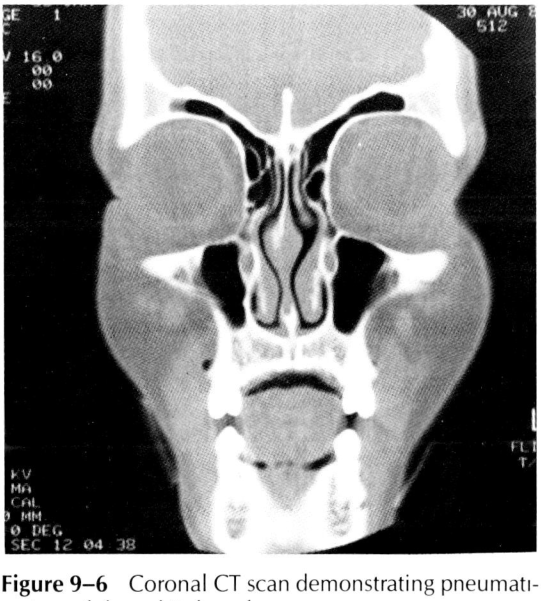

Figure 9–6 Coronal CT scan demonstrating pneumatization of the orbital roof.

Fractures of the superior orbital roof involve the frontal bone and frequently its sinus (Fig. 9–7). It is the posterior frontal sinus wall fracture that has to be specifically evaluated and treated because 50 percent of patients with frontal sinus fractures have dural tears and 30 percent of them have brain lesions.[2,3]

The *medial orbital wall* is jointly formed by the frontal and ethmoid bones which meet at the frontoethmoidal suture. The anterior and posterior ethmoid foramina pass through this suture. A small skeletal contribution comes from the lacrimal bone anteriorly. The medial orbital wall is also known as the lamina papyracea, reflecting its paper-thin consistency (Fig. 9–8). The lacrimal fossa is a concavity within the lacrimal bone at the anteromedial aspect of the orbit. Its boundaries are distinctly formed by the anterior lacrimal crest (a termination of the inferior orbital rim) and by the posterior lacrimal crest (the final medial and inferior extent of the superior orbital rim). It houses the lacrimal sac. Medial to the orbit is the ethmoid labyrinth.

The medial orbital wall is the most frequently fractured structure of the orbital complex. The intraorbital soft tissue (with medial rectus muscle) may herniate medially by the same mechanism that causes orbital floor fractures and is often missed (Fig. 9–9). Intraorbital space is delineated by the ethmoid labyrinth with middle turbinates laterally. The roof is formed by the cribriform plate and superior turbinates (Fig. 9–10).

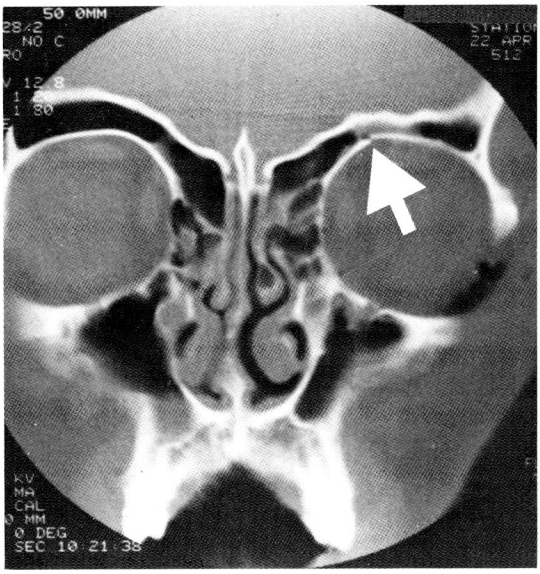

Figure 9–7 Coronal CT scan outlining a fracture of the left orbital roof into the frontal sinus (arrow).

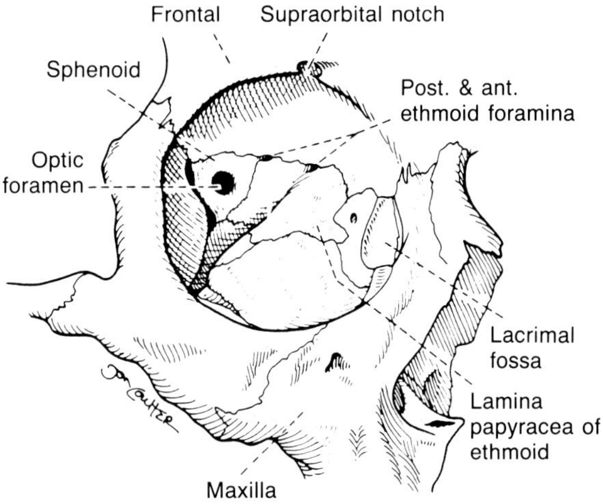

Figure 9–8 Medial orbital wall.

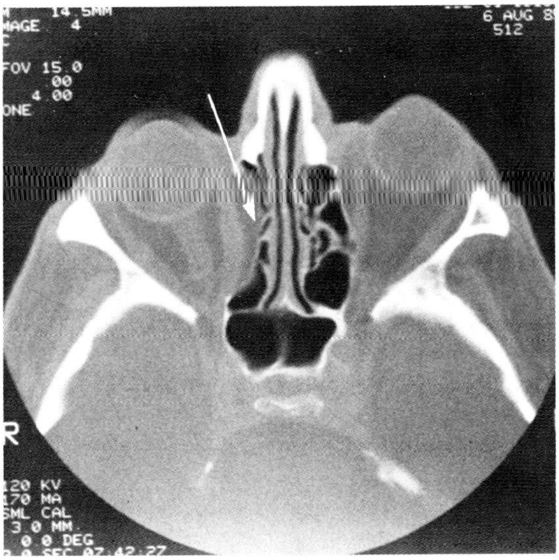

Figure 9–9 Axial CT scan depicting an old fracture of the right medial orbital wall; the proximity of the medial rectus muscle is also seen (arrow).

The junction of the cribriform plate and the roof of the ethmoid is the weakest portion of the roof of the interorbital space. The dura is intimately adherent to the thin bones in that location. Fractures of this area result in frequent loss of the sense of smell and cerebrospinal fluid (CSF) leak.

Associated Injuries

One of the most important steps in evaluating and treating facial fractures is the diagnosis of associated

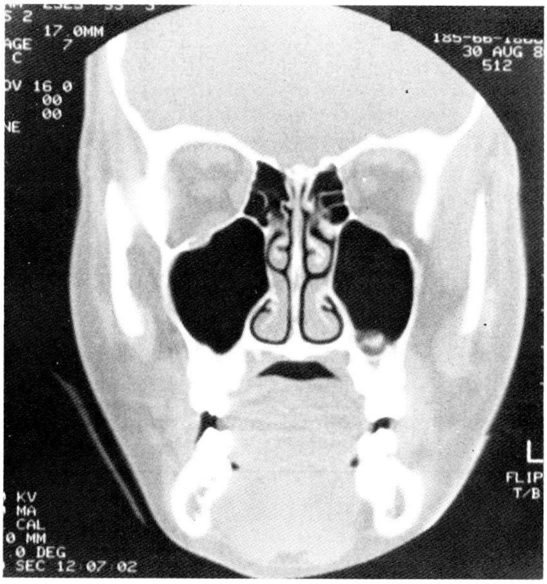

Figure 9–10 Coronal CT scan delineating the interorbital space.

injuries. There is a direct correlation between fractures of high-resistance bones (e.g., supraorbital ridge) and the occurrence (50 percent) of life-threatening injuries (e.g., central nervous system involvement). The high incidence of life-threatening injuries is secondary to the fact that high-resistance bones transmit the injuring force directly to vital structures. Low-resistance bones, on the other hand, collapse and absorb most of the impact. High-velocity accidents (e.g., motor vehicle crashes) have a 60 percent chance of associated injuries, 30 percent of which can be life threatening. In comparison, low-velocity accidents (e.g., assault, fall) cause associated injuries in 14 percent of patients, with only a 4 percent chance of a life-threatening injury.[4]

DIAGNOSIS

The correct assessment of facial injury requires accurate history, clinical examination, and radiographic evaluation at the time of injury, and at frequent intervals afterward if progression of injury is suspected.

The essentials of the *history* would include medical status of the patient prior to the accident and knowledge of the cause of the injury as well as the level of function of vital organs immediately following the injury. The type of injury, the size of the injuring object, and the direction of the injuring force are also helpful to know.

A high-impact force, such as in motor vehicle accidents, is associated with more extensive fractures, as well as with a greater number of associated injuries. Knowledge of the baseline function of vital as well as significant organs (eye, facial nerve) at the time of injury permits the physician a greater degree of clinical judgment when the patient is later seen in the emergency room. It is the stabilization, worsening, or improvement of the individual organ function which gives us valuable information on which we can act and with which we can potentially salvage diminishing sight or treat an expanding central nervous system injury.

Clinical examination assesses function of vital organs (circulatory, respiratory, and central nervous system). The exclusion of associated injuries (extremities and abdomen are the most frequent sites) is an essential part of the initial clinical evaluation. At this point, specific assessment of the naso-orbital fractures is made. There are several basic steps fundamental to all clinical examinations: external observation, palpation, and internal visualization.

External observation evaluates the appearance of the injured area (Fig. 9–11). Swelling with ecchymosis points to a specific site of injury but may mask gross bony displacement. Symmetry of malar eminence, orbital rims, interorbital and interpupillary distance, nasofrontal prominence (altered symmetry and prominence indicates displaced bones), shape of palpebral fissure (change would indicate rupture of canthal ligaments, medial or lateral or both), position of lids as well as of the globe should all be checked. The direction and extent of lacerations are also assessed.

Palpation first verifies findings from external observation (e.g., stability of the orbital and nasal framework, canthal ligaments, globe). The presence of subcutaneous emphysema is ascertained, as well as sensory changes in supraorbital and infraorbital nerve distribution. Ocular and lid movement is checked, as well as the presence or absence of diplopia (Fig. 9–12).

Internal visualization further confirms findings from external observation and palpation. Through-and-through lacerations of the lids are verified. Globe examination should include its position within the orbit in addition to evaluation of the cornea for abrasion or tears, blood in the anterior chamber, pupillary reflex, as well as vitreous, retinal, and disc status. An assessment of visual acuity must be attempted. A slit-lamp evaluation by an ophthalmologist is the most accurate.

Radiographic evaluation of extensive facial injuries should cover three areas: the primary site of

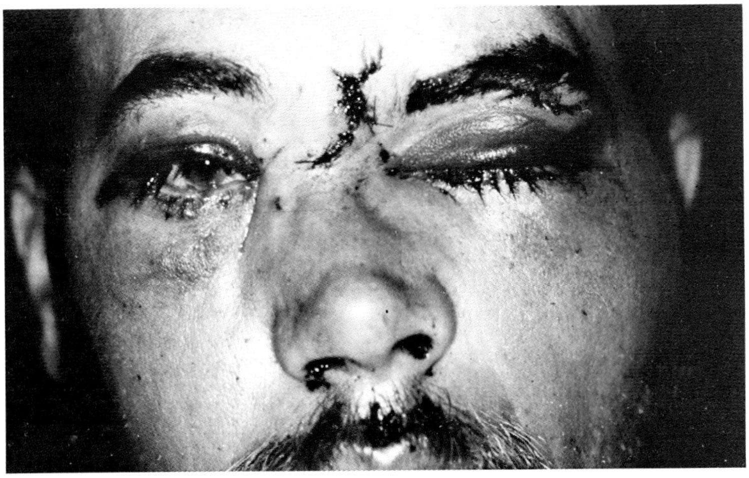

Figure 9–11 Patient who sustained nasoethmoid fracture.

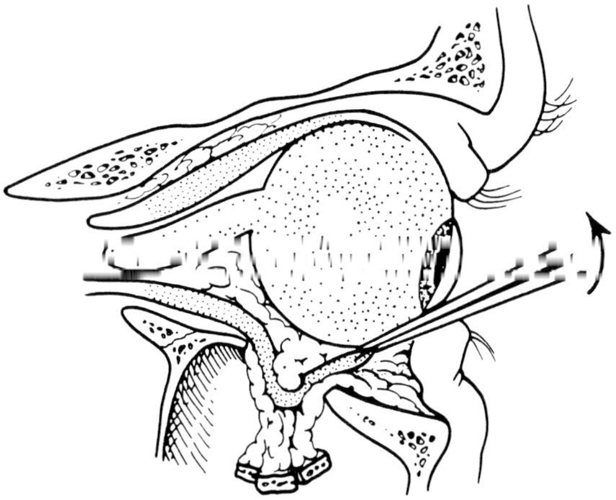

Figure 9–12 Traction test of inferior rectus muscle checks the extent of muscle and globe movement. (Adapted from Converse JM, Smith B, Obear MF, Woodsmith D. Orbital blowout fractures: a ten-year survey. Plast Reconstr Surg 1967; 39:20–36.

injury, cranium, and cervical spine. Given the advent of computerized tomography (CT) and recent advances in the clarity of bone algorithms, the primary method of evaluating facial fractures is now CT scanning. Its ability to give us accurate information in the axial plane and true or reconstructed coronal and sagittal views (Fig. 9–13 A,B) provides the most detailed analysis of fractures and surrounding soft tissues. Three-dimensional reconstructions may also be helpful (Fig. 9–14). In addition to bony alignment, we can evaluate with CT scan the presence of air (Fig. 9–15) or blood in the orbit or intracranial cavity, intracerebral or intraocular fragments or foreign bodies, position of the globe, and the optic nerve and extraocular muscles.

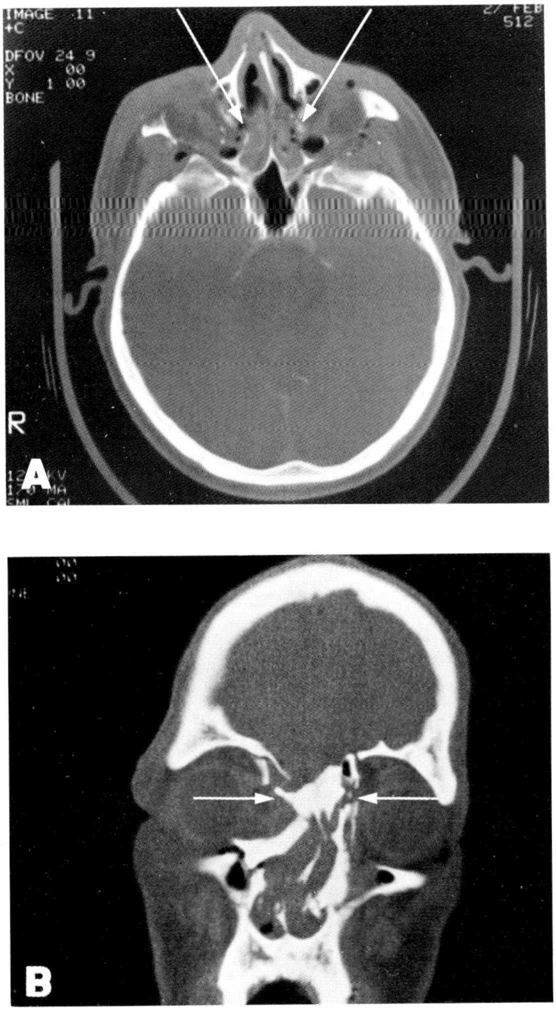

Figure 9–13 *A*, Axial and *B*, Coronal CT scan outlining extensive nasoethmoid and orbital fractures (arrows).

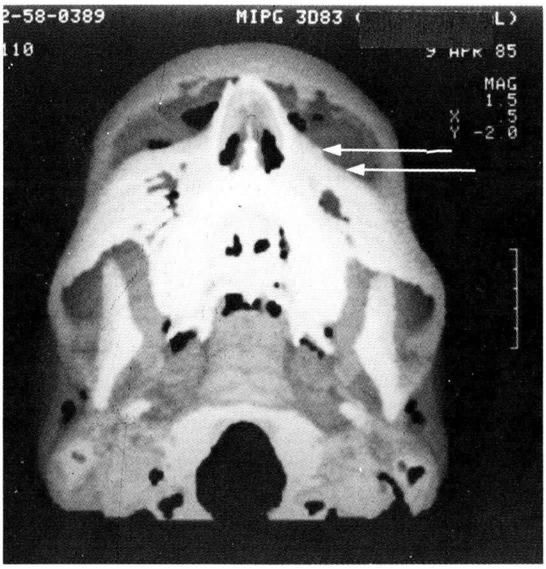

Figure 9–14 Three-dimensional CT reconstruction of an old orbitomaxillary fracture demonstrating an inferior displacement of the left malar eminence (arrows).

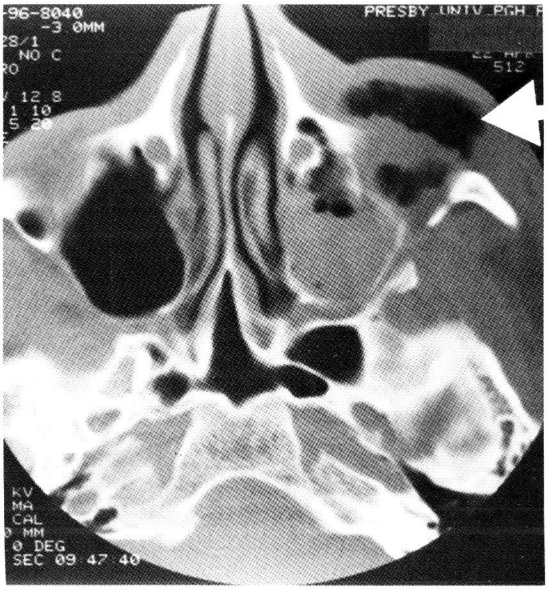

Figure 9–15 CT scan showing air in left orbital soft tissue (arrow).

The presence or absence of normal air contrast in all periorbital sinuses is a valuable guide to sites of additional fractures which cause mucosal hemorrhage and thus air replacement in individual sinuses. Plain radiographs are still useful in evaluation of some facial fractures. For example, the floor of the orbit can be examined by the Waters' view, which demonstrates two parallel lines at the normal orbital floor: first, the most superior, is the orbital rim, and the second is the floor proper; this is due to the concavity of the floor and head-upward rotation during the taking of the Waters' radiograph) (Fig. 9–16). The submentovertex view identifies the maxillary line jointly with lateral orbital projection and the middle cranial fossa perimeter.

TREATMENT

Reestablishment of a normal bony architecture with proper midfacial height, projection, and definition of facial contour lines should be the aim of the repair of nasoethmoid and orbital fractures. This is accomplished by repositioning of displaced bones and their fragments or substitution of missing parts with autogenous bone grafts. This should be done by recreating the main vertical and horizontal support buttresses of the orbital skeleton (the nasomaxillary and the zygomatic frontal

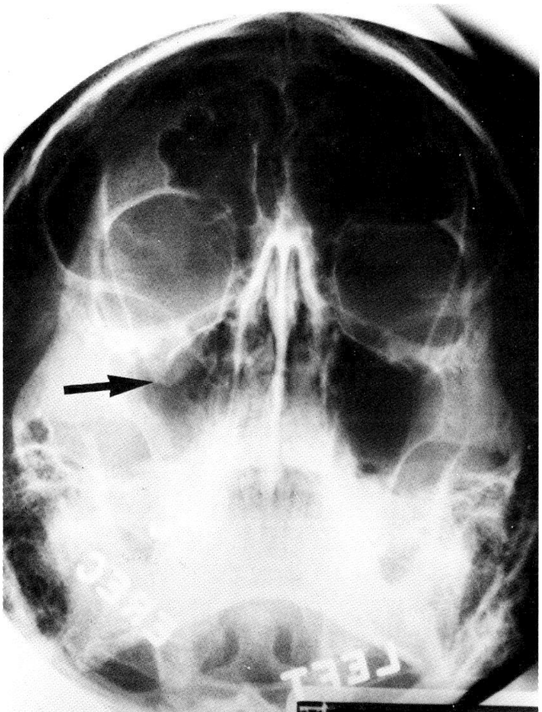

Figure 9–16 Waters' view outlining the two parallel lines of the left orbital rim and floor; a fracture of right orbital floor is seen with herniation of soft tissue into the maxillary antrum (arrow).

struts) as well as the superior and inferior orbital rims. Direct loop wiring or miniplate fixation (Fig. 9–17) ensures stability and should be done from one stable point to another in at least two or possibly three planes. This prevents possible regression or rotation of repositioned bone secondary to soft-tissue pull. In comminuted fractures, the technique of interfragment loop wiring permits salvage of free segments of bone, provided the surrounding soft tissue is adequate and viable.

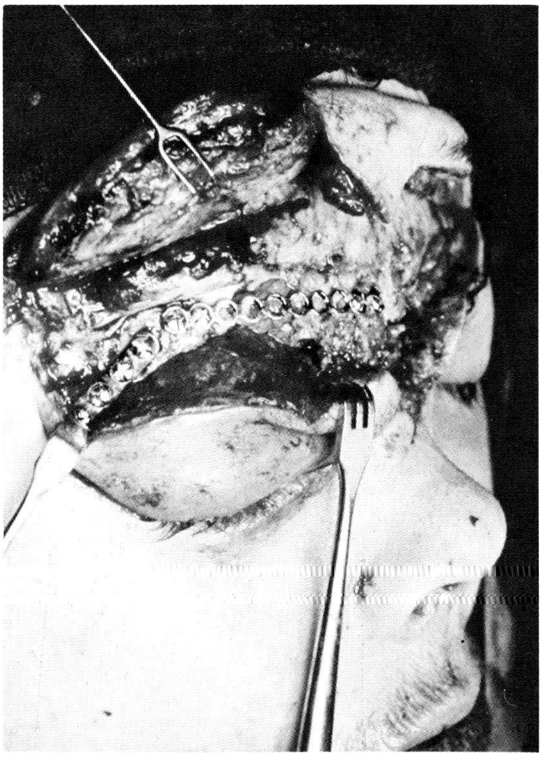

Figure 9–17 Use of miniplates for stabilization of orbital fracture through existing laceration.

Missing or multifragmented segments of bones should be replaced by autogenous bone grafts. The bones can be obtained from either the cranium or chest wall. The availability of contoured cranial bone grafts, which are considered the least resorbable of all free bone grafts, makes the cranial bone graft the first choice for cranio-orbital and nasoethmoid reconstruction.[5] The frequently seen retrusion of nasoethmoid complex into the interorbital space is also handled by direct open reduction, fixation, and/or bone grafting. This gives better results than did previously used headframes for correction of nasoethmoid retrusion.

Alloplastic biomaterials such as acrylic, silicon, polyethylene, and Teflon are seldom used in the acute repair of extensive nasoethmoid or cranio-orbital fractures owing to their potential for subsequent infection and/or extrusion even years after the injury. Only in isolated bony defects of the orbit could such materials be considered.

The surgical approach uses a bicoronal incision with anterior deflection of the frontoparietal scalp (Fig. 9–18). This exposure ensures good access to the roof of the orbit as well as to the naso-orbital region. Also, the frontal bone, its sinuses, and the anterior cranial fossa can be entered simultaneously. The availability of pericranial flap, which can be raised from the undersurface of the bi-

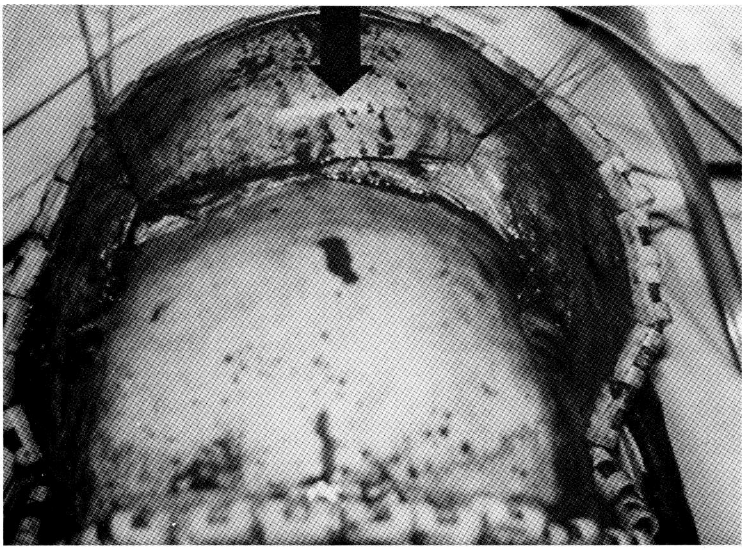

Figure 9–18 A reflected bicoronal flap (arrow) over anterior facial region with an excellent exposure to the anterior cranium.

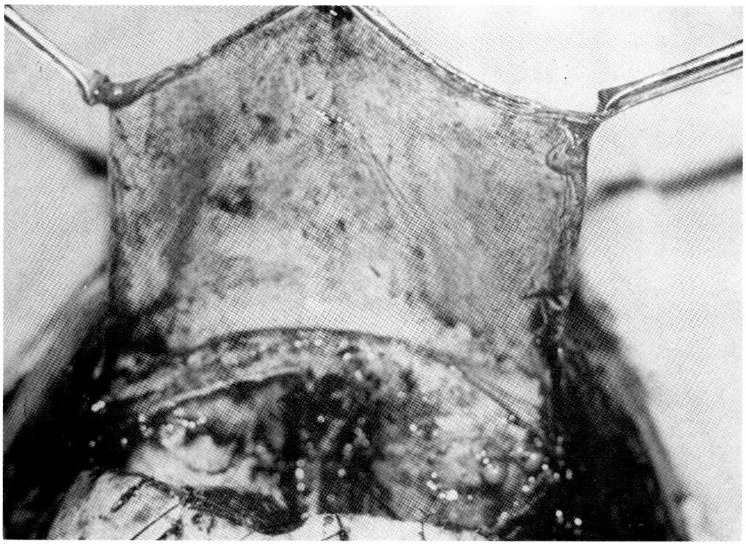

Figure 9–19 A pericranial flap raised over orbital rims and ready for placement between the anterior cranial base and orbitoethmoidal area.

coronal flap and based on one or both of the supratrochlear and supraorbital vessels, offers the opportunity to separate the anterior cranial cavity from the orbit, sinuses, or nasopharynx in cases where these structures are concomitantly involved with the cranial cavity (Fig. 9–19).

Additional approaches are often necessary to secure adequate exposure to the orbit and the nasoethmoid region. They follow the principles of aesthetic facial lines. For access to the orbital floor, the incision of choice is along the natural skin crease, halfway between the ciliary margin and orbital rim, providing excellent visualization of the bones and a satisfactory aesthetic result. The same incision can be used for exploration and repair of the lacrimal sac. Other approaches to the orbital floor, such as the cheek incision and the transconjunctival incision, have been used. A lateral rhinotomy is a time-tested approach to the naso-orbital and nasoethmoid regions which permits direct visualization and repair of intra- as well as perinasal structures (Fig. 9–20).

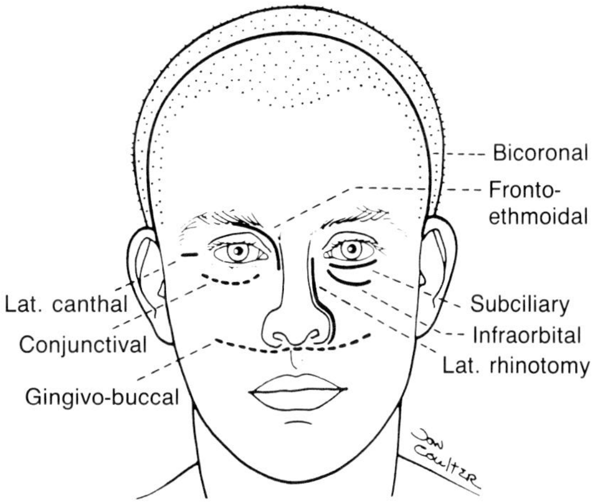

Figure 9–20 Incisions available for direct approach to facial fractures.

Specific Repairs

Canthal Ligaments

In naso-orbital fractures the medial canthus is most frequently displaced laterally (Fig. 9–21*A, B*) causing traumatic telecanthus.[6] (An intact medial canthal ligament can be palpated during a traction test [Fig. 9–22].) The medial canthal ligaments must be repositioned medially and posteriorly; overcorrection is suggested. If the opposite nasoethmoid area is intact, fixation wires can be passed transnasally and affixed to each other (Fig. 9–23). If one or both sides are comminuted, internal fixation to bone grafts spanning the size of each defect can be employed with corresponding medial canthal ligaments attached to them (Fig. 9–24). An external plate fixation would be the third choice, only if internal fixation could not be achieved.

Lacrimal Apparatus

The lacrimal apparatus is almost always involved in nasoethmoid injuries. The nasolacrimal duct, ex-

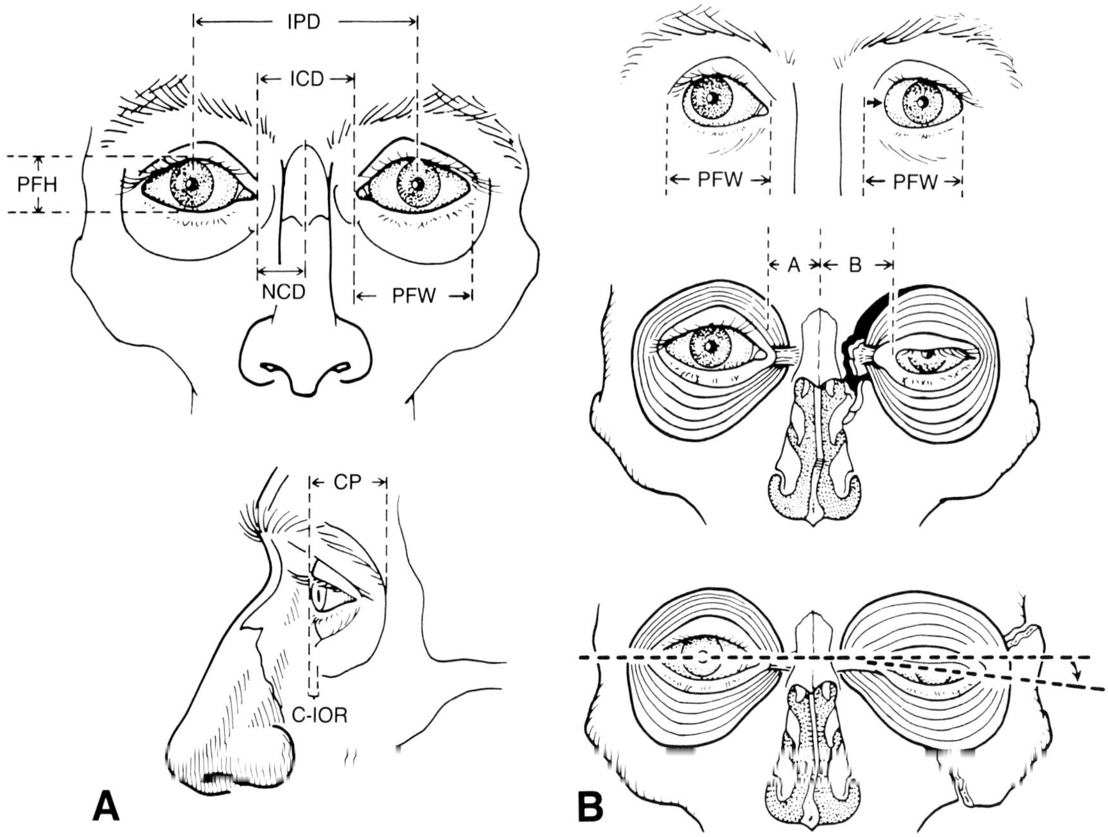

Figure 9–21 *A*, Normal lid position and shape with intact medial and lateral canthal ligaments. PFH = palpebral fissure height; IPD = interpupillary distance; ICD = intercanthal distance; NCD = nasocanthal distance; PFW = palpebral fissure width; C-IOR = cornea/inferior orbital rim distance; CP = cornea/palpebral distance. *B*, Changes in shape and width of palpebral fissure following canthal disruption. (Fig. 21*A* adapted from Marsh JL. Blepharo-canthal deformities in patients following craniofacial surgery. Plast Reconstr Surg 1978; 61:842–853.)

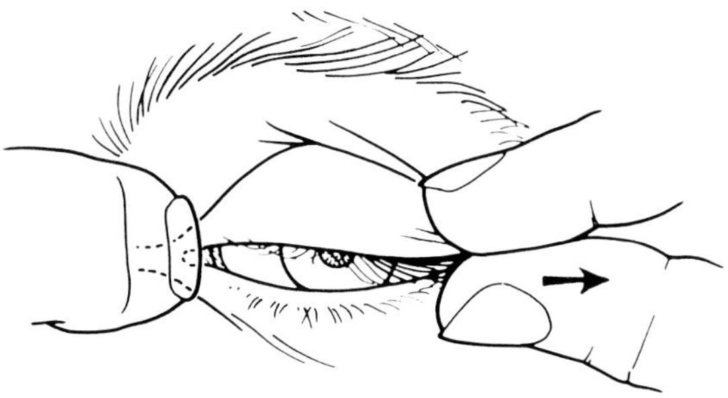

Figure 9–22 A finger palpating the medial canthal ligament during a traction test.

iting under the inferior turbinate, is most frequently obstructed at its exit into the inferior nasal meatus. An avulsion of the medial canthal ligament frequently results in an injury to the canaliculi or the lacrimal sac. A direct repair, under magnification, with placement of a Silastic stent from the punctum to the nose would be the treatment of choice. Special Silastic tubes with a blunt needle are available for such repairs.

Tears

Tears are essential for the health and visual function of the cornea. They provide a gliding surface for eyelids, irrigate the eye, and provide a source of oxygen for the normal cornea as well as white blood cells for an injured cornea. They also distribute antibacterial agents and antibodies, as well as eliminate desquamated epithelium.

Most of the tears ($\geq$90 percent) are secreted from the main lacrimal gland at the rate of 1 to 2 ml per minute. The precorneal and conjunctival volume is about 5 to 10 ml. The precorneal film

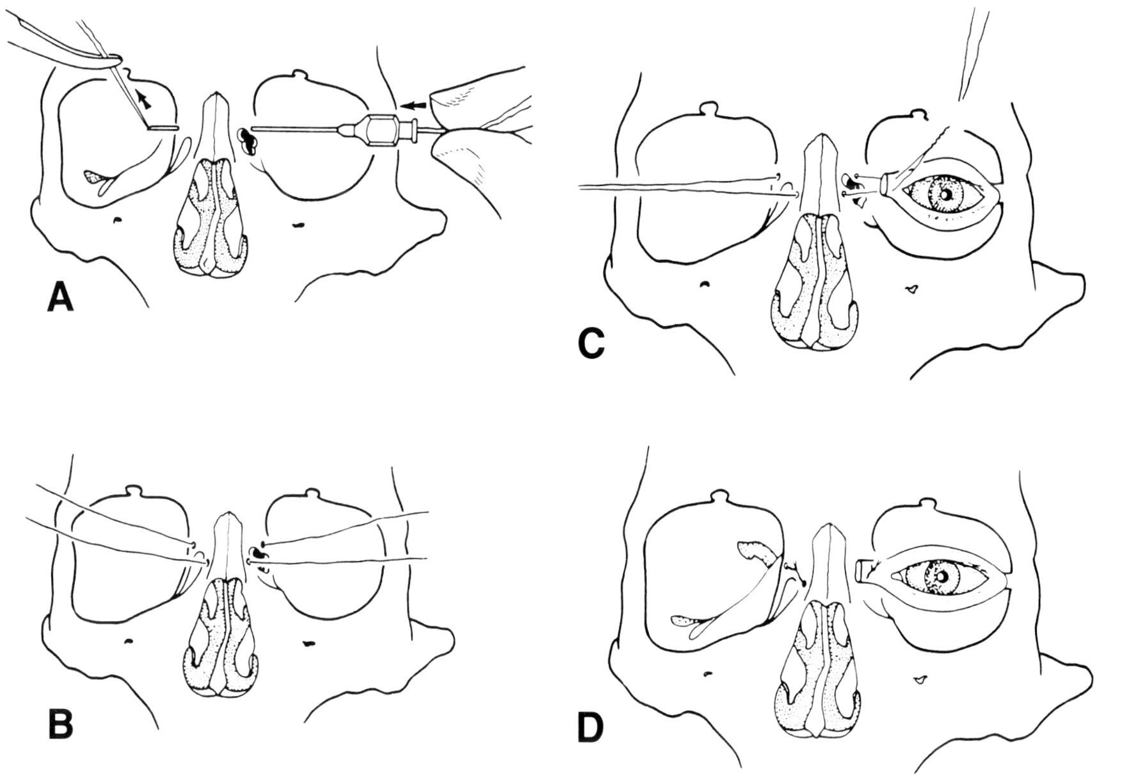

Figure 9–23 Fixation of medial canthal ligament. (Adapted from Tessier P, Callahan A, Mustarde J, Salyer KE, eds. Symposium on plastic surgery in the orbital region. St. Louis: CV Mosby, 1976.)

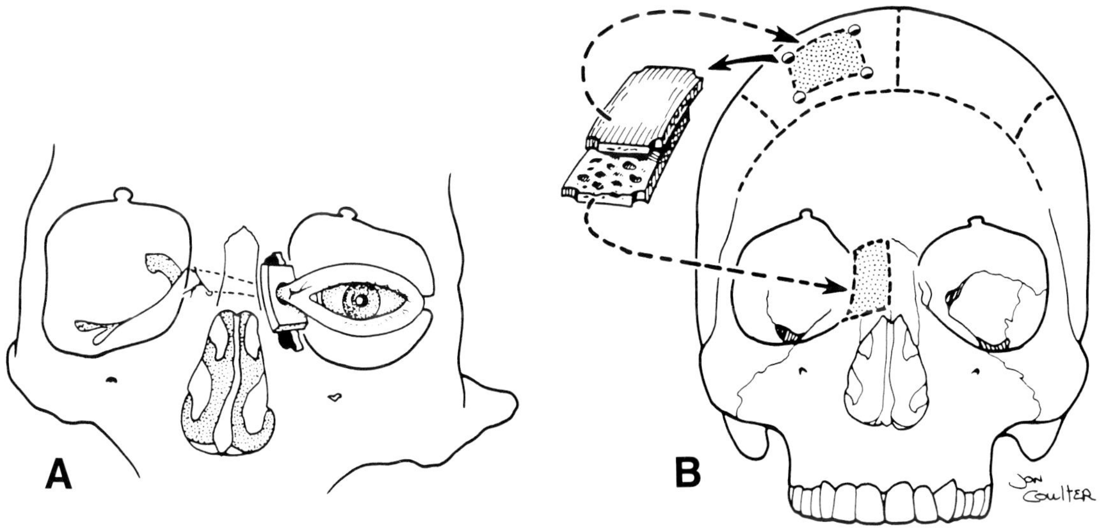

Figure 9–24 *A*, Medial canthal fixation to a bone graft. *B*, Harvesting and placement of cranial bone graft to naso-orbital region. The cranial bone was split and one-half returned to repair the donor site. (Fig. 24*B* adapted from Foster CA, Sherman JE, eds. Surgery of facial bone fractures. New York: Churchill Livingstone, 1987).

is about 5 to 10 μm thick and has three layers: an outside meibomian lipid layer, the middle aqueous zone (the largest), and a thin mucin layer facing the epithelial surface. The balance between secretion and elimination of tears is maintained by the blinking reflex which activates the lacrimal pump (empties the ampulla of the lacrimal sac). The capillary action of the thin lacrimal canaliculi guides tears of the conjunctival film into the lacrimal ampulla. Evaporation accounts for only 10 to 20 percent of tear loss, but without blinking it increases 10 to 20 fold. The anatomy of the lid margin and its close apposition to the globe are essential to a smooth flow of tears toward the point of drainage at the medial canthus. Nasoethmoid fractures with traumatic telecanthus and slackening of the lower lid interfere with tear guidance along lid margin and tear elimination via the lacrimal pump.

Timing of Surgery

There are only a few reasons for an immediate exploration of nasoethmoid or cranio-orbital fractures. Deteriorating vision, CSF leak, and dural or brain herniation would constitute strong indications for rapid repair. In other patients, some delay to permit precise radiographic and patient systemic evaluation, and swelling regression, is beneficial.

COMPLICATIONS

Early Complications

Bleeding occurs with any trauma causing nasoethmoid or orbital fractures. In most patients it is limited to a subcutaneous and intraosseous hematoma. Both the internal carotid artery through the ethmoid arteries and the external carotid artery via the internal maxillary artery and its branches may contribute to acute bleeding in orbital fractures (Fig. 9–25).

Excessive *intraorbital hemorrhage* is manifested by tightness of the orbital soft tissue, limitation of ocular gaze, and possibly even an increase in the intraocular pressure. The acute treatment requires orbital decompression with evacuation of hematoma and coagulation of ethmoid arteries if they are involved. This is done through a medial orbital approach. The status of the visual acuity must be followed at close intervals. Severe *intranasal bleeding* often comes from the internal maxillary system of arteries and in nondisplaced fractures usually requires anterior and posterior

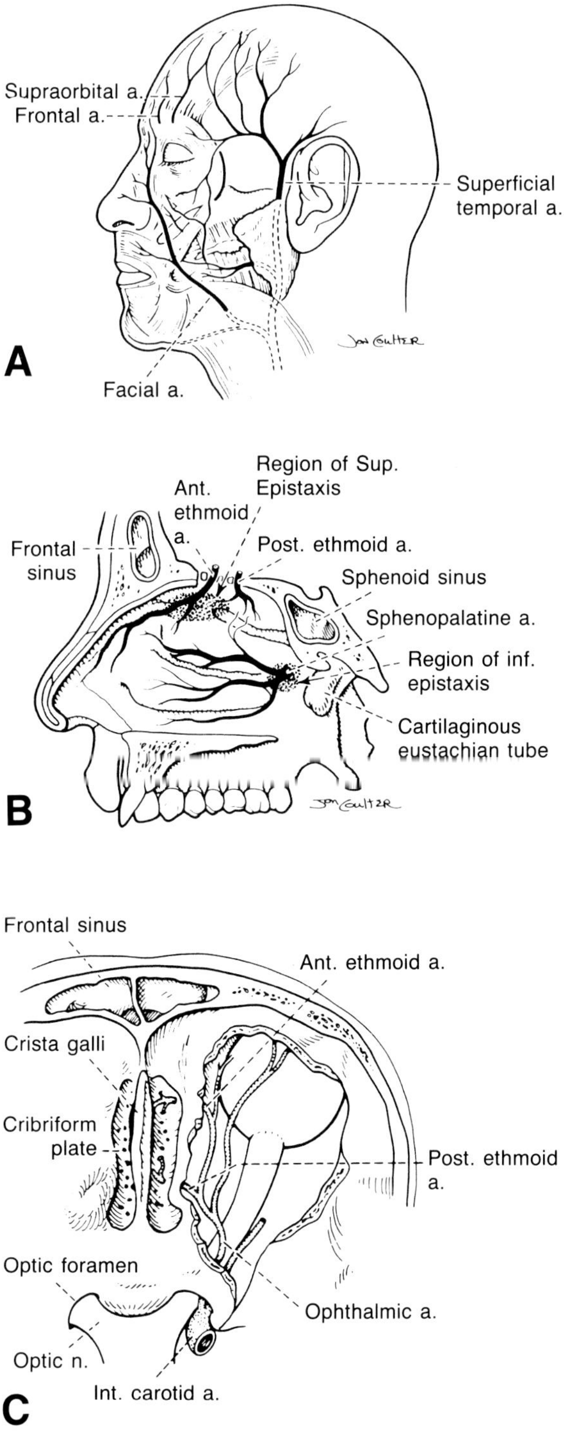

Figure 9–25 Arteries contributing to bleeding in naso-orbital fractures. *A*, External carotid branches. *B*, *C*, Internal carotid branches. (Fig. 25 *B,C* adapted from Montgomery WW, ed. Surgery of the upper respiratory system. 2nd ed. Philadelphia: Lea & Febiger, 1979.)

nasal packing (Fig. 9–26). However, if CSF leak is suspected, nasal packing may significantly increase the chance for retrograde intracranial infection. In such a case, transnasal ligation of the internal maxillary artery would be the treatment of choice.

Infection may develop early or late following nasofrontal or orbital injuries. The incidence, however, is relatively low owing to the excellent vascularity of facial soft tissue and the membranous nature of the facial skeleton. An appearance of infection will therefore raise questions regarding a possible infected hematoma, foreign body, or bony sequestrum; sinus or lacrimal obstruction also should be considered. A detailed CT scan will be helpful. If the cause is an obstruction of drainage, sinus or lacrimal, windowing the sinus or lacrimal sac usually eliminates the possibility of acquiring infection.

Antibiotic coverage should be used in established infections, guided by culture results. The use of antibiotics immediately following trauma should not be routine and should be left to the discretion of the treating surgeon. Fractures communicating with periorbital sinuses, where the possibility of a closed-space infection exists, such as in a frontal sinus and orbit, should be considered for antibiotic prophylaxis. The presence of CSF leak is a definite indication for systemic antibiotics. There is always a potential for masking early signs of meningitis with nonspecific or nontherapeutic antibiotic coverage.

Blindness is a serious complication of orbital trauma as well as orbital surgery. Direct impact may rupture the globe (Fig. 9–27) or interfere with the normal function of the optic nerve through a fronto-orbital impact on the canal or vascular compromise and a direct nerve injury. Recording the status of vision right after the injury and at frequent intervals thereafter gives us invaluable information. Progressive deterioration of visual acuity requires immediate treatment (either ocular or optic nerve decompression if technically feasible, with concomitant systemic steroids).

Diplopia is frequently present in acute orbital injuries and results from intraorbital soft-tissue swelling. The differentiation of soft-tissue and/or muscle entrapment in the fracture can be done by a "traction test." With a local anesthetic, the insertion of the inferior rectus muscle can be picked up in a forceps, and vertical excursion can be checked. In most cases, however, several days of observation, permitting resolution of the swelling, makes the differential diagnosis much easier.

Late Complications

Orbital dystopia is secondary to trauma in about 25 percent of patients (primarily following cranio-orbital fractures) and involves displacement of the orbital soft tissue due to malposition of the entire orbital framework.[7] The correction is best done in two stages: first, the bony orbit and the globe are repositioned following osteotomy and bone graft-

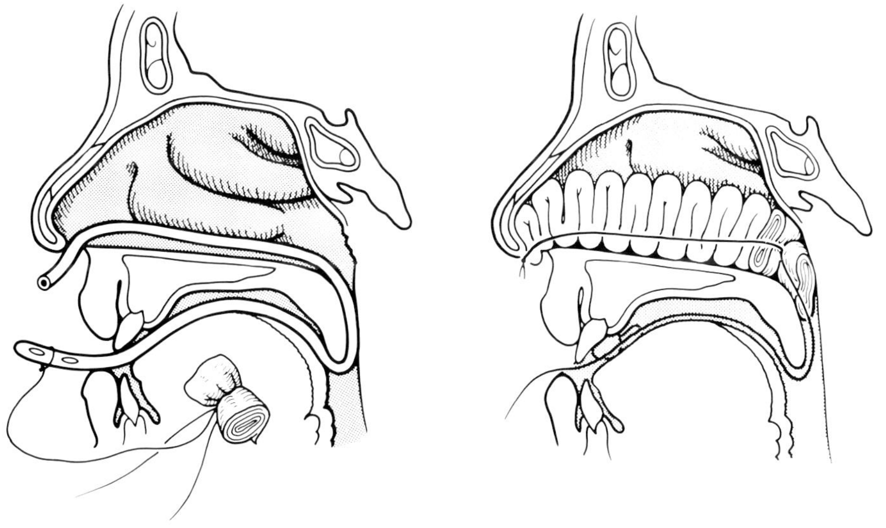

Figure 9–26 Insertion of anterior and posterior nasal packing for epistaxis. (Adapted from Montgomery WW, ed. Surgery of the upper respiratory system. 2nd ed. Philadelphia: Lea & Febiger, 1979.)

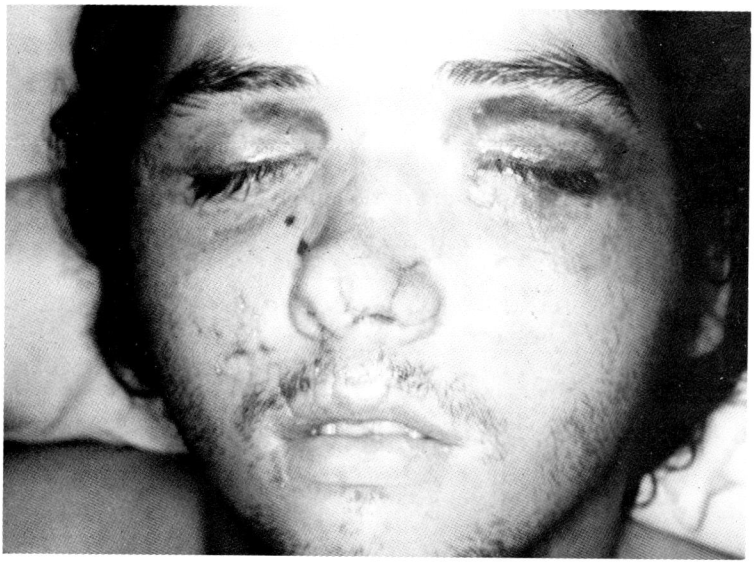

Figure 9–27 Patient who sustained bilateral globe rupture as part of his Le Fort III fracture complex. "Empty orbits" due to absence of globes are seen, as well as traumatic telecanthus.

ing. In the second stage, soft-tissue adjustment is performed, such as canthoplasty and levator shortening.

Enophthalmos results from a discrepancy between orbital bony and soft-tissue volume. Most frequently, an increase in orbital volume occurs due to the displaced orbital floor as well as soft-tissue herniation and late atrophy. All these factors contribute to an enophthalmic orbit (Fig. 9–28). The treatment should reestablish the balance of bony orbit and soft-tissue content. Repositioning of displaced orbital walls or placement of autologous bone grafts can correct the problem. Frequently, two limiting factors are found: (1) an inferiorly displaced orbital roof with corresponding adherence of dura; and (2) the atrophy and fibrosis of orbital soft tissue which does not respond adequately to an attempted repositioning of the globe. Special attention has to be given to the region of the inferior orbital fissure where it is easy for orbital soft tissue to continue to herniate.

Nasolacrimal duct obstruction is found most frequently at the exit of the duct into the inferior nasal meatus. Dacryocystorhinostomy bypasses such an obstruction by connecting the distended lacrimal sac into the nasal cavity. This procedure is indicated if the patient has several episodes of infection in the region of the lacrimal sac or if there is clear demonstration of nasolacrimal duct obstruction on dacryocystogram (Fig. 9–29). The dacryocystogram is done as follows: under topical anesthesia of the conjunctiva, the lower lacrimal punctum is cannulated with a blunt needle probe. A contrast medium is then slowly injected through this probe into the lacrimal drainage system. Tomographic radiographs help to illustrate an existing obstruction. Dacryocystorhinostomy is done through a vertical incision just inferior to the medial canthus; the periosteum of the inferior orbital rim

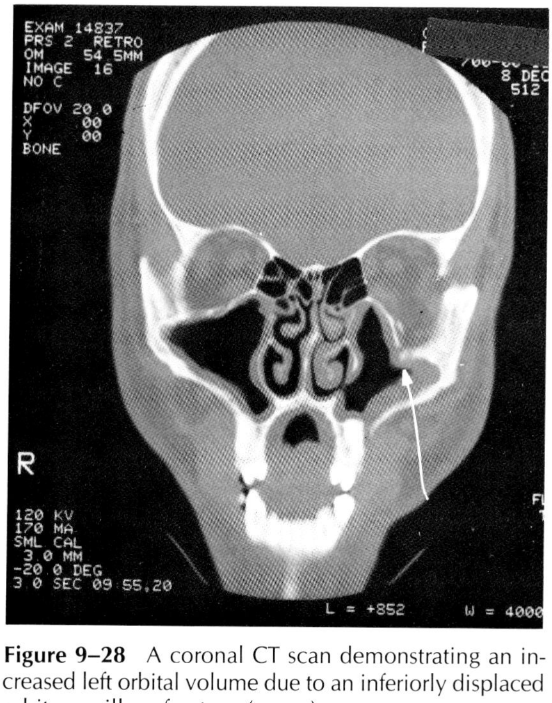

Figure 9–28 A coronal CT scan demonstrating an increased left orbital volume due to an inferiorly displaced orbitomaxillary fracture (arrow).

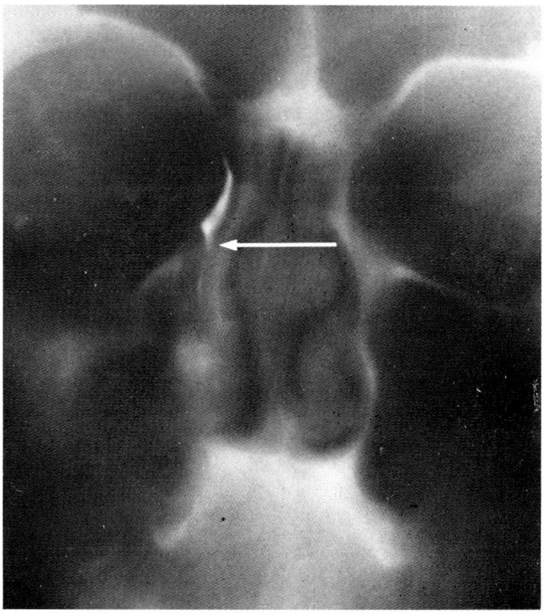

Figure 9–29 A dacryocystogram demonstrating an obstruction of right nasolacrimal duct (arrow).

and the nasal process of the maxilla are reflected. The medial aspect of the inferior orbital rim is removed with a grill for better exposure of the lacrimal sac. A fenestrum is created in the nose through the nasal process of the maxilla. Flaps are created in the nasal mucosa and the wall of the lacrimal sac. They are approximated with absorbable sutures over a silicone stent directed from the lacrimal sac into the inferior meatus of the nose. This is sutured and left in for six to eight weeks (Fig. 9–30).

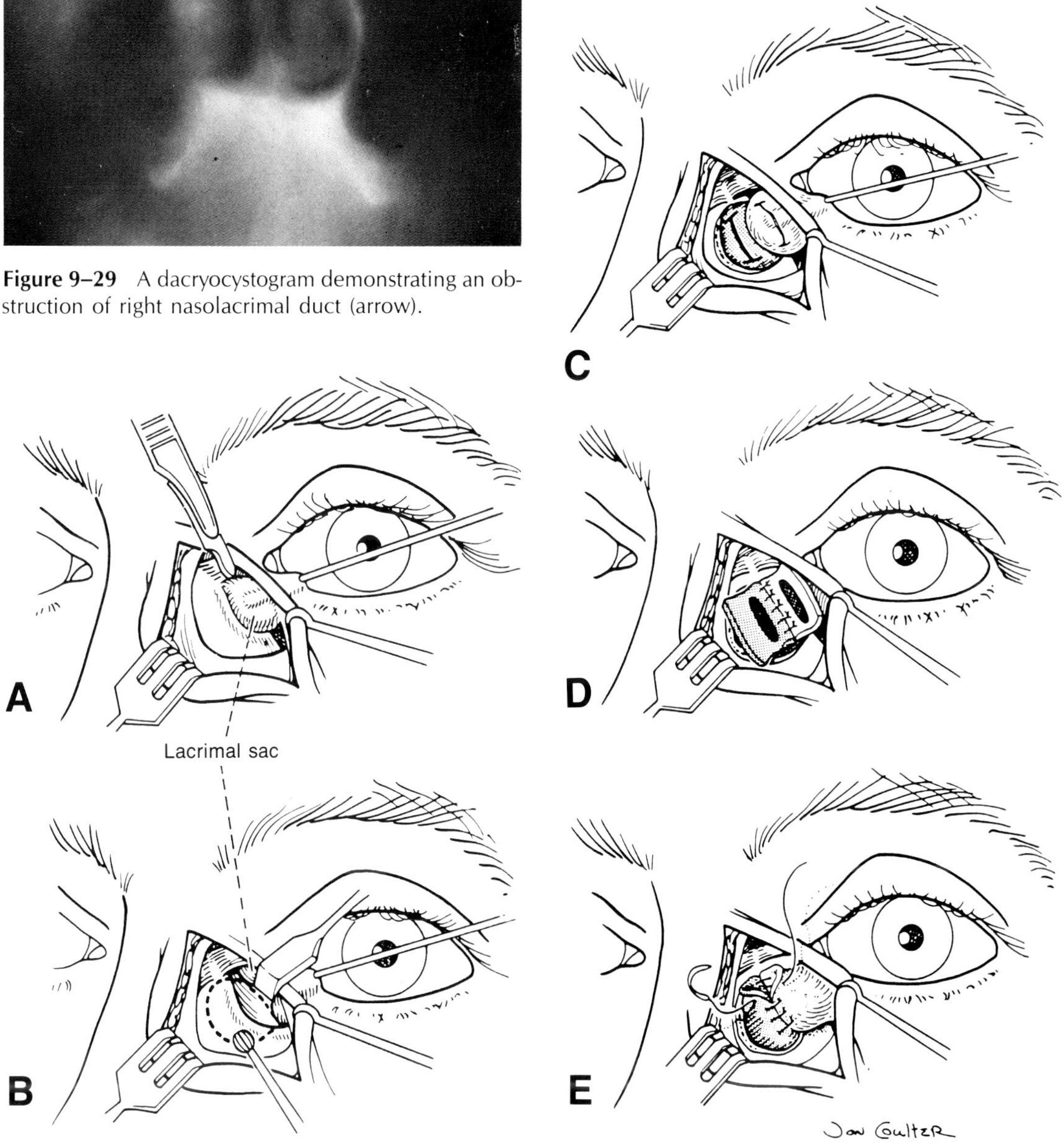

Figure 9–30 Surgical steps performed in dacryocystorhinostomy. (Adapted from Foster CA, Sherman JE, eds. Surgery of facial bone fractures. New York: Churchill Livingstone, 1987.)

Mucocele of the frontal sinus is a rare complication of frontal sinus fractures. The mucosa has to be present in the sinus with concomitant obstruction of the nasofrontal ducts to set the stage for the development of mucocele. The time delay between the injury to the sinus and the development of mucocele may be several years. The patient with a mucocele may demonstrate a mass at the superomedial aspect of the orbit which represents an erosion of the mucocele into the orbit, displacing the globe (Fig. 9–31). A less common presentation is an intracranial infection. The patient with a mucocele may also present with proptosis. Treatment requires removal of the cyst and all the remaining sinus mucosa with the use of a drill and obliteration of the nasofrontal duct with bone graft or fascial graft. Filling the entire sinus cavity with autogenous material such as free fat grafts has been used most extensively (Fig. 9–32).

Another option is to remove the posterior wall of the frontal sinus and permit theoretical expansion of the intracranial contents, brain and dura, into the sinus space. This is not a very effective method. The fibrosis of corresponding dura (from initial injury or subsequent mucocele) may significantly limit the potential for dural expansion. The elected surgical approach elected is done by raising an osteoplastic bone flap or a bifrontal craniotomy if anterior cranial fossa pathology is suspected. The skin incision used for both approaches is a standard bicoronal incision with anterior displacement of the scalp. Another incision that can be used for access to the frontal sinus is a supraorbital rim incision. It permits reasonable access to the frontal sinus and may also be aesthetically acceptable; however, it produces permanent anesthesia of the anterior scalp; eliminates the possibility of pericranial flap usage; and, if the anterior cranial cavity must be entered, it significantly limits the exposure. In an acute phase, when mucocele becomes a pyocele, it should be considered an emergency, and a direct external drainage (via the floor of the frontal sinus) should be considered.

Canthal displacement with orbital fractures may involve medial, lateral, or both canthal ligaments. It is either a ligamentous avulsion, with or without an attached bone, or a displacement of a large fragment of medial or lateral orbital wall. The clinical appearance is that of a rounded and foreshortened palpebral fissure often in association with obstruction of lacrimal drainage. The lower lid, especially in older patients, is unable to maintain an adequate tone and an ectropion often results. Canthoplasty accomplishes repositioning of the canthal ligaments in the vertical as well as the horizontal plane.

The *lateral canthoplasty* is easier to perform (usually more solid bone is available and no other structures are involved, e.g., the lacrimal system medially). The lateral ligament (which has a superior and inferior division) is identified and affixed to a new and more anatomic position on the lateral orbital rim. The repositioning of the entire lateral orbital wall often requires a secondary adjustment of the canthal position. It is done by direct sutur-

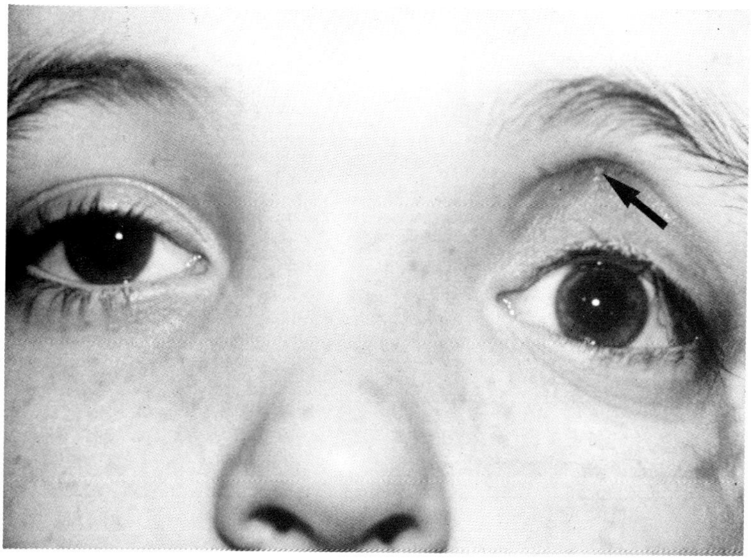

Figure 9–31 Chronic post-traumatic draining mucocele of left frontal sinus with ocular displacement and chronic cutaneous fistula (arrow).

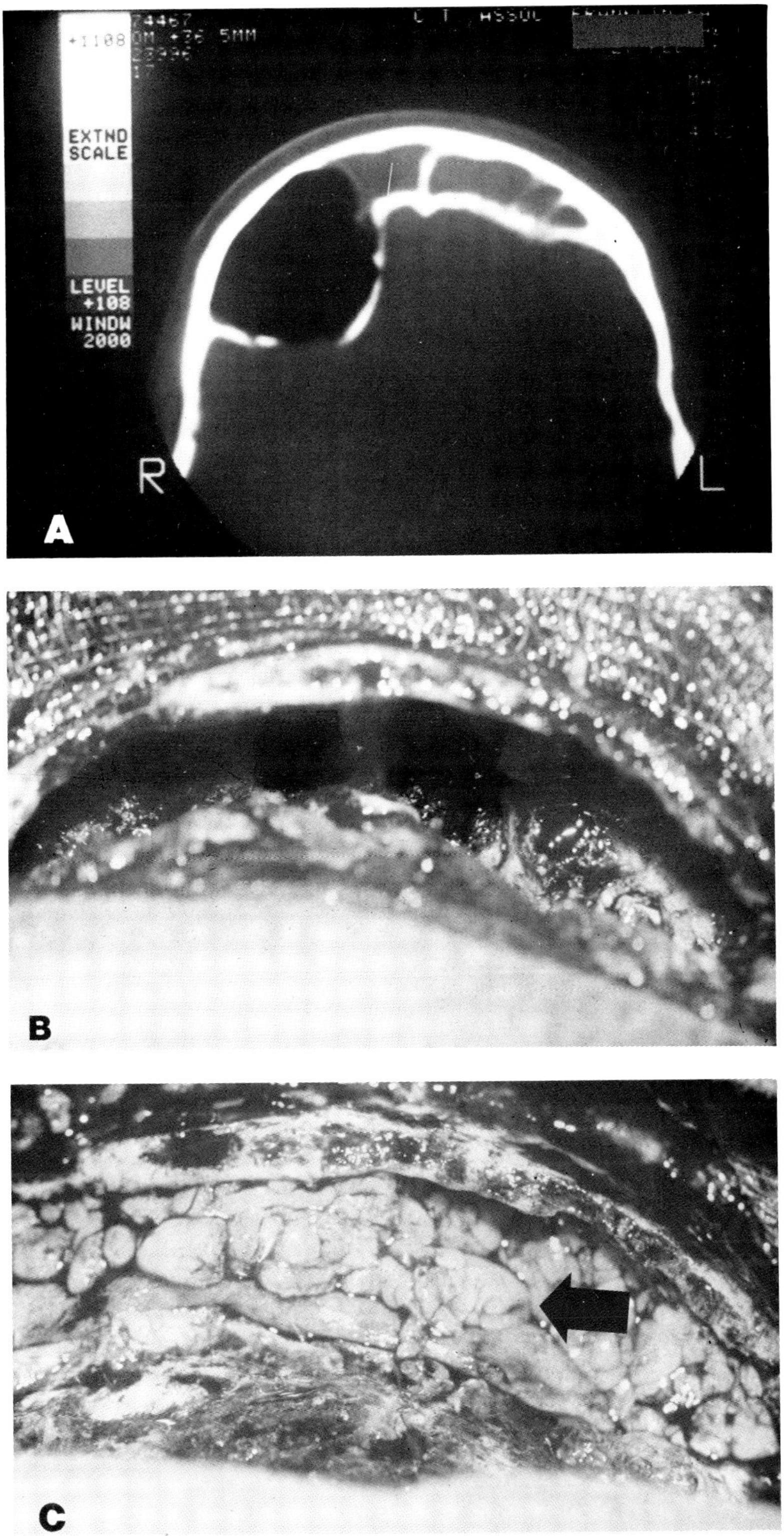

Figure 9–32 *A*, An axial CT scan outlining an extensive frontal sinus mucocele with intracranial erosion on right side. *B*, A view into an exenterated frontal sinus. *C*, Obliteration of the frontal sinus with abdominal fat (arrow).

ing of the ligament to the periosteum or by bringing the ligament into a drill hole in the rim (for more secure fixation) (Fig. 9–33).

The *medial canthoplasty* correction is a more complex procedure and the results are less predictable than with lateral canthoplasty. Therefore, an overcorrection in the superior, medial, and posterior direction is desirable (refer to the description of the acute treatment of nasoethmoid injuries). It is essential that canthoplasty reestablish the tension between the medial and lateral canthal region to maintain apposition of the lower lid to the globe. This is crucial for a normal flow of tears from the superior-lateral production site in the lacrimal gland to the inferior-medial location of the lacrimal draining system. An ectropion or obstruction of the lacrimal drainage causes epiphora and blurred vision. Sometimes, lid shortening should be done in conjunction with lid-canthus repositioning to achieve an aesthetic as well as functional lid-globe relationship. The best place to shorten the lid in a horizontal plane is in the lateral one-third or at the lateral canthus. Realigning the "gray line" of the lid margin with slight eversion and a three-layer closure prevents unsightly lid notching.

Post-traumatic ptosis may result from a reversible neuromuscular injury to the levator complex and therefore a period of several months of waiting is recommended prior to a surgical exploration and levator shortening to determine if spontaneous resolution will ensue. Increasing measurements of the height of the palpebral fissure and an appearance of a supratarsal fold are clues to the returning function of the levator muscle. If it is determined that the levator muscle and/or aponeurosis have been irreparably damaged, a fascial suspension of the lid to the frontalis muscle may provide a surgical option. The disadvantages lie in the fact that most fascial suspensions are static and dynamic reconstruction is only rarely achieved. Therefore, a greater exposure of the cornea, resulting from the static lid suspension, has to be balanced with the desire for lid symmetry. Secondary tightening of the fascial strips into the frontalis muscle should be done with the patient in a sitting position and under local anesthesia to ensure the best chance of accomplishing functional balance.

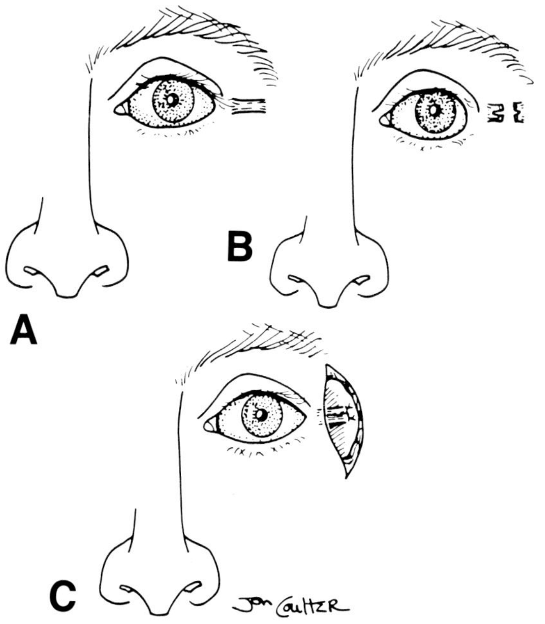

Figure 9–33 Repair of lateral canthus.

Scars may interfere with lid function if they run in a vertical plane. Horizontal scars are more favorable except when they involve the levator aponeurosis or the lacrimal draining system. Medial vertical scars often form a web with or without scar hypertrophy. To change the scar direction, z-plasty is performed and is satisfactory in most cases. If scar hypertrophy persists, even after release of the tension, intralesional injection of steroids is often helpful.

Soft-tissue loss in the orbital region can be compensated for from several sources. The lower lid can be augmented from an upper lid with a skin/muscle uni- or bipedicle flap for small defects (Fig. 9–34). Large flaps can come from the cheek advancement, including temporal and preauricular skin, or from the glabellar and forehead areas. All are well-vascularized flaps that can withstand a great deal of rotation and contouring. However, they all, except for the upper lid flap, have the disadvantage of a skin tissue substitution with lesser quality skin in an area of essential function and aesthetics.

Bone loss can result either from initial loss of substance or from extensive comminution with subsequent devitalization and absorption and secondary infection of bony fragments. An essential missing bone should be substituted with autogenous bone grafts if at all possible at the time of primary repair. Subsequent contraction of soft-tissue in an area missing bony support may prevent secondary bone grafting unless even the soft tissue is augmented or possibly expanded. Osseous resorption is directly related to blood supply of the bone. However, the general vascularity of the facial soft tissue is such that even fragments devoid of periosteum will survive if an adequate repostion-

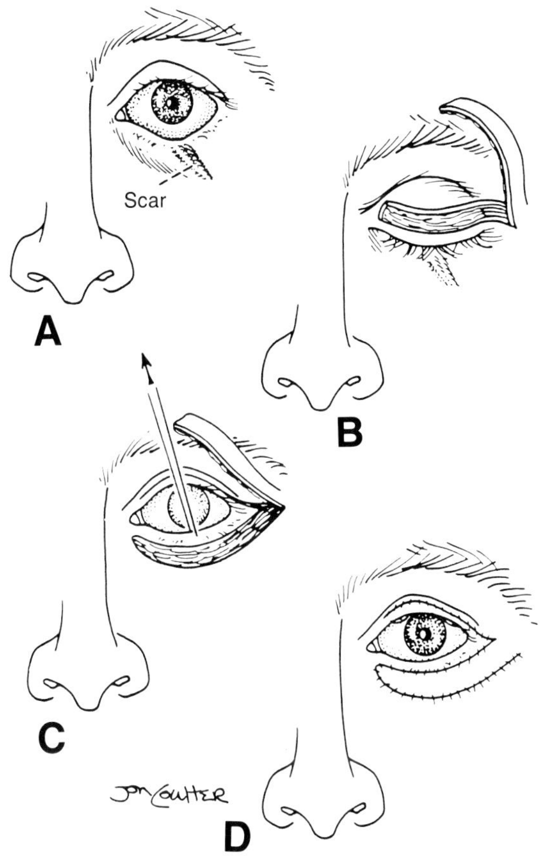

Figure 9–34 Repair of lower lid scar deformity with an upper lid flap.

ing and stability of the fragments is achieved by complete internal fixation. Autogenous bone grafting is the method of choice for bone loss (Fig. 9–35), but acrylic/aluminum cranioplasty may offer a satisfactory result in repair of orbital and cranial defects (Fig. 9–36). *Bony malunions* are infrequent in orbital and nasoethmoid fractures unless they are part of the craniofacial disjunction (Le Fort III) treated with limited fixation. Bone grafting with internal rigid fixation and possibly external stabilization of the entire craniofacial complex would be the treatment of choice. *Malposition of bones* often involves an unreduced or regressed zygomatico-orbital fracture complex. Downward and posterior displacement with inferior rotation of fragments is most frequent. Secondary repair can attempt refracturing of the key fixation points of the deformity (if comminution can be avoided), or direct appositional bone grafting with cranial or rib bone grafts can be performed. In a severe displacement secondary correction may again be limited by the contracted overlying soft tissue.

CSF leak is common following nasoethmoid fractures involving the cribriform plate. The escape of CSF may not be apparent in the acute phase of injury because of the persistent oozing of blood, extra- and intranasally, following trauma. Radiographic evidence of a fracture at the anterior skull base must put CSF leak in the differential diagnosis. A direct surgical approach to the anterior cranial base with dural repair by suturing and/or by using a pericranial patch, as well as repositioning of the

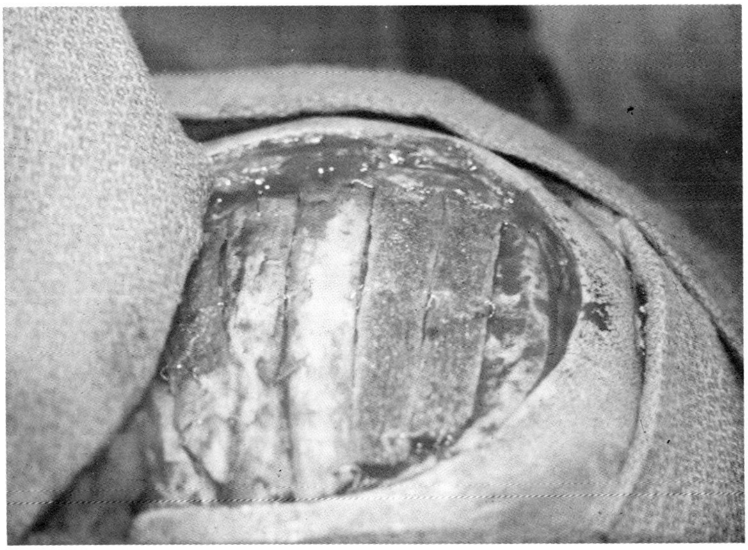

Figure 9–35 Cranio-orbital reconstruction of post-traumatic bone loss with the use of linked split-rib grafts.

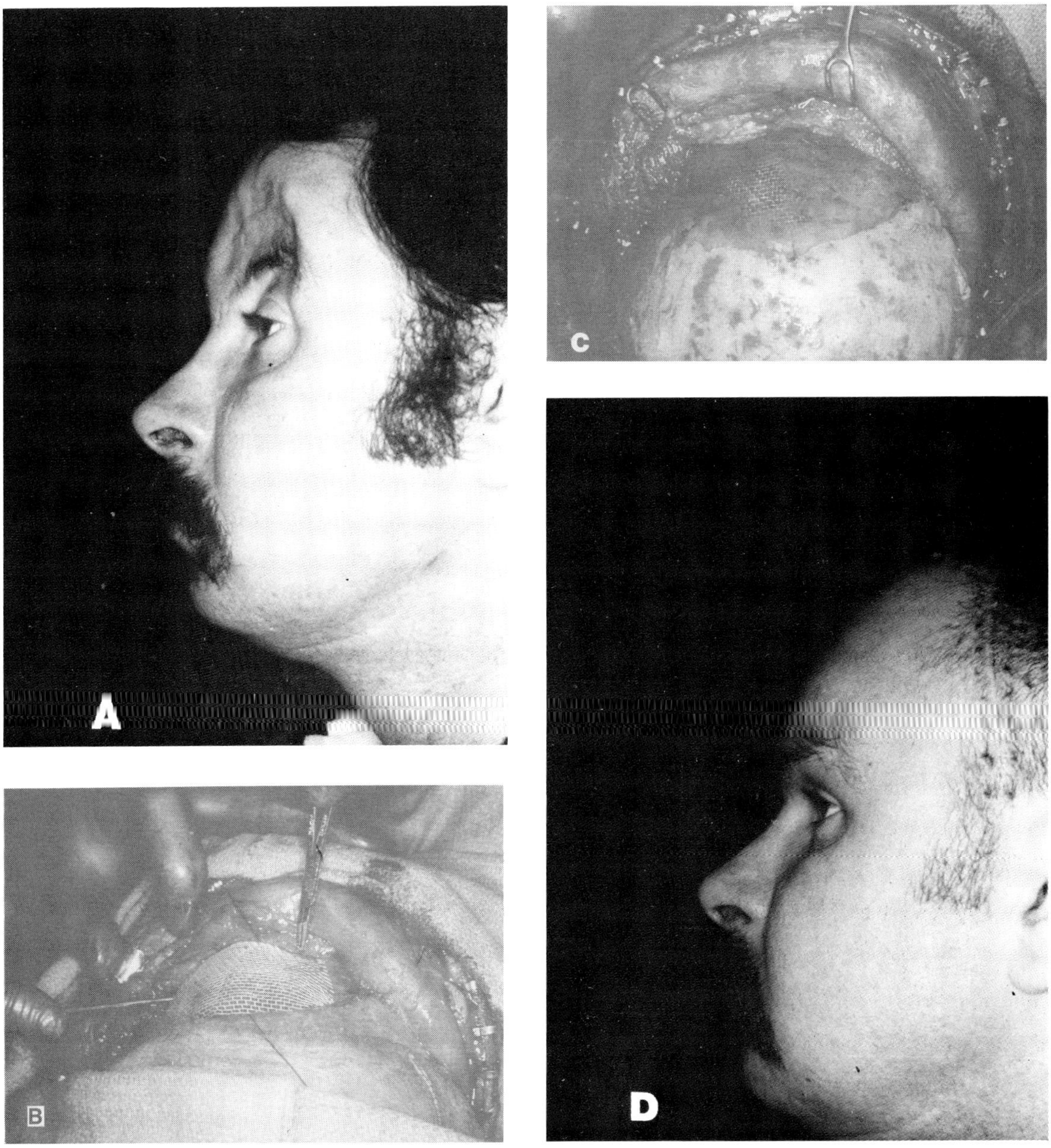

Figure 9–36 *A*, Lateral view of a patient who did not have immediate bone grafting of cranio-orbital fracture; subsequent deformity. *B*, *C*, Reconstruction with aluminum/acrylic cranioplasty. *D*, Postoperative result.

fractured bones have the best chance to stop the leak. If fractures do not need surgical repair but CSF leak is documented, short-term clinical observation (10 to 14 days) may be elected. Historically, most such leaks do cease spontaneously. A recurrent or delayed CSF leak (two to three weeks later) should, however, be considered for surgical repair, because in this category a spontaneous seal is unlikely and the incidence of meningitis rises. The external exit of the delayed CSF leak is seldom in the immediate vicinity of the previous fracture, e.g., the anterior cranial base–sphenoid fractures may drain into the middle ear. Contralateral CSF escape is also possible. All patients with meningitis and a history of cranial base fracture should have CSF leak considered as a possible etiologic agent.

Acknowledgment. The author is grateful to Dr. H. Curtin for the use of CT scans, and to Dr. F. Krebs for Figures 9–11 and 9–17.

REFERENCES

1. Manson P. Some thoughts on the classification and treatment of Le Fort fractures. Ann Plast Surg 1986; 17:356–363.
2. Levine S, Row L, Keane W, Atkins J. Evaluation and treatment of frontal sinus fractures. Otolaryngol Head Neck Surg 1986; 95:19–22.
3. Peri G, Chabannes J, Menes R, et al. Fractures of the frontal sinus. J Maxillofac Surg 1981; 9:73–80.
4. Luce E, Tubb T, Moore A. Review of 1,000 major facial fractures and associated injuries. Plast Reconstr Surg 1979; 63:26–30.
5. Gruss J. Complex nasoethmoid-orbital and midfacial fractures: role of craniofacial surgical techniques and immediate bone grafting. Ann Plast Surg 1986; 17:377–390.
6. Ellis E, El-Attar S, Moos K. An analysis of 2,067 cases of zygomatico-orbital fractures. J Oral Maxillofac Surg 1985; 43:417–428.
7. Horowitz J, Persing J, Winn H, Edgerton M. The late treatment of vertical orbital dystopia resulting from an orbital roof fracture. Ann Plast Surg 1984; 13:519–524.

10
GLOBE INJURY

MARK R. LEVINE, M.D., F.A.C.S.
GILA BUCKMAN, M.D.

The orbit and its contents are frequently damaged as a result of facial trauma. Among 1,436 patients presenting with maxillofacial trauma from 1973 to 1980, 51 percent were referred for ophthalmic examination and 67 percent of these sustained ocular injury.[1] Fifteen to 40 percent of the patients with orbital fractures sustained serious ocular injury,[2–4] including permanent visual loss, persistent hyphema, retinal hemorrhages, macular cysts, corneal-scleral rupture, vitreous hemorrhage, optic nerve changes, central retinal artery occlusion, and retinal detachment. Adnexal injuries are likewise common, with cranial nerve palsy, dacryocystitis, muscle entrapment, telecanthus, and enophthalmos occurring most often.

The high incidence of ocular complications makes an ophthalmic examination mandatory in all cases of orbital fractures. While they do not often alter the type of fracture repair, the results of the eye examination may dictate the timing and appropriateness of the repair, as treatment of certain ocular injuries must be instituted immediately.

Certain aspects of an ocular examination are of critical importance because they have a major bearing on visual prognosis. The proper time for an eye examination is at the initial assessment of the patient's trauma, after life-threatening injuries have been attended to. The eye examination should not be done while the patient is under general anesthesia in the operating room for treatment of associated injuries. It is possible for a retrobulbar hemorrhage to occur following reduction of an ethmoid complex fracture or after repositioning of orbital floor fractures, and in such cases, preoperative documentation is imperative. Traumatic perforations of the globe can lead to the onset of a cataract (sometimes within minutes or hours), and hemorrhage into the vitreous may disperse and cloud the media with equal rapidity. It is important that the first examiner may be the only one able to see the posterior pole of the eye. Such an examination must never be delayed and should be given the appropriate priority. Once opacification of the ocular media occurs, the physician's therapy may have to be performed blindly and the patient may have to go through life in a similar fashion.[5] A discussion of the most common types of ocular injuries follows in anatomic sequence.

MOST COMMON OCULAR INJURIES

Lids and Orbital Areas

To define the basic injuries encountered in this area, we need to take a closer look at the anatomical details of the lids. It is useful to consider the tarsal portion of the eyelids as being composed of an anterior and a posterior lamella. The anterior lamella consists of the skin and orbicularis muscle, while the posterior lamella consists of the tarsus, eyelid retractors, and conjunctiva. Approximately 3 mm above the upper lid margin, the levator aponeurosis has a firm attachment onto the tarsal plate. Higher in the upper eyelid the orbital septum defines the anatomic anterior boundary of the orbit. This relatively inelastic sheet of fibrous tissue originates at the periosteum of the orbital rim and fuses with the levator aponeurosis anywhere from 10 to 15 mm above the superior tarsal border.[6] In the lower eyelid the orbital septum fuses with the inferior retractors and inserts near the base of the tarsus (Fig. 10–1).

Any laceration or break in the skin of the lids or orbit accompanying orbital fractures should be closely examined with regard to direction of the laceration and depth of the wound. If a lid laceration contains fat, the examiner knows that the orbital septum has been perforated. If a perforating instrument or foreign body has penetrated deep enough to pass through the orbital septum, it may well have perforated the oculus.[7]

Visual acuity should be recorded even if only an imprecise determination is possible. This can be done by placing a pinhole over the eye involved and, with the opposite eye occluded, having the patient read a distance visual acuity chart. An alternative approach is to use a magazine or newspaper held at 30 cm (14 inches) from the eye (equivalent to a 20/50 visual acuity near test).

Lacerations involving the superior portion of

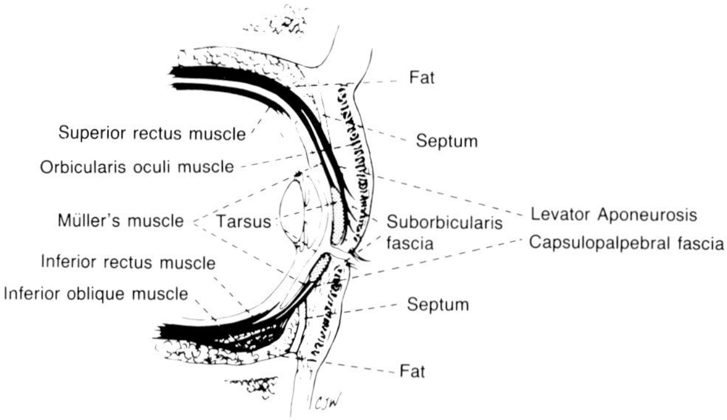

Figure 10–1 Pertinent anatomic structures and their relation to one another.

the orbit, particularly its medial third, may involve the aponeurosis of the levator muscle. Damage to this structure must be recognized and repaired to prevent subsequent ptosis (Fig. 10–2, 10–3).

An injury located in the nasal aspect of the orbit should be evaluated carefully with respect to the lacrimal drainage system. Anteriorly, the medial wall of the orbit is composed of the frontal process of the maxillary bone and the fossa for the lacrimal sac, while posteriorly the major portion of the medial wall consists of the thin and delicate ethmoid bone. Any portion of the lacrimal drainage system (the canaliculi, lacrimal sac, or nasolacrimal duct) may be severed by displaced bone fragments in the naso-orbital region, particularly if Le Fort II or III fractures were sustained. Traumatic telecanthus with lateral displacement of the medial canthi can occur. Although a deferred or missed diagnosis in this area does not have direct visual implications, early repair of these structures can, in many cases, eliminate the need for a more involved and cosmetically less acceptable operation in the future to achieve tear drainage.

Extraocular Muscles

Associated abnormalities that can accompany concussive or penetrating injuries of the orbital areas include dysfunction of the extraocular muscles. In assessing the patient's symptoms, vertical diplopia should not be considered an absolute indication for surgical exploration of the orbital floor. Many patients develop vertical diplopia, both subjective and objective, after blunt trauma to the eye and orbit. Several pathogenic processes may be involved, including hematomas of the extraocular muscles

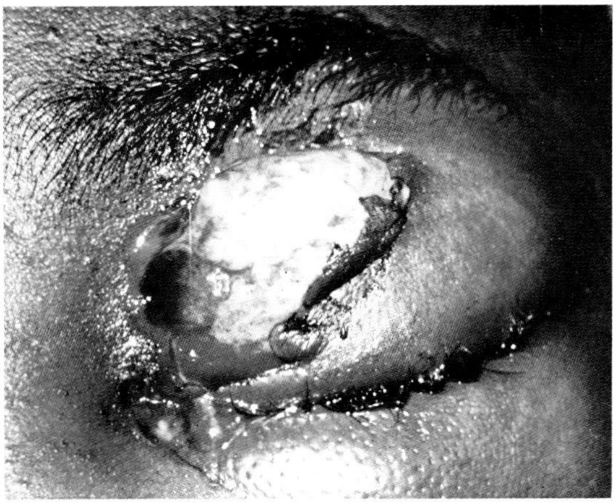

Figure 10–2 Penetrating injury to left upper lid and orbit with protruding orbital fat.

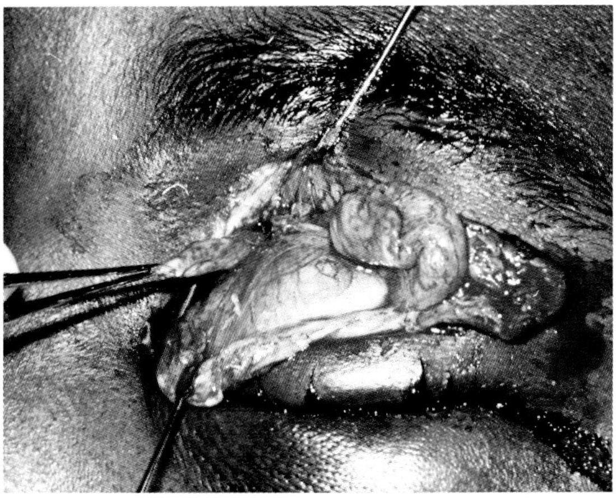

Figure 10–3 Laceration of superior oblique tendon held in forceps, and laceration of levator aponeurosis retracted in double-prong skin hook, exposing tarsal plate.

and neural injury from contusion. Diplopia in these cases may be transient.

The forced-duction test is invaluable in differentiating limitation of motion due to orbital edema, muscle contusion, and nerve damage from limitation caused by incarceration of the inferior muscles in orbital floor fracture. After topical anesthesia, a toothed forceps is used to grab both the conjunctiva and Tenon's fascia at the insertion of the inferior rectus muscle (7 mm below the limbus). The patient is requested to look up, and the examiner rotates the eye upward; if it shows a full range of motility, then there is probably no physical entrapment of periocular tissue at the fracture site. If the affected eye does not elevate with manual force, there should be something restraining the eye, which is usually incarceration of muscle or fat in an open orbital floor fracture.

Conjunctiva

Conjunctival hemorrhage is the most common accompaniment of ocular trauma. The hemorrhage itself is of no consequence. Sometimes, however, the subconjunctival hemorrhage from orbital bleeding is so severe that the conjunctiva prolapses between the lids. The conjunctiva must be kept lubricated or covered with Saran Wrap until the swelling subsides to avoid any ulceration.

Chemosis (edema) of the conjunctiva, with or without hemorrhage, is often a more serious sign. After injury, acute chemosis can be caused by a retained intraorbital foreign body, fracture of the orbit, scleral rupture, scleral perforation, or carotid-cavernous fistula.

Air under the conjunctiva (crepitus) is usually associated with fractures of the lamina papyracea of the ethmoid or paranasal sinuses. The air itself is absorbed and of no consequence. However, the presence of crepitus is an indication for systemic antibiotic therapy to prevent an orbital cellulitis originating from bacteria in the sinuses.

Every conjunctival laceration potentially overlies a scleral laceration or rupture. Associated hemorrhage and edema may conceal the presence of transparent gelatinous vitreous, black uveal tissue, or even retina, any of which may have herniated through a scleral laceration. Consequently, almost every conjunctival laceration deserves careful visual and instrumental exploration.

Cornea

Corneal abrasions are often due to foreign bodies caught under the upper lid. The abrasion may occur coincident with an orbital fracture. This can occur if the patient wore eyeglasses or contact lenses at the time of the initial trauma. The cornea and conjunctival sac should be examined for foreign bodies and epithelial damage. Corneal abrasion produces pain, lacrimation, and blepharospasm, and a drop of topical anesthetic should be instilled prior to examination. If foreign body is not found, fluorescein dye should be instilled and the cornea viewed with a cobalt blue light under a slitlamp. Green dye stains wherever corneal epithelial cells have been damaged or lost because of abrasion.

Corneal lacerations are rarely a complication of orbital fractures. When they do occur, they often accompany more severe intraocular damage and treatment is planned accordingly.

Concussive Injuries to the Anterior Segment—Hyphema

Concussion injuries of the anterior segment are common. The term "hyphema" refers to blood within the anterior chamber; it occurs in nearly 10 percent of patients suffering significant ocular trauma in association with orbital fractures.[1] Some hyphemas fill the entire chamber but most are smaller and settle inferiorly (Fig. 10–4). Resorption usually occurs within the first 5 to 6 days. There is, however, a 9 to 38 percent incidence of rebleeding,[8,9] without concomitant trauma usually seen 2 to 6 days following the initial hemorrhage. Delayed secondary bleeding into the anterior chamber results in a markedly worse prognosis. Eventual visual recovery to an acuity of 20/50 (6/15) or bet-

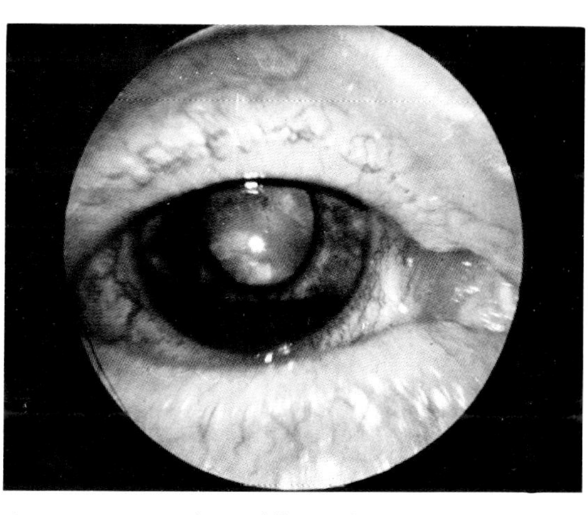

Figure 10–4 Hyphema filling inferior 25 percent of anterior chamber. Cataract also present.

ter occurs in 64 percent of patients with secondary hemorrhage, as compared with 79.5 percent of those in whom no rebleeding occurs.[10]

The major vision-threatening complications of traumatic hyphema are corneal blood staining and optic atrophy secondary to intractable glaucoma. Increased intraocular pressures may accompany hyphemas of any amount and occur in approximately 32 percent of all hyphemas.[11] Highly elevated pressures occur during the acute phase of the hyphema (first 24 hours) and are probably the result of trabecular plugging by the anterior chamber red cells. Intraocular pressure then subsides with recovery of the trabecular meshwork and resolution of the hyphema. Exceptions to this may be seen in patients with total ("eight-ball") hyphemas, either primary or secondary, in whom pressure elevation remains continuously high. When large segments of the anterior chamber angle have been irreparably damaged, the intraocular hypertension continues and intractable glaucoma ensues.

Corneal blood staining, with rare exceptions, occurs in patients with total hyphemas and high intraocular pressures. According to a recent animal study, the earliest pathologic event leading to corneal blood staining in the presence of persistent hyphema and elevated intraocular pressure is endothelial decompensation.[12] Increased intraocular pressure has been hypothesized to drive hemoglobin through the endothelium and Descemet's membrane into the stroma. Stromal dispersion of hemoglobin eventually overwhelms the metabolic capacity of keratocytes to convert hemoglobin to hemosiderin and leads to necrosis of stromal cells and ultimately to complete corneal opacification.

Traumatic Mydriasis and Miosis

A mild inflammation of the iris and ciliary body may follow almost any trauma. The intraocular pressure is usually low at the beginning owing to ciliary body shutdown, and the aqueous humor contains cells and fibrin. More severe trauma can produce dilation or constriction of the pupil. The pupil reacts minimally and is often slightly irregular. A normal consensual response in the opposite eye will reassure the examiner that the optic nerve is normal on the injured side. Traumatic rupture of the sphincter of the iris can produce a peaked pupil and permanent deformity of the pupil. Traumatic disinsertion of the ciliary body is sometimes associated with contusion hyphema.

Angle Recession

Blunt trauma to the globe frequently causes damage to the anterior chamber angle, the most important site of aqueous drainage from the eye. The concussive force produces a cleft in the ciliary body. The recessed trabecular meshwork tends to be disrupted, leaving the ciliary body bare in comparison with other quadrants of the angle or with the angle of the opposite eye. Although angle recessions may occur without anterior chamber hemorrhage, more patients have been observed with coexistent hyphemas. It has been reported that 71 to 86 percent of traumatized eyes with hyphemas have an angle recession.[10,13] Angle recession is recognized as a frequent cause of unilateral glaucoma which may occur 10 to 15 years after the injury. Ocular hypertension at this time behaves and responds very much like that of open angle glaucoma. Eyes with recession greater than 180 degrees are particularly prone to develop glaucoma. Those patients found to have angle recession at the time of injury should be advised to have periodic examinations for the rest of their lives to detect late onset glaucoma.

Lens Subluxation

The zonular fibers that encircle the lens and anchor it to the ciliary body may be broken by blunt trauma. If more than 25 percent of these zonular fibers are broken, the lens is loosened. It may sublux backward into the vitreous cavity, thus deepening the anterior chamber, or it may dislocate anteriorly, causing the anterior chamber to become shallow. Pupillary-block glaucoma may result from incarceration of a dislocated lens in the pupillary space. The lens mechanically prevents aqueous fluid from gaining access to the outflow channels of the eye and causes an acute rise in intraocular pressure.

Cataract

Nonpenetrating concussion injuries to the eye not uncommonly result in permanent lens opacification. The initial lens change is usually in the posterior capsular area and progress is usually gradual. If the globe is perforated and the lens capsule ruptured, an opacity appears at the site of rupture. This usually progresses rapidly to produce an intumescent cataract. However, on rare occasions the lens capsule may heal and the opacity is confined to the region of injury. This may represent a more favorable outcome.

Scleral Rupture

Contusion ruptures of the globe associated with orbital and facial fractures may be direct or indirect. In the direct type the globe rupture is at the point of impact; while in the more common indirect type, rupture occurs at a point remote from the site of impact. Blunt injury perpendicularly directed against the cornea rarely ruptures the globe, since the shock of retrodisplacement is cushioned by the orbital fat and the force of the blow is transmitted to the orbital walls.

Compression trauma, which essentially bursts the eye on impact, is usually directed obliquely, forcing the globe laterally against the unyielding wall. This compression causes precipitous expansion of the eye in a plane perpendicular to the line of impact. The resultant internal pressure causes rupture at an anatomically weak area, such as the thin equatorial sclera or the limbus over Schlemm's canal. The direction of force is upward medially or upward and laterally in most cases of scleral rupture.

The rare concomitant occurrence of rupture and blowout fracture may be the result of two independent forces. The first force compresses the globe against an unyielding orbital wall, causing an increase in intraocular pressure and rupture at an anatomically predisposed area. The second force, directly transmitted by bone conduction through the rigid inferior orbital rim, fractures the thin orbital floor.[14]

A scleral rupture or laceration can be hidden under hemorrhagic or edematous conjunctiva, and occasionally the signs of serious intraocular damage are mild. Rupture is suspected when the anterior chamber is filled with blood, the eye is soft, and there is marked hemorrhagic chemosis of the conjunctiva, sometimes localized to the quadrant, overlying the rupture (Figs. 10–5, 10–6). The anterior chamber may be abnormally deep. The iris or ciliary body may be incarcerated in the wound or prolapsed through it, giving a peaked or pear-shaped pupil. These eyes are by no means beyond salvage, but the more posterior and larger the rupture, the worse the prognosis.

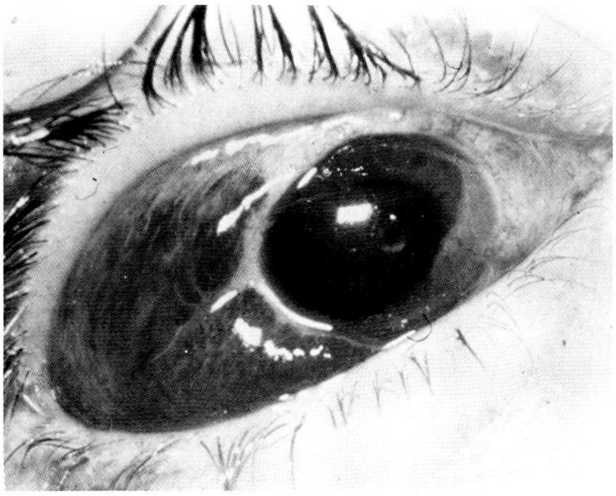

Figure 10–5 Hemorrhagic and edematous conjunctiva hiding a posterior scleral laceration. Eye pressure is soft, the pupil is dilated eccentrically, and there is blood in the anterior chamber overlying the iris.

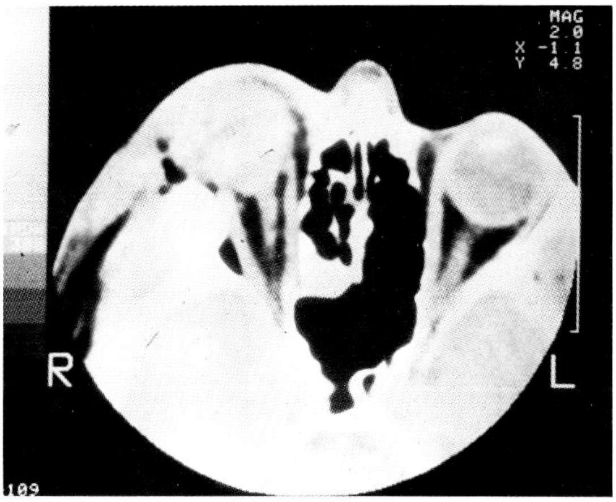

Figure 10–6 Axial CT scan showing a bone fragment of the frontal process of the zygoma rupturing the sclera posteriorly, resulting in the eye seen in Figure 10–5.

Concussion Injuries to the Posterior Segment

Following concussion of the eye, vitreous hemorrhage may result secondary to damage to a retinal or choroidal vessel. Loss of vision may be sudden and profound. Careful examination of the fundus periphery is extremely important because a retinal dialysis may be present in addition to the vitreous hemorrhage. The most common locations for such a break are the inferior temporal and superior nasal quadrants.

Commotio Retinae

Retinal edema is commonplace after direct blows to the eye. Most authors feel that the pathologic process is concussion injury with vasodilation leading to the edema of the retina. In close examination there is edema of all retinal layers with variable amounts of retinal, subretinal, and choroidal hemorrhage (Figs. 10–7, 10–8). Later there may be necrosis and atrophy of the involved layers.

Visual acuity is usually decreased. Funduscopically, there is edema of the posterior pole, nearly always involving the macula with a variable amount of retinal and subretinal hemorrhage, and there may be a cherry red spot. In mild cases there may only be macular involvement with loss of foveal reflex. The edema usually increases over the first 24 hours and then gradually subsides. The prognosis for visual recovery depends on the degree of damage and the recovery may take weeks to months. Visual recovery may be complete; however, impairment is common because of pigmentary disturbances, macular hole, and macular cysts.

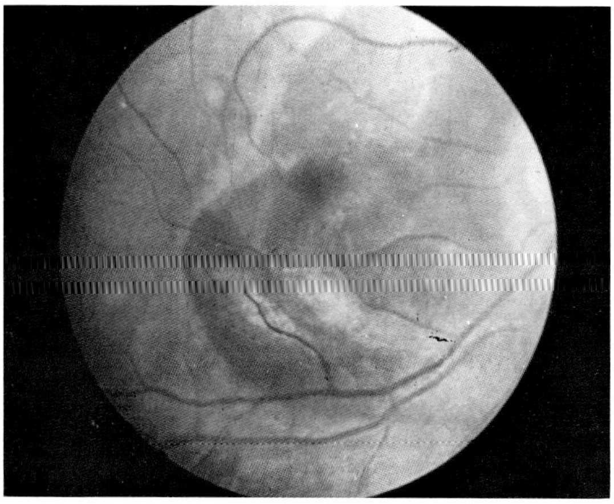

Figure 10–7 Intra- and subretinal hemorrhage and edema obliterating the macula.

Traumatic Macular Cysts and Holes

Macular cysts and holes are not uncommon after blunt trauma, and they also occur after penetrating injuries (Fig. 10–9). On histopathological examination there are cystoid spaces in the retina, especially in the outer plexiform layer of the retina. A typical cyst has only the internal limiting membrane overlying it; if this gives way, a hole is formed. A macular cyst may occur from a few days to several years after injury. There is a variable reduction in visual acuity with a positive central scotoma. The cyst is typically a circular, dark red spot at the fovea, 1/6 to 1/3 DD in size. On examination the differentiation between a cyst and a hole is difficult and is best made with the use of a slit lamp and contact lens. Macular holes are present in 1 to 6 percent of all traumatic retinal detachments but rarely lead to detachment.[15, 16] These lesions lead to permanent loss of central visual acuity in the range of 20/70 (6/21) or better with macular cyst, and 20/200 (6/60) or worse with macular hole.[17]

Chorioretinal Rupture

Chorioretinal rupture is a simultaneous rupture of the retina and choroid, which is frequently seen as a result of a high velocity missile fracturing the orbital wall or striking the globe as a blow without the rupture. The cause of the lesion is probably a combination of mechanical and vascular effects of contusion with subsequent thrombosis and necro-

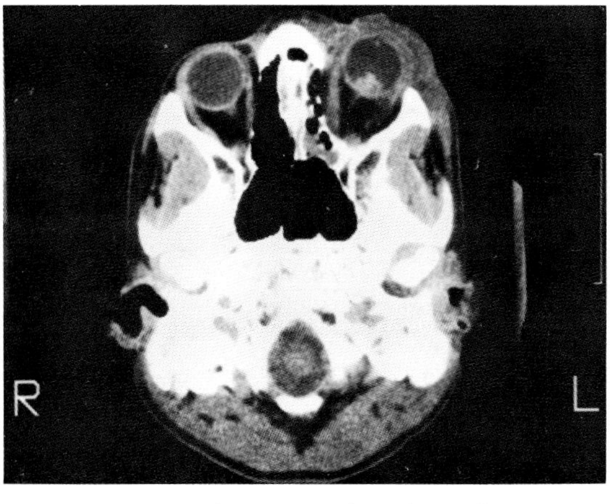

Figure 10–8 Axial CT scan showing a chorioretinal hemorrhage in a patient with a medial wall fracture.

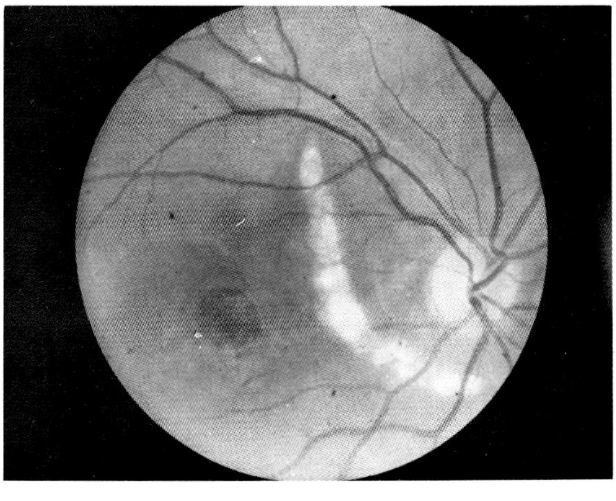

Figure 10–9 Retina with macular hole and choroidal tear through papillomacular bundle.

sis. The unusual problem in these instances is the rapid and extensive development of dense vitreous bands from organization of the vitreous hemorrhage. On histologic examination, in the acute phase there is widespread necrosis of the choroid and retina without perforation of the sclera. In the reparative phase there is extensive glial scarring.

There is usually significant visual loss. Funduscopically, there is severe retinal edema with retinal and choroidal rupture, retinal hemorrhage, and hemorrhage extending into the vitreous. The vitreous is occasionally filled with hemorrhage and the fundus cannot be viewed. Hypotony is the rule, and perforation of the globe should be considered. After healing has occurred, there is a white proliferative glial scar with pigmentary changes. The visual outcome is frequently poor, either from rupture in or adjacent to the macula, or from macular degeneration.

Retinal Detachment

The incidence of retinal detachment in patients who sustained orbital and midfacial fractures varies from 3 to 5 percent.[1,17] A dialysis (tear at the ora serrata) is the most common type of traumatic tear which causes retinal detachment. Dialyses most commonly occur in the inferotemporal quadrant where the globe is exposed and the retina is thinnest due to direct trauma, and in the superonasal quadrant due to the contrecoup injuries. Trauma also produces irregular or angular horseshoe tears at sites of weakness of the retina or in areas of increased vitreoretinal adhesion.

The symptomatology of traumatic retinal detachment depends on the impairment of central visual acuity. Since many of the detachments originate inferiorly, they cause few symptoms. The retinal periphery should be examined carefully with direct ophthalmoscopy. In the majority of patients there is a latent period between injury and detachment (50 percent of detachments develop within 8 months and 80 percent within 2 years).[18,19] Dialyses extending greater than 90 degrees are called giant tears. Such tears are uncommon and difficult to repair.

Central Retinal Artery Occlusion

Central retinal artery occlusion as a result of an orbital fracture is another common finding. However, prolonged compression of the eye from external pressure on the eyelid or from severe intraorbital bleeding may occlude the central retinal artery. A conscious patient may complain of a profound loss of vision that at first is intermittent. A characteristic fundus appearance is seen: a pale optic nerve, narrowed arterioles, and a diffuse retinal whitening causing a cherry red spot at the macula where retinal thinning permits transmission of the normal choroidal circulation. Prognosis is poor with the majority of patients developing optic atrophy.

Optic Nerve Injuries

The most serious complication of orbital fractures is permanent blindness. In the absence of severe injury to the globe, the optic nerve is most frequently involved. The site of injury may be intraorbital, intracranial, or in the optic canal. Up to 5 percent of head injuries may be associated with fractures through the optic canals, and in cases of head trauma with visual loss, canal fractures have been demonstrated in 6 to 92 percent of patients.[20-23]

The forces acting on the optic nerve have been classified into three groups: classic force, shearing forces, and pterygomaxillary force.[24]

A good example of the classic force is a fist striking the globe, where the anterior orbital contents are pushed back into the cone-shaped orbit, producing an elevated intraorbital pressure. The pressure compresses the optic nerve and transient visual loss is noted by the patient. Macular edema may be present and usually the vision returns to normal within a few days.

The shearing force is related to rotational trauma. The skull and optic canal are set in motion by the trauma. The nerve and its attachments receive a shearing, or twisting, effect that may cause damage to the sheath, blood vessels, or nerve itself.

The onset of blindness complicating orbital fractures may be immediate, delayed for hours or days, or postoperative. Some of the factors in the origin of immediate blindness are: (1) intraneural or intrasheath optic nerve hemorrhage; (2) partial or complete tear of the optic nerve (lateral wall fractures are more likely than other orbital fractures to be associated with avulsion of the optic nerve); (3) pressure from the fracture fragments; and, more commonly, (4) contusion necrosis of the optic nerve and chiasm from bony fragments or concussive injury.

Progressive visual loss following trauma is generally due to optic nerve compression from swelling and edema of the nerve. Necrosis and infarction secondary to vascular obstruction may also be significant factors.

Postoperative blindness in the repair of orbital floor fractures has been reported by Nicholson and Couzak to occur in 8.4 percent of patients following the surgical repair of blowout fractures via either a translid approach or the maxillary antrum.[25] Visual loss may be immediate, due to optic nerve injury, or delayed, associated with increased intraorbital pressure due to hemorrhage, edema, or the implant itself. With prompt decompression vision returns in about 50 percent of patients.[24] If the vision does not return, it is assumed that the optic nerve is seriously damaged. The damage to the optic nerve may be produced by the original injury or the subsequent surgery. This may be a difficult question to resolve, particularly if litigation has been started.

Visual function must be recorded immediately after trauma and pupils must be evaluated. An excellent test to evaluate optic nerve injury is the Marcus-Gunn swinging flashlight test. A light is moved from one eye to the other eye and back again. If conduction in the optic nerve is less on one side, then the consensual response of that pupil will be greater than the response to direct light and the pupil on the involved side will appear to dilate as the light is brought from the normal eye to the involved one.

The merits of observing a positive Marcus-Gunn pupil are: (1) the complaint of decreased visual acuity is always identified with the retina or optic nerve; (2) the visual problem is definitely organic (versus functional); and (3) the test is more sensitive than direct-light testing of the pupil in detection of afferent nerve damage. Unilateral loss of vision, various field defects, a positive Marcus-Gunn pupil, and initially normal-appearing nerve head may be indicative of fracture of the optic canal or avulsion of the optic nerve. Optic disk pallor may not be obvious until 2 to 3 weeks after injury. Careful radiographic tomograms are therefore indicated. A computed axial tomogram (CT) with thin cuts 0.5 to 1 mm is usually sufficient to delineate the extent of the fracture.

DIAGNOSTIC METHODS

The most valuable diagnostic studies in patients who have sustained orbital trauma are plain radiographs, CT scans (axial and coronal), and ultrasonography. Any type of orbital fracture can be demonstrated well on plain water projection films in more than 70 percent of the patients, and on tomographic radiographs in more than 95 percent.[26] Fractures involving the orbital rims are best evaluated on frontal projections. Those of the superior rim are uncommon but when present may involve damage to the levator aponeurosis or trochlea of the superior oblique tendon. They may extend upward to involve the orbital roof and are frequently associated with optic canal fractures. Medial rim breaks are frequently found with nasofrontal, nasoethmoid, and nasomaxillary fractures and tend to be of a more complex type. Lateral rim fractures are often associated with floor fractures and usually involve complex tripod or Le Fort III fractures.

Pure blowout of the floor is the most common type of orbital fracture, representing 70 to 75 percent of all orbital fractures.[27,28] The major radiographic signs include fragmentation and disruption of the orbital floor, depression of bony fragments into the maxillary sinus, and soft-tissue prolapse into the sinus. Stereoscopic Waters views, as well as frontal and lateral tomograms, will provide excellent visualization of such fractures (Fig. 10–10). CT scanning with thin cuts is very helpful.

Although pure medial wall fractures can occur, they are most commonly associated with floor fractures and may be seen in more than 50 percent of the patients with antral or distal fractures.[26] Medial wall fractures may be difficult to demonstrate radiographically without tomograms or CT scans. Fractures through the optic canal are difficult to demonstrate radiographically, but they can be well visualized by CT scanning. In four patients studied by Potter and Trokel, all had normal standard canal views, but fractures were evident in all on tomograms.[29] Therefore, any patient suspected of having a canal fracture, but with normal plain

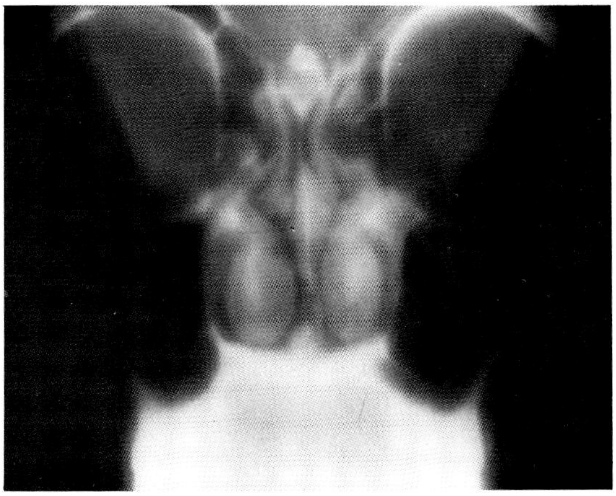

Figure 10–10 Tomogram showing a piece of the floor of the left orbit displaced into the maxillary sinus.

x-ray films of the optic canal, must have hypocycloidal tomograms in the oblique apical projection at 1-mm intervals.

CT is considered to be equal or superior to all other methods of noninvasive diagnostic evaluation. It allows the simultaneous examination of bony structures and associated soft tissues. Orbital scanning should include axial and coronal views, reconstructive or direct, since the latter offer a more accurate determination of spatial relationship within the orbit. Coronal scans are better for viewing entrapped soft tissue and muscle in orbital floor fractures (Figs. 10–11, 10–12). The optic nerve is usually not seen in its entirety because of its sinuous course. The best CT projection is at an axial plane of 20 degrees with the patient looking upward at 40 degrees to the horizontal.[30]

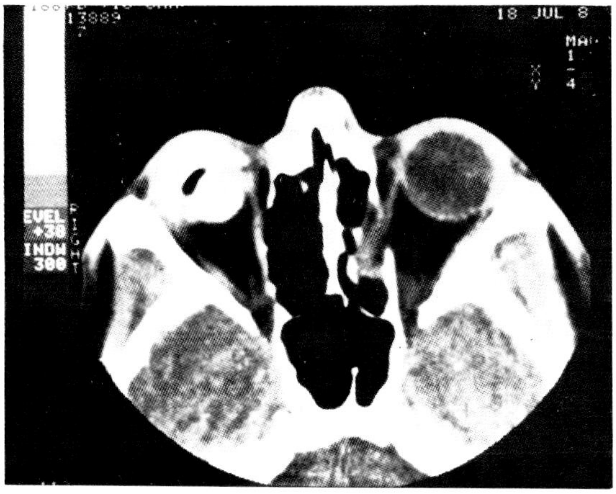

Figure 10–11 Axial CT scan demonstrating entrapment of left medial rectus into the ethmoid sinus. Patient has prosthetic eye on the right.

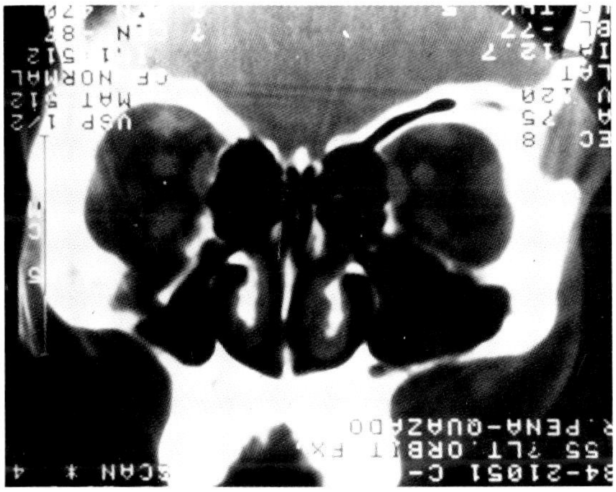

Figure 10–12 Coronal CT scan showing a piece of bone displaced into the left maxillary sinus without entrapment of the inferior rectus.

Sections through the anterior orbit give excellent views of the globe, frontal sinuses, and nasal cavity, allowing one to detect foreign bodies, distorted lenses, and vitreous opacities. On more posterior sections, retrobulbar hematomas may be seen.

The importance of ultrasonography in the evaluation and subsequent management of intraocular injuries cannot be overstressed. While the A-scan provides a one-dimensional picture of the echo amplitude of structures within the globe, the B-scan gives a cross-sectional view of the globe analogous to a histologic cross-section of the eye. Occult structural changes in the globe following contusion and laceration injuries can be well documented using a combined A- and B-scan technique. Despite the presence of hyphema, for example, the depth of the anterior chamber can be precisely measured. An unusually deep chamber may indicate an angle recession. The lens may be dislocated or, in the case of a foreign body or penetrating injury, rupture of the posterior capsule may be seen. In addition to detecting hemorrhage in the vitreous, the density and location of the hemorrhage within the vitreous cavity may be determined. In lacerating injuries, a path of hemorrhage may indicate a posterior perforation site and guide the surgeon to the proper quadrant for exploration. More importantly, retinal detachments hidden behind massive vitreous hemorrhages may be detected early following trauma, thus expediting surgical intervention.[31]

The newest and most advanced diagnostic method in radiology is magnetic resonance imaging (MRI). Using the energy emission of hydrogen nuclei (protons) after a radiofrequency pulse has been applied to a strong magnetic field, MRI is theoretically capable of obtaining soft-tissue resolution equal to the CT scan while showing greater tissue contrast. As in the first generation of CT scanners, improvements in instrumentation will probably lead to further refinement in the quality and accuracy in diagnosis of ocular injuries.

TREATMENT

Once injury to the eye has been evaluated, treatment must be instituted. One of the few emergencies in ophthalmology that requires immediate therapy is occlusion of the central retinal artery, which is a rare sequela of orbital trauma due to severe intraorbital pressure from hemorrhage or edema. A lateral canthotomy and inferior cantholysis should be performed, as well as retrobulbar injection of hyaluronidase to reduce pressure on the globe by dissipating orbital edema or blood. Paracentesis of the anterior chamber is a rapid way to decompress the eye. Intermittent digital massage of the globe is another, slower, means of lowering the intraocular pressure. Intravenous mannitol should be given, if not medically contraindicated. Treatment is effective only in those unusual circumstances when a patient is examined immediately upon loss of vision or when the artery reflects intermittent occlusion by a variable amount of vision. Most patients do not recover vision and go on to develop optic atrophy.

Other injuries associated with orbital fractures which require immediate treatment are penetrating injuries of the globe, pupillary block glaucoma, corneal foreign body, corneal abrasion, acute retinal tears, acute retinal detachment, acute vitreous hemorrhage, and hyphema. Although this group of injuries requires prompt attention, treatment can be instituted within hours rather than minutes; thus there is usually time for adequate examination, unhurried decision making, and optimal preparation of treatment facilities. Definitive diagnosis of orbital floor fracture is not an emergency, and the surgeon often should wait several days for orbital swelling to subside before deciding on management.

Penetrating Injuries to the Globe

A penetrating ocular injury, no matter how severe, requires primary repair. Occasionally salvage is accomplished in the face of seemingly overwhelming odds. However, primary enucleation is justified only when the globe is totally disorganized and the retina has prolapsed. Written consent preoperatively should be given by an alert, sober patient.

When the eye has been lacerated, pressure on the globe must be avoided and surgery not deferred any longer than necessary. Broad-spectrum parenteral antibiotics and topical antibiotic drops should be started promptly, with a protective shield placed over the eye. The operation should be done under general anesthesia to avoid orbital pressure on the globe from a retrobulbar anesthetic.

The principle of ocular wound repair is to try to re-establish the normal contour of the eyeball. Corneal lacerations should be closed with fine suture material such as 10–0 nylon, with the suture loops extending well beyond the area of edema on both sides of the wound. For larger lacerations, the anterior chamber must be re-formed with air or Healon before suturing. Rarely, a partial penetrating keratoplasty may be necessary.

Scleral lacerations are treated in a similar manner and reapproximated with 8–0 silk. Cryotherapy or diathermy should be used to surround the scleral portion of the laceration to create adhesions of the underlying choroid and prevent retinal tears. Loss of scleral tissue can be repaired by means of a patch graft or hinged scleral flap.

If the lens has been injured at the time of penetration and a cataract has formed, lens surgery should be performed at the time of corneoscleral repair. If vitreous loss accompanies lens damage, the treatment should be extracapsular extraction and vitrectomy through a large incision at the limbus or via the pars plana. If the vitreous is undisturbed, flocculent lens material can be aspirated through the corneal wound.

Iris that has been prolapsed should often be excised. Ciliary body, on the other hand, should not be excised unless it is severely traumatized. Such eyes have a guarded prognosis because of ciliary body detachment and traumatic cyclodialysis. Diathermy in the region of the injury may prevent hypotony from occurring. The eye must be evaluated before the tenth postoperative day to decide if the globe is salvageable or if it should be enucleated to minimize the change of sympathetic ophthalmia.

If a scleral laceration is found posterior to the ora serrata (6 mm or more posterior to the limbus) retinal trauma must be assumed. Careful inspection of the retina by indirect ophthalmoscopy may reveal the site of scleral perforation, and cryotherapy may then be applied under direct visualization. Possible consequences of unrepaired scleral perforation include vitreous loss and retinal detachment. Prophylactic scleral buckling for peripheral retinal tears in these cases appears to have substantial merit.

Pupillary Block Glaucoma

Emergency surgical treatment for dislocation of the lens is usually required when the lens is incarcerated in the pupil or entirely within the anterior chamber. Either condition can result in an acute rise in intraocular pressure. Intravitreal dislocation of the lens is a serious complication of ocular trauma but never requires emergency surgery. Initial management of a lens incarcerated in the pupil consists of dilating the pupil in an attempt to break the pupillary block. If this tactic is successful, the lens will fall posterior to the pupillary diaphragm and no surgery is indicated. If the pupil does not dilate, or if incarceration recurs, the lens should be removed and the surgeon should be prepared to perform a vitrectomy if necessary.

Corneal Foreign Bodies and Abrasion

The treatment of corneal foreign bodies is removal, which is achieved by instilling a drop of topical anesthetic followed by a gentle wipe of the cornea with a saline-moistened cotton swab. Deeper foreign bodies may have to be removed in the operating room to prevent collapse of the anterior chamber during the removal procedure. Inorganic, nonferrous particles scattered through the cornea and conjunctiva are better treated conservatively than with meticulous extraction of each particle. With time, remaining particles will tend to come to the surface of the cornea and extrude. Management of corneal abrasions is ointment and a tight pressure patch for 24 hours.

Acute Vitreous Hemorrhage and Retinal Detachment

The initial treatment of acute vitreous hemorrhage is expectant unless a retinal detachment is associated with the hemorrhage. In this case pars plana vitrectomy and a scleral buckle are indicated. When a giant tear of 90 to 180 degrees occurs the patient should be treated by emergency surgery to prevent further extension that would make the surgical prognosis much less favorable. Clinical trials with intraocular silicone oil indicate that unfolding of the retina and reattachment can be achieved in these difficult cases, with improved prognosis.[32]

Hyphemas

Hyphemas should be managed by monitoring the individual hyphema, the intraocular pressure, and clarity of the cornea. Patients should be hospitalized and examined at the slit lamp with applanation tonometry once a day. There are several dilemmas regarding acute management of traumatic hyphemas: whether or not to keep the patient in bed; whether to patch one or two eyes; whether to dilate or constrict the pupil; and whether to use systemic or topical corticosteroids. For each study suggesting the benefits of a particular agent, there is another study demonstrating the lack of effect, or even harmful effects, of that agent. A well-controlled prospective study by Read and Goldberg compared one group treated with bed rest, bilateral patching, and sedation, with a second group treated with ambulation, patching, and no sedation. There was no statistical difference in the rate of rebleeding between the two groups.[11] The data indicate that unilateral shielding of the involved eye is appropriate; at least it is not harmful.

Antiglaucoma medications are indicated for elevated intraocular pressure. Timolol and epinephrine derivatives are effective during the acute rise of intraocular pressure. Acetazolamide (Diamox), 250 mg four times daily, can be added if the pressure remains elevated.

Reports by Yasuna and Romano suggest that systemic steroids reduce rebleeding episodes.[33,34] However, a randomized, double-blind, prospective study by Spoor and colleagues revealed no statistical differences in the rebleed rate between placebo and systemic steroids.[35]

Antifibrinolytic agents in the management of hyphema have been advocated. Based on the assumption that secondary hemorrhage is most likely due to lysis and retraction of the initial blood clot, agents with antifibrinolytic properties, such as aminocaproic acid, would potentially be helpful in reducing the rebleed rate.[36] Based on recent clinical trials, aminocaproic acid, when administered in the dosage of 100 mg per kilogram every 4 hours for 5 days, is safe and effective in reducing the occurrence of secondary hemorrhage.[37]

Indications for surgical intervention are the following: (1) microscopic corneal blood staining; (2) total hyphema with intraocular pressure greater than 50 mm Hg for 5 days, or pressures greater than 35 mm Hg for 7 days (to prevent optic atrophy); (3) total hyphemas present for 6 days with pressures greater than 25 mm Hg (to prevent corneal staining); and (4) hyphema of greater than 50 percent present for more than 9 days.[9,10] Surgical procedures to remove hyphemas include paracentesis, irrigation and aspiration, clot evacuation, and vitrectomy.

Optic Nerve Injuries

The controversy surrounding emergency surgical unroofing of the optic canals after indirect trauma in hopes of preventing edema and necrosis of the optic nerve has not been resolved.[38] Conventional teaching advocates optic canal decompression

11

TRAUMATIC ENOPHTHALMOS

JEFFREY I. RESNICK, M.D.
HENRY K. KAWAMOTO Jr., D.D.S., M.D., F.A.C.S.

Enophthalmos is defined as the reduction in the balance of the orbital contents and orbital volume.

HISTORICAL BACKGROUND

Nearly a century has passed since the first description of post-traumatic enophthalmos. In 1889, Lang[1] reported a case of a 13-year-old who sustained blunt trauma to the right eye, resulting in downward and posterior displacement of the globe. Lang postulated a fracture and depression of the bony orbit and identified the cause of post-traumatic enophthalmos as a discrepancy between the size of the bony orbital cavity and the volume of its soft-tissue contents. Since Lang's report, few reports have been written about the cause and treatment of traumatic enophthalmos, and its correction remains a formidable challenge to the reconstructive plastic surgeon.

Enophthalmos can be perceived clinically when the difference between the anterior position of the globes is greater than 2 mm. In addition, the recessed globe is often inferiorly depressed (orbital dystopia). Enophthalmos can appear immediately after an orbital injury or, in many cases, weeks to months following trauma. For many years enophthalmos was thought to be secondary to orbital floor fractures alone, but computed tomographic (CT) studies have clearly shown that disruption of any of the orbital walls can produce this deformity. The orbital fracture may be an isolated injury or part of a more complex pattern of facial fractures.

Following Lang's description of traumatic enophthalmos, additional insight into the problem was limited until Pfeiffer's[2] 1943 report of 24 cases of orbital fractures complicated by enophthalmos. He felt that orbital fracture resulted in the enlargement of the orbital cavity and the escape of orbital contents, with both factors contributing to the recessed globe. Although Pfeiffer wrote that "treatment to correct the deformity is receiving attention," he minimized the clinical significance of the enophthalmos and offered no specific treatment.

In 1944, Converse[3] reported the first treatment for traumatic enophthalmos. He described a single case that was corrected by placing an iliac bone graft to the orbital floor. By 1950, Converse and Smith[4] were advocating operative treatment of orbital floor fractures with bone grafting.

In 1957, Smith and Regan[5] coined the term "blowout fracture" for an orbital floor fracture associated with an intact orbital rim. They recommended early exploration of all orbital floor fractures to prevent irreversible scarring that would hinder full restoration of function. Blowout fractures have been further classified as "pure" when they involve only the orbital floor, and "impure" when they involve the floor as well as the orbital rim, to aid in diagnosis and treatment.[6] Over the past 30 years there has been a continuous debate in the ophthalmologic and plastic surgery literature concerning the surgical versus the nonoperative treatment of blowout fractures.[7–10] Nevertheless, clinically apparent enophthalmos is an absolute indication for surgical exploration following a pure blowout fracture.

The optimal surgical treatment for the recessed globe has also been a major source of controversy. A variety of autogenous and alloplastic materials have been used in orbital reconstruction. Autogenous materials have included bone, cartilage, dermal fat, and fascia lata.[11–16] Alloplasts or bioimplants that have been described include tantalum, Teflon, polyethylene, methyl methacrylate, glass beads, Marlex mesh, Supramid, different forms of silicone, and dense hydroxyapatite blocks.[17–27] Irradiated cartilage and lyophilized dura homografts have also been tried.[28] Reconstruction with absorbable material such as polyglactin 910 (Vicryl) film and Polydioxanone (PDS) plates has been reported.[29,30] All these materials were used in the acute phase in the hope of preventing the late development of enophthalmos.

ANATOMY

The bony orbit is roughly a pyramid-shaped structure with the optic foramen forming the apex. Portions of seven bones contribute to the orbit (Fig. 11–1). The roof is mainly formed by the orbital process of the frontal bone, with a minor posterior offering from the lesser wing of the sphenoid. The floor is primarily composed of the orbital plate of the maxilla with contributions from the zygoma laterally and the palatine bone medially. The strong lateral wall is made up of the greater wing of the sphenoid and zygoma, while the delicate medial wall is formed by portions of the maxilla, ethmoid, and lacrimal bones.[31] The optic nerve enters the cone in the superior medial recess of the orbit, approximately 45 mm from the inferior orbital rim (Fig. 11–2).[32]

In addition to the bony framework of the orbit, the eye is supported by a complex ligamentous system and by orbital fat. Mustardé[33] emphasized the role of Lockwood's suspensory ligament, which prevents downward displacement of the globe by forming an inferior sling from the medial to the lateral canthus. Anatomic studies by Koornneef[34] have shown that the globe is suspended in a connective tissue framework of fine fibrous septae. This framework, in turn, is suspended from the orbital walls (Fig. 11–3). The fine septae slide upon one [illegible] mal eye movements. It appears that this fine network must be disrupted if displacement of the orbitis to occur.

Finally, the globe is surrounded by fat which is found inside and outside the cone of the extraocular muscles. Removal of extraconal fat (as in cosmetic blepharoplasty) will not lead to enophthalmos, but studies by Manson and associates[35,36] have demonstrated that displacement of intraconal fat will contribute to enophthalmos

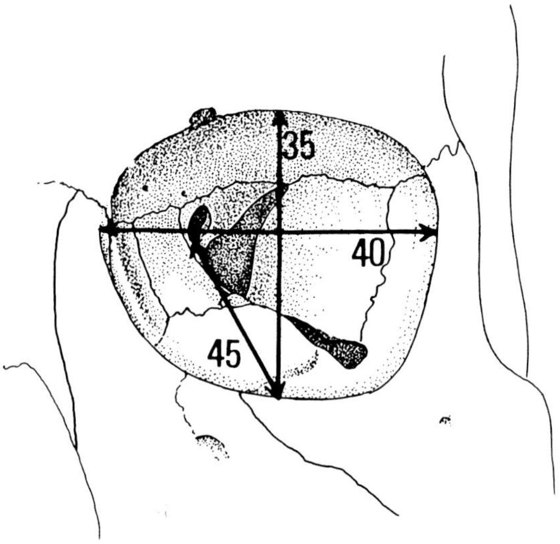

Figure 11–2 Average orbital measurements in millimeters. Optic foramen lies approximately 45 mm from inferior orbital rim.

PATHOPHYSIOLOGY

Many hypotheses have been proposed to explain the discrepancy between orbital bony volume and orbital contents which leads to enophthalmos.[7] These include: (1) herniation of orbital fat into the

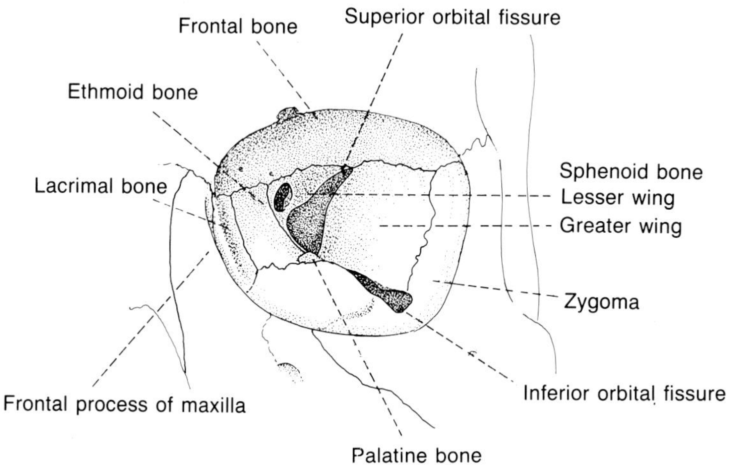

Figure 11–1 Normal orbital anatomy. Note medial and superior location of optic foramen.

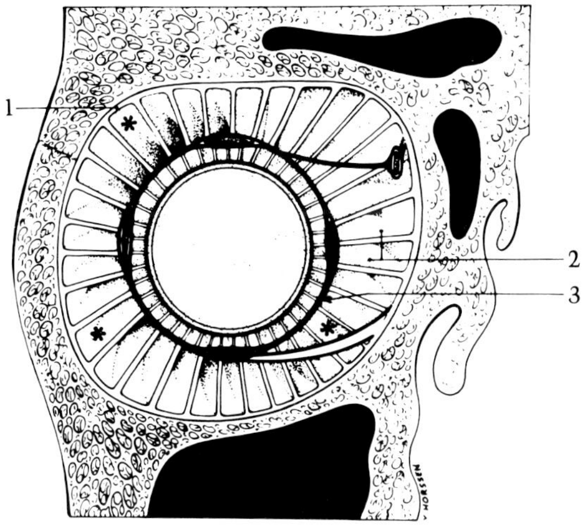

Figure 11–3 Fibrous septae (2) are suspended from orbital walls (1) and surround common muscle sheath (3) of globe. (Reproduced by permission from Koornneef L.[10])

maxillary sinus through torn periosteum and fractured bone; (2) enlargement of the orbital cavity volume by displacement of bony fractures; (3) orbital fat necrosis or atrophy; (4) cicatricial contracture of retrobulbar tissues tethering the ocular globe in a posterior position; and (5) entrapment or fibrosis of extraocular muscles.

Evaluation of enophthalmic patients using the CT scanner has revolutionized our understanding of the pathophysiology of traumatic globe displacement. Bite and colleagues[37] showed that orbital volume is increased in enophthalmos, but the bulk of soft tissue or fat remains essentially unchanged; that is, expanded orbital cavity volume occurs rather than soft-tissue loss or fat necrosis. This study was amplified by Manson and co-workers using CT scanning and anatomic dissections. They verified the displacement of a relatively constant volume of orbital soft tissue into an enlarged bony orbit,[35,36] and they further documented that it is the loss of bony and ligamentous support of the globe that allows gravity and scar contracture to displace and *reshape* the orbital soft tissue. The soft-tissue mass changes from a conical or pyramidal configuration to a more spherical pattern, with the globe sinking posteriorly, inferiorly, and often medially (Fig. 11–4). The orbital volume expansion consistently occurs at the interfaces with the ethmoid and maxillary sinuses (medially and inferiorly), with occasional enlargement in the area of the inferior orbital fissure and the sphenoid bone. With the addition of a zygomatic fracture, the lateral canthal ligament and Lockwood's suspensory ligament are displaced inferiorly and posteriorly. This further accentuates depression and recession of the globe.

It appears then that traumatic enophthalmos is generally not a problem of soft tissue loss, but rather one of increased orbital bony volume. As Tessier and associates have pointed out, "One should not speak of a loss [of fat]. . . . There have been many fewer losses than have been described, but there are many more fractures than have been diagnosed."[38] The essence of correction of traumatic enophthalmos then becomes a matter of restoration of the size and *shape* of the bony orbit.

CLINICAL EVALUATION

In the patient with traumatic enophthalmos, full ophthalmologic evaluation is mandatory. In the acute injury, associated conditions such as globe rupture, optic nerve injury, retinal detachment, hyphema, lens dislocation, corneal laceration, or iritis must be excluded. In established cases of enophthalmos, the eye examination should include assessment of visual acuity, visual fields, extraocular muscle function, and the integrity of the infraorbital nerve. The results of forced duction testing and Hertel exophthalmometry should be recorded. If the lateral orbital rims are intact, corneal projection can be measured from these benchmarks. If the lateral orbital rim is displaced, the patient should be examined from the basal or vertex position using the nasion or intact superior orbital rim as a reference in comparison to the normal eye.

Three to four millimeters of enophthalmos will cause deepening of the supratarsal fold, narrowing of the palpebral fissure, and pseudoptosis of the upper lid. The position of the medial and lateral canthi should be noted, as well as the contour of the malar eminence. Helpful clinical photographs include frontal, lateral, and submental-vertex views.

In the past, radiographic evaluation of the orbit consisted of Waters', Caldwell, and submental-vertex plain views with the addition of tomography when indicated. Because of its superior diagnostic abilities, CT scanning has dramatically improved evaluation of orbital fractures.[39] At present, uniplanar axial scans can be reformatted into coronal, sagittal, and oblique planes.[40] The best views of the orbital floor are generated by a reformatted projection along an oblique parasagittal line connecting the apex of the orbit and the midpoint

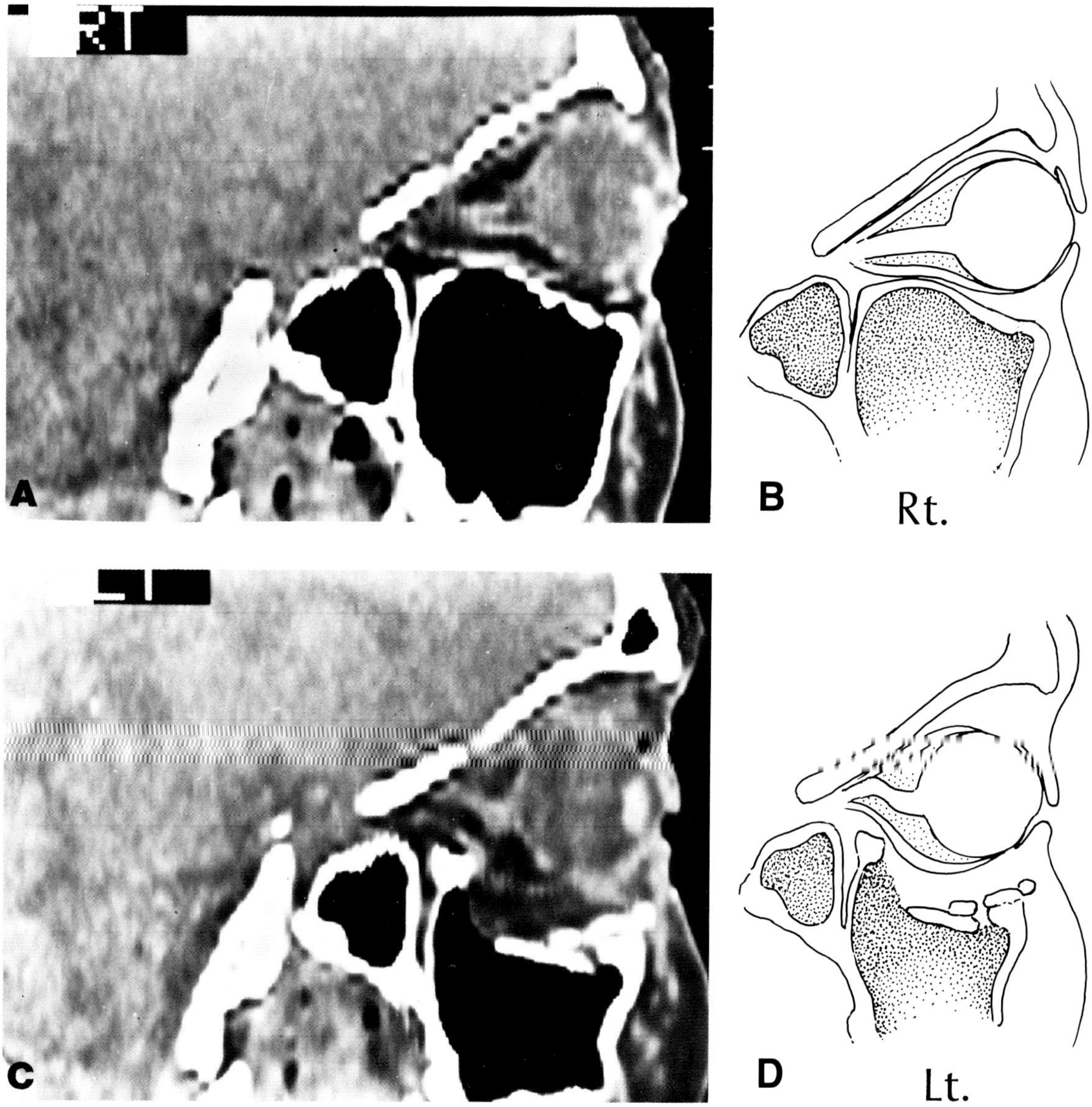

Figure 11–4 Comparison of normal with disrupted orbital floor following repair of displaced zygomatic fracture. *A*, Reformatted CT scan along oblique parasagittal plane showing normal right orbit. *B*, Schematic view of *A* illustrating compound "S" configuration of floor. Note convexity of floor behind globe. *C*, Reformatted study of fractured left orbital floor repaired with silicone implant. Globe is displaced posteriorly and inferiorly with prolapse of orbital contents into maxillary sinus. *D*, Schematic view of injured orbit. Orbital soft tissue mass is more spherical. Note improper placement of orbital floor implant which projects anterior to infraorbital rim and fails to reach posterior edge of fracture and full extent of floor defect.

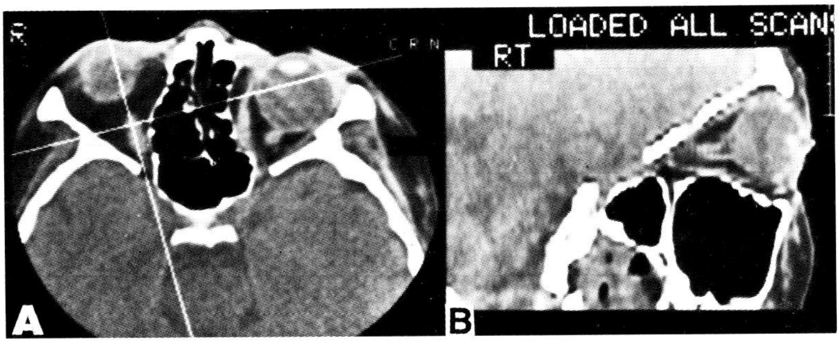

Figure 11–5 CT scan of normal orbit. *A*, Axial view with line connecting apex of orbit and midpoint of globe representing path of oblique parasagittal reformat. *B*, Reformatting of axial scan along oblique parasagittal plane to delineate orbital floor.

of the globe (Fig. 11–5). The medial orbital wall is best assessed on the axial scans. At the present level of refinement, "three"-dimensional CT scans add little worthwhile information, since the thickness of the orbital bones may be less than the interval between the CT slices. This can produce false-positive artifacts.

TREATMENT

As noted earlier, soft-tissue volume in post-traumatic enophthalmos is relatively constant but the orbital cavity is enlarged. Thus, the basis of treatment is restoration of the size and shape of the bony orbit. Tessier and colleagues[41] have noted that the correction of post-traumatic enophthalmos requires: (1) complete subperiosteal dissection to free the periorbita from displaced orbital wall fragments; (2) repositioning of the orbital framework with osteotomies; and (3) reconstruction of the walls and framework by bone grafts.

Alloplastic biomaterials may be used on occasion provided certain conditions are met. There should not be any disruption of the sinus mucosa, substantial volume restoration is not required, and the defect to be spanned should not be large. It is unusual to meet these conditions in the presence of established enophthalmos.

Our choice of grafting material for orbital reconstruction in post-traumatic enophthalmos has been autogenous bone graft. Bone may be harvested from the iliac crest, rib, or outer table of the cranium as cortical or corticocancellous bone. Experimental evidence has shown that cranial bone undergoes less resorption than endochondral bone.[42,43] This has also been our clinical impression, and we now prefer the use of cranial bone graft almost exclusively for orbital reconstruction.

Treatment must be directed at the specific area or areas of injury, whether this be the orbital floor, roof, medial wall, lateral wall, zygoma, or any combination thereof.

Enophthalmos Due to Fractures of the Orbital Floor or Medial Wall

For fractures confined to the orbital floor and medial wall, satisfactory access can usually be gained using a lower eyelid incision with the addition of a medial upper eyelid incision if necessary. A transconjunctival approach can also be considered. A subperiosteal dissection is begun on the intact bone, working toward the defect. The *posterior* edge of the defect *must be identified* or the exploration will be inadequate. The prolapsed soft tissue is returned to the confines of the orbit.

A thin shaving of calvarial bone with the periosteum attached is harvested. The calvarial bone gathered in this manner will be curved by the microfractures that are produced during the removal by the sharp osteotome. The periosteum will hold the microfractured pieces together and also provide a gliding surface (Fig. 11–6) (Tessier P.

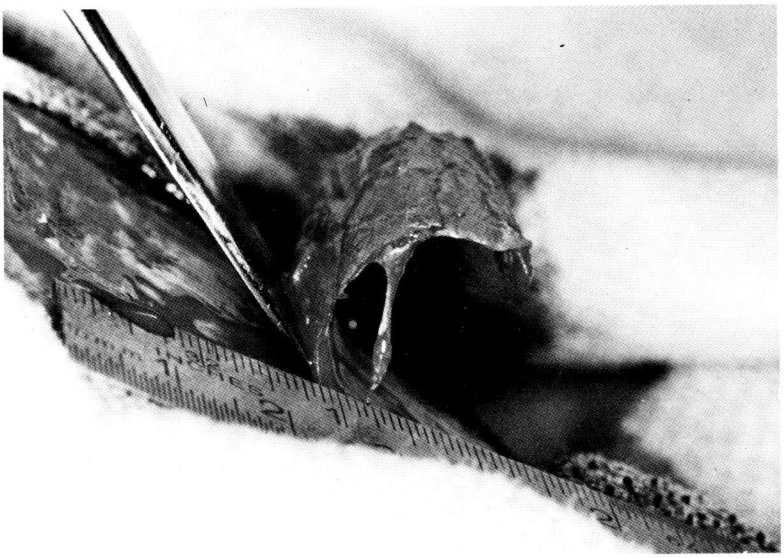

Figure 11–6 Harvesting of thin outer table cranial bone graft shaving. Microfractured bone is held together in satisfactory curve by attached periosteum.

Personal communication, 1974). This bone graft is placed over the defect with the periosteal side facing the orbital contents. Additional pieces of calvarial bone are inserted beneath this graft until the proper level of the wall is achieved (Fig. 11–7).

On occasion, additional exposure of the orbital floor is desirable. The inferior orbitotomy technique provides an unparalleled view of the floor (Fig. 11–8).[44] This technique is useful when the floor defect is large and it is difficult to deliver the herniated orbital tissue from the maxillary sinus. An additional indication for its use is in a patient who has previously undergone reconstructive surgery and has persistent enophthalmos and in whom the dissection to the posterior limits of the defect is arduous and deep.

Enophthalmos Due to a Displaced Zygomatic Fracture

In cases where exposure of the orbital roof or refracture and repositioning of the zygoma is required, a coronal incision is used in addition to the lower eyelid incision. The forehead is reflected in a supraperiosteal plane to a line approximately 1 cm above the superior orbital rim. The periosteum is then incised and the dissection proceeds in the subperiosteal plane into the orbit. The supraorbital and supratrochlear neurovascular bundles are preserved. Laterally, the frontal branch of the facial nerve is protected by staying directly on the deep fascia of the temporal muscle. The dissection extends inferiorly to the zygomatic arch and medially to the lateral orbital rim. The periosteum is incised over these structures and the dissection continues in the subperiosteal plane (Fig. 11–9).[45]

It is of the utmost importance to identify that intact bony edges of the original fracture to ensure that the entire defect is displayed. The periorbita is degloved to the posterior limits of the bony destruction.

If the zygoma is to be repositioned, the attachments of the temporalis and masseter to the zygoma are sharply divided to allow free movement of the zygoma. Additional exposure to the zygomaticomaxillary buttress is attained via an intraoral maxillary vestibular incision. The fracture is then re-created with a reciprocating saw (Fig. 11–10). The orbital framework is anatomically reduced and fixed. Formerly, only interosseus wires were used

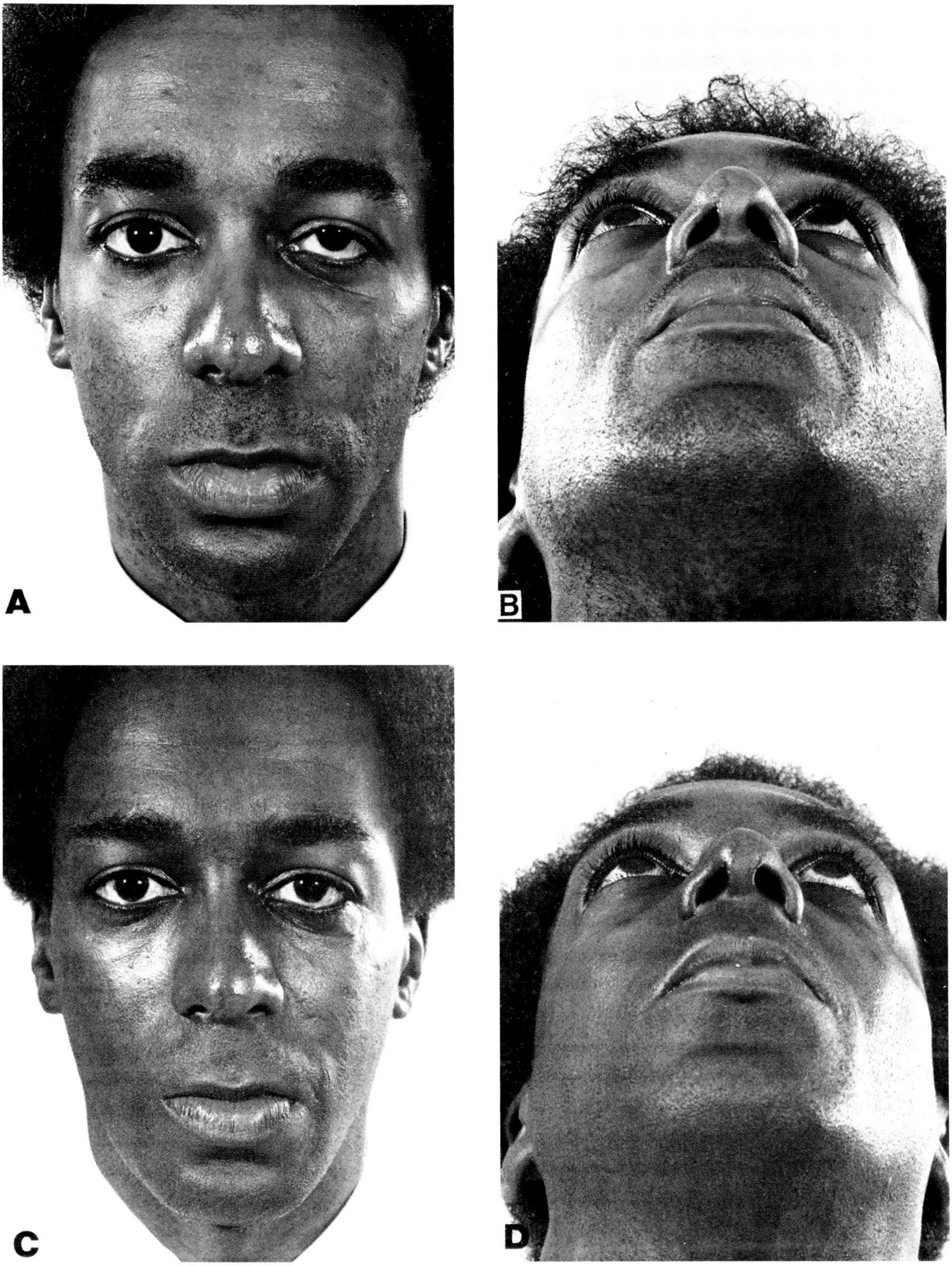

Figure 11–7 Late enophthalmos following multiple previous operations sent for evaluation of absent orbital floor. *A, B,* Preoperative views showing overelevation of globe due to anterior placement of floor implants but persistent enophthalmos because of lack of posterior support. *C, D,* Postoperative result following removal of malpositioned implants and repair of orbit with cranial bone grafts.

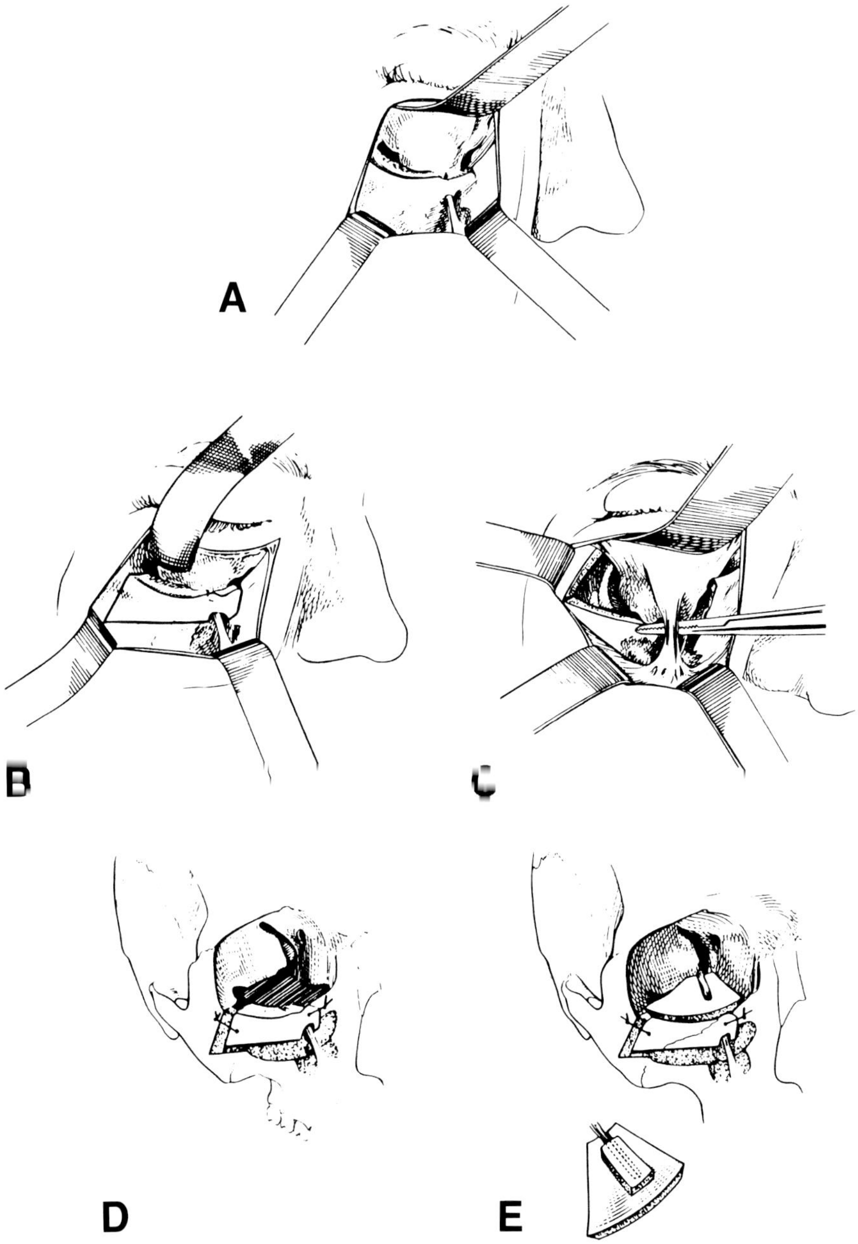

Figure 11–8 Inferior orbitotomy technique of Tessier. *A, B*, Lower eyelid exposure and outline of osteotomy. *C*, Rim removed and freed prolapsed orbital contents about to be returned to orbit. *D*, Replacement of rim segment. *E*, Reconstruction of floor with bone grafts. (Reproduced by permission from Tessier.[44])

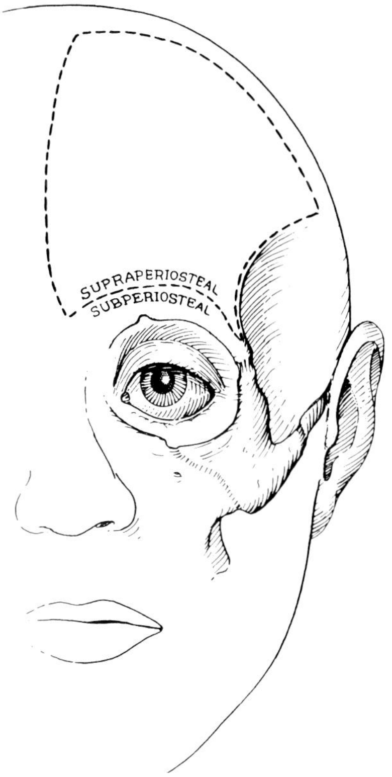

Figure 11–9 Outline of forehead dissection. Coronal flap is reflected in supraperiosteal plane. Approximately 1 cm above superior orbital rim, dissection proceeds in subperiosteal plane to enter orbit. (Reproduced by permission from Kawamoto.[45])

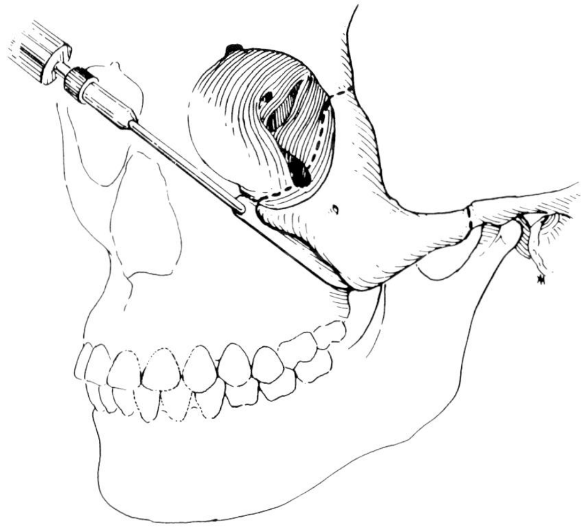

Figure 11–10 Re-creation of zygomatic fracture with reciprocating saw to allow malpositioned fragment to be anatomically reduced. (Reproduced by permission from Kawamoto.[45])

and the zygoma was fixed in an overcorrected superior and medial direction prior to bone grafting.[45] With the advent of miniplate and screw fixation to increase stability, as well as cranial bone grafts which undergo less resorption than endochondral bone, anatomic alignment is attained during the operation and maintained postoperatively. Usually two miniplates will provide adequate fixation.

Defects of the orbital floor, medial and lateral orbital walls, and zygomatic arch along with the inferior orbital fissure are obliterated with autogenous bone graft. To thrust the globe forward effectively, it is absolutely essential that the bone grafts be placed behind the mid-coronal plane of the globe (Fig. 11–11). Bone graft is stacked in layers to allow for slight anterior overcorrection of globe position. The contour of the normal orbital walls must be kept in mind when reconstructing the orbit (see Fig. 11–2), especially the acute superior angulation of the medial orbital floor as it joins the medial orbital wall. The position of the bone graft is usually maintained by closure of the periorbita alone, but interosseus wires may be used if necessary. It is also important to bone graft any defects of the anterior maxilla to prevent late soft-tissue retraction into the gaps and a depressed contour of the cheek.

It is not unusual to find that the pupil is looking downward at the end of the procedure. We feel that this is related to fibrotic shortening of the inferior rectus muscle and is probably one of the major contributors to immediate postoperative diplopia. Fortunately, the extraocular muscles accommodate within a few weeks.

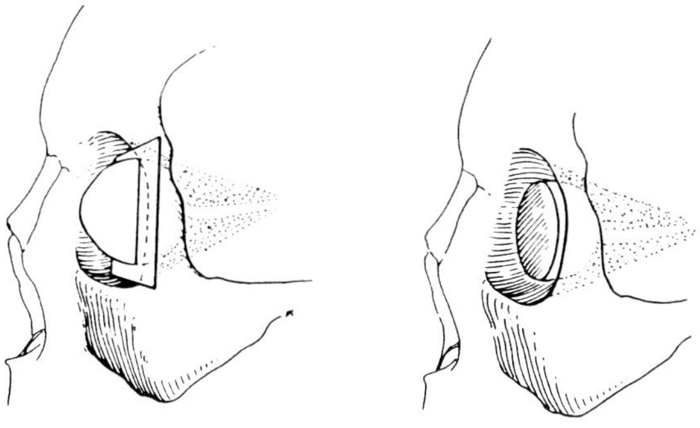

Figure 11–11 Mid-coronal plane of globe nearly coincides with lateral orbital rim. Effective forward projection of globe can only be achieved by placing grafts behind mid-coronal plane and simulating compound "S" curvature of floor. (Reproduced by permission from Kawamoto.[45])

No attempt is made to reattach the masseter to the zygoma because spontaneous attachment will occur. All incisions are closed in the usual manner, and a Frost lid traction suture is placed through the lower lid to prevent ectropion. Ancillary procedures for the correction of lateral or medial canthal position, lid ptosis, or epiphora are performed as needed (Fig. 11–12).

Enophthalmos Due to Loss of Orbital Globe Volume

On rare occasions, enophthalmos is seen when the globe is preserved but its volume is reduced following partial loss of its vitreous. The volume discrepancy can be addressed by inserting bone graft behind the vertical equator of the shrunken globe. A lower eyelid incision can be used to gain access to the areas of interest. The most efficient use of the grafts is to place them along the medial and lateral walls. Additional bone grafts can be inserted beneath the globe to restore its vertical position (Fig. 11–13).

Enophthalmos in the Anophthalmic Orbit

Enophthalmos is commonly noted after orbital enucleation and insertion of a prosthesis. This deformity is usually associated with deepening of the supratarsal fold and ptosis of the upper and lower eyelids.

Vistnes and colleagues have approached the correction of enophthalmos in the anophthalmic orbit using room temperature vulcanized silicone to overcome the volume deficit.[46] They recommend that the correction of lower and upper lid ptosis be deferred until the orbital volume deficit has been addressed. They caution, however, that room temperature vulcanized silicone should not be used in the orbit where globe loss has been secondary to trauma.[47] When portions of the orbital wall are absent as a result of trauma, they should be rebuilt first. Additional bone grafts can then be inserted to project the prosthesis forward and correct the enophthalmos (Fig. 11–14).

POSTOPERATIVE CONSIDERATIONS

Postoperative problems have been minimal. Infection and hematoma are exceptionally rare. Persistent enophthalmos has been encountered, given the difficulty of accurately estimating orbital volume intraoperatively. A second procedure may be required in some patients, and the patient should be informed of this possibility.

A minor displacement of the lateral canthus may not be appreciated preoperatively, but once the enophthalmos is corrected, lateral canthal malposition will become more apparent. Therefore, careful assessment of the position of the lateral canthus must be performed preoperatively, since a lateral canthopexy may be required at the time of enophthalmos correction.

Transient exophthalmos and diplopia are expected and usually resolve within a few months. Occasionally, extraocular muscle surgery will be needed for correction of diplopia. Any secondary operative procedure should be deferred until six months after the initial operation to allow for resolution of edema and maturation of scars.

Weakness of the frontal branch of the facial nerve can be seen following refracture and repositioning of the zygoma. Extreme caution must be exercised in raising the coronal flap, especially over the zygomatic arch where the normal topography may be altered by the original fracture.

Decrease in visual acuity following enophthalmos correction has not been encountered. Thorough understanding of the orbital anatomy, avoidance of excessive and prolonged compression on the globe, careful dissection in the subperiosteal plane of the orbit, and meticulous hemostasis will prevent optic nerve injury.

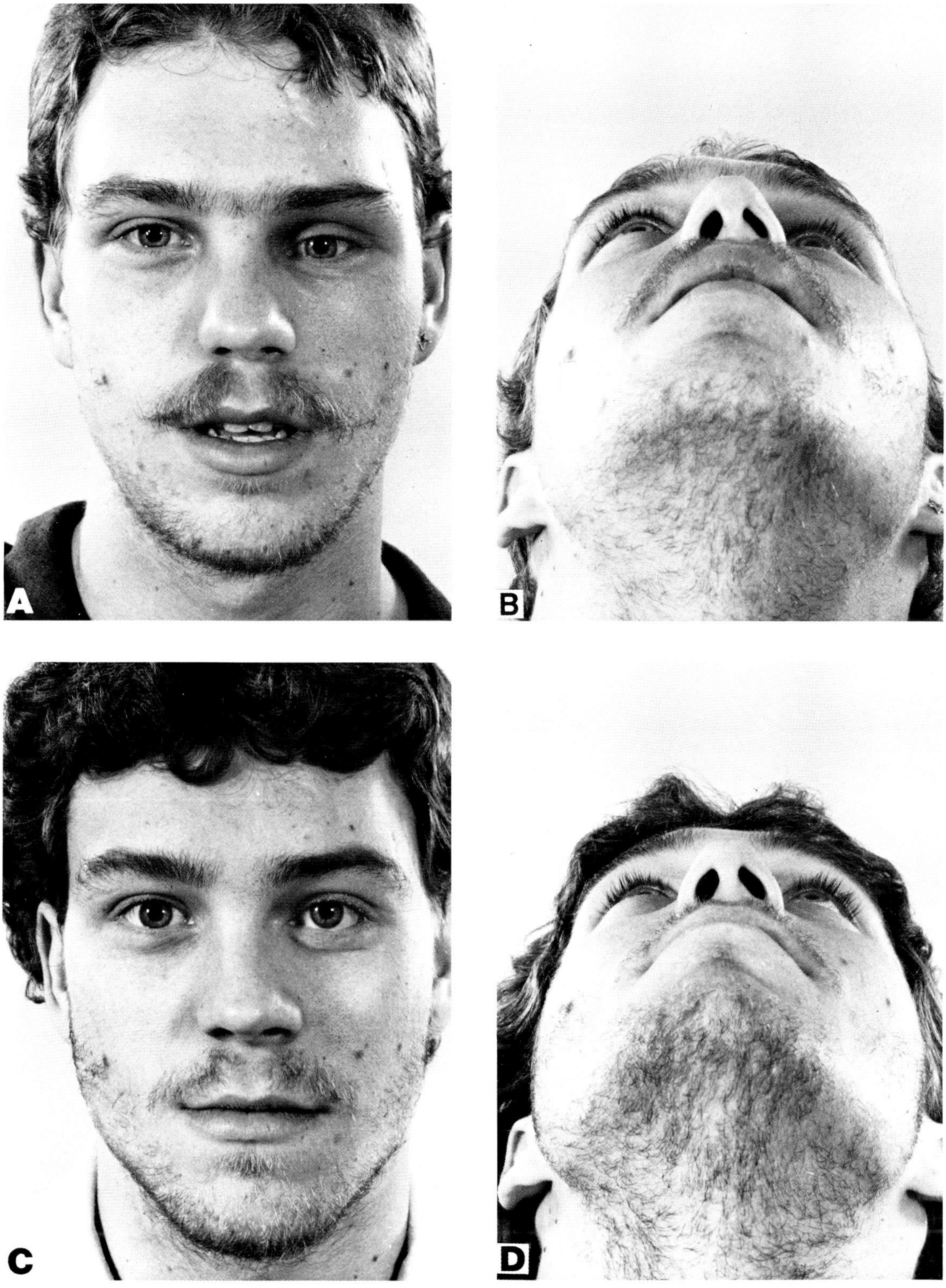

Figure 11–12 Previously treated displaced left zygomatic referred for late enophthalmos and dystopia. *A, B,* Appearance following acute reduction of fracture and insertion of silicone implant. *C, D,* Correction following refracture and repositioning of zygoma and cranial bone grafting of orbital defects.

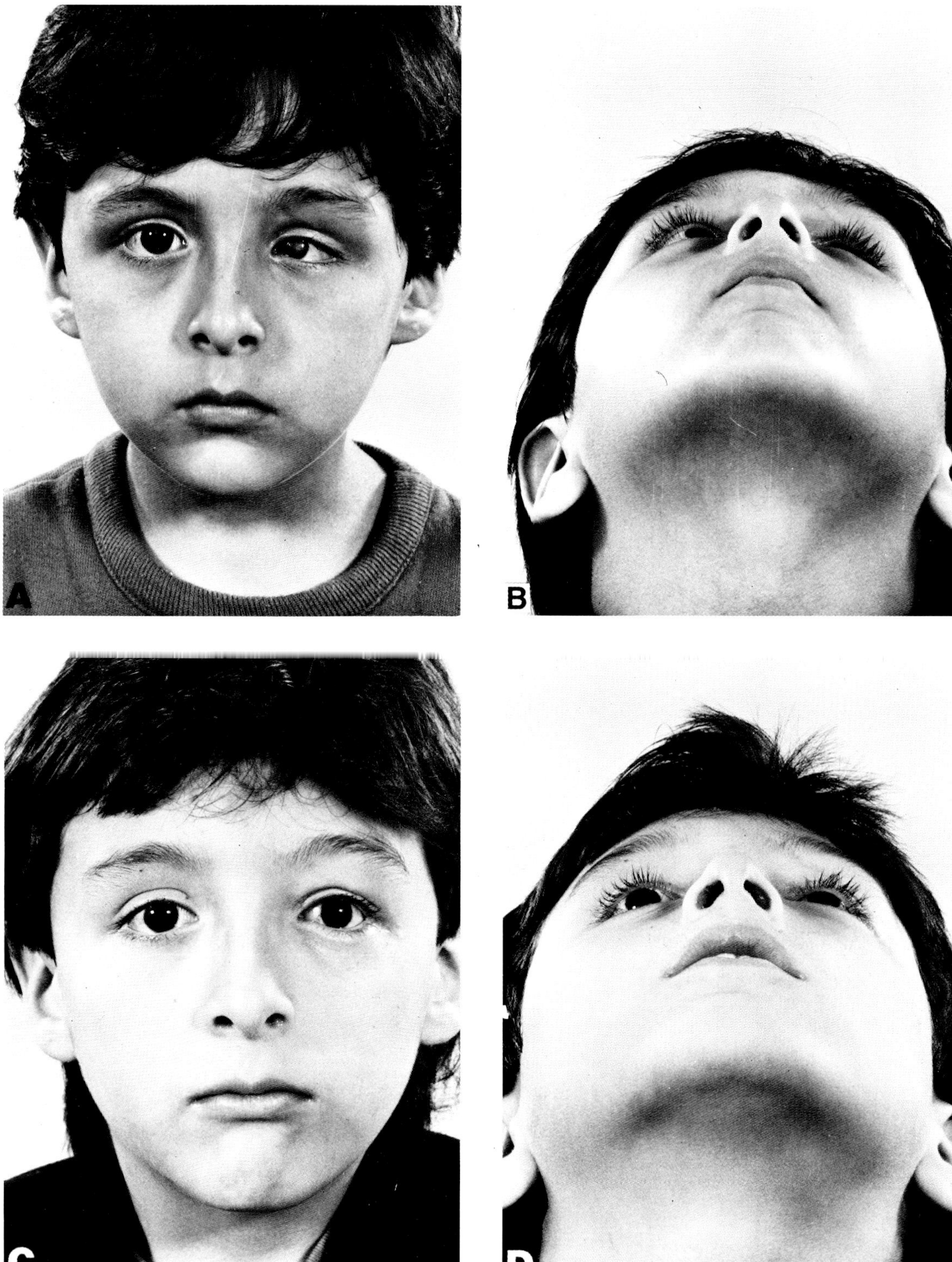

Figure 11–13 Patient with enophthalmos associated with traumatic partial loss of left globe volume. *A, B,* Bony orbital volume is normal but decreased size of globe is responsible for its sunken appearance. *C, D,* Following compensation of volume discrepancy with cranial bone grafts. A second procedure was required to correct upper lid ptosis and lateral canthal position.

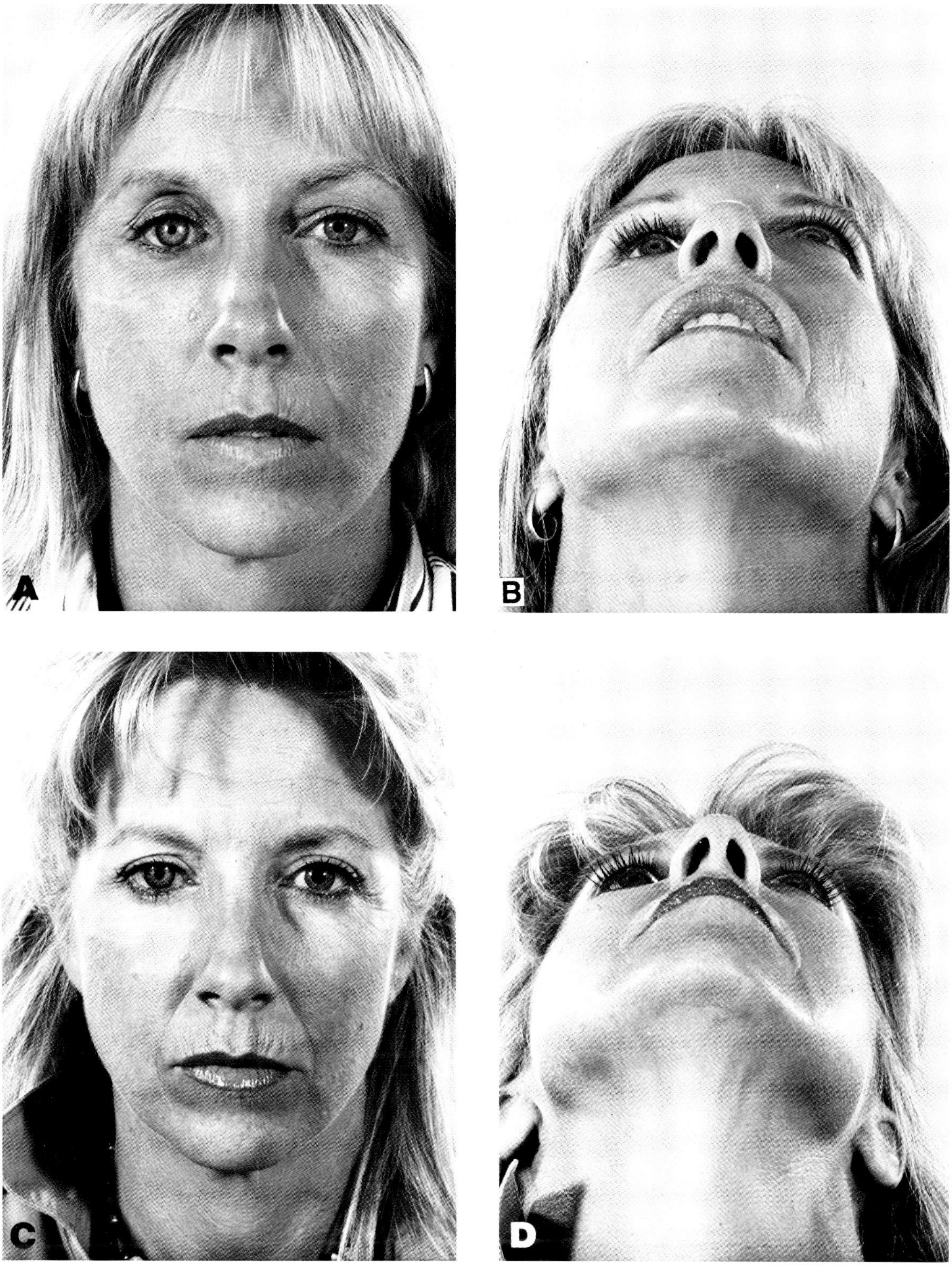

Figure 11–14 Right post-traumatic orbital deformity with loss of globe due to kick by horse. Referred for correction after initial reduction of zygomatic fracture. *A, B,* Anophthalmos camouflaged by large ocular prosthesis. Note deepening of superior palpebral fold and ptosis of upper and lower eyelids. *C, D,* After reconstructing practically entire orbital floor with cranial bone grafts and insertion of thinner ocular prosthesis.

REFERENCES

1. Lang W. Traumatic enophthalmos with retention of perfect acuity of vision. Trans Ophthalmol Soc UK 1889; 9:41–45.
2. Pfeiffer RL. Traumatic enophthalmos. Arch Ophthalmol 1943; 30:718–726.
3. Converse JM. Two plastic operations for repair of the orbit following severe trauma and extensive comminuted fracture. Arch Ophthalmol 1944; 31:323–325.
4. Converse JM, Smith B. Reconstruction of the floor of the orbit by bone grafts. Arch Ophthalmol 1950; 44:1–21.
5. Smith B, Regan WF. Blowout fracture of the orbit. Am J Ophthalmol 1957; 44:733–739.
6. Cramer LM, Tooze FM, Lerman S. Blowout fractures of the orbit. Br J Plast Surg 1965; 18:171–179.
7. Converse JM, Smith B, Obear MF, et al. Orbital blowout fractures: a ten year survey. Plast Reconstr Surg 1967; 39:20–36.
8. Putterman AM, Stevens T, Urist MJ.Non-surgical management of blowout fractures of the orbital floor. Am J Ophthalmol 1974; 77:232–239.
9. Converse JM, Smith B. On the treatment of blowout fractures of the orbit. Plast Reconstr Surg 1978; 62:100–104.
10. Koornneef L. Current concepts on the management of orbital blowout fractures. Ann Plast Surg 1982; 9:185–200.
11. Converse JM, Smith B. Enophthalmos and diplopia in fractures of the orbital floor. Br J Plast Surg 1957; 9:265–274.
12. Converse JM, Cole G, Smith B. Late treatment of blowout fracture of the floor of the orbit. Plast Reconstr Surg 1961; 28:183–191.
13. Smith B, Petrelli R. Dermis fat-graft as a moveable implant within the muscle cone. Am J Ophthalmol 1978; 85:62–66.
14. Stark RB, Frileck SP. Conchal cartilage grafts in augmentation rhinoplasty and orbital floor fracture. Plast Reconstr Surg 1969; 43:591–596.
15. Coster DJ, Galbraith JEK. Diced cartilage grafts to correct enophthalmos. Br J Ophthalmol 1980; 64:135–136.
16. Monasterio FO, Rodriguez A, Benavides A. A simple method for the correction of enophthalmos. Clin Plast Surg 1987; 14:169–175.
17. Sherman AE. Reconstruction of orbital floor defects. Surg Gynecol Obstet 1947; 84:799–803.
18. Quereau JVD, Souders BF. Teflon implant to elevate the eye in depressed fracture of the orbit. Arch Ophthalmol 1956; 55:685–691.
19. Bromberg BE, Rubin LR, Walden R. Implant reconstruction of the orbit. Am J Surg 1960; 100:818–822.
20. Bennett JE, Armstrong JR. Repair of defects of the bony orbit with methyl methacrylate. Am J Ophthalmol 1962; 53:285–290.
21. Ballen PH. Further experiences with rapidly polymerizing methylmethacrylate in orbital floor fractures. Plast Reconstr Surg 1964; 34:624–629.
22. Smith B, Obear M, Leone CR Jr. The correction of enophthalmos associated with anophthalmos by glass bead implantation. Am J Ophthalmol 1967; 64:1088–1093.
23. Hill JC, Radford CJ. Treatment of advancing enophthalmos. Am J Ophthalmol 1965; 60:487–492.
24. Browning CW, Walker RV. The use of alloplastics in 45 cases of orbital floor reconstruction. Am J Ophthalmol 1965; 60:684–699.
25. Borghouts JMHM, Otto AJ. Silicone sheet and bead implants to correct the deformities of inadequately healed orbital floor fractures. Br J Plast Surg 1978; 31:254–258.
26. Kummoona R. Chrome cobalt and gold implant for the reconstruction of a traumatized orbital floor. J Oral Surg 1976; 41:293–299.
27. Zide MF. Late posttraumatic enophthalmos corrected by dense hydroxylapatite blocks. J Oral Maxillofac Surg 1986; 44:804–806.
28. Dingman RO, Grabb WC. Costal cartilage-homografts preserved by irradiation. Plast Reconstr Surg 1961; 28:562–567.
29. Morain WD, Colby E, Stauffer M, et al. Reconstruction of orbital blowout fractures with polyglactin-910 film. Plast Surg Forum 1986; 9:131–132.
30. Holtje WJ. Reconstruction of fractured or resected orbital floors with PDS plates. Plast Surg Forum 1986; 9:277–279.
31. Clemente CD. The neck and head. In: Clemente CD, ed. Anatomy: a regional atlas of the human body. Philadelphia: Lea & Febiger, 1975: Fig. 482.
32. Manson PN, Ruas EJ, Iliff NT. Deep orbital reconstruction for correction of post-traumatic enophthalmos. Clin Plast Surg 1987; 14:113–121.
33. Mustardé JC. The role of Lockwood's suspensory ligament in preventing downward displacement of the eye. Br J Plast Surg 1968; 21:73–81.
34. Koornneef L. Spatial aspects of orbital musculo-fibrous tissue in man: a new anatomical and histological approach. Amsterdam: Swets & Zeitlinger, 1977.
35. Manson PN, Clifford CM, Su CT, et al. Mechanisms of global support and posttraumatic enophthalmos: I. The anatomy of the ligament sling and its relation to intramuscular cone orbital fat. Plast Reconstr Surg 1986; 77:193–202.
36. Manson PN, Grivas A, Rosenbaum A, et al. Studies on enophthalmos: II. The measurement of orbital injuries and their treatment by quantitative computed tomography. Plast Reconstr Surg 1986; 77:203–214.
37. Bite U, Jackson IT, Forbes GS, et al. Orbital volume measurements in enophthalmos using three-dimensional CT imaging. Plast Reconstr Surg 1985; 75:502–507.
38. Tessier P, Rougier J, Hervouet F, et al. Sequelae of orbital trauma. Plastic surgery of the orbit and eyelids. Translated by S. Anthony Wolfe. New York: Masson Publishing USA, 1981:96.
39. Finkle DR, Ringler SL, Luttenton CR, et al. Comparison of the diagnostic methods used in maxillofa-

cial trauma. Plast Reconstr Surg 1985; 75:32–38.
40. Marsh JL, Gado M. The longitudinal orbital CT projection: a versatile image for orbital assessment. Plast Reconstr Surg 1983; 71:308–317.
41. Tessier P, Rougier J, Hervouet F, et al. Sequelae of orbital trauma. Plastic surgery of the orbit and eyelids. Translated by S. Anthony Wolfe. New York: Masson Publishing USA, 1981:99.
42. Zins JE, Whitaker LA. Membranous versus endochondral bone: implications for craniofacial reconstruction. Plast Reconstr Surg 1983; 72:778–784.
43. Kusiak JF, Zins JE, Whitaker LA. The early revascularization of membranous bone. Plast Reconstr Surg 1985; 76:510–514.
44. Tessier P. Inferior orbitotomy: a new approach to the orbital floor. Clin Plast Surg 1982; 9:569–575.
45. Kawamoto HK Jr. Late posttraumatic enophthalmos: a correctable deformity? Plast Reconstr Surg 1982; 69:423–430.
46. Iverson RE, Vistnes LM, Siegel RJ. Correction of enophthalmos in the anophthalmic orbit. Plast Reconstr Surg 1973; 51:545–554.
47. Sergott TJ, Vistnes LM. Correction of enophthalmos and superior sulcus depression in the anophthalmic orbit: a long-term follow-up. Plast Reconstr Surg 1987; 79:331–338.

12

MAXILLARY FRACTURE

DONALD L. LEAKE, D.M.D., M.D., F.A.C.S.

Fractures of the maxilla occur because of motor vehicle accidents, sports and industrial accidents, or falls and altercations. They often are aesthetically deforming and they also may severely compromise function because of the proximity of the maxillary antra, the nasal cavity, and the orbits. The occlusion is also disturbed. Patients with midface trauma are treated initially by any necessary lifesaving procedures, including establishment and maintenance of the airway, control of hemorrhage, and management of intracranial injuries. If the vital signs are stable, the initial assessment of the maxillofacial injury includes a history, clinical examination, and appropriate radiologic studies. When the dentition is not complete, or when there are loose teeth, it is sometimes useful to take impressions of the teeth to fabricate splints. The study models made from dental impressions may also be useful in determining the occlusion. The principles of treatment are the same as for any other fracture of the skeleton, including reduction of the fracture and fixation.

In addition to stabilizing the patient's vital signs, initial therapy of midface trauma includes tracheostomy if indicated, repair of facial lacerations, and temporary stabilization of the dentition if definitive treatment must be delayed.[1,2]

The advent and development of computed tomography (CT) have revolutionized the diagnosis and management of facial fractures. Frontal and cross-table lateral skull radiographic studies are often obtained before cranial CT and may provide enough information for emergency surgery in the rapidly deteriorating patient. In these cases cranial CT is then used in the immediate postoperative period to evaluate head injury or spine injury. CT scans not only delineate bone fractures but also define in a superior way the accompanying soft tissue changes. It is the procedure of choice for detecting cerebral hemorrhage or contusion, and for epidural and subdural hematomas as well as intraorbital hematomas.

PHYSICAL EVALUATION

Patients with maxillary fractures typically have marked facial edema. They are unable to occlude the teeth, which results in lengthening of the middle third of the face, or they may have an overbite deformity. Often there is circumorbital ecchymosis and the nares may be filled with blood clots. There may be sensory loss due to damage to the infraorbital nerve and occasionally a facial palsy secondary to paralysis of the facial nerve. Surgical subcutaneous emphysema may be present when maxillary, nasoethmoidal, or zygomatic fractures result in a tear in the mucoperiosteum and the patient blows the nose after injury.

Palpation is an important element of the physical evaluation of midface fractures. Typically, tenderness and a step deformity may be detected overlying a fracture. Intraorally there may be ecchymosis in the buccal sulci or in the palate. Blood coming from the nasal pharynx may be drawn into the mouth by the patient and it may coat the palate. The occlusion must be carefully evaluated. There may be step defects in the occlusal plane, fractures of the teeth, or luxated teeth. Typically, a downward and posterior displacement of the maxilla results in an open bite due to premature closure of the posterior teeth, a finding that may also occur with fracture-dislocations of the mandibular condyles. A gloved hand should be used to palpate the maxilla. Grasping the premaxilla with the thumb and index finger of one hand while palpating the bridge of the nose in the frontomaxillary region will test the mobility of the maxilla. Putting the thumb and index finger on either side of the buccal aspect of the premolars or molars is also a useful maneuver in diagnosing fractures of the maxilla. Examination of individual teeth with a mouth mirror and dental explorer is appropriate to evaluate the status of the dentition. Fractured crowns often occur in cases of trauma to the maxilla, and in a patient with an apparently abnormal occlusion, careful inspection of the facets of the teeth may be helpful in establishing the normal, pretrauma occlusion of the patient.

TRIMALAR FRACTURES

The zygoma, or malar bone, is usually fractured in conjunction with one or more adjoining bones such as the maxilla, the frontal bone, or the temporal bone. Shortly after the traumatic event, before the anatomy has been obscured by edema, the appearance of the patient provides clues to the lines of fracture. There may be flatness of the face with depression of the malar bone. The interpupillary line is no longer horizontal but will dip toward the fractured side when the palpebral ligament is displaced because of downward rotation of the malar bone. Ecchymosis of the lid, conjunctiva, and sclera may be marked. Pain and trismus occur when the arch is depressed enough to interfere with mandibular opening. When the infraorbital nerve is impinged upon, there will be altered sensation or anesthesia in the upper lip, the lower eyelid, and the lateral aspect of the nose. Diplopia occurs when the fracture is severe and the orbital floor's support for the globe is lost, resulting in partial herniation of the global contents into the maxillary antrum. This is not evident in some patients until after the edema subsides.[3]

Palpation of the orbital rim and the zygomaticofrontal and zygomaticomaxillary sutures may reveal step discrepancies.

Classically, the Waters view, a posteroranterior oblique projection of the face, is used to confirm the diagnosis. The submental-vertical projection is used to evaluate the zygomatic arches (Figs. 12–1 and 12–2). CT scans also delineate these fractures very well and typically are ordered when there is a question of intercranial trauma (Fig. 12–3). Typical findings include step deformities at the infraorbital margin and separation of the zygomaticofrontal sutures. The maxillary sinus usually is clouded because of hemorrhage into the sinus from tears in the antral mucosa.

Treatment of fractures of the zygomatic bones depends on the severity, degree of displacement, and fragmentation. The aim of fracture treatment is to reduce the fractures and stabilize the bone fragments so that form and function ultimately are

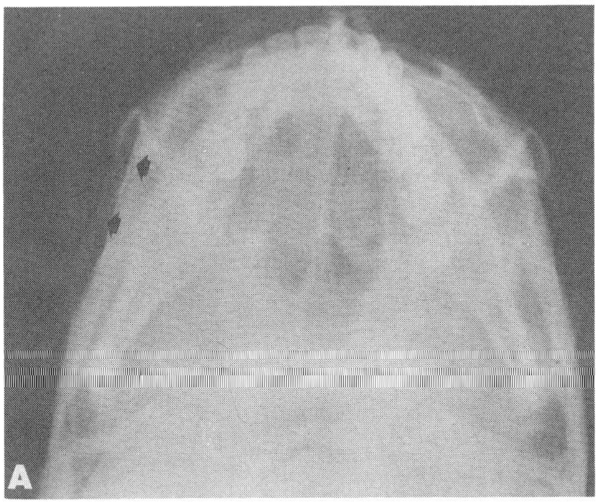

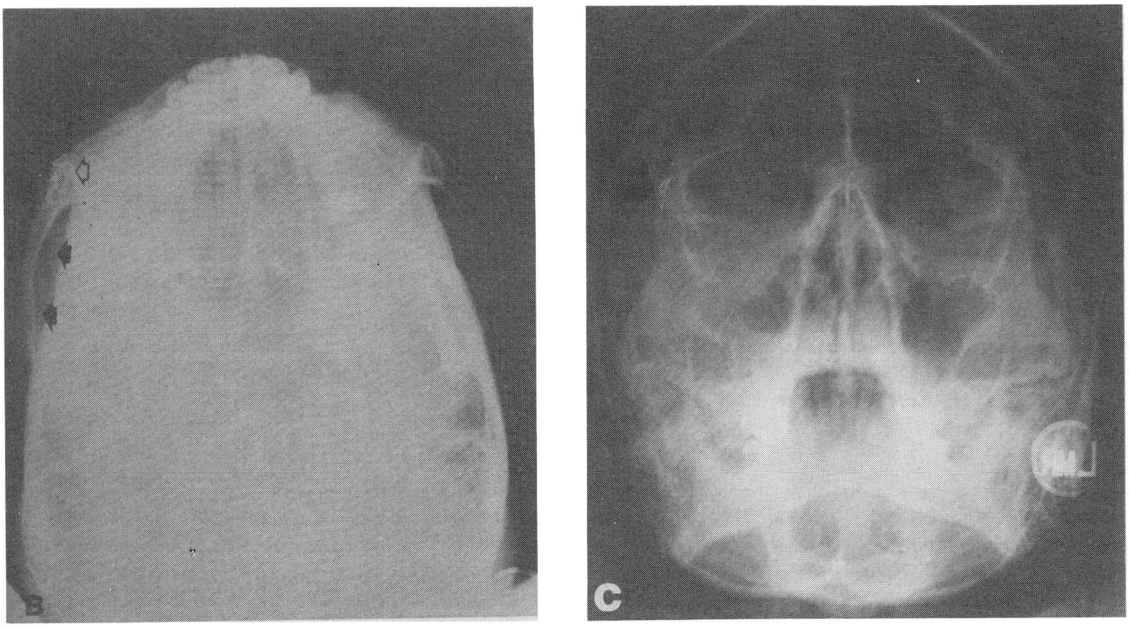

Figure 12–1 *A*, Preoperative, and *B, C*, postoperative views of a right trimalar fracture with a depressed zygomatic arch. The patient was treated by simple elevation through a brow incision and interosseous wire fixation at the frontal zygomatic suture fracture line.

restored. Simple elevation may suffice when the breaks are clean and there is no comminution. Direct, interosseous wiring at one or more points may be required to stabilize the fractures, typically at the frontozygomatic suture and on occasion the infraorbital rims (see Figs. 12–1B and C).

Methods of Reduction

The temporal approach, named for Gillies, is accomplished by making a vertical incision approximately 2 cm long in the direction of the skin lines through the hair-bearing portion of the temple. The incision is carried through the skin, subcutaneous tissues, and the two layers of the temporal fascia to the temporal muscle. A heavy elevator is slipped between the temporal fascia and the muscle into the temporal fossa to the undersurface of the zygoma. Strong leverage can then be used to elevate the bones into position. When the fracture is uncomplicated, the reduction may be accomplished with a resounding pop.

When zygomatic fractures are comminuted, closed reduction is rarely adequate. Open reduction and fixation using interosseous wires may be performed as late as 10 days to 2 weeks after the injury without compromising the result. Occasionally only one incision is required in the lateral end of the brow, accompanied by elevation of the fractured bone into position and stabilization with one interosseous wire. When this is inadequate, an additional incision is made at the inferior margin of the lower lid. The incision is through a skin line and exposes the infraorbital margin and floor of the orbit. The incisions are made through the hair-bearing areas of the brow and shaving is not required—in fact it should be avoided. The area to be incised is generally injected with a local anesthetic containing epinephrine, enough time should be allowed for it to become effective, in order to reduce bleeding during the operation. A drill hole sufficient to allow passage of the appropriately sized wire is placed on either side of the fracture line. Twenty-four- to 26-gauge wires are used for the frontal zygomatic area, 26- or 28-gauge wires for the infraorbital area. The use of a small bone hook or a tracheal hook sometimes is useful in stabilizing the fragments until the wires are tightened. When the zygomatic arch is fractured and unstable following the reduction because of comminution, a slightly curved horizontal incision can be made over the arch to allow direct fixation with interosseous wires.[4–12]

When the orbital floor is severely comminuted, a small, thin bone graft or an alloplastic material such as Silastic, Supramyd, OsteoMesh, or heavily tanned collagen is used to reestablish the orbital floor. Occasionally the addition of packing in the maxillary sinus provides support for the orbital implant; if no fracture exists through which the packing can be placed, a surgical opening, the Caldwell-Luc approach, is made through the lateral wall of the antrum and packing is placed using 1/2-inch selvage gauze permeated with an antibio-

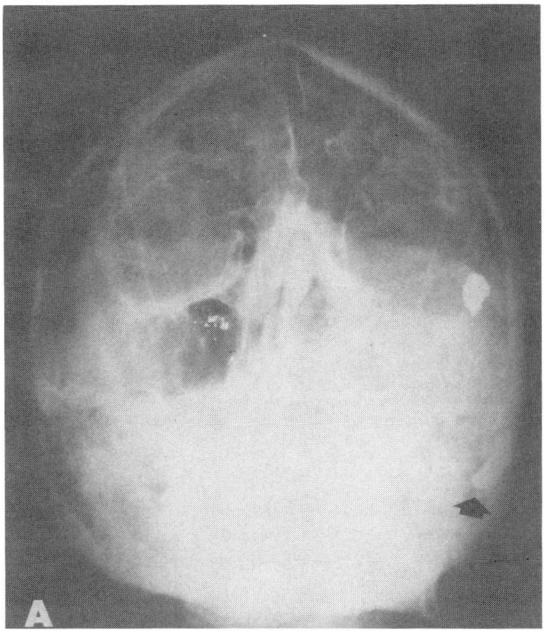

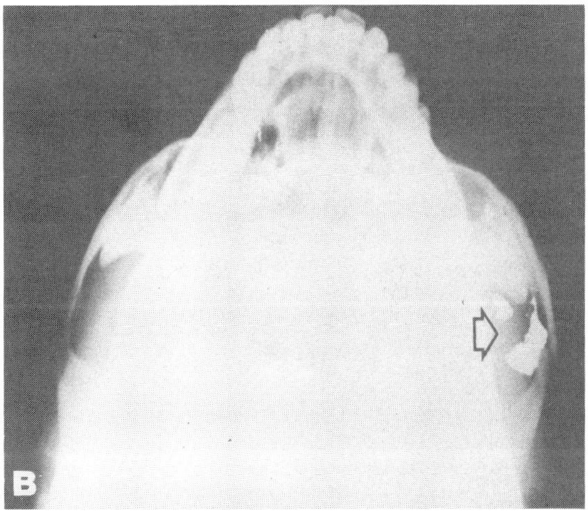

Figure 12–2 *A, B,* Radiographs of a patient with a gunshot wound to the face in which he sustained a fracture of the left zygomatic arch. He was treated by coronoidectomy, removal of the bullet fragments impinging on the mandible, and suture of facial lacerations.

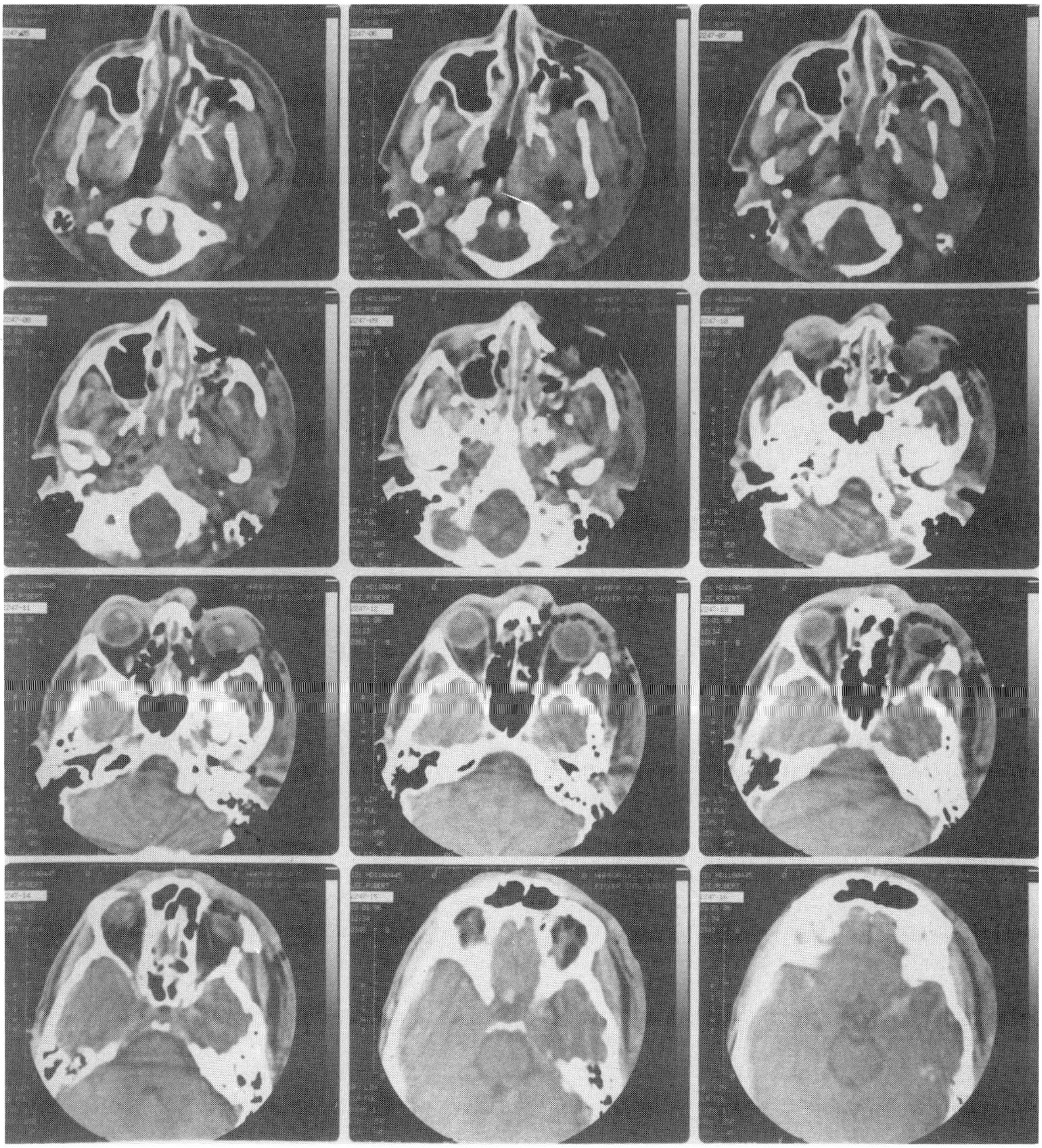

Figure 12–3 Computed tomography scan of a patient with closed head trauma, frontal sinus fracture, and a left trimalar fracture. There were also bilateral fractures of the mandible, one at the left angle and the other a parasymphyseal fracture.

tic salve. An antrostomy is performed beneath the inferior turbinate bone and the end of the packing is brought through this opening into the nasal cavity. The oral wound is closed using resorbable sutures. The packing should be removed within a week to ten days.

CLASSIFICATION OF MAXILLARY FRACTURES

For convenience, maxillary fractures are generally divided according to the level of the fracture and are classified as Le Fort I, II, or III (Fig. 12–4).

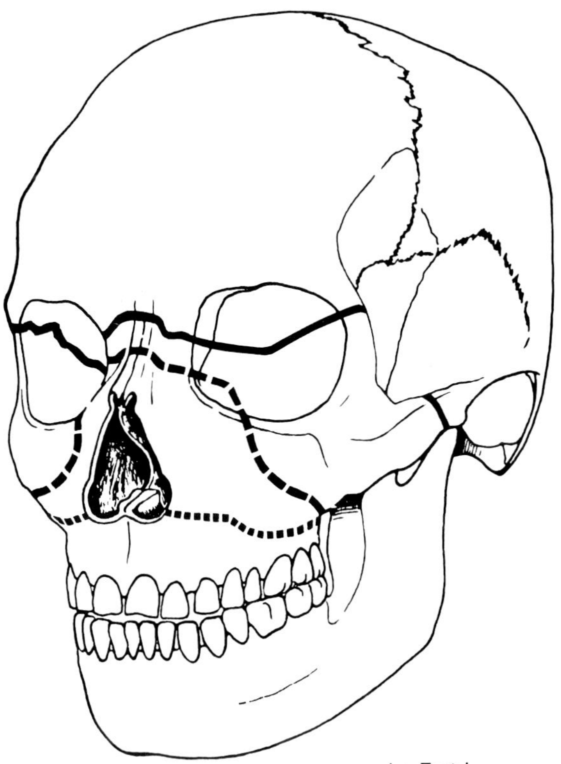

Figure 12–4 The Le Fort lines of fracture.

Le Fort I, a horizontal fracture, is one in which the maxilla is separated from the base of the skull just below the zygomatic process. These fractures are highly mobile and have been termed "free-floating maxillas." The fracture may be unilateral and involve more than a simple alveolar fracture because the midline of the palate is involved in unilateral Le Fort I fractures.

The degree of displacement is variable. Some fractures are free floating but nondisplaced. Others may be severely retruded and depressed in the posterior aspect of the maxilla, causing an open bite deformity. These fractures may be visualized on routine posteroanterior, lateral jaw, and Waters views of the skull as well as by CT scanning.

Le Fort I, the low transverse maxillary fracture, is also called the fracture of Guerin in reference to the French surgeon who initially described it, as well as the designation of one of the lines of weakness described by René Le Fort later on. Le Fort's lines are the ones referred to now. The line of fracture connects the lower end of the nasal cavity with the pterygomaxillary fissure, crossing the facial wall of the maxillary sinus and the posterior lateral wall. Traversing the lateral wall of the nasal cavity, the fracture returns to the nose. The fragment separated by a fracture of this type comprises the vault of the palate, the alveolar processes, and the lower portion of the pterygoid process. Displacement may be backward, lateral, or downward.

Le Fort II, also called a pyramidal fracture, starts from the lower end of the nasal bones, crosses the orbital margin, usually above the nasolacrimal canal, traverses a substantial portion of the orbital floor, and crosses the inferior orbital margin near the zygomaticomaxillary suture. It continues through the infraorbital canal and the anterior and posterior sinus walls. Crossing the posterior pillar of the upper jaw and the pyramidal and pterygoid processes, it reaches the pterygomaxillary fissure and finally returns to the medial orbital margin, traversing the lateral wall of the nasal cavity. These fractured bones may be impacted backward and upward or the fragment may be floating free, dislocated inferiorly, aided by contraction of the pterygoid muscles (Fig. 12–5).

Le Fort III fractures separate the facial skeleton from the neurocranium. These fractures start from the upper part of the nasal bones, cross the orbital margins near the frontomaxillary suture, continue through the ethmoid and lamina papyracea downward and backward and pass below the optic canal, and reach the infraorbital fissure where the line bifurcates. Complete, bilateral Le Fort III fractures result in craniofacial disjunction, leaving the entire bony structure of the face floating free. More often, fractures of the Le Fort III type are unilateral. There are generally three Le Fort III fracture lines as follows: One line traverses upward and forward following the zygomaticosphenoidal suture between the roof and lateral wall of the orbit and crosses the orbital margin near the frontozygomatic suture. The second line runs downward and backward, crossing the upper part of the pterygoid process near its base. The third line involves the zygomatic arch. The second and third lines of weakness roughly outline the strong zygomatic buttress. The first and second lines outline the second fragment, consisting of the upper processes of the maxillary bone and the nasal bones. Between the first line of weakness and the oral cavity a third fragment is found, consisting of the palatine vault, the upper tooth-bearing processes, and the greater part of the pterygoid processes. Facial fractures follow these lines of Le Fort unilaterally or bilaterally partially or in full length, often combining parts of more than one line. In a typical dislocation fracture of the zygomatic bone, the fracture lines follow part of Le Fort II and III lines of weakness.

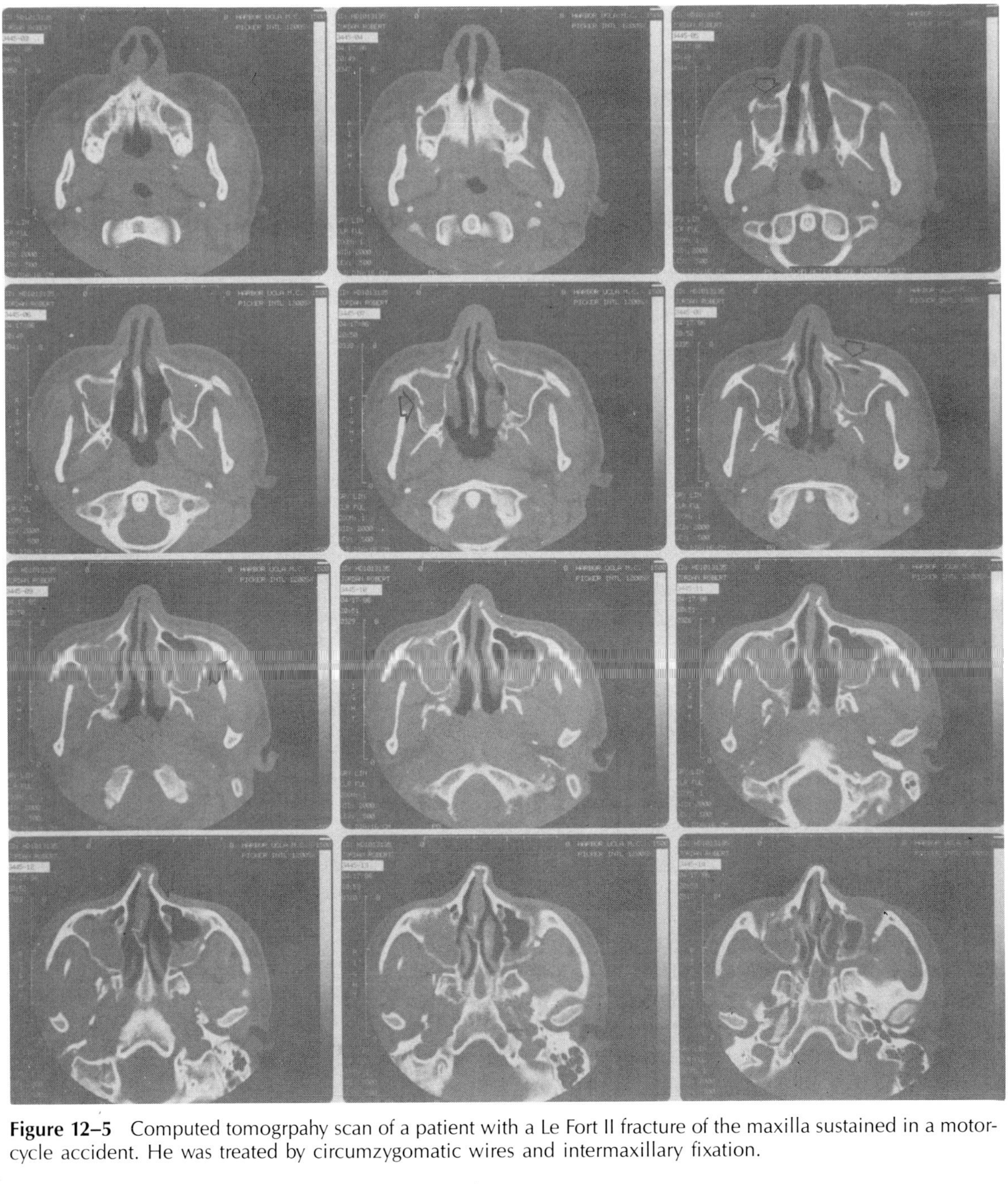

Figure 12–5 Computed tomogrpahy scan of a patient with a Le Fort II fracture of the maxilla sustained in a motorcycle accident. He was treated by circumzygomatic wires and intermaxillary fixation.

Where the bony plates are thin, comminution usually occurs. This is particularly so, for example, in the inferomedial orbital wall, the canine fossa, the posterolateral maxillary sinus wall, and the ethmoid, where the fracture lines frequently bifurcate. Note that both Le Fort II and Le Fort III fractures pass through the orbit (Figs. 12–6, 12–7, and 12–8).[9–12]

CEREBROSPINAL RHINORRHEA

Severe facial fractures may be associated with cerebrospinal rhinorrhea when the perpendicular plate of the ethmoid is forced backward and upward, transmitting the force to the cribriform plate which is fractured upward. Fractures involving a sinus wall of the ethmoid, frontal, or sphenoid si-

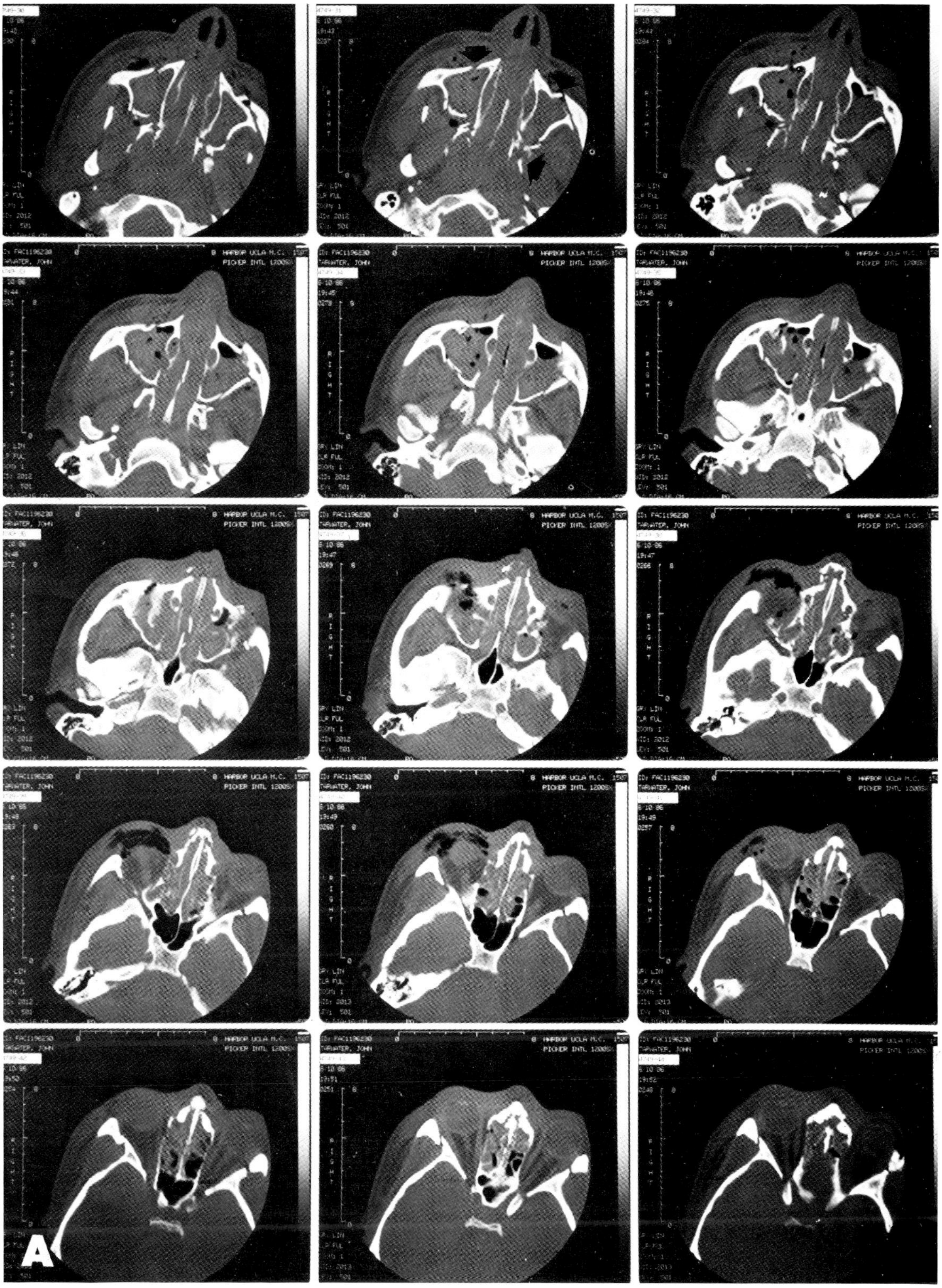

Figure 12–6 *A, B,* Computed tomography scans of a patient who sustained multiple facial fractures including bilateral fractures of the maxillary sinuses that were comminuted and pterygoid plate fractures. Scans show in exquisite detail not only the fractures of the bone but also the alterations in soft tissues secondary to trauma.

Figure continues on following page

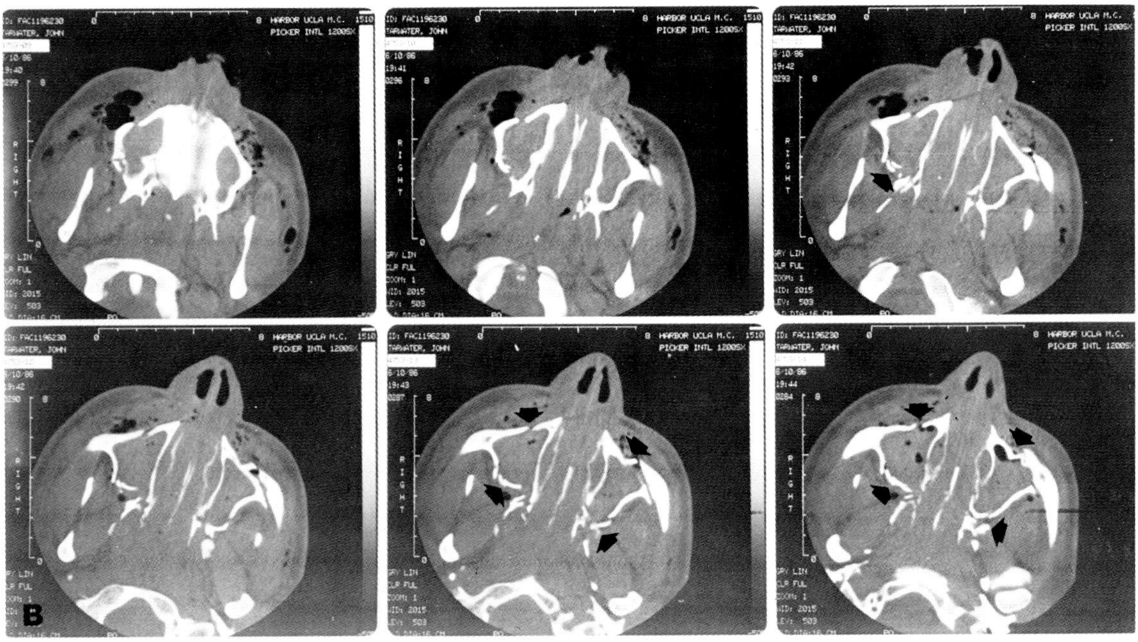

Figure 12–6 Continued.

nus associated with ruptures of the dura also give direct access to the anterior cranial fossa. The cribriform plate may be fractured by direct extension of fractures of adjacent bones or by telescoping fragments of the perpendicular plate of the ethmoid. The dura covering the cribriform plate is thin and is anchored to the bone as it extends along the olfactory nerve. The identity of cerebrospinal fluid (CSF) may be determined by laboratory examination demonstrating the presence of sugar. CSF leakage may be masked by hemorrhage. Temporary intranasal packing with gauze may be appropriate. The patient may complain of a salty taste. X-ray evidence of orbital or intracranial emphysema suggests an association with CSF rhinorrhea. The presence of CSF rhinorrhea is not a contraindication to early reduction and fixation of midfacial fractures; on the contrary, the presence of midfacial bone fragments that move every time the patient swallows or speaks will retard consolidation of the cribriform plate and therefore the dural tears. The successful reduction and fixation of midfacial bone fractures usually results in the cessation of CSF leakage. If it continues, consultation with the neurosurgery service is essential.

DEFINITIVE CARE OF MAXILLARY FRACTURES

The reestablishment of the proper anatomic relations of the bone fragments and of the teeth is achieved in various ways, usually depending on the degree and extent of the fractures. Simple segmental fractures of the alveolar bone are treated by digital manipulation to achieve appropriate reduction and fixation by placement of arch bars or some other form of interdental wiring, or by the use of an acrylic splint. Fractures of the maxillary bone do not affect the orbit and its contents as much as fractures of the zygoma. Maxillary bone fractures are treated primarily by restoration of the proper occlusion of the teeth and the stabilization of the supportive bone. When the fracture is not mobile enough to be reduced with digital manipulation, Rowe disimpaction forceps will be helpful. When a disimpacted maxilla results in an adequate reduction of the fracture lines, simple intermaxillary fixation may be all that is required to secure a proper occlusion. Occasionally, however, interosseous wires or the use of bone plates may be required.

Dentoalveolar fractures often involve fractured

teeth with or without exposure of the pulp. Teeth that are comminuted or fractured must be extracted. Salvageable teeth with pulp exposures should be treated appropriately by root canal or by extraction. Subluxated teeth may require reduction of the alveolar plate and splinting of the teeth. If there is a question about pulp viability, root canal fillings may be deferred until the teeth have become firm in the sockets.

Treatment of Le Fort I, II, and III Fractures

The key to successful treatment of midface fractures involving tooth-bearing bone is to reestablish the occlusion present prior to the trauma. When there are adequate teeth, placement of arch bars and intermaxillary fixation often is all that is required for a Le Fort I fracture. Typically, Le Fort I fractures are reduced by the placement of intermaxillary fixation with 24- or 26-gauge stainless steel wires. If the fracture is old enough to have become fixed, an attempt to disimpact the fracture with disimpaction forceps should be made; if that fails, open reduction exposing the fracture line through a mucosal incision in the buccal sulcus and mobilization with osteotomes may be required. Le Fort II fractures often may be treated the same way.

With Le Fort III fractures and associated fractures of the zygomatic complex and of the zygomatic arch and malar components is achieved with an appropriate elevator, of which there are several: Dingman, Gillies, Bristow, or Rowe. Following disimpaction and reduction of the zygomatic bones, the Le Fort II fracture or the tooth-bearing portion of the upper jaws is reduced by manipulation, by hand, or by disimpaction forceps; if the reduction seems close, often the placement of the intermaxillary fixation wires between the maxilla and the mandibular arch bars perfects the result. Finally, the nasoethmoidal portion is repositioned and secured either by closed or open methods as appropriate.

It is rarely necessary today to use extraskeletal fixation, but it may on occasion provide the best solution for stabilization of multiple fractures. Direct fixation is achieved using intraosseous wires at the frontozygomatic, zygomaticomaxillary sutures, or through the maxillary buttress. Excellent fixation can also be achieved with circum-mandibular wires and suspension wires from stable portions of the midface or from the zygomatic process of the frontal bone running underneath the zygomatic arch and attached by a wire loop running between these two suspension wires, i.e., the

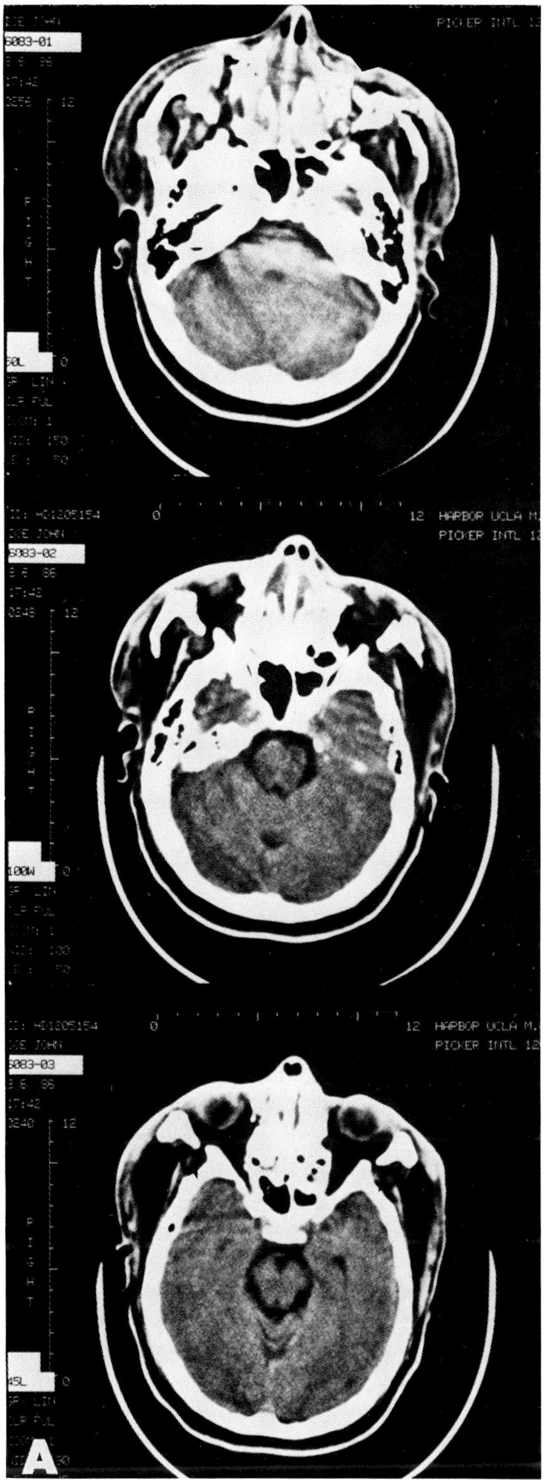

Figure 12–7 *A, B,* Preoperative, and *C,* Postoperative views of a patient who was beaten and sustained severely comminuted fractures of the mandible and the midface through the Le Fort III lines of fracture.

Figure continues on following page

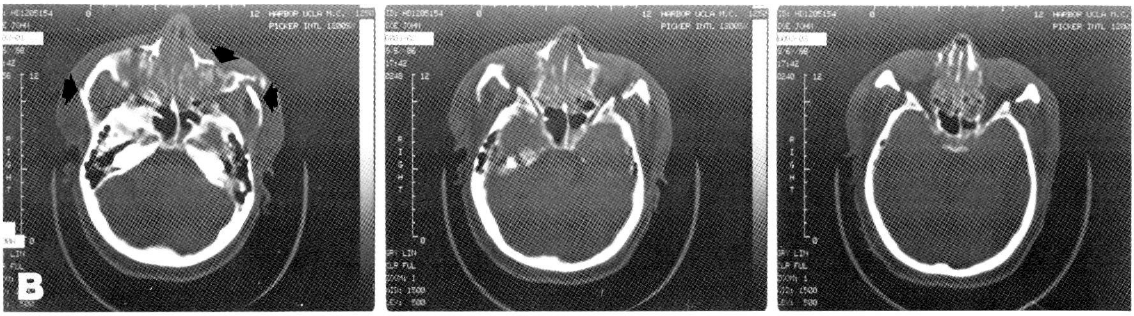

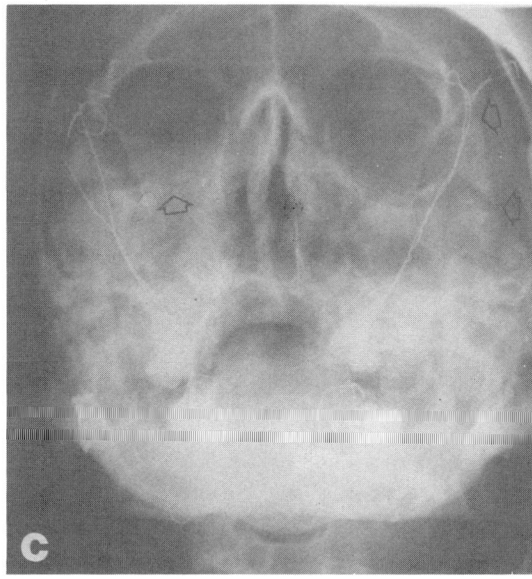

Figure 12–7 Continued.

circum-mandibular wire and the wire suspended from above. Occasionally, a Kirschner wire provides exactly the right degree of immobilization running through the frontal process of the maxilla, through the nasal cavity and the maxillary antrum, and impinging on the contralateral malar bone. Typical suspension wires may run as follows: circumzygomatic, zygomaticomandibular, inferior-orbital border to circum-mandibular, frontomandibular, or pyriform-fossa to the mandibular bone. An important principle in using suspension wires is that the point of fixation must be found in the stable portion of the facial skeleton above the line of fracture. The suspension wires are connected with circum-mandibular wires by wire loops between the suspension wire and the circum-mandibular wire, generally in the mandibular canine region. Thus the fractured middle third of the face is sandwiched between the mandible and the base of the skull. The wires are passed with the aid of awls. Suspension from the upper, lateral border of the orbit is typical. Rarely, inferior orbital border–mandibular wiring is used, through a 3/4-inch incision overlying the orbital rim.

Bone Plating

The use of rigid, but malleable miniplates for osteosynthesis is another useful method for stabilization of fractures of facial bones. They are particularly desirable when they can provide adequate stability, as in mandibular fractures and less often perhaps in maxillary fractures, to avoid intermaxillary fixation. Careful positioning to avoid tooth roots is mandatory. The screws must fit snugly. The question of compressive versus noncompressive plates is, in my view, academic. Clinically, these small plates function in a comparable way. Compression plates have, however, been reported to result occasionally in bone resorption.

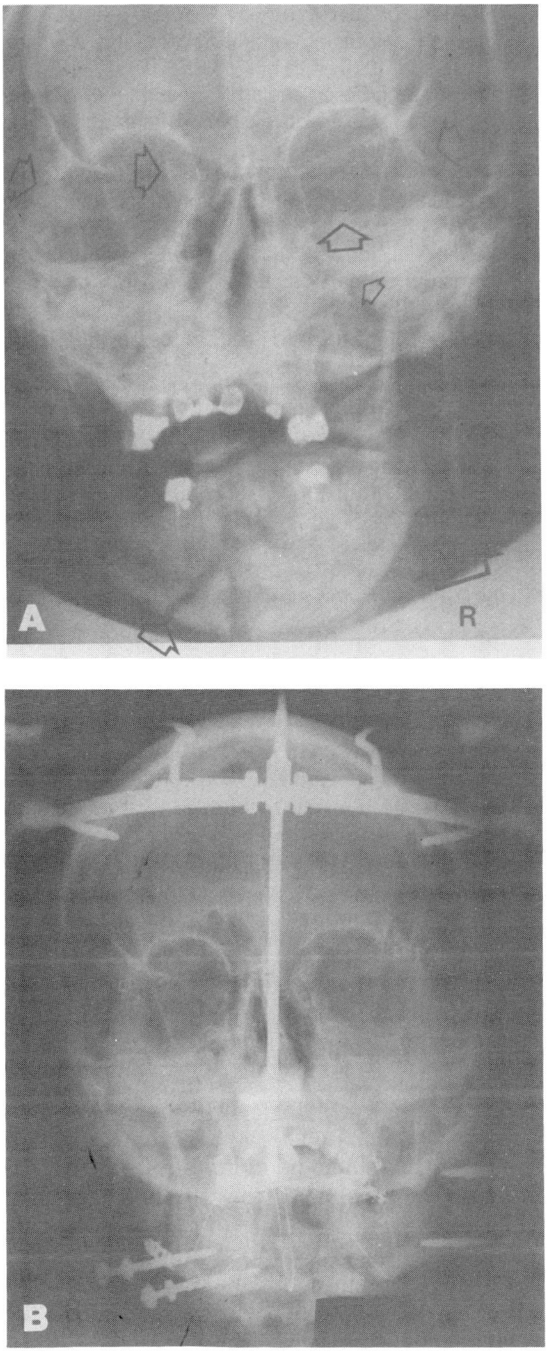

Figure 12–8 *A*, Preoperative, and *B*, Postoperative x-ray films of a patient who sustained a Le Fort II fracture on the right, a Le Fort III fracture on the left including a displaced right trimalar fracture, and a left parasymphyseal and left condyle as well as right angle fracture of the mandible. He was treated with upper and lower acrylic splints, open reduction and internal fixation of the right angle fracture, head frame, and biphase and ASCH plates.

ASSOCIATED FRACTURES OF THE NASAL COMPLEX

Although the nasal bones may have isolated fractures, which will be discussed separately, it is more typical for them to be fractured along with the frontal processes of the maxillae which articulate with the nasal bones on their lateral aspects. There may be associated fractures of the lacrimal bones and the orbital laminae of the ethmoid. Typically the nasal septum is involved and sometimes the septal cartilage is dislodged from its groove in the vomer. In more serious injuries the vomer and the perpendicular and cribriform plates of the ethmoid may also be fractured. These fractures may be associated with cerebrospinal fluid rhinorrhea. The displacement of the fracture is the result of the direction of the blow. Blows from the front or from above tend to flatten the nose with a broadened bridge. The result is an increase in the distance between the inner canthi which suggests an increased separation of the eyes but this, in fact, is an illusion. Blows from the side tend to deviate the nose to one side and may block both nares.

On inspection there is marked edema. There may be bilateral circumorbital ecchymosis and there may also be subconjunctival ecchymosis. Epistaxis is found in the fresh injury, but after the blood has clotted there may be only a discharge of clear serum. When the cribriform plate of the ethmoid has been comminuted, a CSF leak may occur. The patient may complain of a salty taste when the CSF passes backward and down the throat. On palpation, the underlying nasal bones are felt to be mobile and the area is acutely tender. Sometimes sharp step defects can be felt.

Nasal complex fractures may often be reduced under local anesthesia, but general anesthesia is preferred with an endotracheal tube and an adequate throat pack to protect against the inevitable hemorrhage and the possibility of aspiration. Various nasal forceps are available for manipulating the fragments. Ideally, Walsham's forceps are passed in the nostril to reduce the nasal bone and fragments of the frontal processes of the maxilla, and Ashe's septal forceps are then used to reduce the vomer and perpendicular plate of the ethmoid and to reposition the septal cartilage and its groove in the vomer. Finally, the finger and thumb of one hand are used to compress the lacrimal bones in the immediate walls of the orbit on each side to reshape the narrow bridge of the nose. It is important to test for patency of the nares to secure the airway postoperatively. Typically, small splints are placed on either side of the nose to stabilize the head within the joint capsule. Extracapsular fractures involve the condylar neck to the sigmoid notch. Low subcondylar fractures, below the sigmoid notch, are considered to be the same as ramus fractures and are treated as such.

Ramus

Ramus fractures are vertical or horizontal fractures in the area of the sigmoid notch to the angle. They are normally caused by direct trauma to the ramus of the mandible.

Angle of the Mandible

Angle fractures occur within or just anterior to the attachments of the masseter and medial pterygoid muscles. They frequently involve roots of the 12-year molars and/or erupted or unerupted wisdom teeth.

Body

Body fractures occur in the tooth-bearing area, from first premolar through second molar. They are usually caused by a direct blow.

Symphysis and Parasymphysis

Fractures in the midline of the mandible are very uncommon because the bone is thick and muscle attachments provide stability. The force of injury is often deflected to one side or the other of the midline and therefore manifests itself as a parasymphyseal fracture.

The degree and direction of displacement of the fractured mandibular segments depend on a number of factors, including: (1) direction of the injuring blow, (2) relative strength of the mandible in the affected area, and (3) direction of muscle pull. The masseter and medial pterygoid muscles pull the ascending ramus superiorly, anteriorly, and medially; the temporalis pulls superiorly and posteriorly. The suprahyoid muscles (digastrics, mylohyoid, and geniohyoid) pull the anterior mandible inferiorly and posteriorly. Depending on the orientation of the fracture line, muscle pull either has a tendency to approximate the fragments or distract them. Fractures are therefore classified as "favorable" or "unfavorable" in both a vertical and horizontal direction (Fig. 13–2).

Mandibular fractures are also classified as simple or comminuted and closed or compound. Fractures involving teeth are always compound, as the periodontal ligament space is open to the oral cavity.

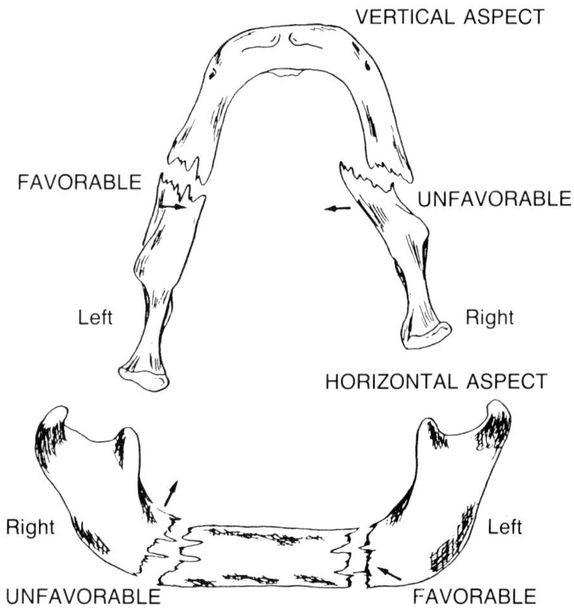

Figure 13–2 Favorable and unfavorable fractures.

DIAGNOSIS

History and Physical Examination

A careful history should be taken from the patient. When possible, the source, direction, and force of the traumatic injury should be determined. *Symptoms* indicating a mandibular fracture include pain, altered occlusion, and paresthesia.

Pain is particularly noticeable on movement of the jaw.

Proprioception in the teeth is extremely acute, and patients become aware of any alteration in the occlusion.

The inferior alveolar nerve is the sensory nerve to all mandibular teeth and associated gingiva, lower lip, and chin. Thus any mandibular fracture occurring proximal to the mental foramen and distal to the mandibular foramen may produce an injury of this nerve. The prognosis for recovery of normal sensation is determined by the degree of displacement and comminution of the fracture. In the lower third molar region, the lingual nerve is closely related to the medial aspect of the mandible, and the long buccal nerve to the lateral surface. In cases of displaced fractures, these nerves may also be damaged. The patient will have paresthesia or anesthesia over the anterior two-thirds of the tongue, in the case of a lingual nerve injury, or the cheek mucosa and corner of the lip, in the case of a long buccal nerve injury.

The physical signs that suggest a mandibular fracture include swelling and ecchymosis, hematoma, trismus, and malocclusion.

Swelling and ecchymosis may occur over the site of direct or "contrecoup" injury. A laceration, abrasion, or soft tissue injury may also be present.

Ecchymosis and hematoma may be present intraorally, on the buccal and/or lingual aspect of the mandible, at the site of fracture. For this reason the tongue must be retracted and a full examination made of the sublingual region.

Trismus is common and is due to a combination of pain and muscle spasm.

In patients with teeth, any degree of displacement of the mandible is accompanied by a change in the occlusion. This is perceived by the patient and is a very important point in the history. A malocclusion may already have been present, and without a perceivable change in occlusion, it may not indicate a fracture. If the patient is unconscious, the presence of a malocclusion can be documented if the wear facets on the maxillary and mandibular teeth do not line up properly when the jaw is closed.

Radiography

At least two radiographs are necessary to assess displacement of a mandibular fracture in three dimensions (Fig. 13–3, 13–4). Standard x-ray views include:

1. Lateral oblique. This view provides excellent visualization of the mandible from the condyle to the mental foramen. It is therefore the radiograph of choice for fractures of the condylar neck, ascending ramus, angle, and body of the mandible.
2. Posteroanterior. A posteroanterior radiograph shows displacement of fractures of the ascending ramus, angle, and body in a lateral or medial direction. In addition, it shows fractures of the anterior mandible and their displacement in a vertical direction. The vertebral bodies are, however, superimposed and they make definition in the anterior region difficult.
3. Townes. A Townes (occipital frontal) or a reverse Townes (frontal occipital) view is useful to demonstrate fractures of the condyle and their displacement in a medial or lateral direction. Since the condyle lies near the center of the skull in the mid-sagittal plane, there is little difference in definition between the two views.
4. Mandibular occlusal. A mandibular occlusal radiograph demonstrates displacement of a symphysis fracture in an anteroposterior direction.

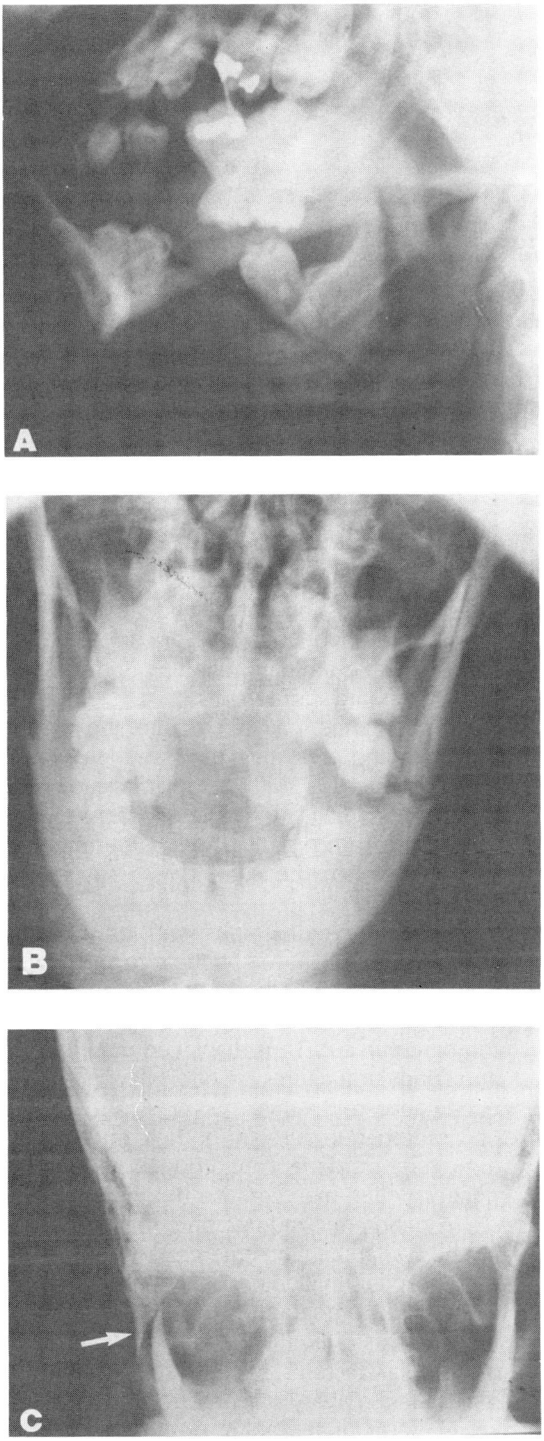

Figure 13–3 *A*, Lateral oblique; *B*, posteroanterior; *C*, Townes views of mandibular fracture.

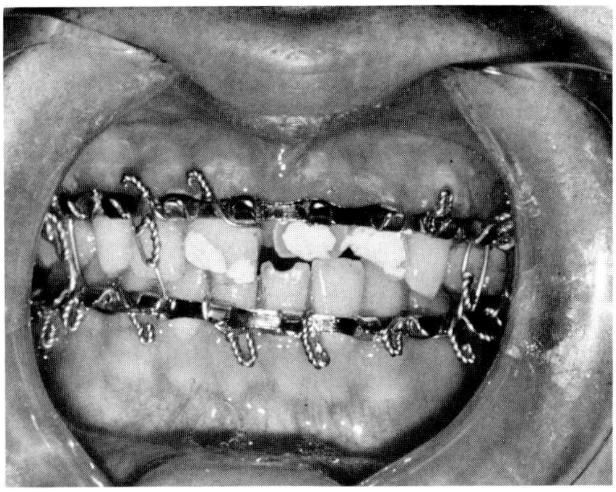

Figure 13–6 Erich arch bar used for mandibulomaxillar fixation.

Fixation Techniques

A variety of techniques are currently used for direct interosseous bone fixation.

Superior Border Wire. In this technique the fracture site is approached intraorally and, after reduction, a 21 gauge wire is placed across the superior border of the mandible. Superior border wiring is most applicable to angle fractures and is often used in conjunction with removal of a wisdom tooth in the fracture line. The wire may be placed through the buccal plate or the external oblique ridge, but where no tooth has been removed or where greater stability is required, the wire is passed through buccal and lingual plates (Fig. 13–7). Intermaxillary fixation, to prevent separation at the lower border of the mandible, is always used in these cases. Though many superior border wires remain in place for life, some are removed because they become extruded through the thin overlying mucosa or exposed under a denture that irritates the overlying mucosa.[8,9]

Inferior Border Wire. An interosseous wire is frequently placed at the lower border of the mandible for fracture fixation. In the posterior mandible, this procedure is carried out through a submandibular incision. Anterior to the mental foramen, a labial sulcus incision may be used to expose the inferior border.

One hole is drilled on each side of the fracture. To provide greater stability in both vertical and horizontal directions, two wires are normally passed: a direct transosseous wire, and a figure-of-eight wire beneath the lower border (Fig. 13–8).

This type of fixation provides good stability at the lower border of the mandible. In the tooth-bearing area a lower border wire may be combined with an arch bar and/or lingual splint at the superior border of the mandible. In such cases only a short period of intermaxillary fixation (two or three weeks) is required. When a lower border wire is placed at the angle or in an edentulous area, four to six weeks of intermaxillary fixation is necessary.

Stable Fixation. *Brons wire.* A type of intraosseous wire fixation stable enough to be used without intermaxillary fixation was described by Brons and Boering in 1970[10]; long-term results were published in 1977.[11] A single wire is inserted through four holes (Fig. 13–9). For maximum stability two holes are placed above the inferior alveolar nerve and two holes below it in the posterior mandible or in edentulous areas. When teeth are present at the fracture site, all four holes are placed below the mandibular canal.

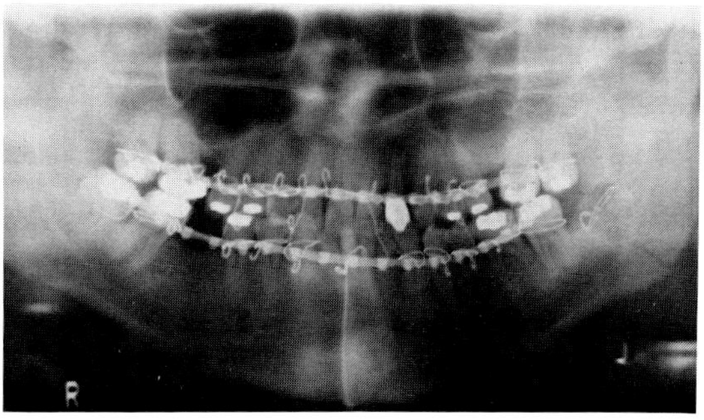

Figure 13–7 Superior border wire used for reduction of a mandibular angle fracture after removal of wisdom teeth.

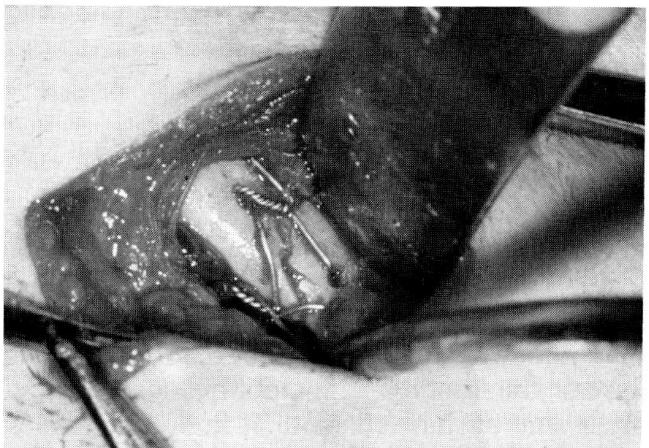

Figure 13–8 Combined transosseous and figure-of-eight wire for stability at the inferior border of the mandible.

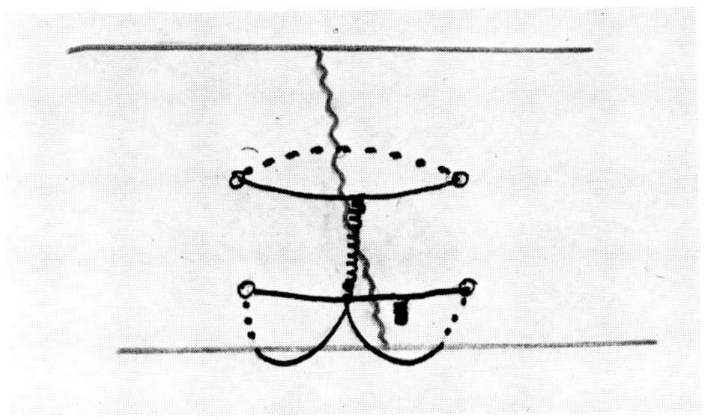

Figure 13–9 Brons wire technique.

Increased stability with this technique is the result of a broader area of fixation and the use of a single, long piece of prestretched wire. Wires loosen primarily because they untwist to a minor extent resulting in increased length. Thus, when a longer wire is used, the percentage of lengthening that occurs from untwisting is decreased. The Brons wire is normally inserted through an extraoral incision; in the anterior part of the mouth an intraoral degloving approach may be used (Fig. 13–10).

Miniplates. Miniplates can also be used to provide stable fixation. The plates are made of stainless steel, Vitallium, or titanium alloys. They can be inserted into the external oblique ridge, via an intraoral incision, for angle fractures. They may also be placed through an intraoral incision in the anterior region of the mandible. In other situations, an extraoral approach is employed. In many cases, a single plate does not give sufficient stability to dispense with intermaxillary fixation, and if rigid stability is required, it is necessary to place two plates across the fracture: one along the buccal aspect of the mandible and one at the lower border (Fig. 13–11). The screws supplied with these plates are normally self-tapping and need to engage only one cortical plate.

Some manufacturers recommend removal of miniplates after a few months, but clinically this rarely seems to be necessary. The most frequent complications are penetration of the inferior alveolar canal by the screws, and infection.

Compression Osteosynthesis. Compression osteosynthesis is intended to provide stable fixation *without* intermaxillary immobilization. It is important to understand that this technique also involves a different concept of bone healing. When fractured bone segments are rigidly approximated (i.e., compressed), such that the gap between the fractured segments is eliminated, there is direct bridging of the fracture with osteocytes. This results in a more rapid union and virtually no callus formation (primary healing).[12] The advantages of primary bone healing are: (1) more rapid fracture union, (2) no callus formation, (3) lower infection rate, and (4) no need for intermaxillary fixation. The two commonly used techniques for compression osteosynthesis in the mandible are compression plates and lag screws.

A compression plate is rigid and has elliptical screw holes. Therefore, when the screws are inserted and tightened, the fractured ends are forced together (Fig. 13–12). Compression plates are large and generally require a long extraoral incision for adequate exposure. The fracture must be accurately and rigidly reduced before the compression plate is applied. The special fracture reduction and holding forceps usually supplied for this purpose may be cumbersome and the operator must become familiar with them.

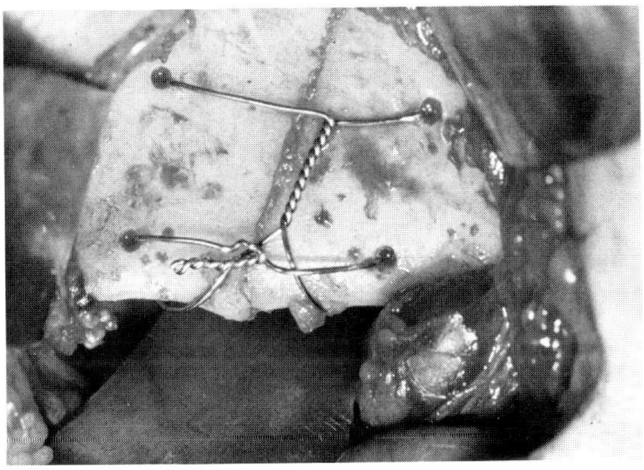

Figure 13–10 Brons wire inserted from extraoral approach.

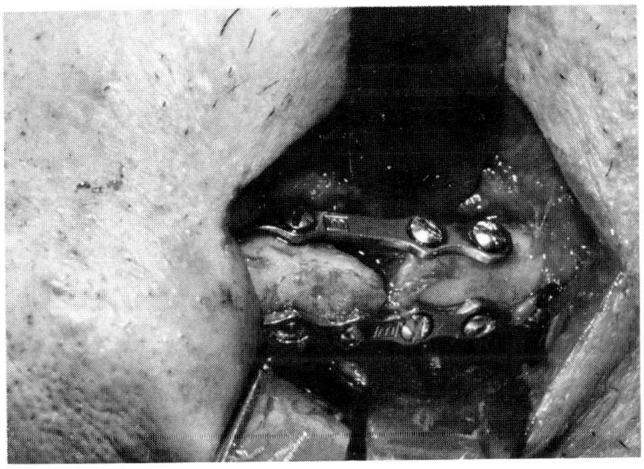

Figure 13–11 A fracture reduced and fixated with two miniplates.

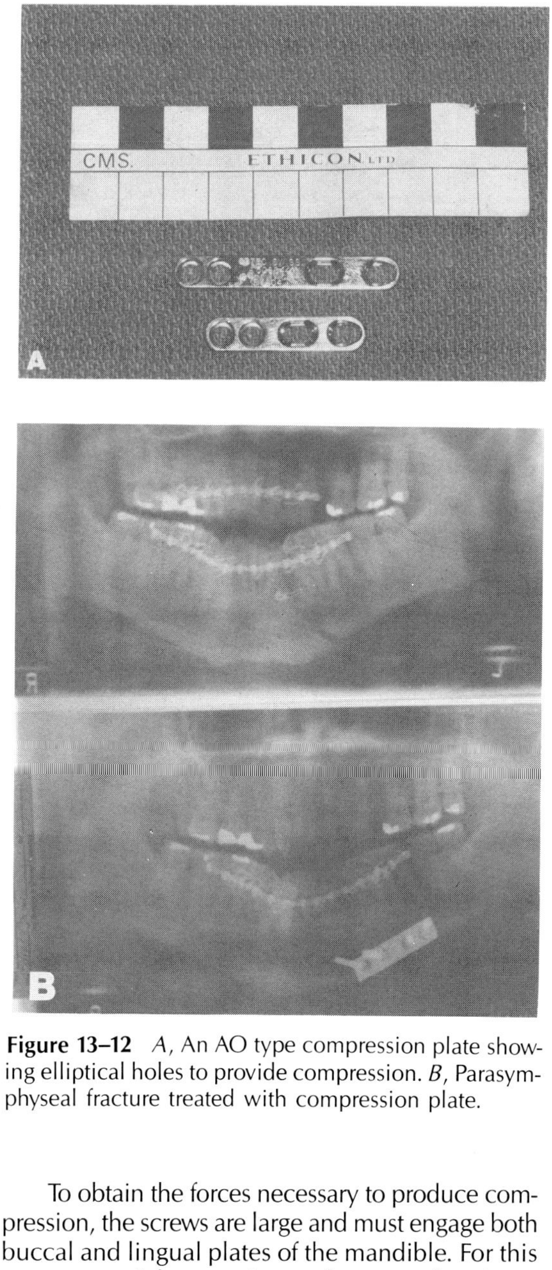

Figure 13–12 *A*, An AO type compression plate showing elliptical holes to provide compression. *B*, Parasymphyseal fracture treated with compression plate.

To obtain the forces necessary to produce compression, the screws are large and must engage both buccal and lingual plates of the mandible. For this reason, special measuring tools are used to determine the appropriate length of screw needed.

If a plate is used to compress the lower border of the mandible, there is a resultant force that causes distraction of the upper border. This distracting force must be counteracted, otherwise occlusal disharmony will result. The upper border, must therefore, be reduced and stabilized separately by means of an arch bar or a separate small plate or wire. Alternatively, a specially designed plate that provides compression in two directions may be used. In this case, both the inferior and superior borders of the mandible are simultaneously approximated. The plate must be contoured to the shape of the defect, otherwise the fracture alignment and thus the occlusion will be altered.

The disadvantages of compression plating include the following: (1) the need for a large extraoral incision, (2) the plates may need to be removed when healing is complete, and (3) unless great care is taken, occlusal disharmony may result.

Lag screws may be used to apply compression across oblique fractures. A large, flat-headed screw engages only the distal portion of an oblique fracture. When the screw is tightened, the proximal and distal portions are therefore forced together. To provide compression, screws with a coarse thread and a diameter of at least 2 mm are required. Lag screws are threaded only in their distal half so that they are free within a hole in the proximal fragment (Fig. 13–13). This is a very quick and easy technique that can be used to great advantage from both intra- and extraoral approaches. It is limited, however, to oblique fractures.

External fixation. This technique is employed when open reduction and direct internal fixation are contraindicated: (1) a continuity defect in the mandible making direct fixation impossible, (2) a badly comminuted fracture where direct fixation is impractical, (3) an infected fracture where direct wiring or plating may aggravate the infection, and (4) an atrophic mandible where extensive periosteal stripping should be avoided.

Two screws with a coarse "wood screw" type thread are inserted on either side of the fracture. They should be divergent, so that the direction of pull required to loosen them will be different for all four screws. The pins are then joined extraorally by means of connecting rods of stainless steel with universal joints or an acrylic bar (Fig. 13–14).

A simple custom-made connector can be constructed by means of a plastic endotracheal tube filled with cold-cured acrylic (Fig. 13–15). In the systems employing connecting rods and universal joints, the fracture can be x-rayed, and, if the fragments are not in proper alignment, adjustments can be made repeatedly until the correct position is reached. This is an alternative not available with some of the cold-cured acrylic systems.

External fixation may need to be supplemented by intermaxillary fixation, because when external fixation is used alone, many mandibular fractures are still subject to movements at the fracture site. The main disadvantages of extraoral fixation are aesthetic: the pins protrude from the cheek for a number of weeks and postoperative puncture marks remain after pin removal.

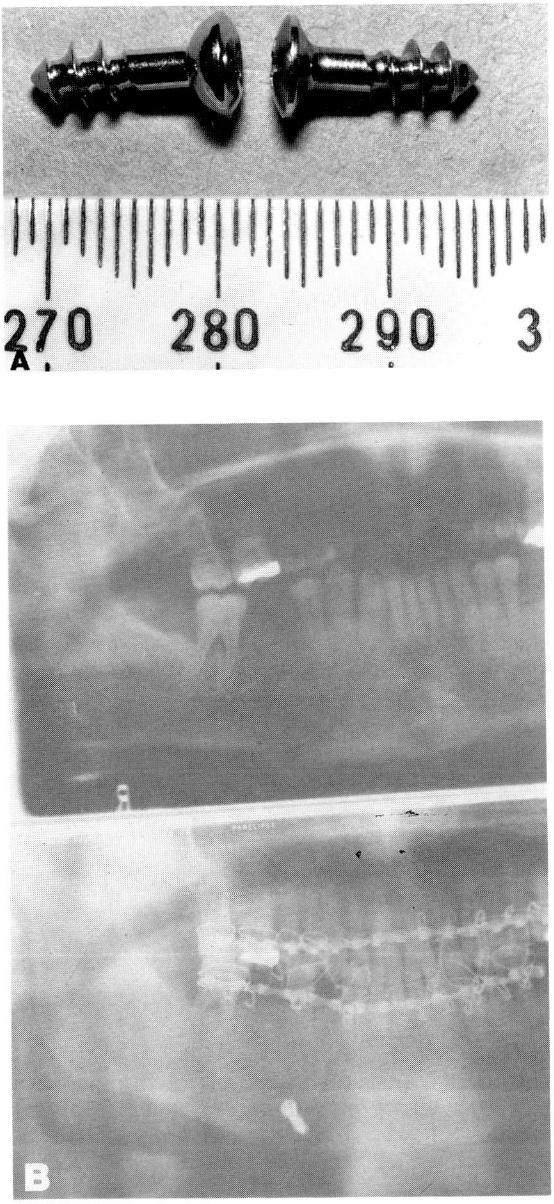

Figure 13–13 *A*, Lag screw technique for oblique fractures. *B*, Oblique fracture treated by lag screw.

Treatment of Specific Fractures

Edentulous Fractures

Fractures of the edentulous mandible present special problems relating to the anatomy and physiology of the edentulous jaw. However, postoperative occlusal disharmonies may not be as important as in the mandible with teeth, since these can generally be corrected by modifying the patient's dentures or constructing new ones. It is important to keep the dentures, if at all possible, since they can be used as a basis for fracture splints.

In the atrophic edentulous mandible, there is evidence that the major blood supply is via the periosteum, and if there is extensive periosteal stripping during fracture reduction, delayed healing and nonunion may result.[13] For this reason, fractures of the edentulous mandible are usually treated by closed reduction. Immobilization of the fracture is achieved by intermaxillary fixation using the patient's dentures or Gunning splints (Fig. 13–16). Fixation may have to be maintained for eight weeks or longer because healing can be slow in the aged and/or atrophic jaw.

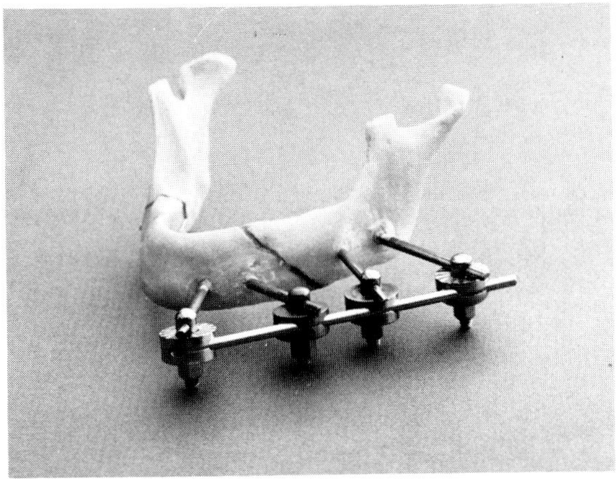

Figure 13–14 Extraoral pin fixation with stainless steel connecting rods.

Fractures of the Ascending Ramus and Coronoid Process

The ascending ramus is protected by the pterygomasseteric sling, which cushions the bone and splints any fracture. Unless a ramus fracture is badly displaced, open reduction is rarely necessary. Closed reduction and intermaxillary fixation alone suffice for treatment.

Fractures of the coronoid process are rare, since the coronoid is well protected by the arch of the zygoma. Isolated coronoid fractures usually do not require treatment even by intermaxillary fixation, since they are well splinted by the musculature. When there is complete separation of the coronoid process from the ramus, it may cause mechanical interference with mandibular movements. The entire coronoid is then removed via an intraoral approach.

lowing infection or inadequate fixation. They can also occur if soft tissue is interposed between the fractured ends during treatment.

The treatment of an established nonunion involves open operation, freshening of the bone ends, cancellous bone grafting if there is a continuity defect, and rigid fixation for 6 to 8 weeks.

Malocclusion

Malocclusion may occur following compression osteosynthesis or any other method of fracture repair in which an accurate occlusion is not obtained. In minor cases, selective grinding of teeth or replacement of restorations may be satisfactory, but in other cases only extraction of teeth or osteotomy can restore the occlusion.

Trismus and Ankylosis

Trismus is not uncommon after prolonged intermaxillary fixation. After release of fixation, active physical therapy may be necessary. Shortwave diathermy or ultrasound might also be effective in relieving trismus caused by muscle spasm. Rarely, surgical excision of fibrous bands may be necessary.

Bony ankylosis may occur following intracapsular fractures in children. The treatment involves aggressive excision of the bony ankylosis. The defect is reconstructed by means of a costochondral rib graft or other suitable bone graft. Some cases of trismus and ankylosis can result from attachment of the coronoid process to the undersurface of the arch of the zygoma. This rare complication can be treated quite satisfactorily by means of coronoidectomy.

Dental Abscesses

Teeth in proximity to the fracture are often devitalized and may become infected if they are not treated endodontically or extracted. The application of arch bars and Ivy loops can also be traumatic to the teeth and periodontium.

REFERENCES

1. Rowe NL, Williams JL. Maxillofacial injuries. Edinburgh: Churchill Livingstone, 1985:1002.
2. Reil B, Krans S. Traumatology of the maxillofacial region in childhood. J Maxillofac Surg 1976; 4:197–200.
3. Kaban LB, Mulliken JB, Murray JE. Facial fractures in children: an analysis of 122 fractures in 109 patients. Plast Reconstr Surg 1977; 59:15–20.
4. Kaban LB, Goldwyn RM. Facial injuries. In: May H, ed. The emergency. New York: John Wiley & Sons, 1984:323.
5. Mulliken JB, Kaban LB, Murray JE. Management of facial fractures in children. Clin Plast Surg 1977; 4:491–502.
6. Neal DC, Wagner WF, Alpert B. Morbidity associated with teeth in the line of mandibular fractures. J Oral Surg 1978; 36:859–862.
7. Juniper RP, Awty MD. The immobilization period for fractures of the mandibular body. J Oral Surg 1973; 36:157–163.
8. Chuong R, Donoff RB. Intraoral open reduction of mandibular fractures. Int J Oral Surg 1985; 14:22–28.
9. Edgerton MT, Hill E. Fracture of the mandible—a series of 434 cases. Surgery 1952; 31:933–950.
10. Brons R, Boering G. Fractures of the mandibular body treated by stable internal fixation—a preliminary report. J Oral Surg 1970; 28:407–415.
11. Van Dijk L, Brons R, Bosker H. Treatment of mandibular fractures by means of stable internal wire fixation. Int J Oral Surg 1977; 6:173–176.
12. Spiessl B. Principles of rigid internal fixation in fractures of the lower jaw. In Spiessl B, ed. New concepts in maxillofacial bone surgery. Berlin: Springer, 1976.
13. Pogrel MA, Dodson T, Tom W. Arteriographic assessment of patency of inferior alveolar artery and its relevance to alveolar atrophy. J Oral Maxillofac Surg 1987; 45:767–769.
14. VanHoof RF, Merkze CA, Stekelenburg EC. The different patterns of fractures of the facial skeleton in four European countries. Int J Oral Surg 1977; 6:3–11.
15. Zide MF, Kent JN. Indications for open reduction of mandibular condyle fractures. J Oral Maxillofac Surg 1983; 41:89–98.
16. Wheat PM, Evaskus DS, Laskin DM. Effects of temporomandibular joint meniscectomy on adult and juvenile primates. J Dent Res 1977; 58:139.

14

MALUNION AND NONUNION

ROBERT A. HARDESTY, M.D.
JEFFREY L. MARSH, M.D., F.A.C.S.

"Many patients present with long-standing post-traumatic structural deformities. In a competitive society, a facial deformity constitutes a definite socioeconomic handicap . . . these individuals are entitled to an attempt at reconstruction."

Reed O. Dingman
American Association of Plastic Surgeons Meeting
May 6, 1950, Washington, D.C.[1]

The primary objectives in reduction of facial fractures are restoration of function and reestablishment of appearance to the premorbid state. This requires protection of vital structures, alignment of altered bony architecture, restoration of dental occlusion, and attainment of proper soft-tissue relationships. Adverse results follow facial fractures when concurrent life-threatening conditions preclude timely definitive intervention or when there is unrecognized injury, misdiagnosis, or unsuccessful initial management.[2-11] The consequences of untreated or inadequately treated facial fractures are usually obvious. Such deformities can limit mastication, cause pain, and alter speech, hearing, or vision.[12-18] In addition, the unfavorable transformation of facial appearance may lead to serious social and emotional problems.[19,20] Post-traumatic facial deformities are some of the most challenging problems confronting the reconstructive craniofacial surgeon.

This chapter discusses our approaches and those of others to revisional surgery for deformities that result from malaligned or nonunited facial fractures. The initial pages review pertinent factors in bone biology, clinical evaluation, diagnostic imaging, and pretreatment planning. The remainder deal with specific anatomic areas of fracture using representative case examples. For the sake of clarity and brevity, details of standard surgical techniques are not included but rather principles, rationales, and applications to clinical situations are presented.

HISTORICAL PERSPECTIVE

The oldest known human malar fracture is on the skull of the Shanidar I Neanderthal (*Homo sapiens neanderthalensis*) (Fig. 14–1).[21] This specimen, approximately 50,000 years old, is an adult male who is thought to have died between 35 and 40 years of age. Sometime prior to death, he presumably sustained a blow to the left side of the head which resulted in fractures of the zygoma and frontal bone. He survived the injury, and the malar fracture healed in a malunited position with characteristic flattening and orbital distortion. Details of his medical treatment are, of course, unknown.

The first known recorded complication of a

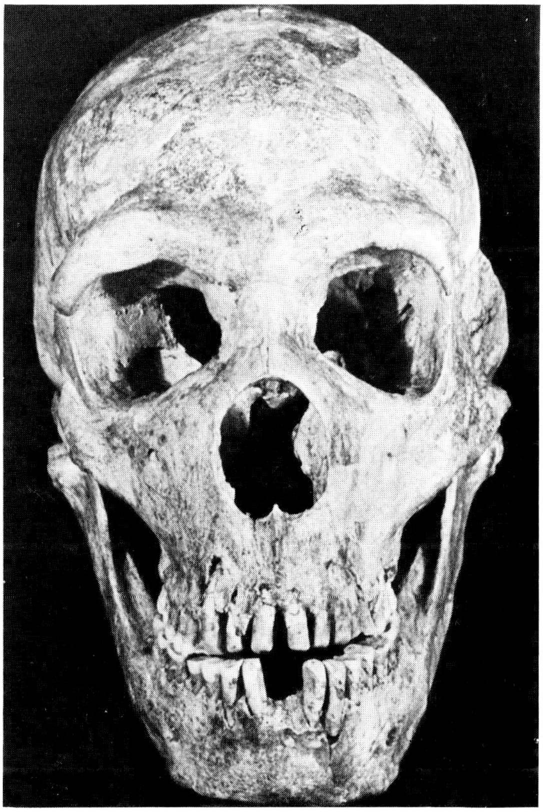

Figure 14–1 Shanidar I Neanderthal skull with malunion of the left zygoma. (Courtesy of E. Trinkaus and M.R. Zimmerman.[21])

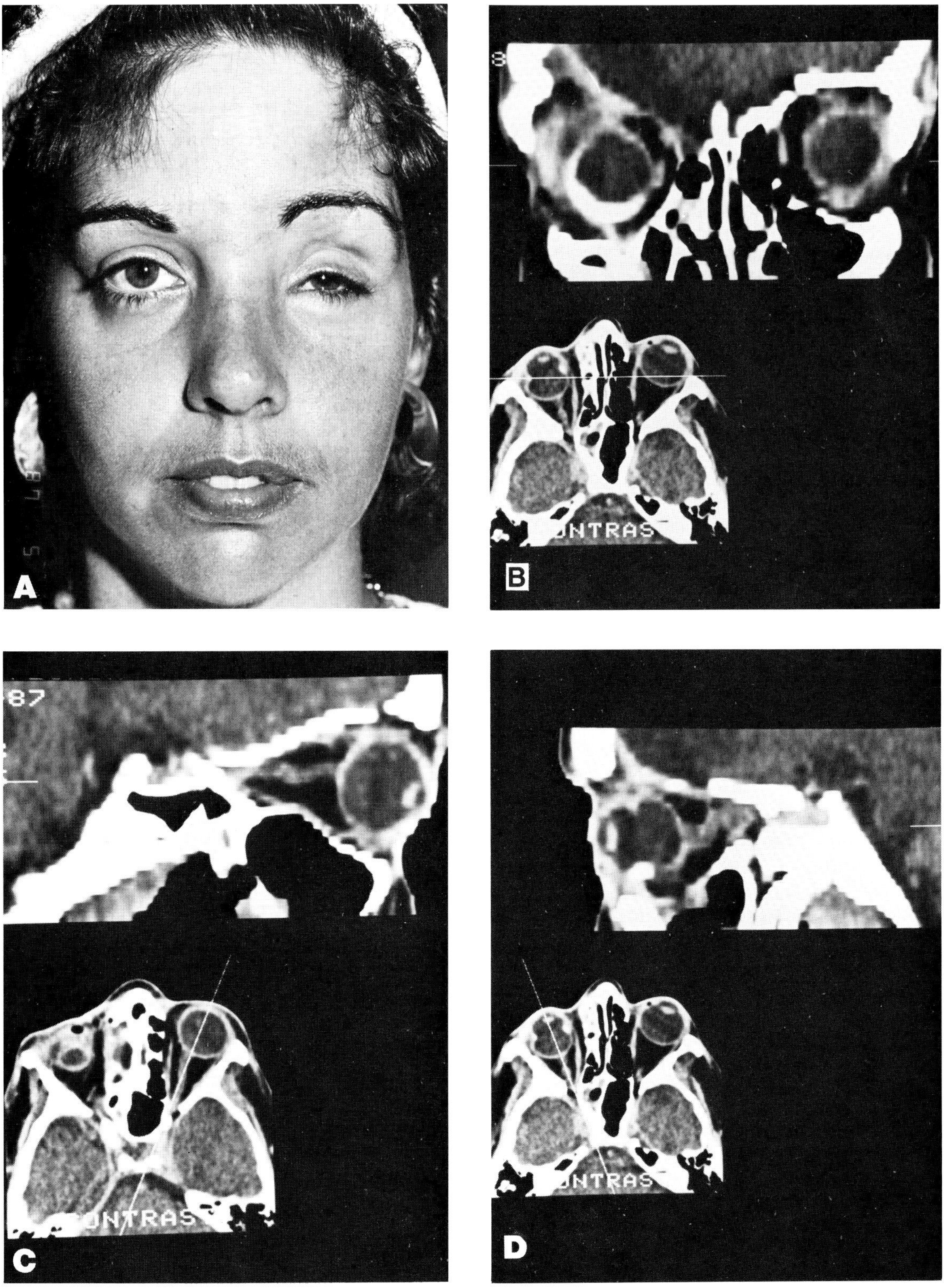
A
B
C
D

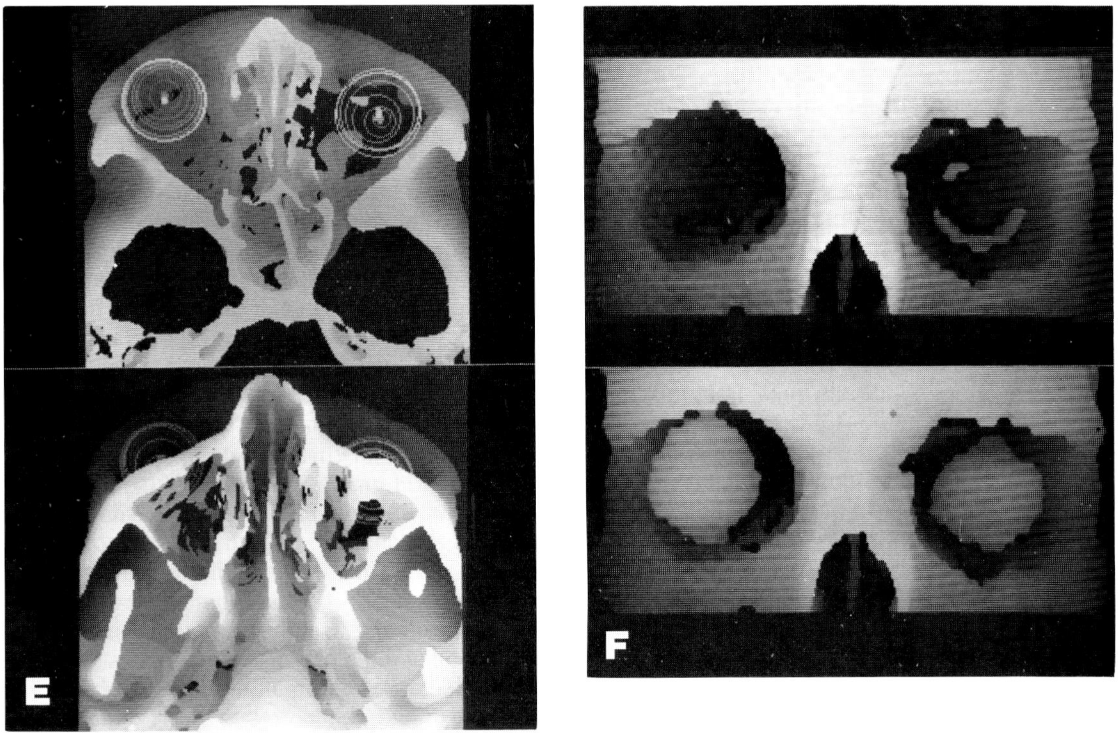

Figure 14–2 Radiographic evaluation of a 29-year-old woman with post-traumatic deformities 7 months following open reduction/internal fixation of a left frontal depressed skull fracture sustained in an automobile accident. A "blow-out" fracture of the orbital floor was diagnosed initially but not treated. *A*, Frontal photograph demonstrating depression of the left forehead and brow and marked enophthalmos with deep superior palpebral fold and pseudoptosis of the upper eyelid. *B*, Direct axial (bottom) and reformatted coronal (top) CT scan images. The axial image, at the level of the ocular lenses, documents left enophthalmos, compression of the left ethmoid sinuses, and clouding of the left sphenoid sinus. The transverse white line indicated the plane through which the coronal reformat was reconstructed. On the coronal image, the roof and floor of the right orbit are intact as is the air-filled antral cavity. The roof of the left orbit is absent; the floor of the left orbit is displaced caudally into the antrum. The excess whiteness about the left globe is a scleral band. *C*, Longitudinal orbital image[40] of the right orbit. The white line on the direct axial image (bottom) indicates the plane through which the reformat is reconstructed. The longitudinal orbital image documents normal anatomy of the floor of the anterior fossa (orbital roof), floor of the orbit, and maxillary antrum. *D*, Longitudinal orbital image[40] of the left orbit. The cranial and orbital cavities are in continuity because of the absence of the roof of the orbit. The ventral portion of the floor of the orbit is absent as well. The globe is enophthalmic with characteristic telescoping of the optic nerve. *E*, Frontal three-dimensional osseous surface reformats (Vannier-Marsh[118] method) of the skull with and without globe opacification. Step-off of the left orbital rim and depression of the left orbital floor are visible. The scleral band is visible within the globeless left orbit. *F*, Axial sectioning of the globe opacification three-dimensional images are useful for clarification of the relationships between the globes and adjacent bones. The top image, an axial cut through the equator of the globes, is viewed cephalad from the plane of section. The malunion of the left superior orbital rim is evident as compared to the contour and position of the right rim. The osseous defect in the roof of the left orbit appears as a black void. The left globe sits more posteriorly in its orbit than the right. The bottom image, an axial cut through the mid-antra, also is viewed cephalad. The enophthalmos is more evident on this image because the inferior orbital rims and anterior maxillary walls are relatively symmetric. The medial wall of the left nasal cavity is displaced into the cavity as a result of the ethmoid "blow out." The displacement of the left orbital floor into the antrum is indicated by increased whiteness as compared to the right floor: the gray scale is depth encoded, with white closest to viewer, black farthest away.

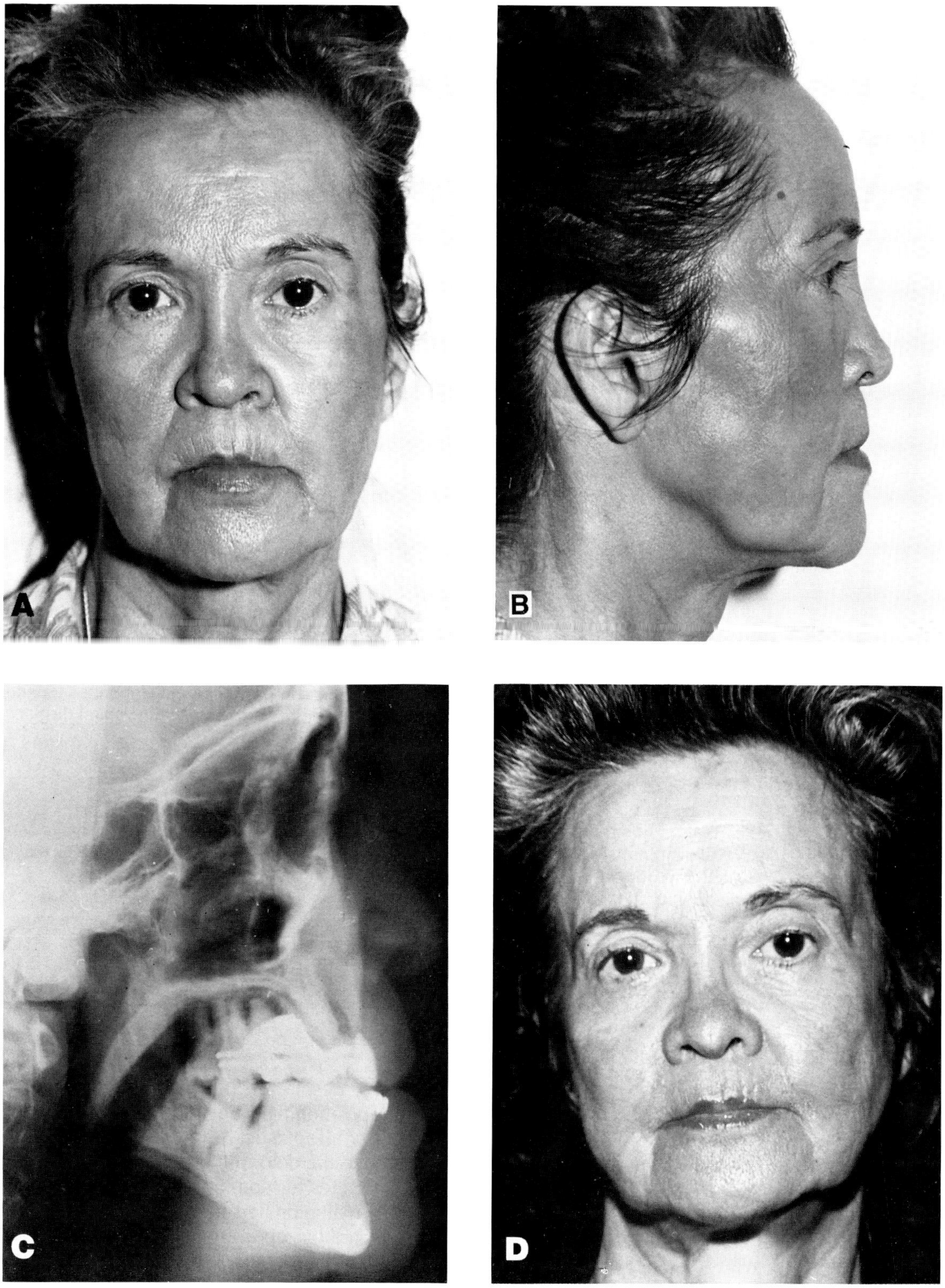

Figure 14–4 *See legend on opposite page.*

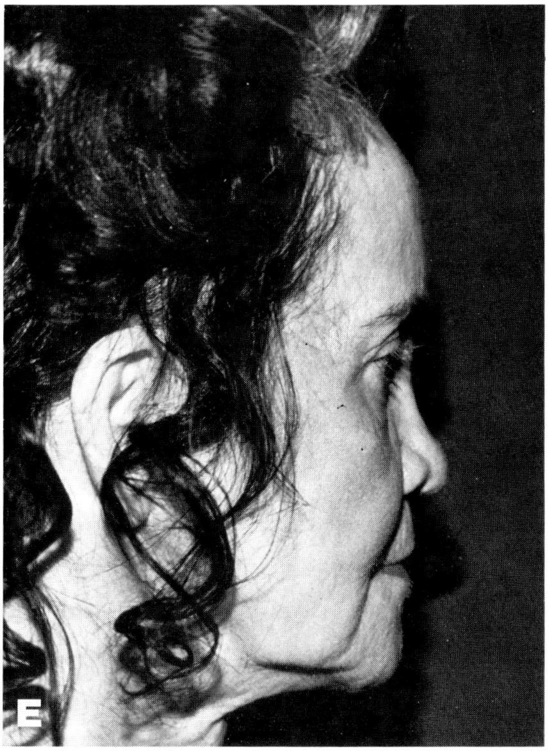

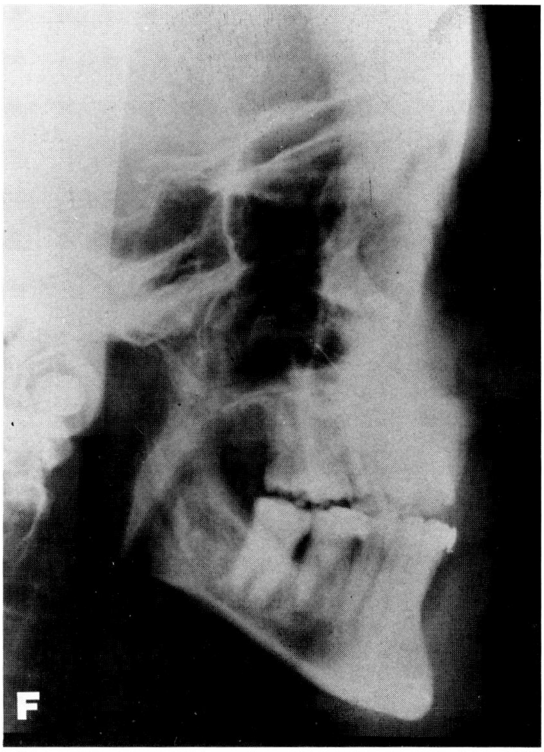

Figure 14–4 *A, B,* Fifty-eight-year-old woman after Le Fort III fracture managed with intermaxillary fixation and Adams suspension wire. The profile is concave with relative mandibular prognathism, steep mandibular plane, and elongation of facial height. The upper lip is posterior to the lower lip. There is a complete dental cross-bite. *C,* Lateral cephalometric radiograph that documents maxillary retrusion and profile deformities. There is a class III molar relationship. *D, E,* Photographs 3 years following Le Fort I type maxillary osteotomy with correction of deformities noted preoperatively (*A*). The nose also has been revised. *F,* Lateral cephalometric radiograph 3 years following Le Fort I type maxillary advancement. Note the changes in molar relationship, soft-tissue profile, and mandibular plane compared to preoperative view (*B*).

the early fibrous union with an elevator, scalpel, chisel, or osteotome. The zygoma then is mobilized using a variety of techniques, e.g., those of Gillies, Dingman, Keen, or Lathrop.[93,125] We find the Rowe zygoma elevator useful in these circumstances. The freed segment must sit passively in the desired position. After anatomic reduction is attained, stable fixation is required to prevent postreduction axial rotation.[37] The use of miniplates for rigid internal fixation have yielded results superior to those of wire fixation in our laboratory investigation.[151] Recent independent experimental evidence contrasting and comparing fixation techniques (wire versus miniplate) and number of fixation points (1 to 3) has documented a greater degree of stability with miniplate usage and multiple fixation points.[152]

Reduction of a zygoma malunion more than 6 weeks after injury may be difficult. Bone healing resulting in firm union is variable. Children and healthy young adults heal faster whereas elderly or debilitated patients achieve consolidation later (see Table 14–3). Combinations of bone healing, resorption, and recontouring of the fracture segments make it difficult to reduce the malunion adequately and obtain proper relationships in late cases.[93] Therefore, alternative plans for reduction including possible osteotomies and grafting should be considered. Prior to making osteotomies, the degree of comminution of the zygomatic complex and adjacent bones, the extent of sinus involvement, and the amount of bone graft required are evaluated. The irregular resorptive remodeling of bone healing may obscure the precise location of old fracture lines. As a result, anatomic reduction and stabilization of the mobilized segment may be difficult. Thus, bone grafting is often necessary in late reconstructions. After obtaining adequate exposure, direct mobilization of the malunited segments is attempted prior to osteotomy. Insertion of an elevator or small osteotome into the fibrous union may facilitate mobilization. If unsuccessful, the preplanned osteotomy is performed to allow repositioning of the malunited bone. When contour deformity persists after reduction, autologous bone grafts (rib, iliac crest, or calvarial sources) and shaping burrs are used to resolve asymmetry.[148,149,153–155] Since resorption of onlay bone is unpredictable, slight overcorrection is recommended. After reduction of the bone, the orbital contents and blepharocanthal structures are inspected for soft-tissue asymmetries.[147] When there is persistent lateral canthal displacement following repositioning of the lateral orbital rim, a periosteal pennant flap, containing the lateral canthal tendon in its base, is elevated and fixed, medially to laterally, through a hole in the rim to correct the malpositioned canthus.[10,101]

Alloplastic materials usually are reserved for "touch-up" procedures following secondary osseous reconstruction. The principal advantages of alloplasts are decreased patient morbidity, less surgery, unlimited supply, and stable volume and shape.[156–158] The disadvantages include dislodgement, exposure, bony erosion, and an increased risk of infection.[159–162] The soft-tissue dissection, periosteal stripping, and osteotomy needed to reduce old malunited fractures may compromise the vascular supply to both the zygoma and overlying soft tissue. Since successful use of alloplastic implants requires an adequate cover of well-vascularized soft tissue, we prefer to perform alloplastic augmentation subsequent to the autogenous reconstruction. This approach seems to enhance precision contouring and placement and decrease the chance of infection and extrusion.

Maxilla

Correction of defects which result from fractures of the maxilla is challenging and perplexing. Given its central location, the maxilla articulates with most of the other facial bones and its dentition occludes with that of the mandible.

The indications for surgical treatment of malunited maxillary fractures are both functional and aesthetic. Functionally, maxillary deformity may impair mastication, speech, ventilation, and even vision.[163–166] Disruption of the premorbid dental relationship may lead not only to occlusal difficulties but also to temporomandibular joint dysfunction. In addition, these fractures often are associated with intracranial injury and its related morbidity. The aesthetic consequences of maxillary malreduction include alterations in the appearance and position of the lips, nose, and cheeks (see Fig. 14–4). Surgical correction of maxillary malunion is indicated and performed to restore proper dental alignment and mastication, to correct airway obstruction, and to normalize the appearance. It is important, prior to embarking on any surgical procedure, that realistic goals and results be understood by the patient and his family. Despite "new techniques and advances," optimal reconstruction may take staged consecutive procedures.[143,167]

Classically, maxillary fractures have been divided into Le Fort I (dentoalveolar), Le Fort II (pyramidal), and Le Fort III (craniofacial disjunction) types.[25] Pooled data from various series indicate that the relative frequency of Le Fort fractures in descending frequency is: Le Fort II, I, and III in the ratio of 8:7:1.[4,168] Most midfacial fractures seen today are the result of high-velocity trauma. These fractures often are not isolated Le Fort types and seldom are symmetric. Thus, the majority of maxillary fractures do not conveniently fall into one of these classification categories. Nonetheless, the Le Fort system of maxillary fracture classification persists without an obvious replacement. It is important to think of the Le Fort Roman numerals as generic rather than anatomically exact labels.

Malunited maxillary fractures, in patients who have undergone primary fracture treatment, usually occur because of insufficient duration of immobilization, incomplete reduction, unrecognized associated facial fractures, or overzealous compression fixation.[37,169] Other factors that contribute to inaccurate anatomic reduction include comminuted mandibular fractures, edentulous alveoli, and associated skull fractures. Because of the abundant blood supply to midfacial bones, true nonunion of opposed bone in this area is rarely seen.[147] Nonunion, when it occurs, often results from the exclusive use of intermaxillary fixation without stabilization of the midface. Persistent motion at the maxillary fracture site leads to eburnation and architecturally unstable fibrous union.[10,152,170]

The amount of aesthetic deformity and functional disharmony associated with malunited maxillary fractures varies depending on the pretrauma facial relationships and the degree of secondary displacement. The usual profile of a patient with an untreated maxillary fracture with malunion is an elongated concave contour with a relatively prognathic appearance of the nondisturbed mandible (see Fig. 14–4). The presumed mechanism for this "classic" deformity is unopposed action of intact medial pterygoids which retrude the maxilla. This results in a retropositioned maxillary dentition which, having created a reduced interocclusal space in the region of the maxillary tuberosity, produces an anterior open bite.

In contrast, when the maxillary fracture has been treated, especially with suspension wires, the resultant deformity often includes midface shortening with loss of anterior projection and segmental horizontal retrusion between the maxillary alveolus and the bony orbits.[37] Experimental evidence from rhesus monkeys suggests that midfacial elongation does not occur following Le Fort I fractures treated without vertical suspension wires.[34,171]

Formulation of a reconstructive plan for maxillary malunions begins with a thorough physical evaluation with documentation of soft- and hard-tissue abnormalities. Standard anteroposterior and lateral cephalometric x-ray films are obtained for both treatment planning and serial comparisons pre- and postoperatively.[108] Preoperative planning based on standard cephalometric x-ray films can be difficult in complex, combined Le Fort fractures because of overlapping structures and distortion of standard anatomic landmarks. In addition, the extent of fracture, the amount of comminution, the displacement, and the degree of rotation of segments cannot be accurately determined from only an anteroposterior and lateral format. In such cases, high-resolution, narrowly collimated axial CT scanning with three-dimensional reformats is done. This sophisticated computer-assisted imaging allows better understanding of the fracture complex and thus, a more complete diagnosis and treatment plan (Fig. 14–5). Life-size reformatted bony images and models can be constructed to assist in preoperative planning.

After accurately defining the anatomy of the traumatic deformity, definitive treatment plans are made. Restoration of premorbid occlusal relationships is of paramount importance in the reduction of maxillary fractures. However, assessment of the

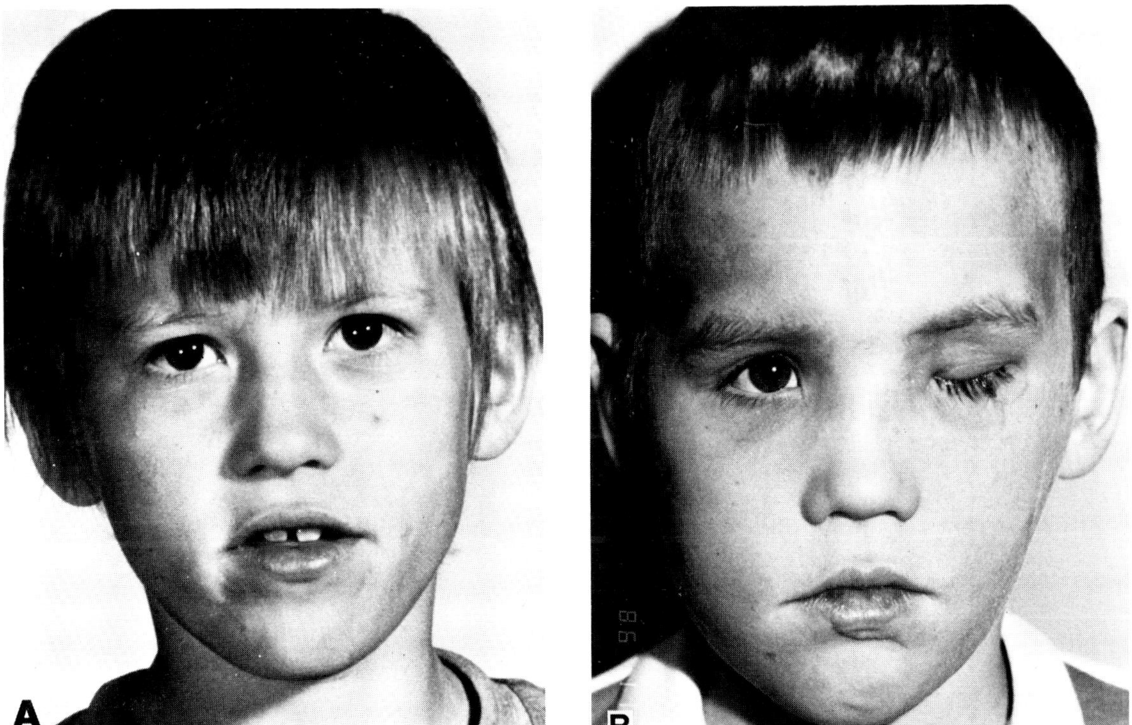

Figure 14–5 Evaluation of a 10-year-old boy with malunion comminuted Le Fort III and mandibular fractures using three-dimensional osseous surface reformation from CT scans (Vannier-Marsh method).[118,119] *A*, Pretrauma photograph. *B*, Two months after trauma. Acute management consisted of frontal craniotomy and intermaxillary fixation for 4 weeks. There is left upper eyelid ptosis and enophthalmos, telecanthus, flat nasal bridge, and asymmetry of the mid- and lower face.

Figure continues on following page.

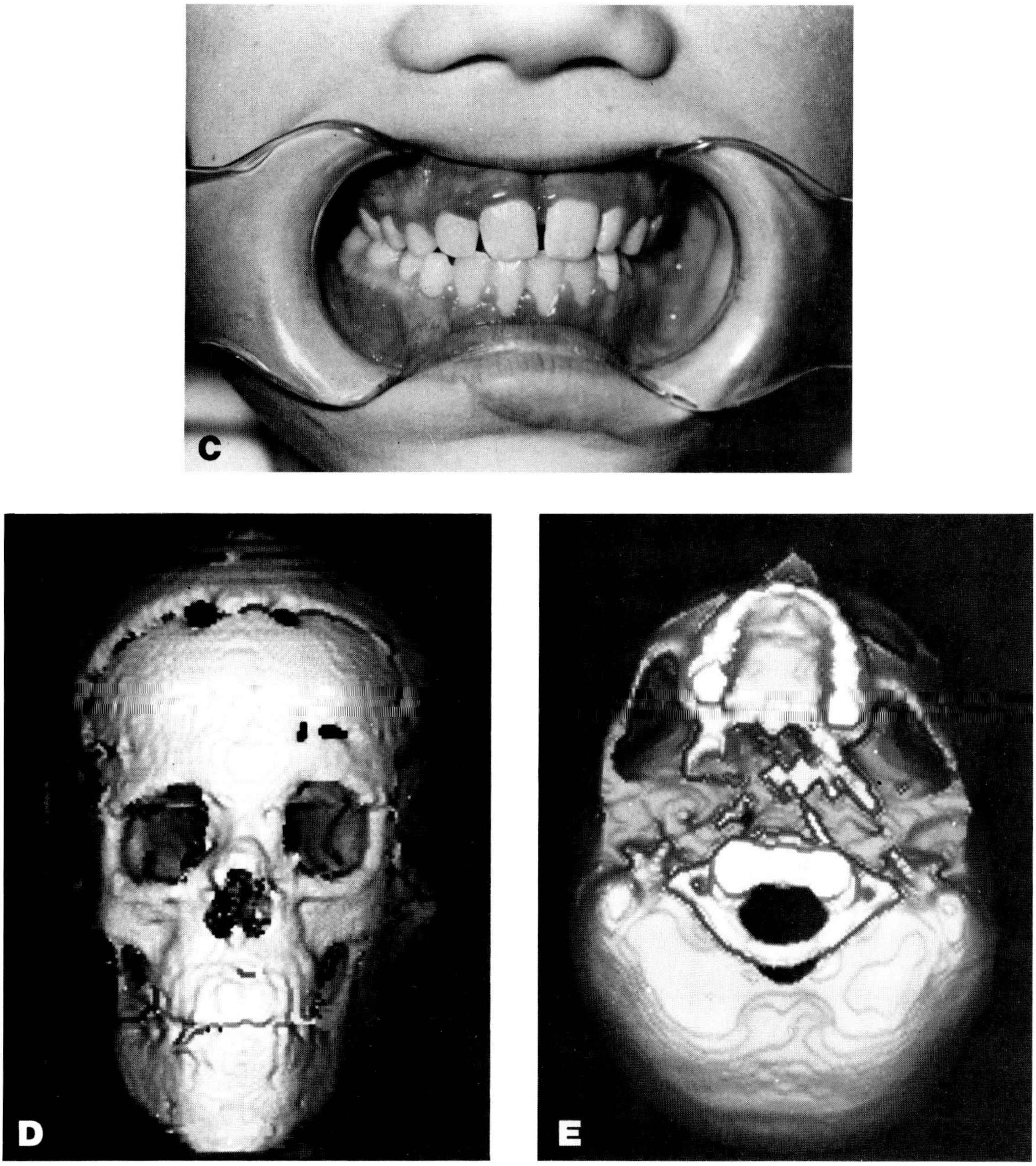

Figure 14–5 Continued. *C*, Dental occlusion 2 months after trauma. Rotation of the right and left maxillary alveoli can be appreciated by comparing the incisor mesial angulation to the vertical diastema visible in *A*. The mandibular incisal midline is shifted to the right of that of the maxilla. There is a left buccal cross-bite. *D*, Frontal three-dimensional osseous surface reformat from CT scan (the image is of poor quality owing to motion artifact). The frontal craniotomy defect is visible. There is step-off at the zygomaticofrontal articulations. The nasoethmoid is broad. The entire midface is shifted to the left of the midsagittal plane of the skull. The zygomas are asymmetric. The mandible is shifted to the right with lateral projection of the left condyle. *E*, Bottom three-dimensional osseous surface reformat from CT scan. The maxilla is rotated clockwise off the midsagittal plane of the skull. The left pterygoid plates are shattered. The left zygoma is displaced dorsally and rotated about the bizygomatic axis, the cephalad aspect ventrally, and the caudad aspect dorsally. The zygomatic arches are asymmetric with the left being foreshortened and displaced mesially.

premorbid occlusion may be difficult because of displacement of fracture segments, avulsed or fractured teeth, or both.

Dental study models are obtained in all patients scheduled for revisional midface surgery. These models are essential for determining proper occlusal relationships, planning osteotomies, and constructing dental splints.[172,173] The models also serve as a permanent pretreatment record. Interdental splints and appliances are especially important in management of edentulous patients and those selected patients who require prosthetic splints for proper intermaxillary fixation. A close working relationship with a maxillofacial prosthodontist facilitates construction of accurate dental splints. Sophisticated preoperative plans and complex intraoperative osteotomies are for naught if an ill-constructed splint precludes attainment of satisfactory occlusion. In contrast, appropriate use of splints, when indicated, can simplify surgical technique and decrease patient morbidity.[174]

Standardized photographs are also an important aspect of preoperative evaluation and planning.[94,96] When camouflage procedures are planned, a full-face moulage can quantitate alloplastic needs and allow fabrication of custom implants. New three-dimensional modeling technology, based upon CT scans, further extends the ability of surgeons to obtain custom implants and prostheses. The combination of photographs, dental models, facial impressions, and sophisticated radiographic imaging in conjunction with detailed physical examination allows effective evaluation of bony and soft-tissue defects and formulation of an accurate reconstructive plan.

When the deformity resulting from maxillary malunion is without a functional component and a satisfactory occlusal relationship has been maintained, camouflage of the defects rather than "anatomic" reconstruction may be indicated. Autogenous grafts of hard and soft tissues, alloplastic onlay implants, or alloplastic inlay prostheses may give satisfactory aesthetic results in such cases. The advantages and disadvantages of autogenous versus alloplastic material were discussed earlier in this chapter. Our preference usually is to use autogenous material.[10,149,154,175] While some alloplastic materials seem to be contraindicated in the management of acute injuries, e.g., methyl methacrylate, others, such as metallic internal fixation devices, are well tolerated. Other alloplastic materials, especially those with tissue bonding, may be indicated in reconstructive cases when nasal, sinus, and oral mucosas are intact or can be repaired easily.

The choice of reconstructive surgical maneuver depends upon the location, severity, and type of fracture. Often, a combination of refracturing, autogenous grafting, and camouflage procedures is used.[176] When there is a substantial defect or functional problem, the best solution is refracture with anatomic reduction and stable internal fixation with miniplates, bone grafts, or both. Alloplastic materials for augmentation or recontour are reserved for secondary "touch-up" procedures.[177] The time span between initial injury or initial treatment and secondary revisional surgery dictates the use of certain surgical procedures. Within the first 4 weeks after injury, malunion of the maxilla can usually be mobilized by digital manipulation. An impression tray containing dental compound may be used to obtain a firm atraumatic grip of the maxillary dental alveolus to facilitate mobilization. Between 4 and 12 weeks following injury, increasing force is needed to mobilize fractured segments. Sophisticated yet cumbersome traction devices have been used successfully in the past to realign the maxilla preoperatively.[178] The stubborn, adherent, malunited maxilla often can be mobilized intraoperatively during this period using maxillary disimpaction forceps. When the maxilla is comminuted or the palate fractured, these instruments become ineffective. Fractures that are more than 12 weeks old usually cannot be mobilized by the above techniques and therefore require osteotomy for repositioning.[169,179]

Prior to the reintroduction of the elective Le Fort III type osteotomy by Tessier, the only operative management proposed for the "dishface" defect of a malunited maxillary fracture was onlay bone grafting and camouflage techniques.[180] Today, the popularization of craniofacial surgery techniques of coronal incision, intra- and extracranial osseous exposure, and fixation methods, as well as advances in anesthesia allow safe, direct, anatomic correction of these severe complex deformities. The basic surgical principle to be followed is correction of the functional anatomic defect by controlled osteotomies or fractures for mobilization stabilized by rigid internal fixation. When properly conceived and correctly executed, standard craniofacial procedures can reposition the retruded maxilla, restore dental occlusion and establish a more natural appearance. Concomitant nasal reconstruction and onlay bone grafting may be necessary. Subsequent alloplastic implants, soft-

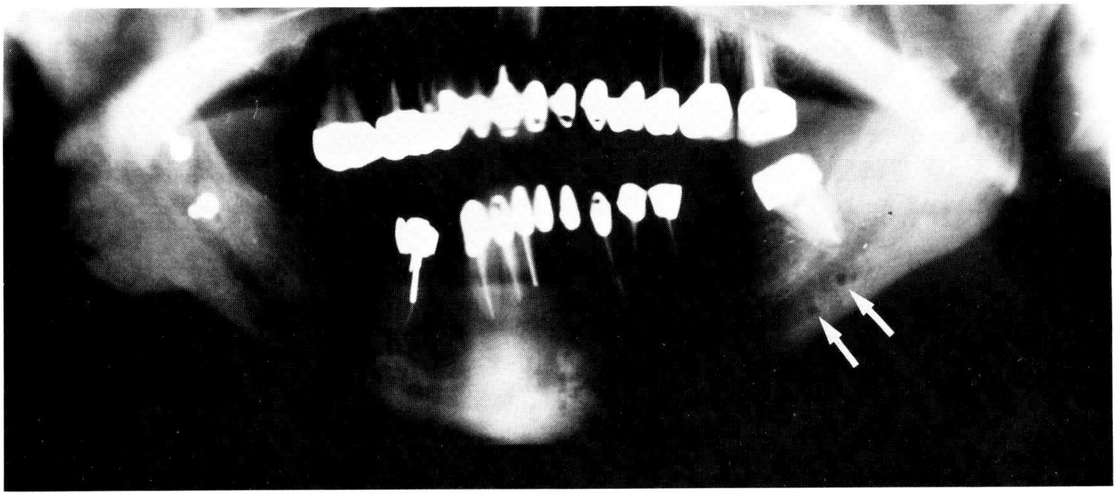

Figure 14–7 Panoramic radiograph of a 39-year-old woman 10 months following intraoperative comminution of the left mandibular ramus during sagittal split osteotomy. The patient complained of lower facial asymmetry and osseous movement at the angle of the left mandible. The rigid internal plate fixation used for the left ramus has been removed but the screw holes (arrows) can be seen transgressing the alveolar nerve canal (the patient lost sensation on the left). The inferior fixation screw on the right ramus is precariously close to the nerve.

be superior to cortical bone in rate of vascular invasion, degree of incorporation, and appositional bone formation.[203] Probably of more critical importance than donor site are the condition and preparation of the recipient bed. Control of infection, appropriate débridement, adequate soft-tissue envelope, and rigid fixation are all prerequisites for successful bone grafting.[72,148,204]

In addition to evaluation of the osseous mandible, the skin and soft tissues of the lower face are assessed carefully. Soft-tissue scarring resulting from the initial trauma, the primary treatment, or secondary complications may create a less than optimal environment for attainment of operative exposure, manipulation of bone fragments, or as a recipient site for bone graft incorporation. Contracting scar tissue along with muscle pull may prevent accurate intraoperative positioning or subsequently displace the realigned fragments. "Undermining" and "relaxing incisions" may be helpful intraoperatively but if not supported with rigid internal fixation, relapse may occur quickly.

After completion of the physical examination and review of radiographs, we routinely consult with our dental colleagues, the orthodontist and prosthodontist. A complete evaluation of the entire stomatognathic system, which includes dental study models, is carried out by each of the subspecialists. These additional assessments provide important adjunctive options for treatment of difficult secondary problems. To achieve optimal results, the efforts of the craniomaxillofacial surgeon, the orthodontist, and prosthodontist must be coordinated. Working together, they can restore optimally the dental occlusion, temporomandibular joint function, and the pretraumatic facial appearance.[205–207]

In addition to standard mandibular radiographs (anteroposterior and lateral cephalometric, mandibular series, and orthopantographic images), special radiographic views (obliques, temporomandibular joint, arthrography, bone scans) are obtained when indicated. We have found high-resolution CT scanning with three-dimensional surface reformats useful in evaluation of and planning for complicated secondary mandibular revision surgery (Fig. 14–8). Reconstructed images can be viewed from any position. On such images, symmetry is readily appreciated and can be analyzed quantitatively. Using different "windowing" techniques on the axial CT scans, osseous and fibrous unions can be differentiated (Fig. 14–9). Planes of disruption, extent of fractures, soft-tissue interposition into the fracture, and bone fragment position not only can be visualized but their relationship to each other better comprehended with computer-assisted imaging.

The treatment plan is formulated upon the collation of the findings of the physical examination, photographs, dental models, radiographic images, and specialty consultations. Treatment options include surgery, orthodontics, prosthetic devices, or

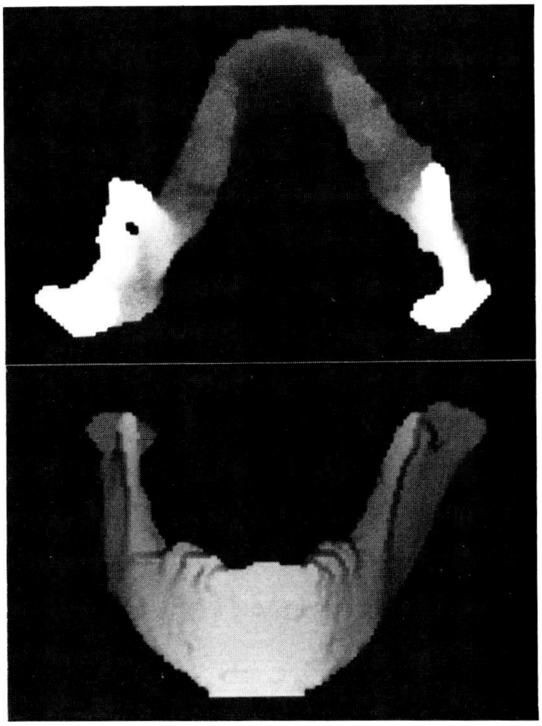

Figure 14–8 Disarticulated mandible three-dimensional osseous surface reformats[118] from CT scans of patient in Figure 14–5. The mandibular body was oriented to the malreduced maxilla via interdental fixation. It is unclear whether the initial trauma, subsequent soft-tissue tensions, or a combination thereof produced the abnormal relationship between the rami and body.

a combination thereof.[208] Osteotomy is necessary to reposition malaligned fragments that have progressed to osseous union. Autogenous bone grafting and rigid internal fixation plates are used for stabilization and to bridge bony gaps. Orthodontic management can provide detailing of the occlusion. Prosthetic devices can restore or stabilize damaged teeth and provide an immediate foundation for secondary procedures.[172,209] Our integration of these different modalities is addressed below for three general types of secondary mandibular fracture management: delayed union or nonunion, malunion, and temporomandibular joint ankylosis.

The symptoms of delayed union or nonunion of the mandible vary from minimal discomfort to total incapacitation. Nonunion usually presents as abnormal mobility and pain following initial treatment of a mandibular fracture. Nonunion can result in a reduced caloric intake and subsequent malnourishment. The most common causes of nonunion are poor immobilization and inadequate reduction.[71] Increased incidences of mandibular nonunion have been correlated with postoperative trauma, intraoral reduction, osteomyelitis, and the edentulous patient[64,210] Factors not felt to be associated with nonhealing of the mandible were sex, age, cause of the fracture, site of injury, timing of treatment, periosteal stripping, general health of the patient and general status of the teeth. Mandibular fractures are usually architecturally stable at 6 weeks after reduction, provided additional secondary trauma is not encountered. In some centers, recurrent trauma accounts for up to 20 percent of the mandibular nonunions. The adverse effect of subsequent injury is substantial for up to 1½ years following fracture.[62,64,210,211]

Delayed union exists when there is movement of the mandibular fragments in all planes after 6 weeks of immobilization. When intermaxillary fixation is used exclusively as a technique in reduction and delayed union occurs, the prognosis is not good. In such cases, an additional 2 weeks of fixation is recommended provided there are no signs of infection and the pretraumatic occlusal relationship exists. The patient is re-evaluated 2 weeks later. At that time, fixation is released and the jaw reexamined. The decision to continue with intermaxillary fixation and serial examinations is one of clinical judgment and must be balanced against the effects of prolonged immobilization upon the temporomandibular joints. When after 2 months the mobility of the segments has not significantly decreased or when follow-up x-ray films exhibit a pattern of eburnation, further improvement is unlikely. The arbitrary but clinically relevant term of "nonunion" now applies.[61] Once the diagnosis of nonunion has been firmly made, prolonged immobilization cannot be expected to lead to osseous union. Autogenous bone grafts and concomitant rigid fixation are necessary for restoration of bony continuity. Techniques of fixation and grafting include onlay and inlay bone grafts with wire fixation, alloplastic preformed trays filled with cancellous bone chips, rigid metallic bone plates with screw fixation, and external fixation devices.[212] Additional immobilization can be obtained through dentures, Gunning splints, and intermaxillary fixation.[62] Whatever the method of fixation used, immobility of all fracture segments is essential for successful bony healing. Our preference is for rigid internal fixation with autogenous bone grafts as needed.

Obvious causes of nonunion which manifest themselves early, such as gross infection and chronic osteomyelitis, should be managed aggres-

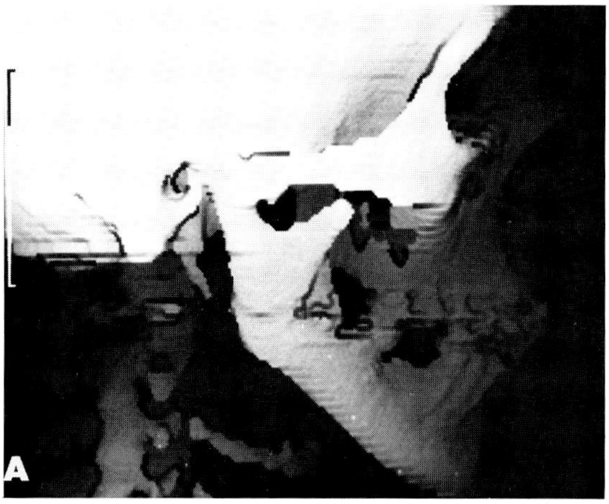

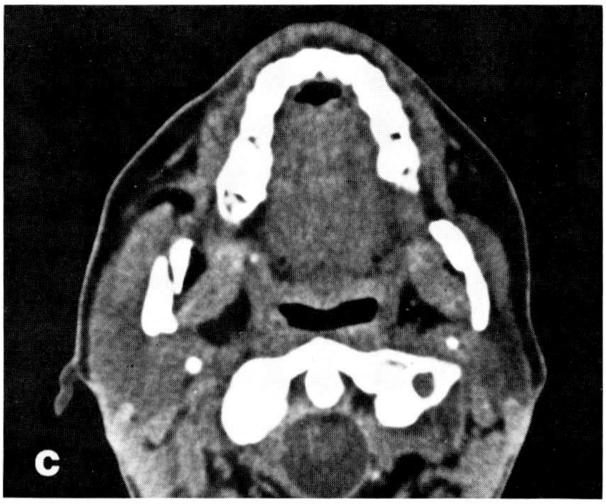

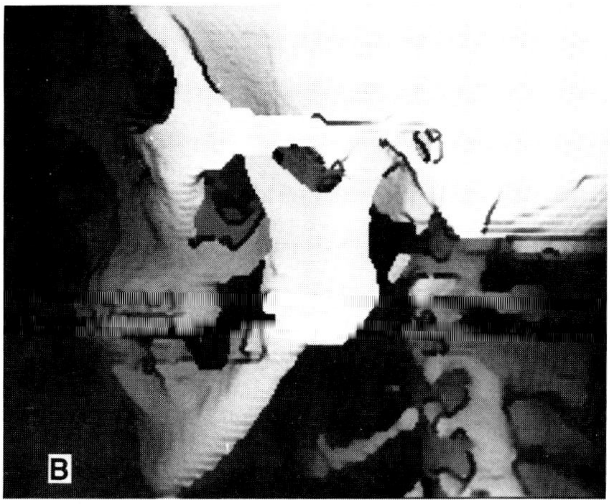

Figure 14–9 Computer-assisted diagnostic imaging of the mandibular nonunion in Figure 14–7. *A*, Right lateral three-dimensional osseous surface reformat[118] from CT scans. Continuity of the mandibular ramus, angle, and body is present. *B*, Left lateral. There is a discontinuity of the inferior border of the mandible anterior to the angle. While these images demonstrate the asymmetry of the mandible, they cannot clarify the nature of the union of the fragments. *C*, Direct axial CT scan at level of maxillary alveolus. Both mandibular rami are visible. The solid white of the right ramus implies osseous union of the sagittal split. The lucency between the lateral and medial fragments of the left ramus indicates a fibrous malunion.

sively.[199] While radiographic evaluation is obtained to monitor the resolution or progression of the nonunion, radiographs are poor temporal and quantitative indicators. Once the diagnosis of nonunion has been made, systemic antibiotic administration is initiated and the patient taken to the operating room for bone biopsy, cultures, and a thorough débridement of the fracture site. Any devitalized teeth at the fracture site are extracted. Traditionally, all internal alloplastic hardware was removed and the mobile fragments stabilized with an external fixation device. While such devices are cumbersome, they allow establishment of a relatively accurate osseous relationship and immobilization of bone fragments without the attendant morbidity of long-term intermaxillary fixation.[209] Of interest, however, are recent reports discussing successful management of infected mandibular fractures without removal of the rigid internal fixation plates.[60,142] This approach echoes that often used in compound limb fractures. After resolution of the infection, if sufficient quantity and quality of bone exist and there is adequate immobilization, osseous union occurs.

However, when substantial bone was removed during débridement or significant resorption with eburnation of the bone ends has taken place, bone grafting is needed in addition to rigid internal fixation to achieve bony union. Probably of more critical importance than the bone graft donor site are the condition and preparation of the recipient bed. Control of infection, appropriate débridement, adequate soft-tissue envelope, and rigid fixation are all prerequisites to successful bone grafting.[213,214]

While malunion most commonly is a sequela of untreated fractures, it also may occur in treated patients. Certain fractures are predisposed to malunion because of their location and degree of angulation.[141,215] In such fractures, the muscles of mastication distract the fragments. (Such fractures are referred to as "unfavorable" while those in which the muscle forces impact the fragments are called "favorable.") In initially treated patients, most cases of malunion result from either inadequate reduction or inadequate immobilization of the fracture. The indications for treatment of a malunited fracture depend on the patient's symptoms. Malunion of the edentulous patient may be managed simply by adjustment of dentures.[208,216] In the partially dentulous patient, extraction of a few diseased teeth with a dental bridge constructed to compensate for the malalignment is not only expeditious but also avoids surgical risk and morbidity.[217] In contrast, osteotomy and osseous realignment often are necessary for restoration of facial symmetry, correction of occlusion in the dentulous patient, repositioning of the mandible, and correction of temporomandibular joint disharmony.

Successful surgical planning is based upon a combination of physical examination, x-ray films, and dental models. After establishing the pretraumatic occlusion with the dental models on an articulator, registration and lingual splints are fabricated. At surgery, the site of malunion usually is approached percutaneously and the fracture site mobilized. The registration splint is inserted and the patient restored to the premorbid occlusion with wire intermaxillary fixation between the arch bars. The fracture site is reinspected, fragments adjusted as needed and rigid internal fixation applied. We prefer heavy mandibular compression or reconstruction plates for the mandible rather than miniplates. Following successful plate fixation, the wire intermaxillary fixation and registration splint are removed. The lingual splint is inserted and secured to the mandibular arch bar and teeth. Upon completion of insertion of the lingual splint, the fracture site is reinspected and the wounds closed. Thus, the patient recovers in the perioperative period without intermaxillary fixation. When the occlusion remains stable, no other intermaxillary fixation is needed and the patient is discharged to be examined on a weekly basis as an outpatient. However, if the occlusion begins to relapse or if satisfactory occlusion could not be maintained prior to discharge from the hospital, the patient is placed in intermaxillary elastics and examined weekly.

The temporomandibular joint is a complex articulating system between the skull base and the mandible. There is a significant mandibular growth site in children immediately beneath the articular surface of the condylar head. Nonetheless, experience has shown that the majority of fractures in this region when treated in closed fashion, even when accompanied by angulation or displacement, heal with satisfactory functional results in spite of poor anatomical alignment and irrespective of patient's age.[67,105,218] Untoward sequelae of condylar neck or head fractures, however, do occur and constitute one of the most difficult problems for the maxillofacial surgeon.[62,219–224]

When the traumatic episode occurs during mandibular development, the condylar growth site may be disturbed resulting in cessation of downward and forward advancement of the mandible. In unilateral cases, this produces a progressive shift of the lower face and mandibular incisal midlines toward the side of injury (Fig. 14–10). In bilateral cases, retrognathia width with open bite develops (Fig. 14–11).[68,105,225] Similar findings have been observed in subhuman primate experimental models of condylar fractures.[104,226,227] In addition, maxillary alveolar bone deformity, growth impairment, and occlusal plane can be seen in severe cases.[228,229] It is not known whether the mandibular shift, the atrophic ramus, or the retrognathia occurs from growth site disturbances or from an inability to place normal functional strains on the growing bone.[68,107,229–231]

The ultimate complication of a malunited condylar fracture is joint ankylosis (see Fig. 14–11). Ankylosis is characterized clinically by progressive trismus which results in an interincisal distance of less than 5 mm. Difficulties in mastication, speech, and breathing have been reported secondary to ankylosis.[62,232,233] Temporomandibular joint ankylosis may be due to pathological fibrotic changes, either within the joint capsule or outside the joint in adjacent tissues, which result in restriction of the normal mobility of the mandible. While intraarticular ankylosis is more common, when left unattended for a prolonged time, secondary extracapsular fibrosis in surrounding tissues develops. Extraarticular fibrosis, which produces a functional pseudoankylosis, can arise from a variety of conditions including, infrequently, zygomatic arch fractures.[9,24,26,34,38,43,44,61,68,70,74,90,91,140,143,151,153,158,164,165,169,184–186,193,204,206,213,214,224,232,234,235,237] In such cases, adhesions usually occur between the temporalis-coronoid complex and either the zygomatic arch or the maxilla.[135,235,236] The diagnosis is made from a history of an isolated zygomatic fracture, normal-appearing radiographs of the temporomandibular joint without displacement or disruption of the joint capsule, and progressive jaw immobility. Nonsurgical treatment is usually unsuccessful. Transoral coronoidectomy followed intraoperatively by gentle but forceful mobilization

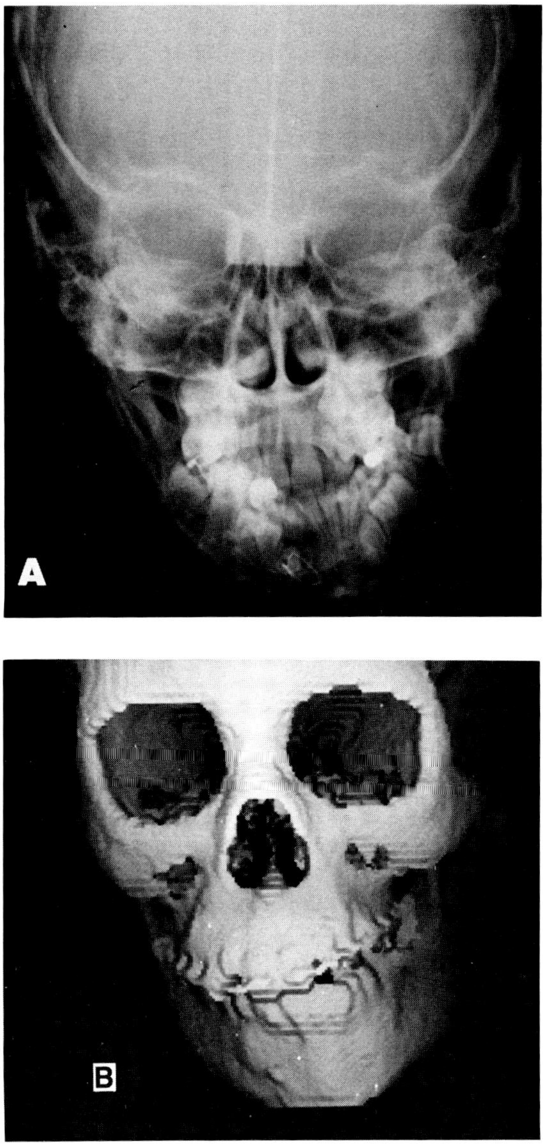

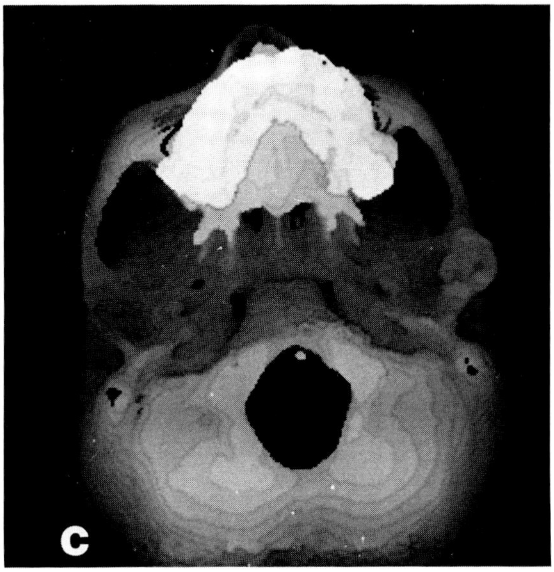

Figure 14–10 An 8½-year-old girl 6 years following right parasymphyseal and left condylar neck mandibular fractures. Initial treatment consisted of open reduction/wire internal fixation of the parasymphyseal fracture with a brief period of intermaxillary fixation followed by a nonchew diet. Facial asymmetry and painful chewing were first noted 1½ years after injury. Orthodontic elastic and functional appliance therapies failed to reverse or halt the progressive deformity. *A*, Cephalometric skull roentgenogram demonstrating mandibular asymmetry. Details of the left temporomandibular joint are unclear. *B*, Frontal three-dimensional osseous surface reformat[118] from CT scan. The occlusal cant with hypoplasia of the left maxilla and the deformity at the root of the left zygomatic arch are appreciated more easily on this image than in *A*. *C*, Bottom three-dimensional osseous surface reformat[118] from CT scan. There is hyperostosis at the anterolateral aspect of the left glenoid fossa. This is the region of the post-traumatic ankylosis. The asymmetries of the maxillary alveoli, zygomas, and zygomatic arches are secondary to the ankylosis.

of the mandible is the initial treatment of choice. Intensive active dental exercises should follow. True temporomandibular joint ankylosis in children can result from many causes. Trauma and infectious or inflammatory conditions are the most common causes, in that order. The standard hypothesis for the development of traumatic ankylosis postulates that bleeding around and within the joint stimulates abnormal fibrosis thereby destroying the meniscus and obliterating the joint space. In other cases, infection or autoimmune conditions may trigger this proliferative process.

Management of condylar fractures in children has been a controversial subject.[68,104,105,188,225,231,237] Clinical experience and serial longitudinal radiographic findings, substantiated by experimental studies, argue that condylar fractures, even with deviation or displacement, undergo resorption and recontouring with long-term morbidity. Closed reduction with short-term intermaxillary fixation and early active range of motion seem to ensure the best outcome.[67,104,218,220,226,227,237] Nonetheless, absolute criteria for open reduction of condylar fractures in both adults and children have

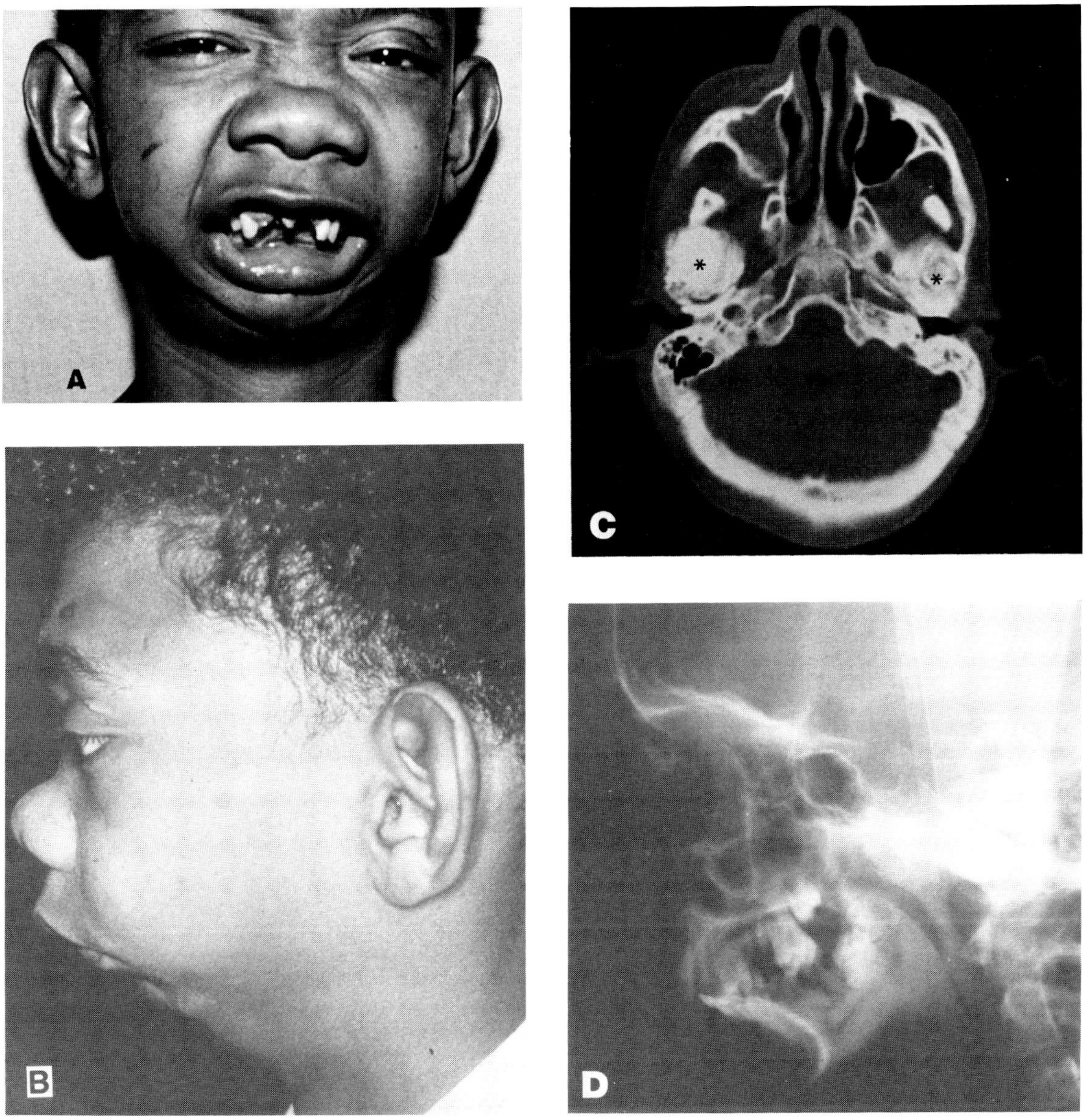

Figure 14–11 *A, B,* A 14-year-old boy with retrognathia and bilateral temporomandibular joint ankylosis 12 years after bilateral mandibular condylar fractures. *C,* Direct axial CT scan through level of temporomandibular joints. There is bilateral hyperostosis in the region of the joints (asterisks) which is consistent with bony ankylosis. *D,* Preoperative lateral cephalometric roentgenogram.

Figure continues on following page.

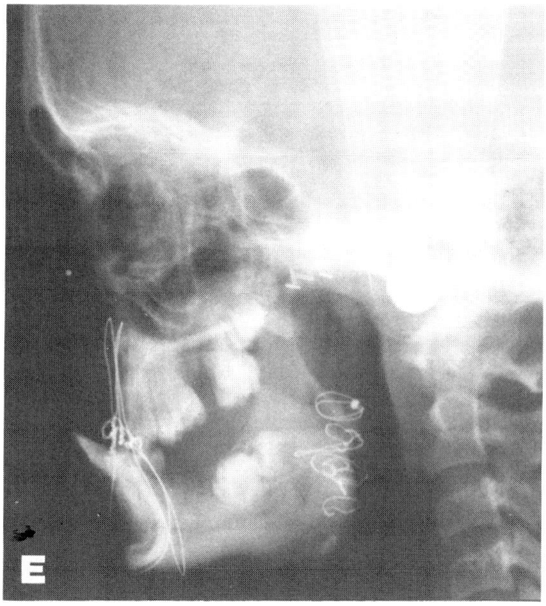

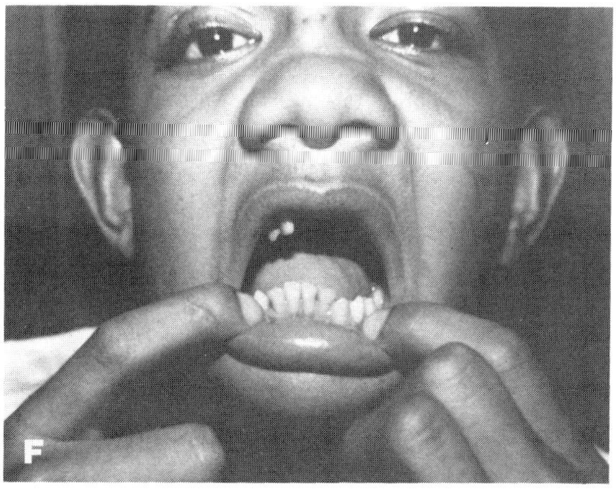

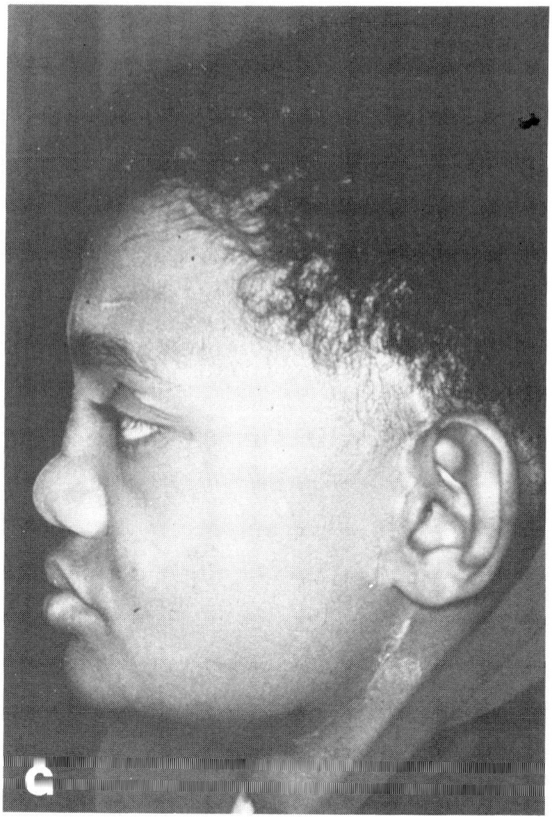

Figure 14–11 Continued. *E*, Postoperative cephalometric roentgenogram. The condyles and coronoid processes were resected, the mandible advanced, and new condyles and rami reconstructed with autogenous costochondral grafts. Postoperative oral opening (*F*) and profile (*G*).

been proposed. These include: (1) displacement of the condyle into the middle cranial fossa; (2) inability to obtain adequate occlusion by closed reduction; (3) lateral extracapsular displacement of the condyle; and (4) invasion of the joint space by a foreign body.[237a]

Treatment of true temporomandibular joint ankylosis requires re-creation of a joint mechanism and restoration of dentoskeletal harmony. Interposition arthroplasty, using a wide variety of substances between the glenoid fossa and the mandibular condyle remnant, has been practiced for many years.[238] In the adult, alloplastic joint arthroplasty has become popular. Ramus osteotomy or bone grafting also may be indicated to restore skeletal symmetry.[239] If the ankylosis occurred in childhood, maxillary osteotomy may also be necessary to level the occlusal plane of the untreated adult (see Fig. 14–10). In the growing child, we the use of autogenous tissue (costochondral graft) to alloplastic implants.[155,238,240,241] Prior to undertaking this reconstruction, dental models are obtained, registration splints created, and orthodontic brackets applied. A neocondyle is constructed out of the cartilage and bone of the sixth or seventh rib contralateral to the side of the ankylosis. If three-dimensional CT scan images have been obtained, a life-size model based on the contralateral condyle can be constructed and used as a guide during surgery. The pathological condyle and coronoid process are excised through a standard Risdon external incision. The teeth are then placed into occlusion and intermaxillary fixation secured. The costochondral graft with its carved neocondyle is inserted into the glenoid fossa and visually inspected for fit. While we do not use any fixation for the neocondyle, others have advocated this maneuver.[242] The bony caudal portion of the transferred rib is then fixed, with lag screws if possible rather than wire, to the ramus and body. We have not attempted microvascular transfer of toe joints or iliac bone nor have we used nonvascularized toe or sternoclavicular joint grafts in these cases.

The fate of nonvascularized costochondral grafts for condyle reconstruction varies from resorption to overgrowth. In the majority of cases, however, there will be minimal to moderate growth.[48] Therefore, during the initial consultation with the patient or the parents, the erratic growth potential and possible need for additional surgery should be discussed. The possibility of growth in autogenous grafts outweighs the nonexistent growth potential of alloplastic material when determining the treatment course for children with ankylosis.

CONCLUSION

The late results of untreated or inadequately treated facial fractures are generally obvious. When less than optimal results occur after initial treatment or complications result in malaligned or nonunited fractures, a comprehensive analysis of the entire pathological process is mandatory prior to revisional surgery.

Management of these difficult problems requires an in-depth understanding of why the untoward events occurred. This is predicated upon a basic understanding of bone healing, a complete and well-documented physical examination, a thorough understanding of the radiographic deformity and a contemporary knowledge of surgical instrumentation and techniques.

Successful surgical correction of acquired complex craniofacial deformities requires reconstruction of bony architecture, normalization of soft-tissue irregularities, and restoration of premorbid dental occlusion. A realistic, expeditious, and definitive therapeutic plan of action, based upon biologic and surgical principles, must be formulated to achieve these ends.

REFERENCES

1. Dingman RO, Harding RL. The treatment of malunion fractures of the facial bones. Plast Reconstr Surg 1951; 7:505–519.
2. Converse JM, Smith B, Woodsmith D. Deformities of the midface resulting from malunited orbital and nasoorbital fractures. Clin Plast Surg 1975; 2:107–130.
3. Georgiade G, Riefkohl R, Serafin D, Georgiade N. A silent but lethal injury associated with facial trauma. Plast Reconstr Surg 1981; 67:665–667.
4. Gwyn PP, Carraway JH, Horton CE, et al. Facial fractures: associated injuries and complications. Plast Reconstr Surg 1971; 47:225–230.
5. Luce EA, Tubb TD, Moore AM. A review of 1,000 major facial fractures and associated injuries. Plast Reconstr Surg 1979; 63:26–30.
6. McCoy FJ, Chandler RA, Magnan LG. An analysis of facial fractures and their complications. Plast Reconstr Surg 1962; 29:381–390.
7. Ord RA, Awty MD, Pour S. Bilateral retrobulbar hemorrhage: a short case report. Br J Oral Maxillofac Surg 1986; 24:1–6.
8. Press BH, Boies LR, Shones AR. Facial fractures in trauma victims: the influence of treatment delay on ultimate outcome. Ann Plast Surg 1983; 11:121–124.
9. Schultz RC. Facial injuries from automobile accidents: a study of 400 consecutive cases. Plast Reconstr Surg 1967; 40:415–425.
10. Tessier P. Complications of facial trauma: principles of late reconstruction. Ann Plast Surg 1986; 17:411–420.
11. Van Hoof FH, Merkx CA, Stekelenberg EC. The different patterns of fractures of the facial skeleton in four European countries. Int J Oral Surg 1977; 6:3–11.
12. Afzelius L, Rosen C. Facial fractures: a review of 368 cases. Int J Oral Surg 1980; 9:25–33.
13. Babajews A, Williams J. Blindness after trauma insufficient to cause bony injury: case report and review. Br J Oral Maxillofac Surg 1986; 24:7–11.
14. Bergstrom L, Hemenway WG. Parotid-antral fistula. Complications of facial fracture. Arch Otolaryngol 1971; 519–520.
15. Jurkiewicz MJ, Nickell WB. Fracture of the skeleton of the face: a study of diagnosis and treatment based on twelve years' experience in the treatment of over 600 major fractures of the facial skeleton. J Trauma 1971; 11:947–958.
16. Kreidler JR, Koch H. Endoscopic findings of maxillary sinus after middle face fractures. J Maxillofac Surg 1975; 3:10–14.

17. Lunden K, Ridell A, Sandberg N, Ohman A. 1,000 maxillofacial and related fractures at the ENT Clinic in Gothenburg: a two-year prospective study. Acta Otol 1973; 75:359–361.
18. Zachariades N. Laryngeal incompetence following facial trauma. J Oral Maxillofac Surg 1985; 43:638–639.
19. McCoy FJ. Late results in facial fractures. In: Goldwyn R, ed. Long-term results in plastic and reconstructive surgery. Vol 2. Boston: Little, Brown, 1980:485.
20. Moore FT, Ward TG. Complications and sequelae of untreated fractures of facial bones and their treatment. Br J Plast Surg 1949; 1:257–267.
21. Trinkaus E, Zimmerman MR. Trauma among the Shanidar Neanderthals. Am J Phys Anthropol 1982; 57:61–76.
22. Lipton JS. Oral surgery in ancient Egypt as reflected in Edwin Smith papyrus. Bull Hist Dent 1982; 30:108–113.
23. Gahos F, Ariyan S. Facial fractures: Hippocratic management. Head Neck Surg 1984; 6:1007–1013.
24. Rowe NL. The history and treatment of maxillofacial trauma. Ann Royal Coll Surg Eng 1971; 49:329–349.
25. Le Fort R. Experimental study of fractures of the upper jaw: part I and II. Rev Chir Paris 1901; 23:208–227, 360–379.
26. Rowe NL. The evolution of treatment of maxillofacial injuries. In: Rowe NL, Killey HC, eds. Fractures of the facial skeleton. 2nd ed. Edinburgh: E & S Livingstone, 1968:825.
27. Ivy RH. Evaluation of advantages in the treatment of jaw fractures since 1941. Plast Reconstr Surg 1968; 42:472–476.
28. Adams WM. Internal wiring fixation of facial fractures. Surgery 1942; 12:523–527.
29. Adams WM, Adams LH. Internal wire fixation of facial fractures: a 15-year follow-up report. Am J Surg 1956; 92:12–19.
30. Altonen M, Ranta R, Ylipaavalniemi P. Midface deviation due to mandibular fractures. (An experimental study with clinical comparison.) J Maxillofac Surg 1978; 6:143–147.
31. Furnas DW. Transverse maxillary osteotomy for malunion of maxillary fractures. Plast Reconstr Surg 1968; 42:378–383.
32. Manson PW, Hoopes JE, Su CT. Structural pillars of the facial skeleton: an approach to the management of Le Fort fractures. Plast Reconstr Surg 1980; 66:54–61.
33. Yee KF, Cravens J, Kotler R. Traumatic ophthalmoplegia: a complication of fractures of the zygomaticomaxillary complex. Review of etiology with report of an unusual case. Laryngoscope 1975; 85:570–575.
34. Sofferman RA, Danielson PA, Quatela VA, Reed R. Retrospective analysis of surgically treated Le Fort fractures. Arch Otolaryngol 1983; 109:446–448.
35. Gruss JS. Nasoethmoid-orbital fracture: classification and role of primary bone grafting. Plast Reconstr Surg 1985; 75:303–308.
36. Kellman RM. Repair of mandibular fractures via compression plating and more traditional techniques: a comparison of results. Laryngoscope 1984; 94:1560–1567.
37. Manson PN, Crawley WA, Yaremchuk MJ, et al. Midface fractures: advantages of immediate extended open reduction and bone grafting. Plast Reconstr Surg 1985; 76:1–10.
38. Spiessl B. Principles of rigid internal fixation in fractures of the lower jaw. In: Spiessl B, ed. New concepts in maxillofacial bone surgery. Berlin: Springer Verlag, 1976:21–51.
39. Artzy E. Display of three-dimensional information in computed tomography. Comput Graphics Image Proc 1979; 9:196–198.
40. Marsh JL, Gado M. The longitudinal orbital CT projection: a versatile image for orbital assessment. Plast Reconstr Surg 1983; 71:308–317.
41. Marsh JL. Vannier MW, Bresina S, Hemmer KM. Applications of computer graphics in craniofacial surgery. Clin Plast Surg 1986; 13:441–448.
42. Prichard JJ. The general histology of bone. In: Bourne GH, ed. The biochemistry and physiology of bone. 2nd ed. New York: Academic Press, 1972:1.
43. Sevitt S. Bone repair and fracture healing in man. London: Churchill Livingstone, 1981.
44. Rhinelander F, Phillips R, Steel W, Beer J. Microangiography in bone healing. J Bone Joint Surg 1968; 50A:784–800.
45. Frankel VH, Nordin M. Biomechanics of whole bones and bone tissue. In: Frankel VH, Nordin M, eds. Basic biomechanics of the skeletal system. Philadelphia: Lea & Febiger, 1980:15.
46. Burstein AH, Zika JM, Hieple KG, Klein L. Contribution of collagen and mineral to the elastic-plastic properties of bone. J Bone Joint Surg 1975; 57A:956–961.
47. Huelke DF, Harger JH. Maxillofacial injuries: their nature and mechanisms of production. J Oral Surg 1969; 27:451–460.
48. Manchester WM. The long-term results in immediate reconstruction of the mandible and temporomandibular joint by free bone grafting. In: Goldwyn R, ed. Long-term results in plastic and reconstructive surgery. Vol 1. Boston: Little, Brown, 1980:439.
49. Pensler J, McCarthy JG. The calvarial donor site: an anatomic study in cadavers. Plast Reconstr Surg 1985; 75:648–651.
50. Naham A. The biomechanics of maxillofacial trauma. Clin Plast Surg 1975; 2:59–64.
51. Gentry LR, Manor WF, Tursk PA, Strother CM. High resolution computed tomographic analysis of facial struts in trauma: normal anatomy. Am J Radiol 1983; 140:523–532.
52. Gentry LR, Manor WF, Turski PA, Strother CM. High resolution CT analysis of facial struts in trauma. 2.Osseous and soft tissue complications. Am J Radiol 1983; 140:533–541.

53. Kramer IRH. The structure of bone and the processes of bone repair. In: Rowe NL, Killey HC, eds. Fractures of the facial skeleton. 2nd ed. Edinburgh: E & S Livingstone, 1968:615.
54. Weiss L. Static loading of the mandible. Oral Surg Oral Med Oral Pathol 1965; 19:253–262.
55. Bourne GH. In: Bourne GH, ed. The biochemistry and physiology of bone. Vol I–IV. New York: Academic Press, 1977.
56. Tonna EA, Cronkile EP. Cellular response to fracture study with tritated primidine. J Bone Joint Surg 1961; 43:352–361.
57. Cohen L. Methods of investigating the vascular architectures of the mandible. J Dent Res 1959; 38:920–931.
58. Cohen L. Venous drainage of the mandible. Oral Surg 1959; 12:1447–1449.
59. Cohen L. Further studies into the vas architecture of the mandible. J Dent Res 1960; 39:936–946.
60. Tu HK, Tenhulzen D. Compression osteosynthesis of mandibular fractures: a retrospective study. J Oral Maxillofac Surg 1985; 43:585–589.
61. Rowe NL. Nonunion of the mandible and maxilla. J Oral Surg 1969; 27:520–529.
62. Mathog RH, Rosenberg Z. Complications in the treatment of facial fractures. Otolaryngol Clin North Am 1976; 9:533–552.
63. Boyne PJ. Osseous healing after oblique osteotomy of the mandibular ramus. J Oral Surg 1966; 24:125–133.
64. Mathog RH. Non union of the mandible. Otolaryngol Clin North Am 1983; 16:533–547.
65. Thoma KH. Treatment of ununited and malunited fractures. J Oral Surg 1956; 14:93–108.
66. Fortunato WA, Fielding AF, Guernsey LH. Facial bone fractures in children. Oral Surg 1982; 53:225–230.
67. Kaban LB, Mulliken JB, Murray JE. Facial fractures in children: an analysis of 122 fractures in 109 patients. Plast Reconstr Surg 1977; 59:15–20.
68. Schultz RC, Meilinan J. Facial fractures in children. In: Goldwyn R, ed. Long-term results in plastic and reconstructive surgery. Vol 1. Boston: Little, Brown, 1980:458.
69. Paterson CR, MacLennan WJ. Bone disease in the elderly. In: Hall MR, ed. Disease management in the elderly, Vol 3. New York: John Wiley & Sons, 1984:17.
70. Spencer H, Kramer L, Osis D. Factors contributing to calcium loss in aging. Am J Clin Nutr 1982; 36:776–781.
71. Bone RC, Davidson TM, Nahum AM, Dahlberg R. Mandibular trauma: secondary problems in reconstruction. Laryngoscope 1977; 87:909–916.
72. Boyne PJ. Physiology of bone and response of osseous tissue drying and environmental changes. J Oral Surg 1970; 28:12–16.
73. Altner PC, Grana L, Gordon M. An experimental study on the significance of muscle tissue interposition on fracture healing. Clin Ortho 1975; 111:269–273.
74. Schmitz JP, Hollinger JO. The critical size defect as an experimental model for craniomandibulofacial nonunions. Clin Orthop 1986; 205:299–308.
75. Janecka IP. Maxillofacial infections. Clin Plast Surg 1979; 6:553–573.
76. Kerley TR, Mader JT, Hulet WH, Schow CE Jr. The effect of adjunctive hyperbaric oxygen on bone regeneration in mandibular osteomyelitis: report of case. J Oral Surg 1981; 619–623.
77. Kanis JA. Osteomalacia and chronic renal failure. J Clin Pathol 1981; 35:1295–1307.
78. Newcomer AP, Hodgson SF, McGill DB, Thomas PJ. Lactose deficiency: prevalence in osteoporosis. Ann Intern Med 1978; 59:218–220.
79. Nordin BEC, Crilly DA, Smith DA. Osteoporosis. In: Nordin BEC, ed. Metabolic bone and stone disease. New York: Churchill Livingston, 1984:35.
80. Loftus MJ, Peterson LJ. Delayed healing of mandibular fracture in idiopathic edema. Oral Surg Oral Med Oral Pathol 1979; 47:233–237.
81. Paganiui-Hill A, Ross RK, Gerkins VR, et al. Menopause estrogen therapy and hip fractures. Ann Intern Med 1981; 95:28–31.
82. Jowsey J, Delenbeck LL. The importance of thyroid hormones to bone metabolism and calcium homeostasis. Endocrinology 1969; 85:87–95.
83. Ilacqua JA, Murphy JB. Management of osteomyelitis and nonunion of the mandible in a patient with progressive systemic sclerosis. J Oral Maxillofac Surg 1986; 44:561–563.
84. Teitelbaum SL. Pathological manifestations of osteomalacia and rickets. Clin Endocrinol Metab 1980; 9:43–62.
85. Jha GJ, Deo MG, Ramalingaswami V. Bone growth in protein deficiency. Am J Pathol 1967; 53:1111–1121.
86. Cannell H, Boyd R. The management of maxillofacial injuries in vagrant alcoholics. J Maxillofac Surg 1985; 13:121–124.
87. McDade AM, McNical RD, Ward-Boothe P, et al. The aetiology of maxillofacial injuries with special reference to the abuse of alcohol. Int J Oral Surg 1982; 11:152–155.
88. Actasolo K, Aro H. Irradiation induced hypoxia in bones and soft tissues: an experimental study. Plast Reconstr Surg 1986; 77:257–267.
89. Gren N, French S, Rodriguery G, et al. Radiation induced delayed union of fractures. Radiology 1969; 93:635–641.
90. Shimanovskaya K, Shiman AD. In: Radiation injury of bone. New York: Pergamon Press, 1983:24, 129.
91. Starceski PJ, Blatt J, Finegold D, Brown D. Comparable effects of 1800 and 2400 rad (18- and 24 GY) cranial irradiation on height and weight in children treated for acute lymphocyte leukemia. Am J Dis Child 1987; 141:530–552.

92. Vaughan JN. The effects of radiation on bone. In: Bourne GH, ed. The biochemistry and physiology of bone. Vol IV. New York: Academic Press, 1977:485.
93. Gillies H. The diagnosis and treatment of residual traumatic deformities of the facial skeleton. In: Rowe HL, Killey HC, eds. Fractures of the facial skeleton. 2nd ed. Edinburgh: E & S Livingstone, 1968:523.
94. Davidson TM. Photography in facial plastic and reconstructive surgery. J Biol Photogr Assoc 1979; 47:59–64.
95. Farkas LG, Bryson W, Tech B. Is photogrammetry of the face reliable? Plast Reconstr Surg 1980; 66:346–355.
96. Zarem HA. Standards of photography. Plast Reconstr Surg 1984; 74:137–144.
97. Hakelius L, Poten B. Results of immediate and delayed surgical treatment of facial fractures with diplopia. J Maxillofac Surg 1973; 150–154.
98. Jabaley ME, Lerman N, Sanders HJ. Ocular injuries in orbital fractures: a review of 119 cases. Plast Reconstr Surg 1975; 56:410–417.
99. Zachariades N, Vairaktaris E, Papavassiliou D, et al. The superior orbital tissue syndrome. J Maxillofac Surg 1985; 13:125–128.
100. Marsh J. Blepharocanthal deformities in patients following craniofacial surgery. Plast Reconstr Surg 1978; 61:842–853.
101. Marsh JL, Edgerton MT. Periosteal pennant lateral canthoplasty. Plast Reconstr Surg 1979; 64:24–29.
102. Mohr RM. Diagnostic and therapeutic considerations in trauma involving the orbit. In: Jacobs JR, ed. Maxillofacial trauma: an international perspective. New York: Praeger, 1983:78.
103. Perino KE, Zide MF, Kennebrew MC. Late treatment of malunited malar fractures. J Oral Maxillofac Surg 1984; 42:20–34.
104. Boyne PJ. Osseous repair and mandibular growth after subcondylar fractures. J Oral Surg 1967; 25:300–309.
105. Lyons Club (members of). Fractures involving the mandibular condyle: a post treatment survey of 120 cases. J Oral Surg 1947; 5:45–73.
106. Manson PN, Gruss A, Rosenbaum A, et al. Studies on enophthalmos: II. The measurements of orbital injuries and their treatment by quantitative computed tomography. Plast Reconstr Surg 1986; 77:203–214.
107. Proffit WR, Vig KW, Turvey TA. Early fracture of the mandibular condyles: frequently an unsuspected cause of growth disturbances. Am J Orthod 1980; 78:1–24.
108. Ferraro JW, Gerggren RB. A precise method for determination of displacement in fractures of the midface. Plast Reconstr Surg 1972; 50:447–451.
109. Marsh JL, Vannier MW, Gado M, Stevens WG. In vivo delineation of facial fractures: the applications of advanced medical imaging technology. Ann Plast Surg 1986; 17:364–376.
110. Noyek AM, Kassel EE, Wortzman G, et al. Contemporary radiologic evaluation in maxillofacial trauma. Otolaryngol Clin North Am 1983; 16:473–508.
111. Johnson DH Jr. CT of maxillofacial trauma. Radiol Clin North Am 1984; 22:131–144.
112. Manfredi SJ, Mohammand RR, Sprinkle PM, et al. Computerized tomographic scan findings on facial fractures associated with blindness. Plast Reconstr Surg 1981; 68:479–490.
113. Marsh JL, Vannier MW. The "third" dimension in craniofacial surgery. Plast Reconstr Surg 1983; 71:759–767.
114. Marsh JL, Vannier MW. Surface imaging from computerized tomographic scans. Surgery 1983; 94:159–165.
115. Marsh JL, Vannier MW, Stevens WG, et al. Computerized imaging for soft tissue and osseous reconstruction of the head and neck. Clin Plast Surg 1985; 12:279–291.
116. Marsh JL, Vannier MW, Knapp RH. Computer assisted surface imaging for craniofacial deformities. In: McCoy FJ, ed. The year book of plastic and reconstructive surgery. Chicago: Year Book Publishers, 1986:63.
117. Glenn WV, Johnston RJ, Morton PE, Dwyer SJ. Image generation and display techniques for CT scan data. Thin transverse and reconstructed coronal and sagittal planes. Invest Radiol 1975; 10:403–416.
118. Vannier MW, Marsh JL, Warren JO. Three dimensional CT reconstruction images for craniofacial surgical planning and evaluation. Radiology 1984; 150:179–184.
119. Vannier MW, Conroy GC, Marsh JL, Knapp R. Three dimensional cranial surface reconstruction using high resolution computed tomography. Am J Phys Anthropol 1985; 67:299–311.
120. Dingman RO. Symposium: malunited fractures of the zygoma, repair of the deformity. Trans Am Acad Ophthalmol Otolaryngol 1953; 57:887–896.
121. Larsen OD, Scand Tomsen M. Zygomatic fractures. II. A follow-up study of 137 patients. Scand J Plast Reconstr Surg 1978; 12:59–63.
122. Bertin PM, Clark DP, Tomaro AJ. Latent papilledema: complication of a zygomaticomaxillary complex fracture. J Oral Surg 1981; 39:629–633.
123. Bodner L, Taicher S, Shteyer A. Traumatic bony exostosis in the infratemporal fossa. J Oral Maxillofac Surg 1982; 40:179–180.
124. Butt WD. Blindness following reduction of a malar fracture. Ann Plast Surg 1979; 2:522–524.
125. Ellis E, Attar A, Moos KF. An analysis of 2,067 cases of zygomatico-orbital fracture. J Oral Maxillofac Surg 1985; 43:417–428.
126. Finlay PM, Ward-Booth RP, Moos KF. Morbidity associated with the use of antral packs and external pins in the treatment of the unstable fracture of the zygoma complex. Br J Oral Maxillofac Surg 1984; 22:18–23.
127. Godoy J, Mathog RH. Malar fractures associated

with exophthalmos. Arch Otolaryngol 1985; 111:174–177.
128. Kawamoto HK Jr. Late post traumatic enophthalmos: a correctable deformity? Plast Reconstr Surg 1982; 69:423–432.
129. Kurzer A, Patel MP. Superior orbital fissure syndrome associated with fractures of the zygoma and orbit. Plast Reconstr Surg 1979; 64:715–719.
130. Lederman IR. Loss of vision associated with surgical treatment of zygomatic-orbital floor fracture. Plast Reconstr Surg 1981; 68:94–95.
131. Lund K. Fractures of the zygoma: a follow-up study on 62 patients. J Oral Surg 1971; 29:557–560.
132. Morris TA, Booth RP. Delayed spontaneous retrobulbar hemorrhage. A case report. J Maxillofac Surg 1985; 13:129–130.
133. Nordgaard JO. Persistent sensory disturbances and diplopia following fractures of the zygoma. Arch Otolaryngol 1976; 102:80–82.
134. Ord RH, El Attar A. Acute retrobulbar hemorrhage complicating a malar fracture. J Oral Maxillofac Surg 1982; 40:234–236.
135. Warson RW. Pseudoankylosis of the mandible after a fracture of the zygomaticomaxillary. A report of case. J Oral Surg 1971; 29:223–224.
136. Wood GD. Blindness following fracture of the zygomatic bone. Br J Oral Maxillofac Surg 1986; 24:12–16.
137. Knight JS, North JF. The classification of malar fractures: an analysis of displacement as a guide to treatment. Br J Plast Surg 1961; 13:325–339.
138. Kristensen S, Tverteras K. Zygomatic fractures: classification and complications. Clin Otolaryngol 1986; 11:123–129.
139. Kruger E, Schilli W, Worthington P. Midface fractures involving the orbit and blow-out fractures. In: Luhr HG, ed. Oral and maxillofacial traumatology. Vol 2. Chicago: Quintessence Publishing Co, 1986:197.
140. Rich JD, Zbylski Jr, La Rossa DD, Cullington JR. A simple method for rapid assessment of malar depression. Ann Plast Surg 1979; 3:151–152.
141. Dingman RO, Natvig P. Surgery of the facial skeleton. Philadelphia: WB Saunders, 1964:1.
142. Becker HL, Homburg-Scar FR. Treatment of initially infected mandibular fractures with bone plates. J Oral Surg 1979; 37:310–313.
143. Rowe NL. Complications arising in the treatment of fractures of the middle-third to the facial skeleton. In: Rowe NL, Killey HC, eds. Fractures of the facial skeleton. 2nd ed. Edinburgh: E & S Livingstone, 1968:451.
144. Pospisil OA, Fernando TD. Review of the lower blepharoplasty incision as a surgical approach to zygomatic-orbital fractures. Br J Oral Maxillofac Surg 1984; 22:261–268.
145. Gerlock AJ, Sinn DP. Anatomic, clinical, surgical, and radiographic correlation of the zygomatic complex fracture. Am J Roentgenol 1977; 128: 235–238.
146. Manson PN, Clifford CM, Su CT, et al. Mechanisms of global support and post traumatic enophthalmos. I. The anatomy of the ligament sling and its relation to intramuscular cone orbital fat. Plast Reconstr Surg 1986; 77:193–202.
147. Rabuzzi DD. Revision surgery of malaligned midfacial fractures. Otolaryngol Clin North Am 1974; 7:107–117.
148. Dingman RO. The use of iliac bone in the repair of facial and cranial defects. J Plast Reconstr Surg 1950; 6:179–195.
149. Tessier P. Autogenous bone grafts taken from the calvarium for facial and cranial applications. Clin Plast Surg 1982; 9:531–568.
150. Holtman BB, Wray RC, Little AG. A randomised comparison of four incisions for orbital fractures. Plast Reconstr Surg 1981; 67:731–734.
151. Rinehart G, Marsh JL. Presented at the annual Meeting of the American Society for Plastic and Reconstructive Surgeons. Atlanta, GA, November 1987.
152. Manson PN, Solomon G. Compression plates in mid-face fractures. Presented at Northeastern Society of Plastic Surgeons Meeting, Baltimore, MD, September 26, 1986.
153. Spear SL, Wiegering CE. Temporal fossa bone grafts: a new technique in craniofacial surgery. Plast Reconstr Surg 1987; 79:531–534.
154. Tessier P. Anesthetic aspects of bone grafting to the face. Clin Plast Surg 1981; 8:279–301.
155. Wolfe SA, Kawamoto HK. Taking the iliac bone graft. Am J Bone Joint Surg 1978; 60:411.
156. Block MS, Zide MF, Kent JN. Proplast augmentation for post traumatic zygomatic deficiency. Oral Surg Oral Med Oral Pathol 1984; 57:123–131.
157. Kent JN, Westfall RL, Carlton DM. Chin and zygomatico-maxillary augmentation with proplast: long-term follow-up. J Oral Surg 1981; 39:912–919.
158. Schultz RC. Facial reconstruction with alloplastic material. Surg Annu 1980; 12:351–388.
159. Jobe R, Iverson R, Vistnes L. Bone deformation beneath alloplastic implants. Plast Reconstr Surg 1973; 51:169–175.
160. Lilla JA, Vestries LM, Jobe RP. The long-term effects of hard alloplastic implants when put on bone. Plast Reconstr Surg 1976; 58:14–18.
161. Wolfe SA. Correction of a persistent lower eyelid deformity caused by a displaced orbital floor implant. Ann Plast Surg 1979; 2:448–451.
162. Wolfe SA. Correction of a lower eyelid deformity caused by multiple extrusions of alloplastic orbital floor implants. Plast Reconstr Surg 1981; 68:429–432.
163. Gatot A, Tovi F, Moshiashvili A. Periorbital cellulitis: presenting feature of undiagnosed old maxillary fracture. Int J Pediatr Otorhinolaryngol 1986; 11:129–134.
164. Reynolds JR. Late complications versus method of treatment in a large series of mid-facial fractures. Plast Reconstr Surg 1978; 61:871–875.
165. Steidler NE, Cook RM, Reade PC. Residual (complications) in patients with major middle third facial fractures. Int J Oral Surg 1980; 9:259–266.

region; other investigations even reported that biting forces of up to 1,000 Newton are possible. It was also clearly shown by Champy and Lodde[24] that physiologically coordinated muscle functions produce tension forces at the upper border of the mandible and compressive forces at the lower border. In the case of a fracture these forces cause distraction and displacement of the fragments of the mandible.

In the maxilla and the midface, there are practically no muscle insertions to be considered, and the chewing function produces lesser forces. On the other hand, the bones of the maxilla are much thinner compared with the mandible. On the average, the outer cortex of the lower jaw is 3 to 5 mm thick, is reinforced laterally by the oblique line, and is thicker in the chin region. In general, therefore, the bone of the mandible is strong enough to allow a stable screw fixation at practically all places. The maxilla, on the other hand, is very thin, with the facial wall of the maxillary sinus being an average of only 0.85 mm thick. This is too thin a wall for stabilization by even the smallest bone screw.

Investigations carried out by Ewers[25] demonstrated that a bone thickness of 2 mm is sufficient to anchor bone screws, and that the periorbital bone structures are between 3 and 6 mm thick, which are strong enough for bone plating. In the maxilla, however, there are only two areas where bone plates can be securely applied: the paranasal bone struts and the alveolar zygomatic crest. Investigations carried out by Paulus[26] at the Swiss Institute of Bone Research clearly showed that bony union occurs much faster in the maxilla with miniplates than with wire osteosynthesis. The cranial bone, however, is always thick enough to support bone screws, and there are obviously no tension or torsion forces to be considered.

The biophysical requirements of the osteosynthetic material can be clearly stated: it must be totally inert and well tolerated by the human organism; it must be miniaturized and still strong enough to withstand bending and torsion forces up to 1,000 Newton; it must have elasticity high enough to allow a close coaptation to the bony surface without deformation or fracture; and it should be manufactured at a reasonable price.

Most developers of miniplate systems chose an alloy of chrome, nickel, and molybdenum or vitallium because this material was already being used successfully by orthopedic surgeons. Recently, systems manufactured of titanium—which has the important advantage of the highest biologic tolerance—have also been available.[27,28] The other alloys are also well tolerated; since they result in a light metallosis of the adjacent tissues and since an allergy to nickel may develop, the removal of these osteosynthesis materials is recommended. However, there is general agreement that titanium can be left in place because it is well tolerated.

The configuration of the bone plates is also different in the various systems. The systems of Champy (Strasbourg system) and of Heinl (Wurzburg system) provide a design that is narrower in the region of the screw holes (Fig. 15–1). The other systems have rectangular oblong plates that vary in length and shape (Fig. 15–2). However, the thickness of the miniplates differs only slightly, generally measuring 0.9 to 1.1 mm. The width is generally 6 to 8 mm, and the length ranges from 2 to 10 cm. Only the Luhr and the Swiss AO set have oblique gliding holes for dynamic compression (Fig. 15–3); all other miniplate systems have abandoned the compression principle. In all systems, the miniscrews are manufactured of the same metal material as the plates to avoid any oxidation or corrosion. The screws are mostly self-tapping and their length ranges from 3 to 15 mm. Usually, the screw thread has a diameter of 2 mm with a thread core of 1.6 mm, and each turn of the screw leads to 1 mm penetration into the bone. The Steinhauser system has, in addition, "emergency screws" which are 2.2 mm in diameter. These are recommended for use when the regular screw has not got a sufficient grip any more and is loose; then the larger screw can again get a good grip. While the screw heads of most systems have a single slot or cross slots, the Steinhauser set has a hexagonal shape that permits a more secure fit on the screwdriver (Fig. 15–4). Usually, each system has one set of compatible plates and screws, whereas the Steinhauser titanium set contains plates of two differ-

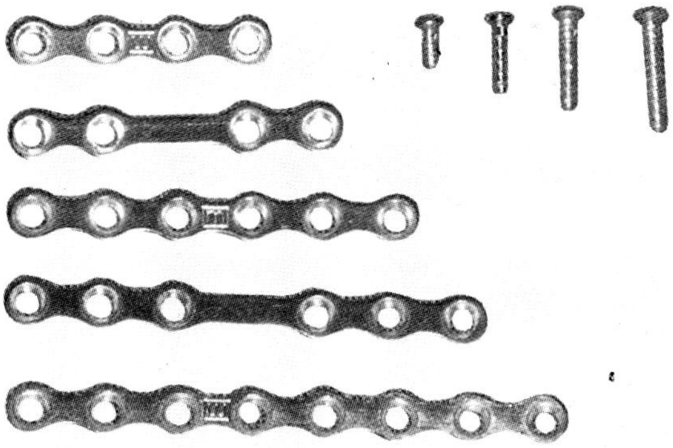

Figure 15–1 The Strasbourg miniplate set; plates and screws are manufactured of an alloy of chrome, nickel, and molybdenum.

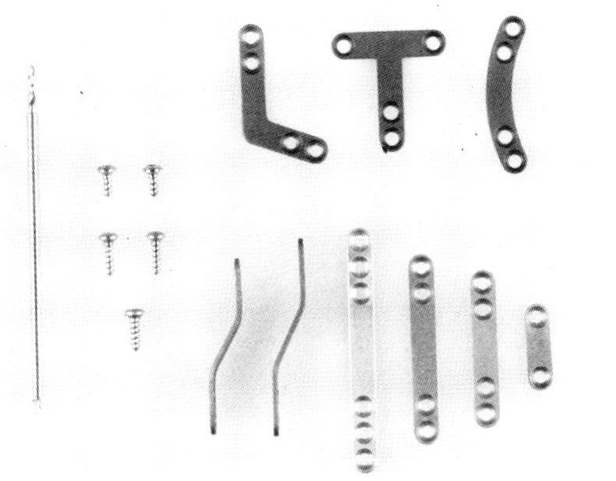

Figure 15–2 The Steinhauser miniplate set manufactured of technically pure titanium with two different degrees of hardness: a softer one for maxilla and a harder one for mandible. The screws are 2.0 mm and 2.2 mm in diameter, respectively.

ent hardnesses. The mandibular plates are harder (Vickers hardness [VH] 250) and their tensile strength is higher to withstand the higher load of the mandible. On the other hand, the plates which are employed on the maxilla and midface should bend more readily for better adaptation to the irregular bony surface of this region and are softer (150 VH) (Fig. 15–5). Since the plates of the two hardnesses are different colors, the plates can be easily distinguished. The self-tapping screws with the hexagonal heads are the same hardness for both types of plates (about 250 VH).

TECHNIQUE OF MINIPLATE OSTEOSYNTHESIS

In general, the miniplate osteosynthesis is an easy procedure and only a few basic principles have to

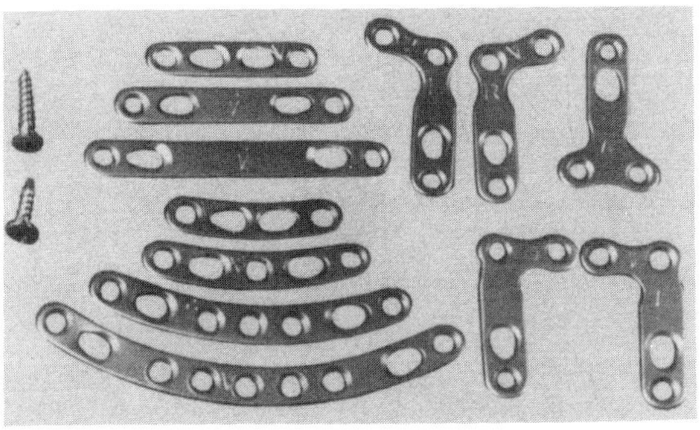

Figure 15–3 The Luhr miniplate system with eccentric gliding holes for compression osteosynthesis.

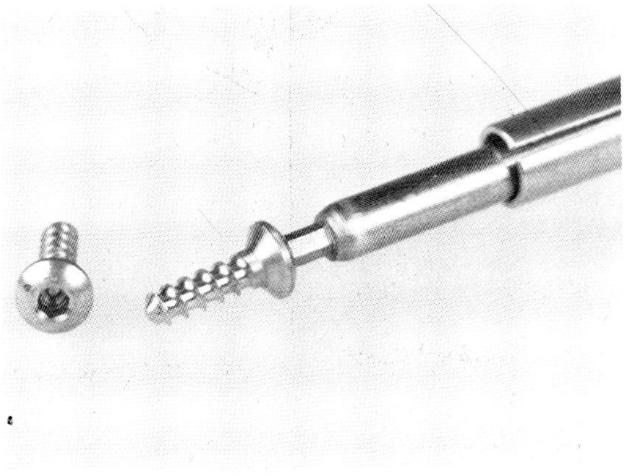

Figure 15–4 The Steinhauser titanium screws have a hexagonal head to permit a secure fit on the screwdriver.

be considered. Very few instruments are necessary for the application of these miniplates (Fig. 15–6). Naturally, a proper reduction of the fragments is the first step in the treatment. The occlusion then has to be established precisely and the jaw secured by intermaxillary fixation. It would be a big mistake to apply the plate prior to this intermaxillary fixation for there is great likelihood of malocclusion. Even in edentulous cases, we prefer to estab-

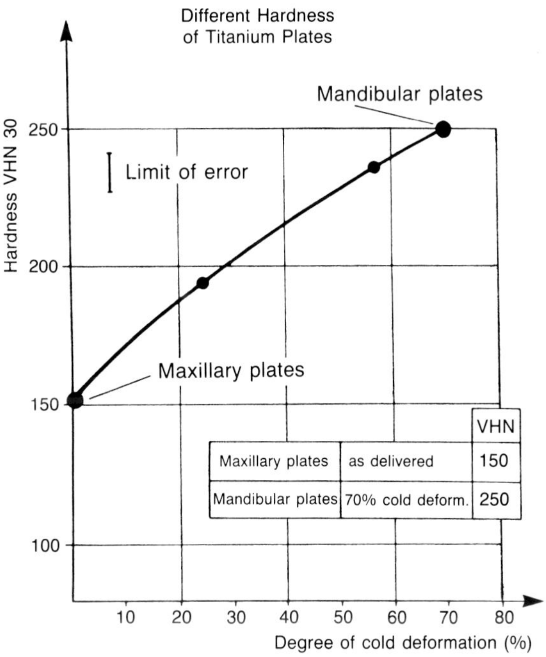

Figure 15–5 The table shows the differently hard plates for maxilla and mandible of the Steinhauser titanium miniplate set.

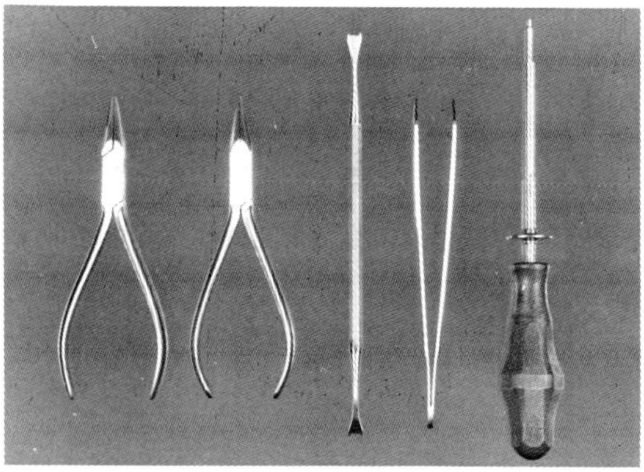

Figure 15–6 Instruments for miniplate application: two modeling pliers, plate-holding fork, plate-holding forceps, screwdriver.

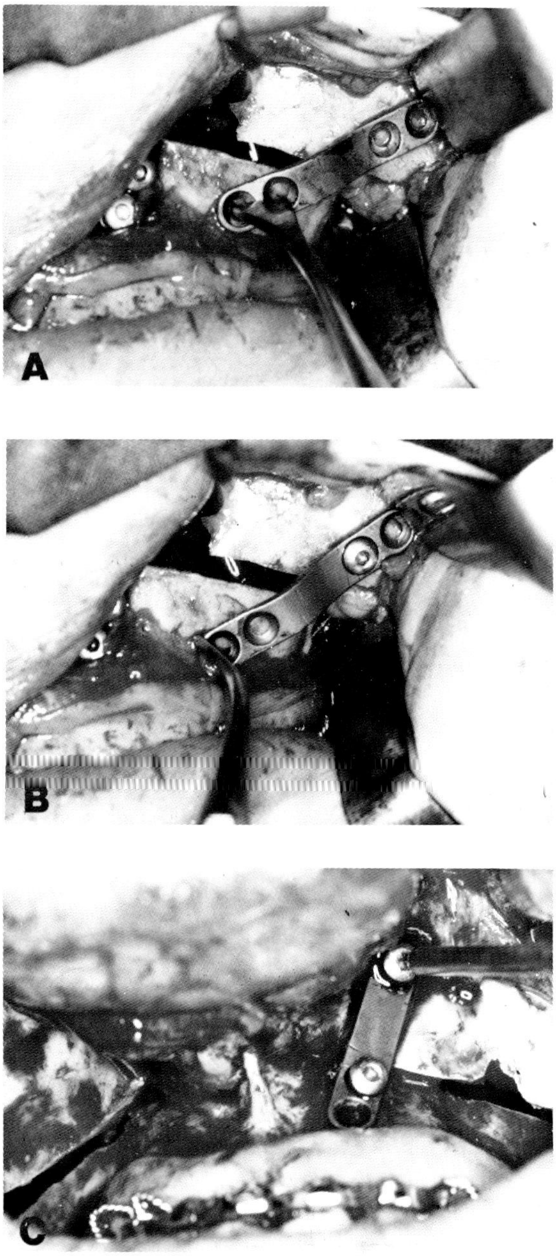

Figure 15–7 Procedure of Steinhauser miniplate application in the maxilla. *A*, The holding fork secures the position of the plate. *B*, One screw is already placed, now the second hole will be drilled. *C*, The second screw is tightened and the remaining holes can be drilled and screws placed.

lish a proper occlusion with the aid of the patient's denture or with splints made in the laboratory.

With the use of two modeling pliers or levers, the selected plate is bent and adapted to the bone surface. This procedure may be time consuming, particularly in areas where the bone surface is not even, as for example with osteotomies for repositioning of the maxilla or mandible. In these instances, we recommend preformed plates.[29] Another possibility is to use a malleable template to determine the exact plate configuration.[23] Care should be taken that the drill holes are at least 5 mm away from the fracture line to prevent splintering of the bone. In comminuted fractures, longer plates should be used with six or more screws.

Although it does not make a difference which hole is drilled first, it is important that the plate be held securely in place with the holding forceps or the holding fork. Then one drill hole is made with the drill held in a perfectly perpendicular direction to the surface of the bone. Also the hole should be drilled at a slow speed and with generous irrigation during the whole drilling process to prevent thermal damage to the osteocytes. Then, the screw, with the appropriately selected length (mostly 6 or 8 mm), is securely placed in a precisely perpendicular fashion. The screw should be tightened with moderate force, because *excessive tightening produces microfractures* within the drilled hole in the bone. Another hole is drilled on the opposite side of the fracture (or osteotomy line) and the second screw is placed. Finally, the remaining holes are drilled and screwed (Fig. 15–7).

Every plate should be fixed with at least two screws for each fragment. If a screw fails to gain a secure grip because it is too close to the fracture line or because the bone wall is too thin, the position of the plate must be changed to get a new purchase of bone. In this situation an "emergency screw" with a 2.2 mm diameter (Steinhauser) can also be used. When all the plates have been placed, the intermaxillary fixation is released and the occlusion is checked for proper fit. If the bite is not perfect, the plates must be removed again, the bone fragments repositioned, and the plates precisely rebent and resecured. If some of the old drill holes are to be reused, then the wider 2.2 mm screws should be inserted (or the 2- to 4-mm screws when vitallium plates are employed). One principle of miniplate fixation that must be especially emphasized is the correct fitting of the miniplates across the fracture site or osteotomy site. If the fit is not perfect, the tightening of the screw will displace the fragment and lead to occlusal disturbances or other undesired skeletal shifts. Therefore, particular attention must be paid to secure a perfect surface adaptation of the plates.

FRACTURES OF THE MANDIBLE

Historically, when fractures began to be stabilized with plates, the mandible became a favorite site for this technique. The reason for this was that the mandible was easily accessible through an intraoral, as well as an extraoral approach, and because its cortex was particularly strong. Furthermore, the shape of the outer surface of the mandible is not too sharply bent and permits a proper adaptation of the plates. However, there are some anatomic limitations to plate fixation as a result of the deep location of the roots of the teeth which come rather far down, particularly in the region of the canine teeth, as well as the mandibular canal which runs underneath the apices of the molar teeth to the mental foramen. Thus, osteosynthesis carries a certain risk of tooth root or nerve injury if proper attention is not given to these structures.

According to the investigations of Champy and Lodde,[13] bending moment forces were found throughout the body of the mandible which increase as one proceeds from the front of the mandible back to the angle. These forces go up to 600 Newton and correspond to the masticating forces. In addition, torsion forces were found anterior to the canine teeth which rise to a maximum of 1,000 Newton in the region of the symphysis. Therefore, these authors concluded that the ideal line for osteosynthesis in the mandible is just underneath the apices of the teeth, which is lower in the front and higher in the molar and retromolar region. In the case of the mandible, the plating should be performed along the broad surface of the external oblique line in the region of the angle; and further forward, it should be located immediately below the dental roots and above the mandibular foramina. In addition to this subapical plate, a second plate would be necessary along the lower border of the front of the mandible to prevent the exertion of the torsion forces in this region.

Although we acknowledge the investigations and the findings of Champy and Lodde,[13] we do not insist on carrying out these steps quite precisely. Our experience with miniplating of more than 300 mandibular fractures within the last 5 years has clearly shown that the fractures heal well, even when the plates are not applied along the absolutely ideal "osteosynthesis line" (Fig. 15–8). We have found that in the treatment of fractures of the angle of the mandible, plating the upper border alongside the external oblique line is an excellent method. This operation can be performed easily through the intraoral approach and the application of the plate is simple and fast. Also, the intraoral approach is preferable for fractures of the horizontal ramus and the chin (Fig. 15–9). However, we would not hesitate to add a plate through the extraoral approach, if an open wound is present.

Fractures of the ascending ramus of the mandible present more difficult problems. Plating is possible in the lower and middle part of the ramus (Fig. 15–10), but this requires a combined intraoral and extraoral approach. The fracture is exposed and repositioned from the intraoral approach, and the plate is secured from there. Then the drill, the screws, and the screwdriver are introduced transbuccally and the plate is fastened with direct visual control of the reduction of the fragments. However, we do not recommend plating condylar neck fractures because the exposure through the intraoral approach is very difficult. Coming from the extraoral approach, the small proximal fragment needs

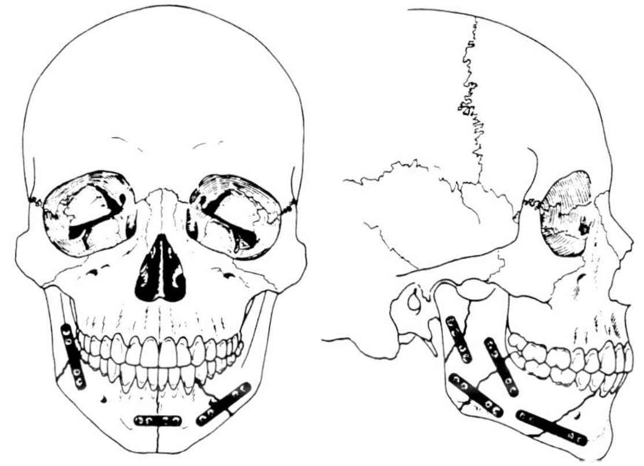

Figure 15–8 Areas of miniplate application in the mandible.

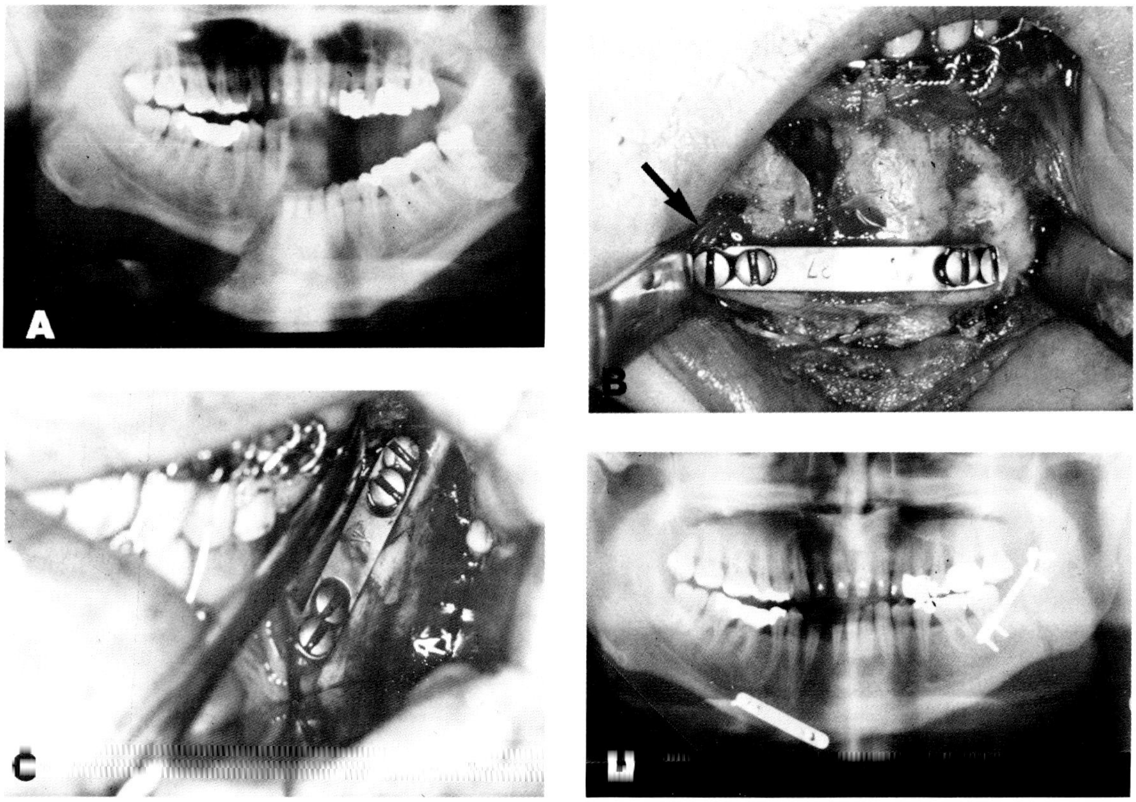

Figure 15–9 Miniplate fixation in a bilateral mandibular fracture. *A*, Severe displacement of the paramedian fracture, and moderate displacement of the angular fracture. *B*, The paramedian fracture is stabilized with a plate (Luhr) underneath the mental foramen (arrow). *C*, A plate (Luhr) is placed alongside the external oblique line. *D*, Postoperative situation after fracture reduction and miniplate fixation. For positioning the plate in the mandibular angle the screws are placed more obliquely to avoid damage to the roots of the molar teeth.

to be denuded of its periosteum which can easily lead to a resorption of the condyle. We think that condylar fractures are best managed by conservative treatment with 1 to 2 weeks of intermaxillary fixation followed by functional exercises.

When there are two or more fractures of the mandible, it is especially important to first obtain proper dental occlusion by intermaxillary fixation. The osteosynthesis is performed in the tooth-bearing portion of the jaw and then the posterior region. For example, in a paramedian and an angular fracture, the paramedian fracture would be plated first. In this way, occlusal disturbances can be avoided.

FRACTURES OF MAXILLA AND MIDFACE

In contrast to the application of bone plates for the mandible, it took quite a while before plates were used for the maxilla and midface. The first reports were exclusively for trauma cases.[10–12,14–16,30] Several years later miniplate osteosynthesis was advocated also for stabilization of midfacial osteotomies.[17,18,21]

The reason that plate fixation of the maxilla and midface was not considered a good method of treatment for quite a long time was the concern over the stability of the screws in these rather thin bones. However, investigations carried out by Ewers[25] showed that the bones of the orbital margin, the region of the zygomatic buttress, and the edge of the piriform aperture are thicker than 2 mm and, therefore, strong enough to support the firm grip of the screws. Also, the alveolar-zygomatic crest usually permits the application of plates (Fig. 15–11), and only the bone of the anterior or lateral wall of the maxillary sinus is too thin for rigid fixation.

The application of plates is much more favorable for Le Fort I osteotomies than for fractures because there are usually no scattered bony fragments

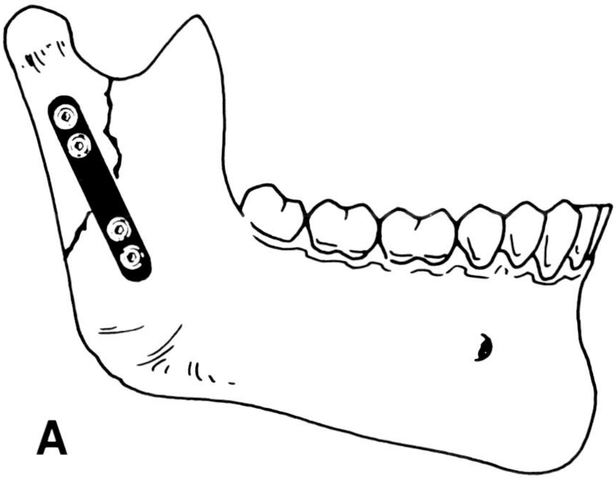

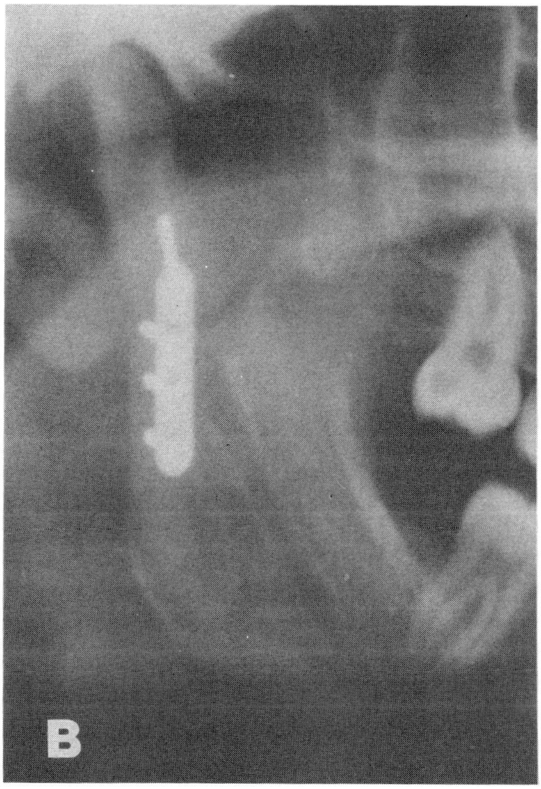

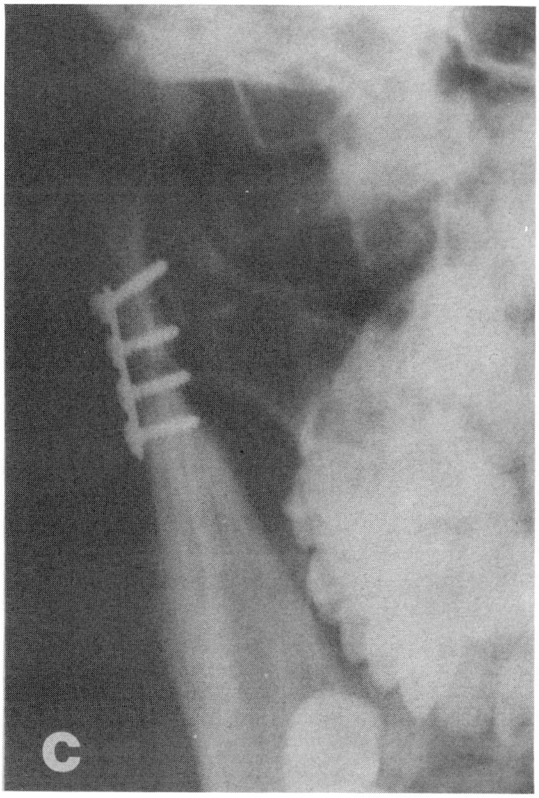

Figure 15–10 Plating of a deep condylar fracture. *A*, Schematic representation of plate position. *B*, Lateral radiographic view of the miniplate position. *C*, The same case in a posteroanterior radiographic view.

to prevent a stable positioning of the plate (Fig. 15–12). If the bone of the alveolar zygomatic crest or the margin of the piriform aperture is broken into several small pieces, suspension wiring should be performed. In sagittal fractures of the maxilla, the medial fracture line can be bridged with a miniplate on the lower margin of the piriform aperture; in addition, a plate can be placed on the alveolar-zygomatic crest, as is done in a typical Le Fort I fracture.

The miniplates can be securely positioned (we try placing four plates) (Fig. 15–13). The intermaxillary fixation that was established prior to the application of the plates should then be removed. If the intermaxillary fixation is left in place, the screws anchored in these rather thin bones would become loosened by the muscular forces from the lower jaw.[31] If, however, there is a comminuted fracture of the maxilla without sufficient stable fragments of bone, frontozygomatic suspension wiring should be performed and the intermaxillary fixation should be left for 3 weeks.

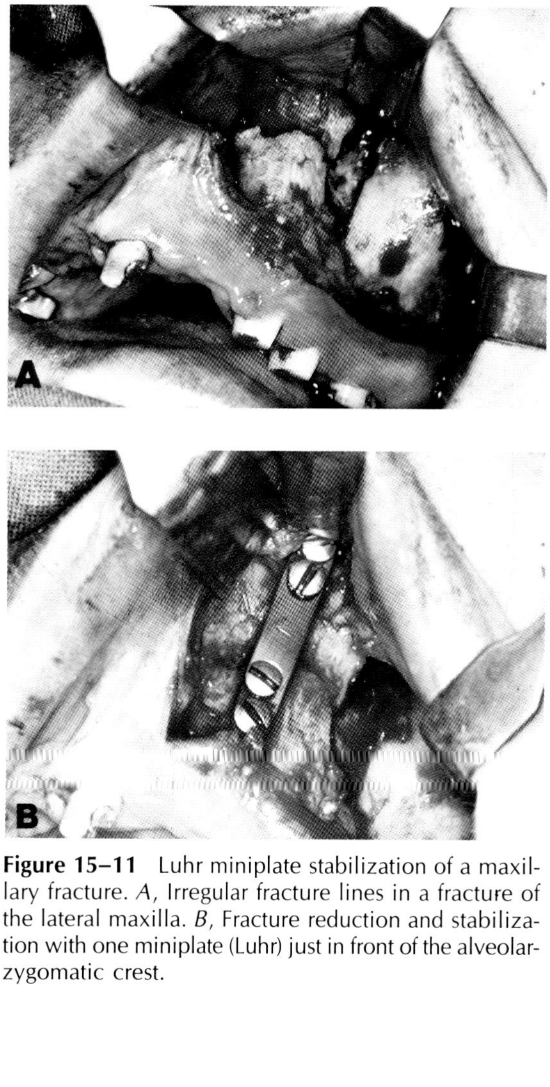

Figure 15–11 Luhr miniplate stabilization of a maxillary fracture. *A*, Irregular fracture lines in a fracture of the lateral maxilla. *B*, Fracture reduction and stabilization with one miniplate (Luhr) just in front of the alveolar-zygomatic crest.

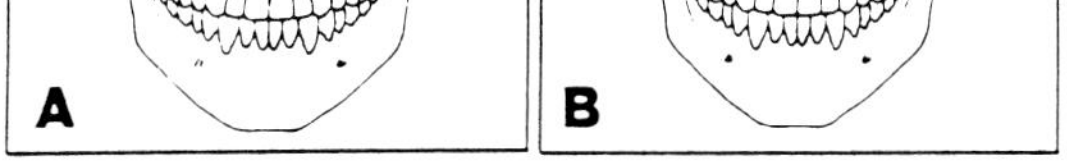

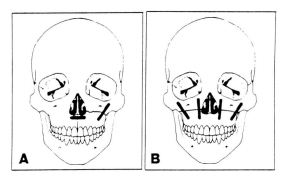

Figure 15–12 Suitable places for bone plate fixation in the maxilla. *A*, Sagittal fracture (unilateral Le Fort I). *B*, Le Fort I fracture or osteotomy. The plates are applied to the zygomatic buttresses and the edges of the piriform apertures of the nasal cavity where the bones are the thickest.

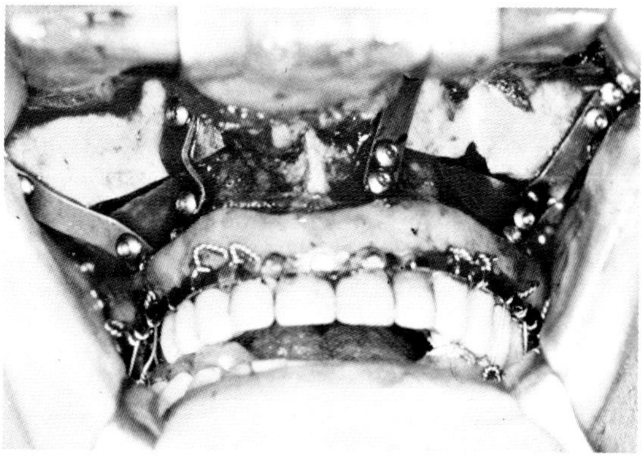

Figure 15–13 Miniplate fixation of a Le Fort I type osteotomy; four miniplates (Steinhauser) secure the advanced maxilla.

Fractures of the classic Le Fort II pattern are relatively rare. They can be stabilized with two plates on the lower orbital margin as recommended by Schilli and Niederdellmann.[32] Nevertheless, we prefer to employ four plates because this provides far more stability. In these Le Fort II osteotomies, miniplates can be securely applied on the body of the zygoma and on the upper margin of the piriform aperture (Fig. 15–14). In addition, the frontonasal junction may be utilized for additional stability which might be necessary when a Le Fort II advancement procedure is also carried out.[29] This can be done either with one miniplate or with wires suspended from the glabella to permit a certain degree of forward traction of the osteotomized midfacial bony structures (Fig. 15–15).

In the Le Fort III fracture, with the whole midfacial structure separated from the base of the skull, miniplating is an ideal method of treatment. The plates can be securely fastened on the frontozygomatic buttresses, as well as the frontobasal junction (Fig. 15–16). In these areas, the bone is also thick enough to permit the use of the longer screws of 8 mm or more. Naturally, this method of miniplate fixation can also be applied in Le Fort III osteotomies. In these instances, we prefer to use a T-shaped plate in the center, which is easy to place, if the coronal incision is used to give an excellent exposure.

COMMINUTED FRACTURES

As is well known, midfacial fractures do not always follow the classic Le Fort fracture lines. This depends on the severity and the direction of the force

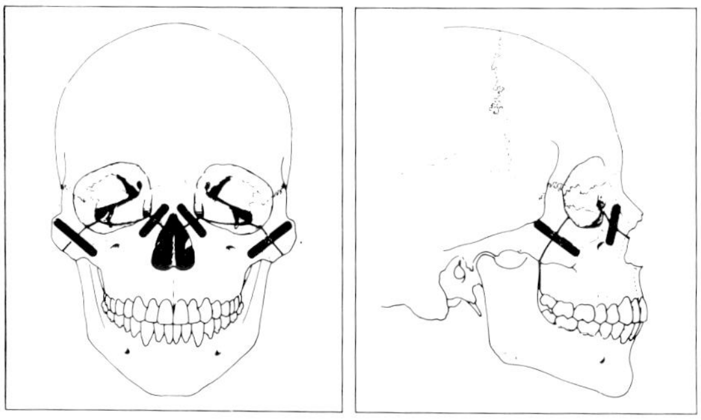

Figure 15–14 Miniplate application in a Le Fort II type osteotomy on the body of the zygoma and on the nasal bones.

that hits the facial bone structures. Therefore, the types of fractures can vary considerably, and the treatment of each can be very different. As an example, there can be a classic Le Fort fracture line on one side of the face, whereas on the other side, the bony walls and pillars may be broken into many comminuted pieces. This means that quite often miniplate osteosynthesis must be combined with other treatments, such as direct wire osteosynthesis or craniofacial suspension (Fig. 15–17). This can also be the case when a combination of a Le Fort III and Le Fort I fracture has occurred. The upper bony pillars are strong enough to support miniplates, but in the maxilla no bone is available that is sufficient for plating. In this instance, a combination of bone plating and craniofacial suspension is also indicated (Fig. 15–18). In all these instances, where additional suspension wires are used, intermaxillary fixation should be left in place for up to 3 weeks. However, there is still an advantage to the use of miniplate fixation because the intermaxillary fixation and suspensory wires can be removed earlier than the 4 to 6 weeks necessary with other treatment methods.

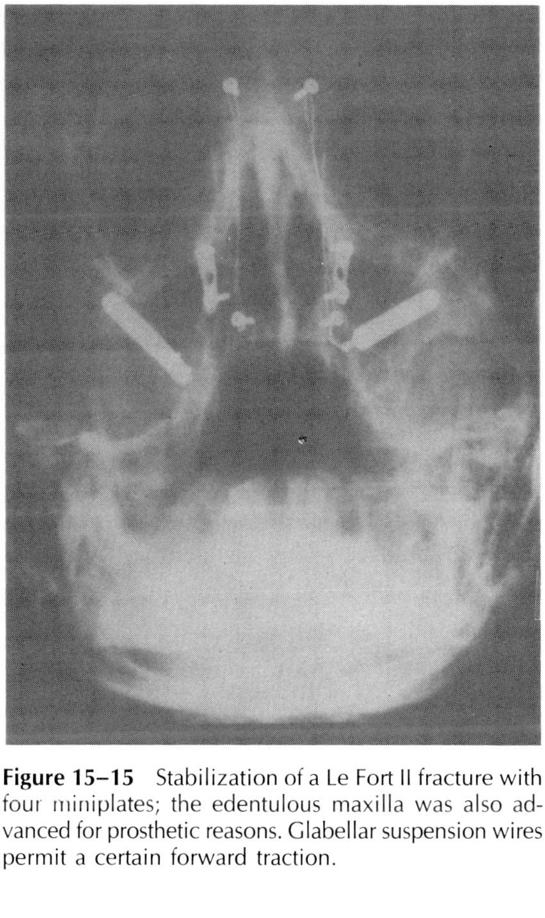

Figure 15–15 Stabilization of a Le Fort II fracture with four miniplates; the edentulous maxilla was also advanced for prosthetic reasons. Glabellar suspension wires permit a certain forward traction.

FRACTURES OF THE ZYGOMATIC COMPLEX

As was stated by several authors,[14,16,31] miniplate osteosynthesis is the method of choice for zygo-

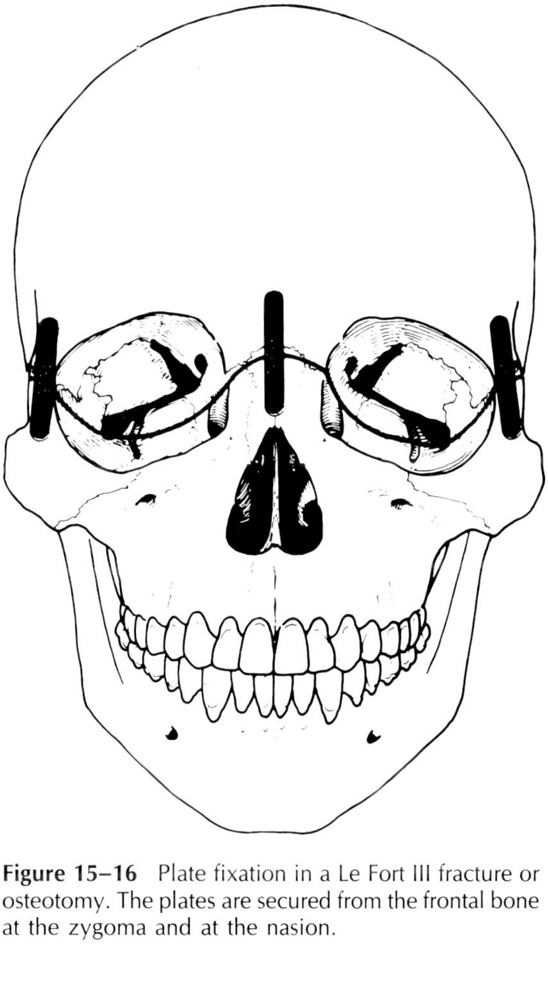

Figure 15–16 Plate fixation in a Le Fort III fracture or osteotomy. The plates are secured from the frontal bone at the zygoma and at the nasion.

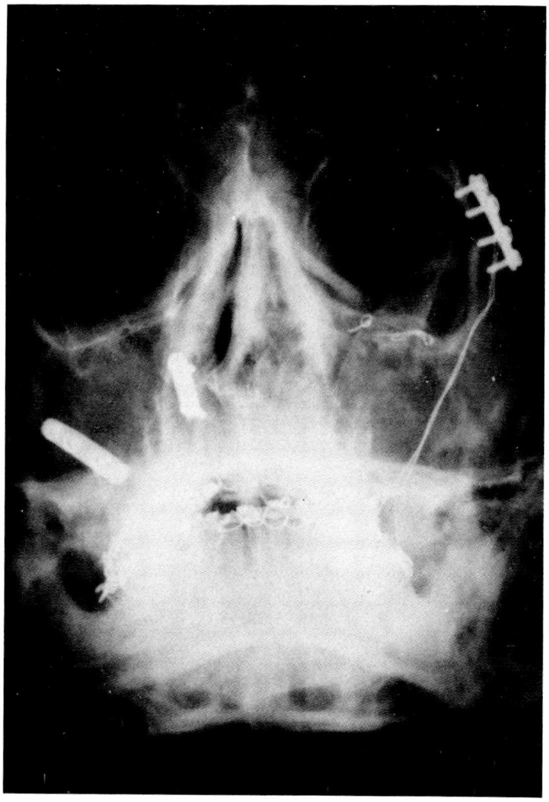

Figure 15–17 Combination of bone plates and suspension wires in a Le Fort I fracture, plus zygomatic fracture. It was possible to stabilize only the zygoma and one side of the maxilla with plates. The remainder was stabilized by wires.

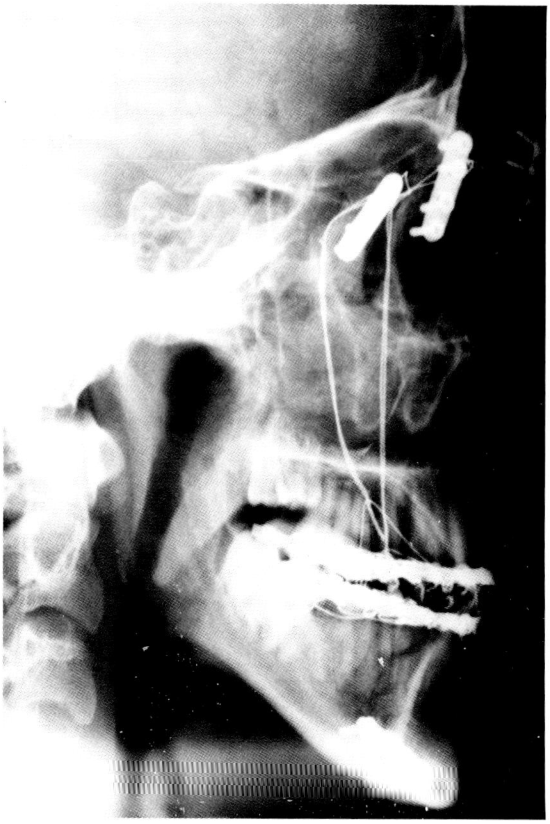

Figure 15–18 Combined Le Fort III and Le Fort I fracture. Only the strong upper bony pillars allow plate application, whereas the Le Fort I fracture is fixed with suspension wires.

matic fractures. We completely agree with this statement because the fixation on the frontal bone buttress and the strong frontal process of the cheekbone is absolutely reliable and has a high loading capacity. A miniplate anchored with four screws at the frontozygomatic suture region guarantees three-dimensional stability (Fig. 15–19). Thus, there is no possible backward or downward rotation of the cheekbone, which is very important for aesthetic reasons. Also, since a denuding of the inner aspect of the orbit is not necessary for plating, the troublesome wire-cathing of soft tissues is avoided, which makes the operation faster and less traumatic.

Quite often the orbital floor is involved in zygomatic fractures. If this is the case, a revision is always indicated. Normally, the bony orbital rim is identified from an infraorbital incision. From there, the orbital floor can be easily inspected. If there is a defect in the orbit floor, we prefer reconstruction with lyophilized dura[33] or with autogenous bone grafts in larger defects. When there is still a step-off or a discrepancy of the infraorbital rim, we may place a thin wire osteosynthesis there (Fig. 15–20). For this procedure, the supraorbital plate must be loosened again, otherwise a proper repositioning in the infraorbital region may not be possible.

The infraorbital rim can also break into several pieces, which makes an exact repositioning practically impossible. Such comminuted fractures may also cause defects in the continuity of the infraorbital margin. In these instances, a second miniplate which is placed just alongside the rim is recommended (Fig. 15–21). For fixation of the plate, 6-mm screws are preferable. Since the covering skin is relatively thin in this region, removal of this plate is recommended even when titanium plates were used.

In severe displacement of the zygoma, an intraoral inspection and reduction might be necessary. Similar to a Le Fort I fracture, the relatively

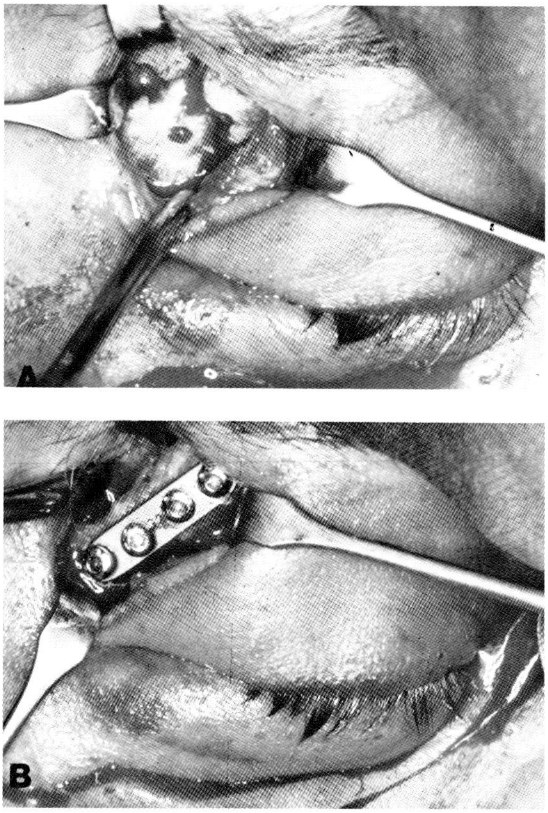

Figure 15–19 Stabilization of a zygomatic fracture with Steinhauser miniplates. *A*, The dislocation of the fronto-zygomatic junction is clearly visible. *B*, The bony plate guarantees stability of the zygomatic bone.

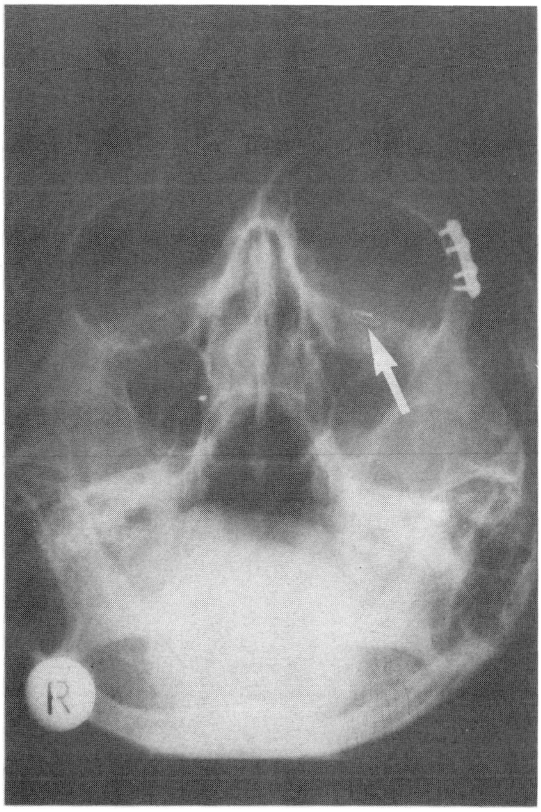

Figure 15–20 Combination of bone plating of the supraorbital fracture line, and wire osteosynthesis of the infraorbital (arrow) fracture line following reduction of the cheekbone and inspection of the orbital floor.

thick pillar of the alveolar-zygomatic crest can serve as the support for a miniplate (Fig. 15–22). It is our experience that it does not matter if the screw ends penetrate into the maxillary sinus. In more than 100 cases of Le Fort I osteotomies stabilized with miniplates, no infection of the maxillary sinus has been observed.

It is also possible to put a miniplate on the fractured zygomatic arch. However, we have found this unnecessary because the repositioning with a sharp hook or an elevation from an incision in the hairline of the temple (Gillies approach) is usually sufficient. However, in Le Fort III osteotomies, the gap in the zygomatic arch following a forward advancement of this segment can be bridged by straight miniplates, which can also provide a rigid fixation of the bone grafts.[23]

We reviewed about 300 cases in which miniplates were applied for stabilization of osteotomized facial bones; the infection rate in these patients was published by Paulus and Hardt[34] and it was found that infections occurred only a few times in trauma cases. In osteotomies, the infection is practically negligible; we had a maxillary sinusitis only once.

FRACTURES OF THE CRANIUM

Fractures of the cranium can ideally be fixed with miniplates. Since there are no regular fracture levels as in the midface, the traumatic force can cause many different fracture lines (Fig. 15–23). The supraorbital margin can be stabilized by one or more miniplates without major problems (Fig. 15–24). Also, fractures in the different regions of the cranial bone, which are mostly reduced from a coronal incision, can be plated without difficulties. Naturally, bone trepanation and the repair of dural defects may be required first. Then the fragments of the cranium which consist of rather thick bone can be stabilized with multiple miniplates, if this is required.

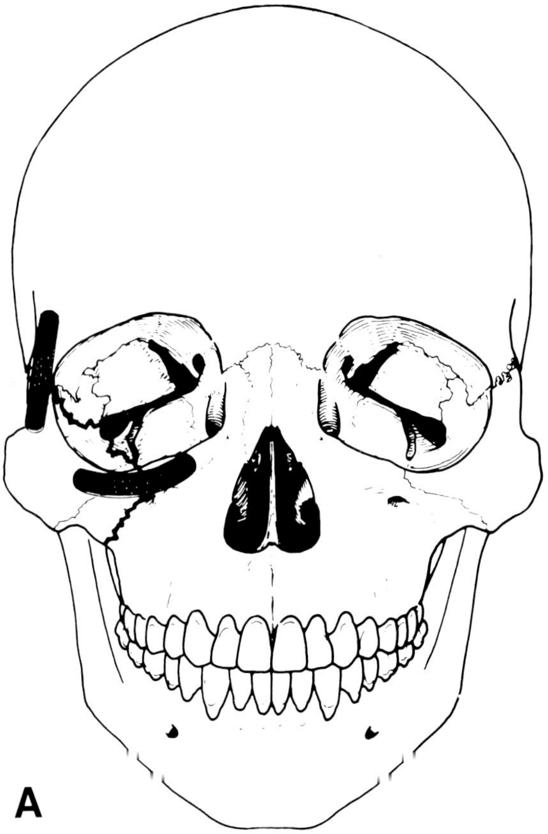

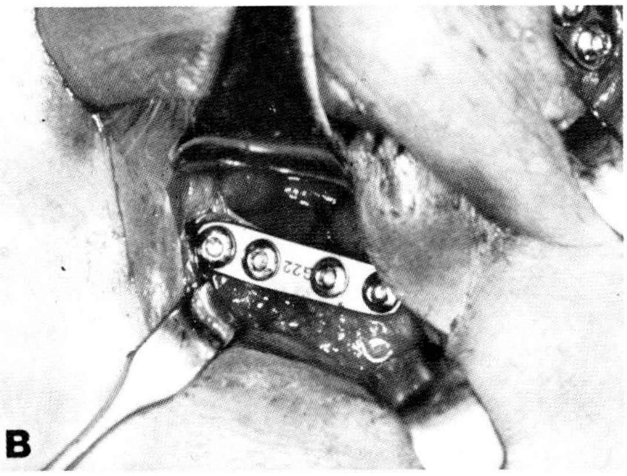

Figure 15–21 Fracture of the zygomatic bone with a bony deficit along the infraorbital rim. *A*, Schematic representation of the position of the Steinhauser plates. *B*, A miniplate bridges the deficit of the infraorbital rim.

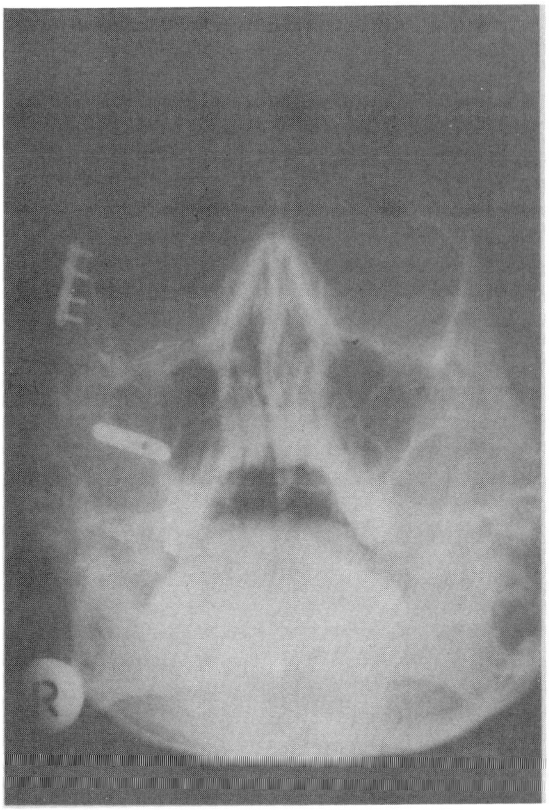

Figure 15–22 In addition to the supraorbital plate, an intraorally inserted miniplate stabilizes the severely dislocated zygomatic alveolar crest.

A whole selection of curved or straight miniplates of various lengths is available for application at almost every part of the cranial bone (Fig. 15–25).

In craniofacial osteotomies for correction of skull deformities, which are mostly carried out in infants, it is essential to select shorter screws (Luhr, 3 mm); this allows application to bones as thin as an infant's skull. Thus, protrusion of the screw intracranially can be avoided.[23]

COMPLICATIONS

Complications following miniplate osteosynthesis occur rather infrequently. However, there are a few principles that must be observed during plate application, otherwise the results can be unfavorably influenced.

Disturbances of the occlusion can lead to disorders of masticatory function and even lead to severe pain in the temporomandibular joint region. The main reason for this annoying complication is an improper occlusal fixation of the fragments during plate application. If the occlusion cannot be re-established properly by manual repositioning, or if preoperative deformities of the jaws do not allow setting into a normal occlusion, cast models should be taken prior to reduction. These

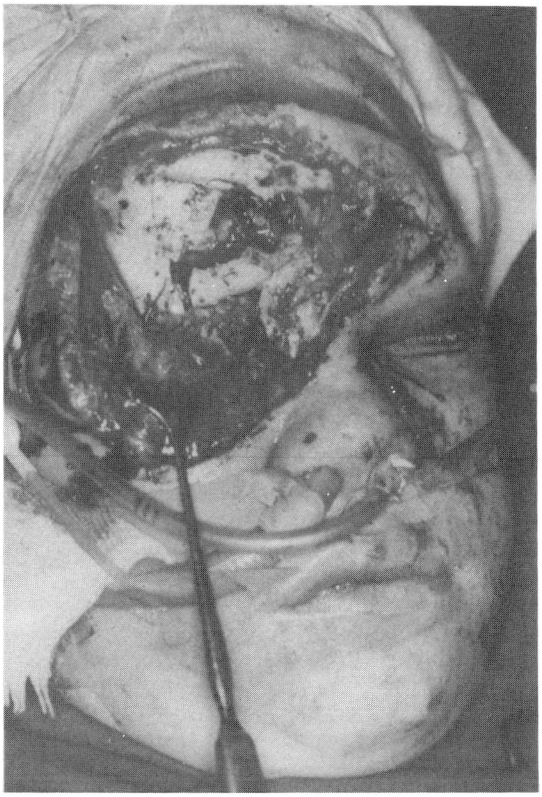

Figure 15–23 Surgical exposure of a comminuted fracture of the frontal cranial bone.

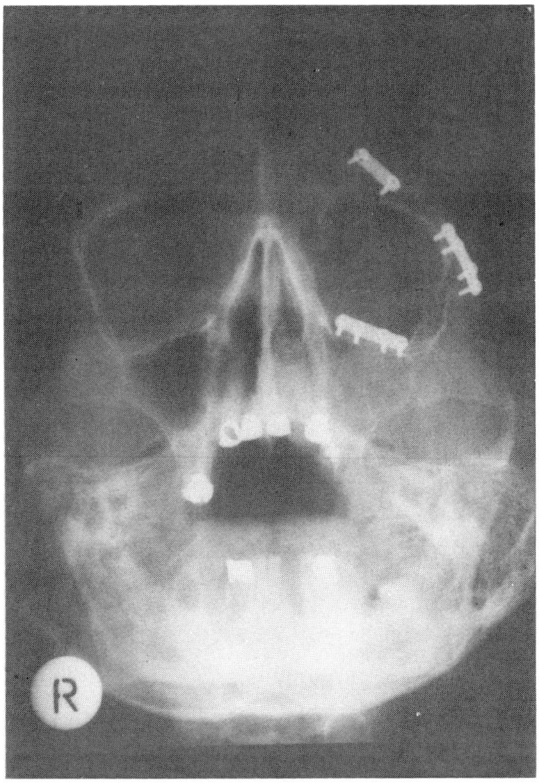

Figure 15–24 Fixation of multiple periorbital fractures with miniplates.

models must be sectioned according to the localization of the fractures. Usually, it is possible to find the former occlusion which can then be compared with the situation during the surgical repositioning of the fractured jaw. As was already mentioned, securing of the occlusion during surgery by intermaxillary wiring prior to the plating is important. When the occlusal disturbance is minimal, it can be compensated for by selective filing of the teeth. If the errors are larger, however, a new osteosynthesis must be performed.

An *inadequate fit* of the plates can also cause postoperative malocclusion. If the fit of the plates across the fracture or osteotomy site is not perfect, tightening of the screws will move the fragments. When tooth-bearing sections are involved, occlusal disturbances will occur. In other regions of the facial bones, e.g., in the area of the malar bone, a displacement due to an incorrect fit of the plate may lead to an aesthetically unpleasant result. Therefore, particular attention must be paid to perfecting the bending of the plates. In this connection, one particular situation should be mentioned: a bilateral condylar fracture with an additional midline fracture of the mandible regularly results in a retrusion of the lower jaw, an open bite deformity, and a widening of the mandibular arch. Even when two miniplates are applied on the buccal surface of the mandible, there can still be an opening of the fracture gap on the lingual surface (Fig. 15–26). In this instance, the plates must be deliberately overbent and the body of the mandible must be compressed during plate application. If this is

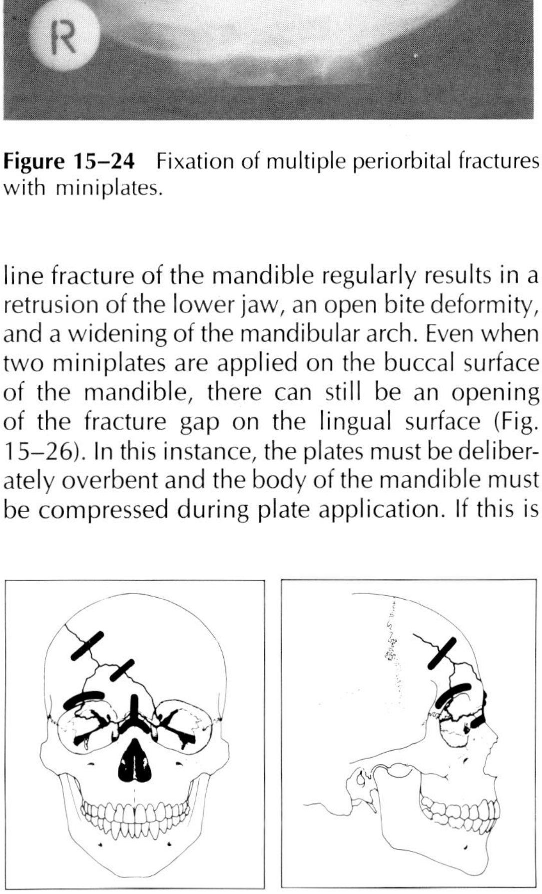

Figure 15–25 Miniplates of different shapes can be used for stabilization of cranial fractures.

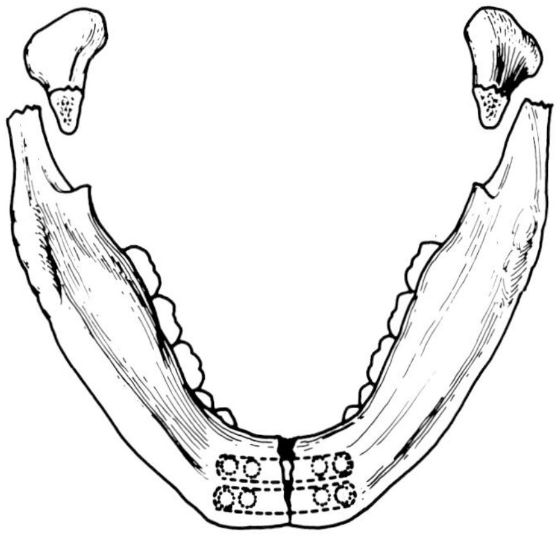

Figure 15–26 In a triple fracture of the mandible, the plate placed on the buccal surface cannot avoid a gap on the lingual surface at the midline. Overbending of plates is recommended in this situation.

not performed, a mandibular deformity will result which is too broad and has a crossbite in the molar region.

It is our experience that the rate of *infection* is very low. In other studies, Champy and colleagues[35] reported on 1,000 cases of miniplate osteosynthesis with incidences of 3.2 percent of local abscess formation and 0.7 percent osteomyelitis of the fracture site. Beals and Munro[23] did not find any infections in the application of 200 plates in different types of midfacial osteotomies. We also found practically no infections in our elective osteotomy cases. Even when the screws were penetrating into the maxillary sinus, which is mostly the case in Le Fort I osteotomies, the sinus clears up a few weeks postoperatively and is translucent again before plates are removed (Fig. 15–27). In trauma cases, the situation with regard to infection is somewhat different. There is always the problem of tooth particles to be found in the fracture line. If these are not removed, an infection will occur. Also, a nonerupted wisdom tooth, close to the fracture site, must be taken out before a plate is placed (Fig. 15–28).

Another cause for infection can be inadequate immobilization of the fragments. This can be the

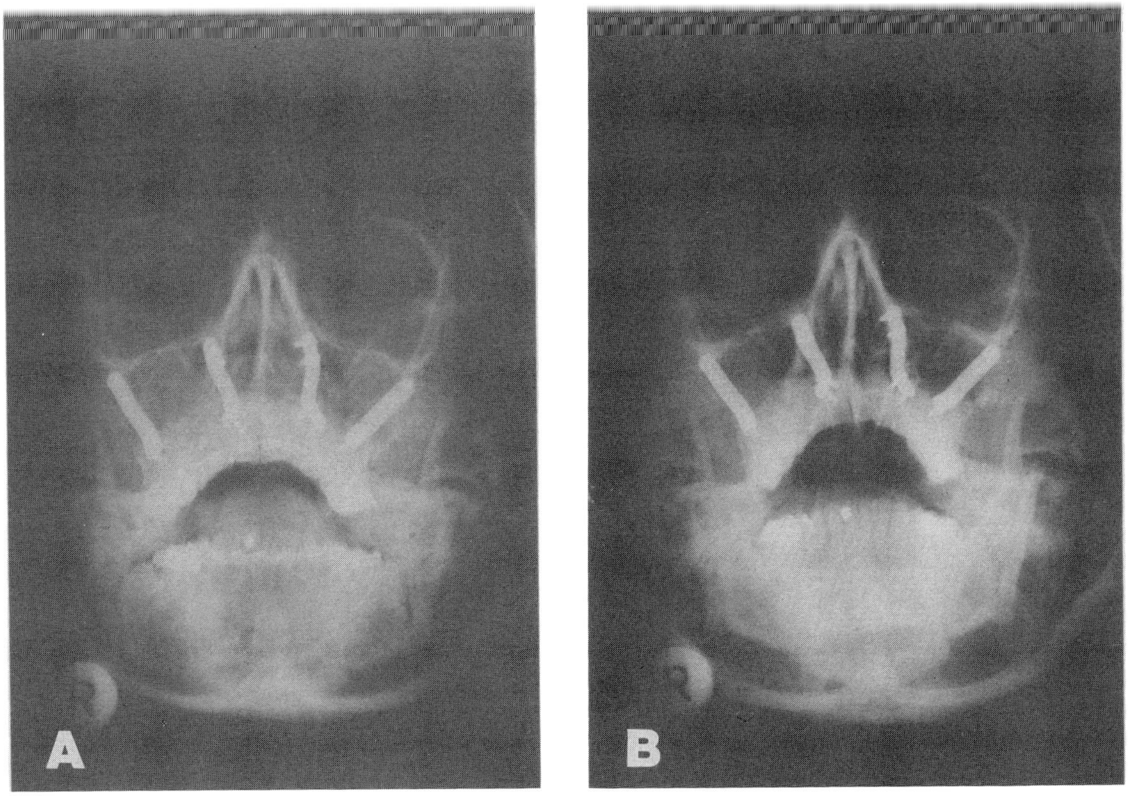

Figure 15–27 Miniplate application in a Le Fort I type osteotomy. *A*, Cloudy maxillary sinus immediately following surgery. *B*, Three months postoperatively, both sinuses have cleared up again.

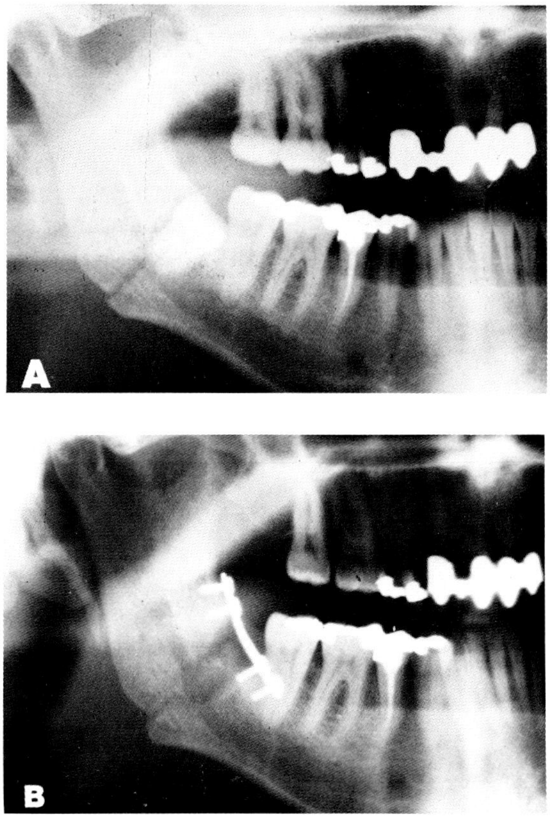

Figure 15–28 Tooth within the fracture line. *A*, The unerupted wisdom tooth is at the fracture line. *B*, Following tooth removal, a miniplate is placed on the lateral oblique line.

case in comminuted fractures of the mandible, in partially edentulous regions when no splints or dentures are available for proper reposition, and also when the biomechanical principles are disregarded. If the plates are outside the regular osteosynthesis line or if only one screw is used for fragment fixation, a postoperative dislocation can occur. Particularly in the mandible, where muscle attachments can cause undesirable motion, a dislocation can lead to delayed infection with subsequent osteomyelitis of the fracture site. If this is the case, the plates must be removed, the site drained, and intermaxillary fixation must be applied for several weeks (Fig. 15–29).

An *exposure* of the screw or plate can occur in the first postoperative days due to suture dehiscence, or later, to delayed wound healing. If there is an early dehiscence, we recommend suture

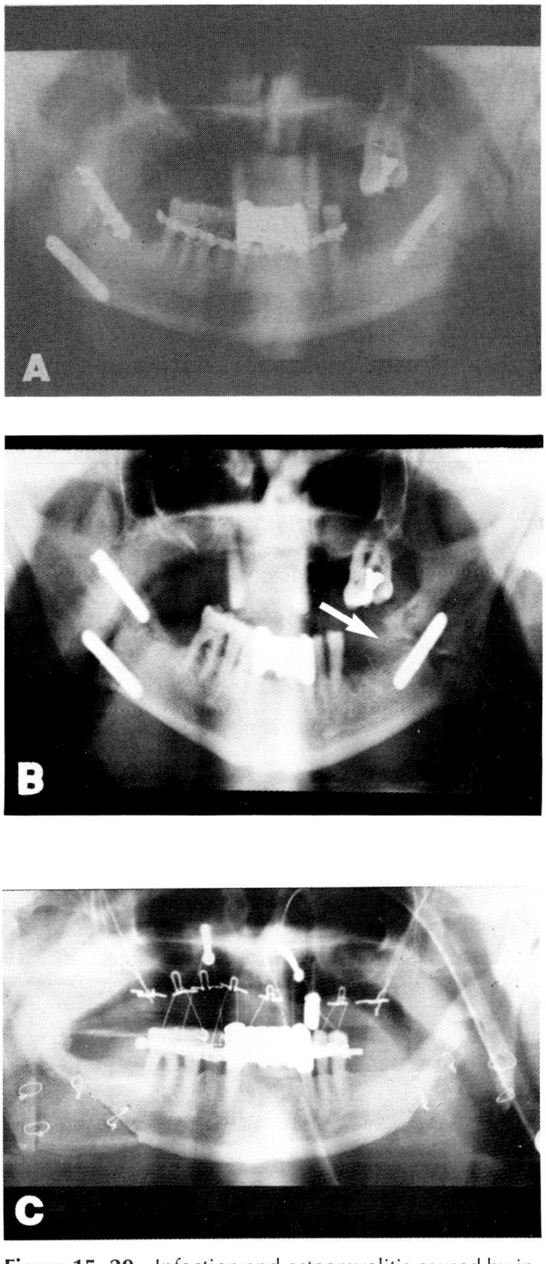

Figure 15–29 Infection and osteomyelitis caused by insufficient stabilization of the fragments. *A*, In a bilateral fracture of the angle, the necessary stability could not be achieved with miniplating. *B*, In spite of miniplate fixation of the upper border, the dislocation of the proximal mandibular fragment is clearly visible (arrow). *C*, Following plate removal, intermaxillary fixation is applied for 6 weeks. The fragments are fixed with wires and bone grafts, resulting in healing and union of the mandible.

removal, cleaning with diluted hydrogen peroxide, and wound dressing with iodoform Vaseline gauze. Normally, this open wound treatment will lead to a normal union of the fracture site provided there is an appropriate fixation of the fragments. When a plate becomes exposed at a later point in time, we still do not remove the plate at this stage because there is usually no inflammatory reaction in the surrounding tissues and the patient has no complaints (Fig. 15–30). One can wait, without concern, until the healing of the fracture site is completed, which is normally the case after 6 to 9 months. Then the plate can be easily removed to allow proper coverage with the healing mucosa.

Since the apices of the teeth sometimes come close to the osteosynthesis line, *injuries of the tooth roots* are possible. This is particularly a danger in the posterolateral region of the mandible and in the area of the canine teeth in the upper and lower jaws. Therefore, care should be taken when the drill holes are made. In the upper and lower front, the roots can be identified and protected more easily, whereas in the posterior mandibular region, where the cortical plate is rather thick, the position of the root tips cannot always be located. Here the drill holes should be made according to the recommendation of Champy and colleagues below the alveolar crest at a distance approximately twice the height of the crown of the tooth.

The *removal of the plate* cannot be considered as a complication, if it is done electively. Since the incompatibility or even allergy to alloys which contain nickel has been recognized, most surgeons recommend the removal of the osteosynthesis material, when the bone healing is completed. We have also found signs of incompatibility in a few patients which was manifested by slight pain, moderate swelling, and general discomfort. These complaints disappeared when the screws and plates were removed. For some years now we have used titanium plates and screws, and we have found no signs of incompatibility so far. We presume that this material can be left in the human body permanently, but the period of observation is still too short to make a definitive statement.

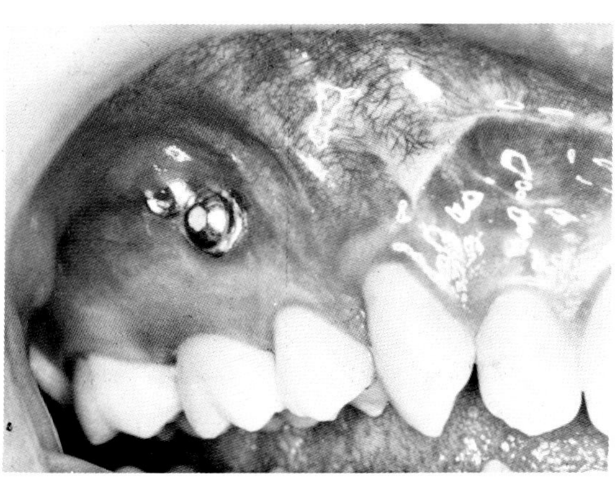

Figure 15–30 Exposed Steinhauser plate in the maxillary region. There is no sign of inflammatory reaction of the surrounding tissue.

REFERENCES

1. Christiansen GW. Open operation and tantalum plate insertion for fracture of the mandible. J Oral Surg 1945; 3:194–204.
2. Thoma K. Oral surgery. Vol 1. 2nd ed. St. Louis: CV Mosby, 1952.
3. Shira RB. Open reduction of mandibular fractures. J Oral Surg 1954; 12:95–111.
4. Reichenbach E. Zur Frage der operativen Knochenbruchbehandlung im Bereich des Gesichtsschädels. Dtsch Zahn Mund Kieferheilk 1953; 17:220–243.
5. Pini CE. Syntheses metalliques avec plaquettes vissées dans le fractures de la mandibule. Rev Fr Odont-Stomatol 1959; 6:814–821.
6. Hoffer O, Arlotta P. Behandlung von Unterkieferbruchen mit Metallplättchen. Dtsch Zahnärztl Z 1961; 16:667–668.
7. Battersby TG. Plating of mandibular fractures. Br J Oral Surg 1966; 4:194–201.
8. Müller ME, Allgower M, Willenegger H. Technik der operativen Frakturbehandlung. Berlin: Springer, 1963.
9. Pape HD, Herzog M, Gerlach KL. Der Wandel der Unterkieferfrakturversorgung von 1950-1980 am Beispiel der Kölner Klinik. Dtsch Zahnarztl Z 1983; 38:301–308.
10. Michelet FX, Festal F. Osteosynthese par plaques vissees dans les fractures de l'etage moyen. Sci Recherche Odonto-Stomat 1972; 2:4.
11. Peri G, Jourde J, Menes R. Des trous surtout pour reconstruire certains segments du squeletter facial. Ann Chir Plast 1973; 18:170–173.
12. Souyris F, Caravel JB. Osteosynthese par plaques vissées en chirurgie maxillo-faciale et cranio-faciale. Ann Chir Plast 1974; 19:131–137.
13. Champy M, Lodde JP. Syntheses mandibulaires. Localisation des syntheses en fonction des contraintes mandibulaires. Rev Stomatol 1976; 77:971–976.
14. Harle F, Duker J. Miniplattenosteosynthese am Jochbein. Dtsch Zahnärztl Z 1976; 31:97–102.
15. Schilli W, Niederdellmann H, Harle F. Schrauben und Platten am Mittelgesicht und orbitaring. Fortschr Kiefer Gesichtschir 1977; 22:47–49.
16. Luhr HG. Stabile Fixation von Oberkiefermittelgesichtsfrakturen durch Mini-kompressionsplatten. Dtsch Zahnärztl Z 1979; 34:851–860.
17. Horster W, Reychler H. Correction du profil dans

les sequelles de fentes labio-palatines. Par avancée du maxillaire superieur et rhinoplastie simultanée. Ann Chir Plast 1979; 23:145–148.
18. Harle F. Le Fort I osteotomy (using miniplates) for correction of the long face. Int J Oral Surg 1980; 9:427–432.
19. Horster W. Experience with functionally stable plate osteosynthesis after forward displacement of the upper jaw. J Maxillofac Surg 1980; 8:176–181.
20. Drommer R, Luhr HG. The stabilization of osteotomized maxillary segments with Luhr miniplates in secondary cleft surgery. J Maxillofac Surg 1981; 9:166–169.
21. Steinhauser EW. Bone screws and plates in orthognathic surgery. Int J Oral Surg 1982; 11:209–216.
22. Frost DE, Koutnik AW. Alternative stabilization of the maxilla during simultaneous jaw-mobilization procedures. Oral Surg 1983; 56:125–131.
23. Beals SP, Munro JR. The use of miniplates in craniomaxillofacial surgery. Plast Reconstr Surg 1987; 79:33–38.
24. Champy M, Lodde JP. Etude des contraintes dans la mandibule fracturée chez l'homme. Rev Stomatol 1977; 78:545–551.
25. Ewers R. Periorbitale Knochenstrukturen und ihre Bedeutung Für die Osteosynthese. Fortschr Kiefer Gesichtschir 1977; 22:45–46.
26. Paulus GW. Die Knochenbruchheilung am Oberkiefer bei Verwendung von Miniplatten. Erlangen: Med Habil Universität, 1986.
27. Heinl T, Neumayer B. Vorschlag für die analytisch begründete Konstruktion einer Osteosynthese-miniplatte aus Titan. Biomed Technik 1986; 31:303–307.
28. Steinhauser EW. A new titanium miniplate system for maxillofacial and craniofacial osteosynthesis (abstr). Presented at the International Congress of Plastic Surgery, New Delhi, 1987.
29. Steinhauser EW. Variation of Le Fort II osteotomies for correction of midfacial deformities. J Maxillofac Surg 1980; 8:258–264.
30. Champy M, Lodde JP, Wilk A, Grasset D. Plattenosteosynthesen bei Mittelgesichtsfrakturen und Osteotomien. Dtsch Z Mund Kiefer Gesichts-Chir 1978; 2:26–29.
31. Schwenzer N, Kruger E. Midface fractures. Oral and maxillofacial traumatology. Vol 2. Chicago: Quintessence, 1986.
32. Schilli W, Niederdellmann H. Internal fixation of zygomatic and midface fractures by means of miniplates and lag screws. Chicago: Quintessence, 1986.
33. Luhr HG. Lyophilisierte Dura zum Defektersatz des Orbitabodens nach Trauma und Tumorresektion. Med Mitt (Melsungen) 1969; 43:233.
34. Paulus GW, Hardt N. Miniplattenosteosynthesen bei traumatologischen sowie korrektiven Operationen im Kiefer- und Gesichtsbereich. Schweiz Mschr Zahnheilk 1983; 9:705–712.
35. Champy M, Pape HD, Gerlach KL, Lodde JP. The Strasbourg miniplate osteosynthesis. Chicago: Quintessence, 1986.

16

IMMEDIATE BONE GRAFTING OF MAXILLOFACIAL INJURIES

ROBERT L. WALTON, M.D., F.A.C.S.
GREGORY L. BORAH, D.D.S., M.D.

Extensive trauma to the facial skeleton commonly results in comminuted and compound fractures of the maxilla, zygomatic complex, nasal ethmoidal complex, and frontal bones. These panfacial injuries, the result of high-energy impact, are usually unstable and cause significant facial deformity. Simple realignment of the fracture segments is often insufficient to provide for stable union of large stress-bearing components of the facial skeleton. In addition, bone segments that are contaminated or lost at the time of injury may require replacement with adequate bone stock. Patients with these injuries are candidates for immediate bone grafting at the time of definitive facial fracture management.

PRINCIPLES

Immediate bone grafting at the time of operative reduction of the facial fracture serves to restore lost bone stock and provide stability between segments of the maxillofacial skeleton and the craniofacial base. Bone grafts can also be used to reconstruct specialized parts such as those supporting overlying facial and cranial soft tissues (e.g., nose, orbital floor, frontal bone).

The three primary support columns of the maxilla are the pyriform (or nasomaxilla), zygomaticomaxillary, and pterygomaxillary buttresses. The pyriform buttress extends from the supradentoalveolar complex adjacent to the upper cuspid teeth along the lateral nasal wall and pyriform aperture to connect the maxilla to the nasal process and frontal-glabellar portion of the skull. The zygomaticomaxillary buttress extends from the alveolar portion of the maxilla in the posterior molar region up to the body of the zygomatic bone. The posterior, pterygoid buttress of the maxilla extends from the medial posterior aspect of the hard palate through the pterygoid plates to the sphenoid bone (Fig. 16–1).

These maxillary buttresses form the supporting framework for the nasomaxillary sinuses and the floor of the orbit. They serve to distribute force from the maxillary dentition to the cranial base. Restoration of these buttresses is an essential component in achieving long-term stability of fractures of the maxilla and particularly the teeth-bearing components.

Primary consideration is given to reconstruction of the anterior pyriform and zygomaticomaxillary buttresses which are easily accessible from an intraoral approach. Reconstruction of the

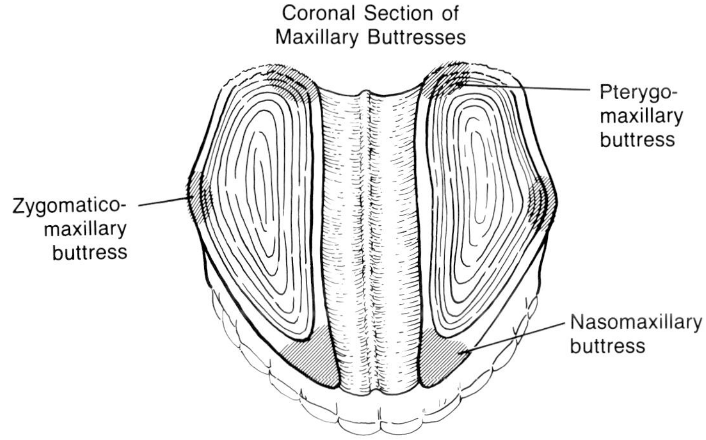

Figure 16–1 Cross section of maxillary buttresses. This section of the maxilla demonstrates the bony pillar buttresses that provide the principal support for the maxilla and its attachments to the base of the skull. Areas of greatest bone thickness are highlighted.

pterygomaxillary buttresses is usually not undertaken because of the posteromedial position of this disruption. Generally, satisfactory position and stabilization of the maxilla can be obtained with reconstruction of the four anterior and lateral buttresses alone.

Significant disruptions of the orbit, including the medial or lateral walls, or orbital floor can be treated with immediate bone grafting. Bone grafts are placed and secured to support the orbital contents allowing the eye to rest in a normal anatomic position. Loss of frontal or lateral cranial vault structures such as the anterior frontal sinus wall or segmental defects of the calvarium can be reconstructed with immediate bone grafting to effect a one-stage repair of a complex injury.

Immediate bone grafting of the mandible is performed less commonly because of the adequacy of thick bicortical bone in the mandible. In those patients with significant bone loss and collapse of the mandibular arch, however, bone grafting can be undertaken at the time of initial repair. Wounds must not be significantly contaminated and adequate soft tissue must be present (or provided) for coverage. Survival of bone grafts in the mandible as well as in the other regions of the maxillofacial skeleton depends upon the surrounding soft-tissue envelope for provision of blood supply and the necessary support for bone growth.

It is impossible to eliminate all bacterial contamination from the site of facial bone fractures, and therefore all bone grafting in the maxillofacial skeleton is technically considered to be contaminated. However, the excellent blood supply in this region works to reduce the potential for infection. Bone grafts will heal satisfactorily in areas where at least one cortex is covered by adequate soft tissue, except in the mandible. Exposed bone graft in the mandible has a high incidence of infection and graft loss. Replacement of bone grafts over frontal and maxillary sinuses without mucosal lining on one side can be accomplished without complication in the vast majority of patients. Mucosal regeneration over an exposed bone scaffold appears to proceed unimpeded. The mucosa may then serve to supply vascular ingrowth to the underlying bone graft.

CLINICAL APPROACH

Essential to management of maxillofacial fractures is a careful and accurate assessment of the injured parts. Thorough examination of the intraoral and extraoral structures with careful palpation for step deformities, malocclusion, and open injuries will provide an initial impression of the overall extent of the patient's injuries. Beyond the physical examination, a full facial series of plain radiographs concludes the initial screening examination. Computed tomography (CT) of the cranial vault and brain structures for evaluation of hematoma and brain contusion can be extended through the midface and mandible region to assess the extent of the maxillofacial fractures. While the protocol for facial CT scanning varies with each trauma center, effort should be made to obtain facial CT studies at the time of the cranial evaluation. These patients not infrequently will be admitted to the Intensive Care Unit and may be less suitable for extensive diagnostic radiographic study later. Early assessment of facial injuries will allow for adequate planning followed by the scheduling of definitive facial skeletal repair (see chapter 5 entitled *Diagnostic Imaging*).

Severe intracranial, intrathoracic, intraabdominal or associated orthopedic injuries will necessitate prioritization of the maxillofacial injury. In these cases early stabilization and soft-tissue wound closure preclude definitive fracture management. Patients with high-velocity injuries to the face which require immediate bone grafting will frequently have intracranial injuries requiring careful assessment and intervention prior to undertaking repair of maxillofacial structures.

Once the patient has been stabilized and is cleared for an operative procedure, he is brought to the operating room. Anesthesia may be provided via a nasotracheal approach under direct visualization or by temporary cricotracheotomy when indicated. If the patient is to be ventilated for long-term sequelae of neurologic injury, a tracheostomy is employed.

The overall goals for management of facial fractures are: (1) to reconstitute the cranial vault and provide protection for the brain, (2) to provide stable anatomic occlusal relationships between the maxilla and the mandible, (3) to restore contour and support for the eyes and nasal structures, and (4) to provide mobility for the mandible and support for the intraoral structures.

To achieve these goals bone grafts may be indicated. All four areas are equally important. Life-threatening conditions are resolved first, followed by attention to function and aesthetics in that order (see chapter 2 entitled *Trauma Victim Management*). The sequence of bony repair may be modified by the extent of injury to each of these associated areas. In patients with severe anterior cranial vault fractures or avulsions, attention is initially directed toward reconstituting the cranial vault with split-rib or split-calvarial grafts from uninvolved areas of the cranium. Once the continuity of the skull has been re-established, the facial bones can be stabilized to the newly reconstructed cranial vault. If the cranium is intact and the orbital structures are aligned, attention is first directed to the mandibular/maxillary complex so that adequate occlusal relationships can be re-established. The bones of the mandible and maxilla are then aligned to achieve optimum occlusion and the entire mandibular/maxillary complex is fixed to the supporting structures of the upper face.

Areas of thin bone are prone to comminute, making reduction and stabilization difficult if not impossible. Because of this tendency, the upper midface is a common site for immediate bone grafting. Access to the fracture is gained through a bicoronal approach which provides excellent visibility and exposure to the frontal, supraorbital, nasal, and zygomatic regions through a single aesthetically acceptable incision.

Bone grafting of the upper midface usually involves reconstruction of a frontal defect, restoration of the nasal root, and re-establishment of the supraorbital rim and the medial or lateral orbital walls. Each one of these areas can be reconstructed with grafts of rib, iliac crest, or calvarial bone. Clinical experience suggests that the latter is most suited for grafting of the facial skeleton because of excellent "take" and less tendency to resorb. The size and shape of the defect will also dictate the site of bone graft harvest.

In frontal sinus defects, our basic philosophy is to perform a facsimile reconstruction of the sinus vault. In these cases drainage of the reconstruction via the nasofrontal duct or intersinus septum is of paramount importance. Cranialization of the frontal sinus may be performed if the midfrontal region has been severely comminuted or destroyed, as seen in blast or other high-velocity injuries. In unilateral defects, contour re-establishment is facilitated by using the opposite normal side as a model for reconstruction. Stabilization by complete immobilization of the bone grafts is achieved by using interosseous wires and/or noncompression plates (Fig. 16–2).

Both techniques are effective, but the former is easily adapted to a variety of situations and requires less rigorous experience. Miniplate fixation is an excellent method for internal rigid fixation of bone but requires stable stock support, extensive dissection, and hands-on experience for optimal results. Attention for detailing the approach should be directed when grafts are used in static and dynamic areas of the facial skeleton.

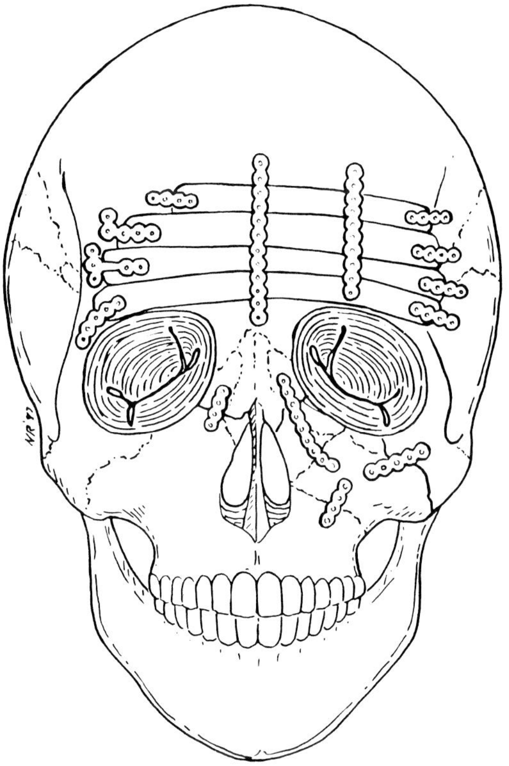

Figure 16–2 Rigid plate fixation of bone grafts for reconstruction of the forehead and upper midface. Noncompression plate fixation provides an extremely stable structural element for alignment and maintenance of bone grafts placed to reconstruct large areas of bony defect. This provides a more stable framework than can be normally achieved with simple wiring alone.

Bone grafting to a nasal cavity or sinus generates risk of exposure and infection with possible loss of the graft. In these cases, coverage of the bone graft on at least one side is mandatory for "take" of the graft. If this is performed in conjunction with rigid fixation, graft infection or resorption is an unlikely complication.

Approach to the maxilla is most easily achieved through a buccal sulcus incision that extends from the retromolar region of the maxilla circumferentially to the opposite retromolar region. The incision is carried down through the mucosa to the periosteum. Mucoperiosteal flaps are then created to expose the underlying abnormality of the pyriform aperture and zygomaticomaxillary buttress regions. Care should be taken at the pyriform apertures to preserve the nasal mucosa lining, as this may be important in providing graft vascularity. Subperiosteal dissection in the retromolar region will prevent herniation of the

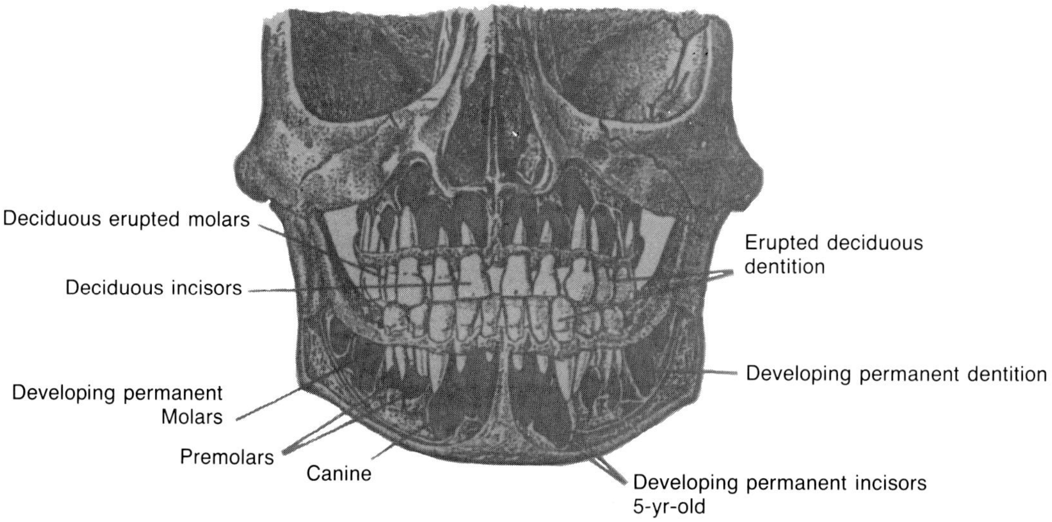

Figure 17–1 Mixed dentition. Only the deciduous dentition is fully erupted in both mandibular and maxillary alveolar arches. The permanent developing dentition lies lingual or palatal to the erupted deciduous teeth. The majority of the alveolar bony area in both the mandible and maxilla is occupied by the erupted deciduous teeth and the developing follicles of the permanent dentition at age 5 years.

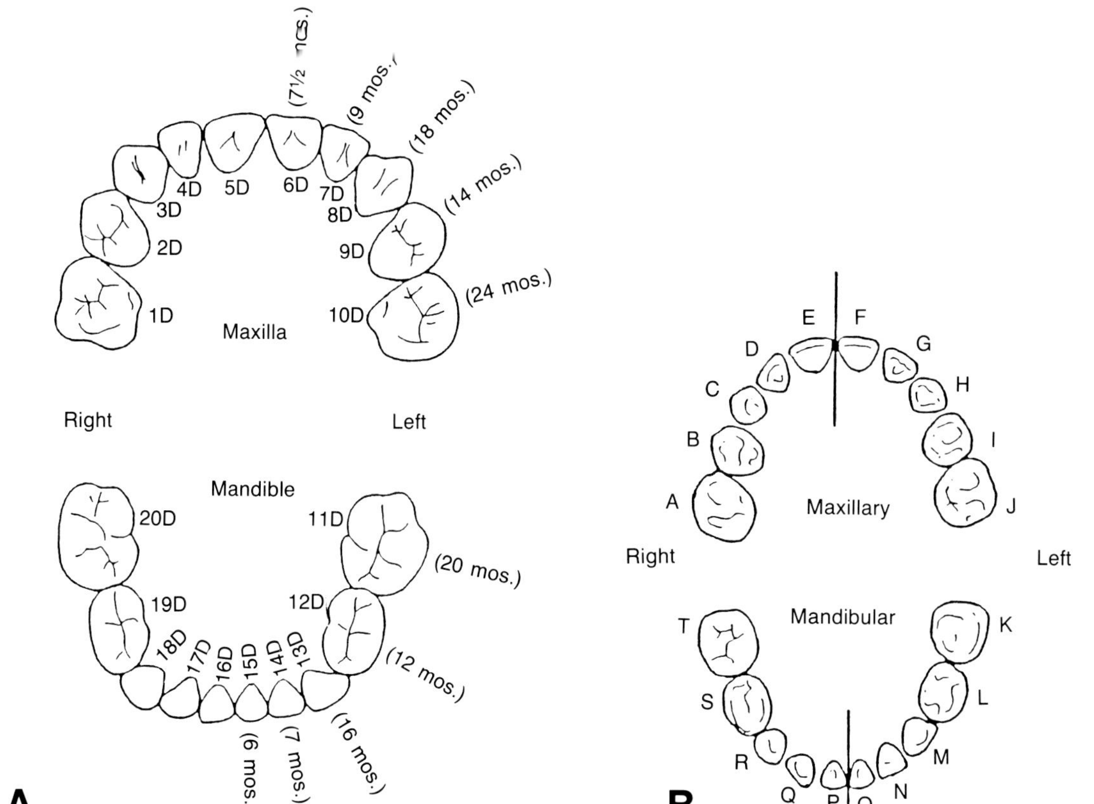

Figure 17–2 Primary dentition. *A*, Diagram of maxillary and mandibular primary dental arches.

Legend continues on opposite page

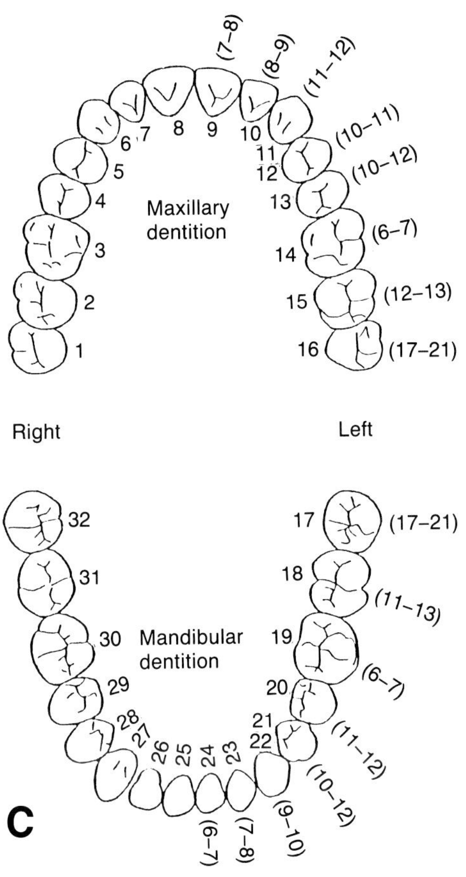

Figure 17–2 Continued. The numbers in parentheses indicate the ages at which each tooth may be expected to emerge into the oral cavity. The numbers 1D through 20D inside the arches indicate one of several ways in which the teeth may be coded (rather than named) for purposes of record-keeping. Starting at 1D, the teeth are right second molar, first molar, canine, lateral incisor, and central incisor (which is 5D). The remaining teeth are similarly coded. *B*, Another method of diagramming the deciduous dentition by quadrants using capital letters of the alphabet i.e.:

A→E F→J
T←P O←K .

E represents the upper *right* deciduous central incisor and K represents the *left* second deciduous molar. *C*, An illustration of the occlusal and incisal surfaces of the maxillary and mandibular permanent dental arches. The numbers in parentheses indicate the usual ages at which each of the teeth emerge into the oral cavity. The numerals 1 to 32 inside the arches indicate the universal numbering code (frequently used) for purposes of record-keeping. Starting at the maxillary right (of the subject) third molar, which is number 1, the numbers extend through consecutive teeth to the maxillary left third molar, number 16, then continue from the mandibular left third molar, number 17, to the mandibular right third molar, number 32.

EMERGENCY ROOM ASSESSMENT

Emergency treatment of children with maxillofacial injuries demands that the examining physician be particularly adept in ascertaining an adequate airway and noting the possible presence of foreign materials that might obstruct the laryngotracheal airway. The amount of edema that occurs following maxillofacial trauma rapidly increases, but if examination is early enough, one can assess the airway with minimal difficulty. Certainly, if the mandible is fractured and comminuted, examination can be painful to the patient. To gain full cooperation of the child is rather difficult, and at times it may be necessary to use a short-acting sedative which should not interfere with assessment of injury to the brain. Removal of any accumulated blood or vomitus in the hypopharynx is of paramount importance. Once the airway is cleared, because there can be increasing local swelling, it may be necessary to place an oral airway in position and position the patient prone with the head turned to the side. It is vital to check for possible cervical spine injury before moving the patient. When there is marked edema of the tongue in an uncooperative patient, it may be necessary to place a traction suture of heavy silk, nylon, or Prolene through the anterior tongue under local anesthesia to open the laryngotracheal airway and facilitate removal of foreign bodies or dental fragments.

It is better to intubate the patient rather than to perform a tracheostomy, if at all possible. Tracheostomy should be a last resort used only if all other means of maintaining airway have failed. In the young child, a tracheostomy contributes greatly to morbidity, and its weaning and removal can be a long-term process. It is advantageous to examine the acutely injured child without the parents being present because it is often easier to establish rapport, gain control, and secure the child's confidence on a one-to-one basis.

X-RAY STUDIES

The x-ray views that provide the most diagnostic information on injuries of the maxillofacial skeleton are the Waters views, Panorex dental film, and computed tomographic (CT) scan (Fig. 17–3). The right and left lateral oblique and anteroposterior views of the jaws in the open position provide added information and include views of the first and second cervical vertebrae along with the odontoid process. The odontoid process can also be visualized in a reverse Waters x-ray view (Fig. 17–4). A chest roentgenogram, along with lateral and anteroposterior views of the cervical spine, is most important and should be taken in every case. The CT scan, which is often ordered by the neurosurgical consultant, can provide meaningful information in midfacial as well as mandibular fractures and should be obtained at 2 to 3 mm cuts, if possible.

ASSOCIATED INJURIES

One must be on the alert for associated injuries to the cervical, thoracic, and lumbar vertebrae as well as to the abdominal viscera and particularly to the skull and brain. In the McCoy and associates series,[5] 41 percent of patients had associated skull fractures. The overall incidence of associated injuries, other than the soft-tissue facial wounds, was noted to be 57 percent, with concussions in 31 percent and cerebrospinal fluid (CSF) rhinorrhea in 14 percent. Extremity fractures appeared in 9.3 percent of all maxillofacial injuries in children, and closed chest trauma was apparent in 5.8 percent. Internal abdominal injuries appeared in 2.3 percent and blinding ocular injuries occurred in 3.6 percent. In the patients described by Kaban and colleagues,[3] 29 percent had associated injuries other than facial wounds (Table 17–1).

Where the maxillary antrum has been partially or almost completely pneumatized in the older child, unilateral nasal bleeding may indicate the presence of a malar bone fracture on the ipsilateral side of injury. CSF rhinorrhea would indicate the communication of a nasofrontal fracture within the subarachnoid space. This can occur in a Le Fort II and Le Fort III type of maxillary fracture or a high nasal fracture through the cribriform plate of the ethmoid bone. Clear fluid may drain from the nose and can be distinguished from mucus by its protein and sugar content, which can be tested by a "Clinistick."

SIGNS AND SYMPTOMS

The clinical manifestations of fractures involving the mandible, maxilla, and the malar-orbital segments are the same for children as they are for adults. Pain and tenderness over any facial bone with the appearance of ecchymosis should arouse suspicion of possible fractures in that area. The presence of diplopia, which is difficult to elicit in the very young child but can be tested for in

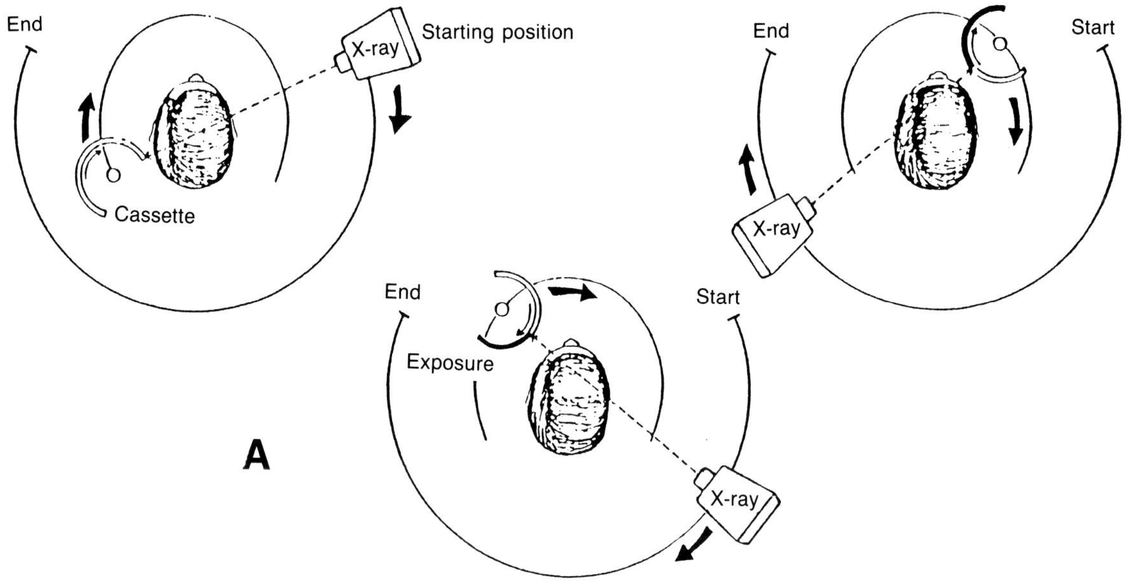

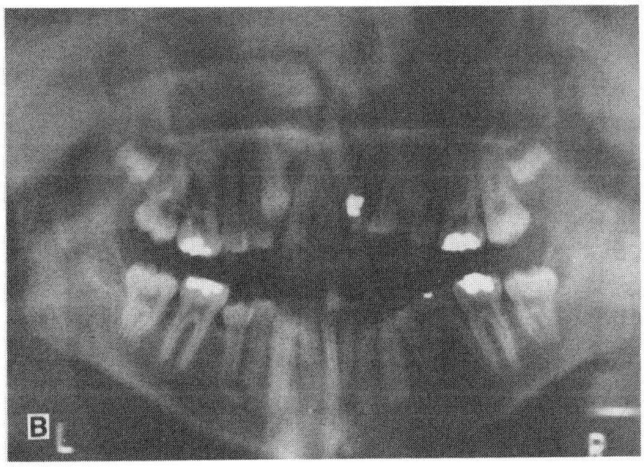

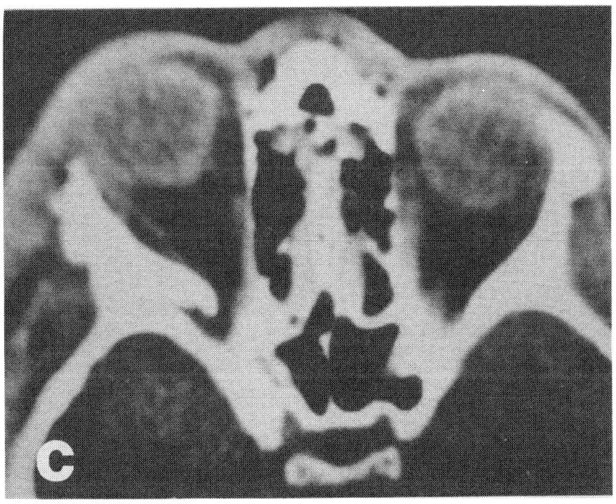

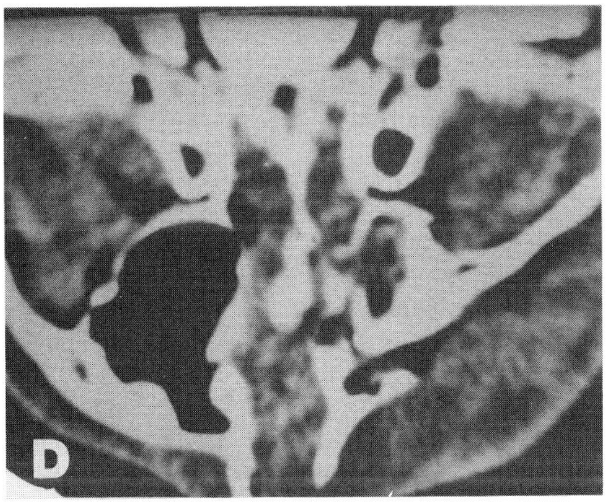

Figure 17–3 *A*, Diagrammatic representations of x-ray penetration in exposing orthopantographic (Panorex) film. X-ray beam and film cassette maintain 180-degree angle throughout the procedure. As both x-ray beam and cassette revolve around patient, cassette rotates secondarily, exposing film as it turns. When an entire revolution is made, a panoramic view of the mandible is exposed. This x-ray study provides a single view of teeth and supporting structures in sharp focus from one temporomandibular joint to the other. *B*, Panorex view of mandible and maxilla with entire dentoalveolar area. Note lower right deciduous 2nd molar and erupting permanent maxillary canine teeth. *C, D*, Computed tomographic scan views to delineate the fractured segments of the maxilla and medial ethmoid-orbital walls.

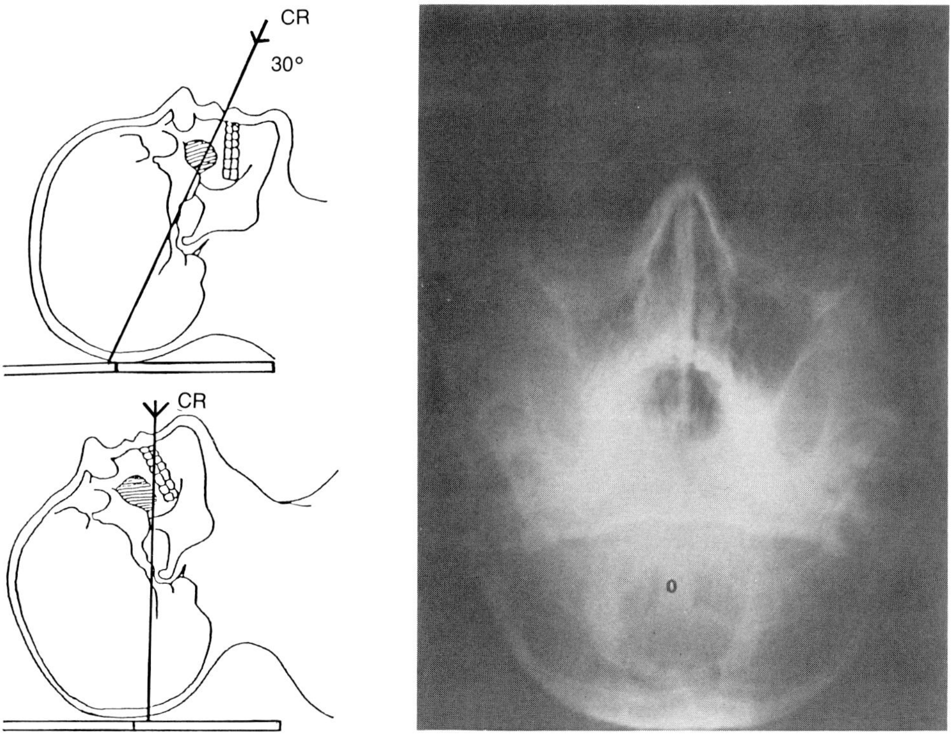

Figure 17–1 Reverse Waters mento-occipital position. The reverse Waters projection gives a view of the facial bones similar to the Waters view except for greater magnification of the facial bones due to increased part-film distance. Fractures of the orbits, maxillary sinuses, zygomatic bones, and zygomatic arches are clearly shown. The odontoid process of the first cervical vertebra can also be visualized (0).

TABLE 17–1 Associated Injuries in the Pediatric Patient with Facial Fractures

Overall incidence of associated injuries	57%*
(other than soft-tissue facial wounds)	29%**
Skull fractures	41%
Concussions	31%
Cerebrospinal fluid rhinorrhea	14%
Extremity fractures	9.3%
Closed chest trauma	5.8%
Internal abdominal injury	3.6%

* Data from McCoy et al.[5]
** Data from Kaban et al.[3]

children 6 years and older, along with enophthalmos and entrapment, would indicate fractures of the orbital floor. Inability to open or to close the jaws into satisfactory occlusion should arouse suspicion of fractures involving the maxilla, the mandible, and malar bones. The actions of the muscles of mastication on the fragments involved in the line of fracture are the same for a child as they are for an adult. Hence, fractures involving the mental foramen area, and a contrecoup fracture involving the ascending ramus or condyle on the opposite side would demonstrate definite displacement of these fragments when opening and closing functions of the mandible are tested. The actions of the masseter-pterygoid sling along with the action of the external pterygoid muscle produces definite positions of mandibular displacement. The muscles of mastication are all innervated by the fifth nerve, and the origin and insertions of these muscles should be thoroughly understood by all who treat facial bone fractures (Fig. 17–5).

Evaluation of occlusal relationships is necessary to determine whether the patient is occluding in the same relationship that was present in the preinjury state. This demands that occlusal relationships be thoroughly understood. The combined deciduous and erupting permanent dentitions, or mixed dentition, have occlusal relationships that can be complicated. A Class I occlusal relationship has the same general first molar relationship in both deciduous and permanent dentitions (Fig. 17–6).

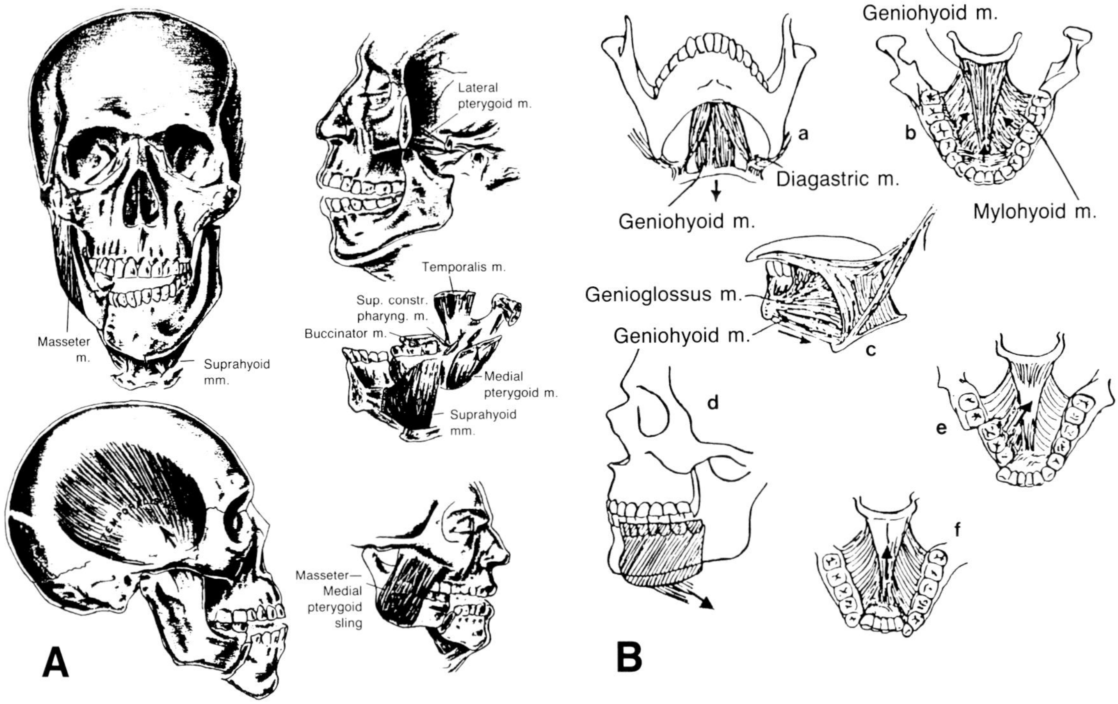

Figure 17–5 *A*, Muscles of mastication and their actions on the mandible. *B*, The suprahyoid muscles. Arrows indicate the direction of muscle pull and displacement of fragments in mandibular fractures.

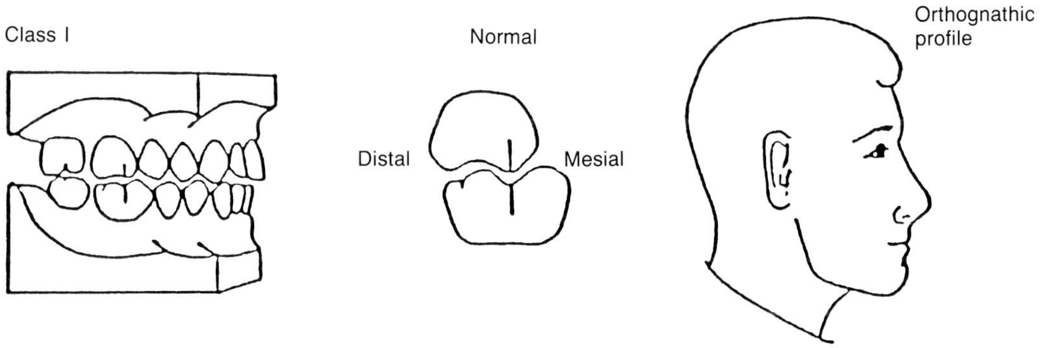

Figure 17–6 Class I occlusion. First molar relationship. (The mesial buccal cusp of the maxillary first molar articulates with the mesial buccal groove of the mandibular first molar.)

Once the injured child has been stabilized and the airway assured, one must question the parents as to the child's past dental treatment and contact the child's dentist or pedodontist. Dental records of occlusal relationships and the teeth that were present or absent prior to injury should be requested for review. In the older or teenage child, when midface hypoplasia or an open-bite deformity might have been present prior to injury, it is most important that this be known and documented prior to reduction and fixation of facial bone fractures. Understanding the relationships between the posterior teeth and the anterior teeth as well as the differences between a Class I, Class II, and Class III occlusion (Fig. 17–7) is most helpful in determining which facets or marks of erosion one must consider when moving bony fragments into proper mandibular and maxillary occlusal relationship.

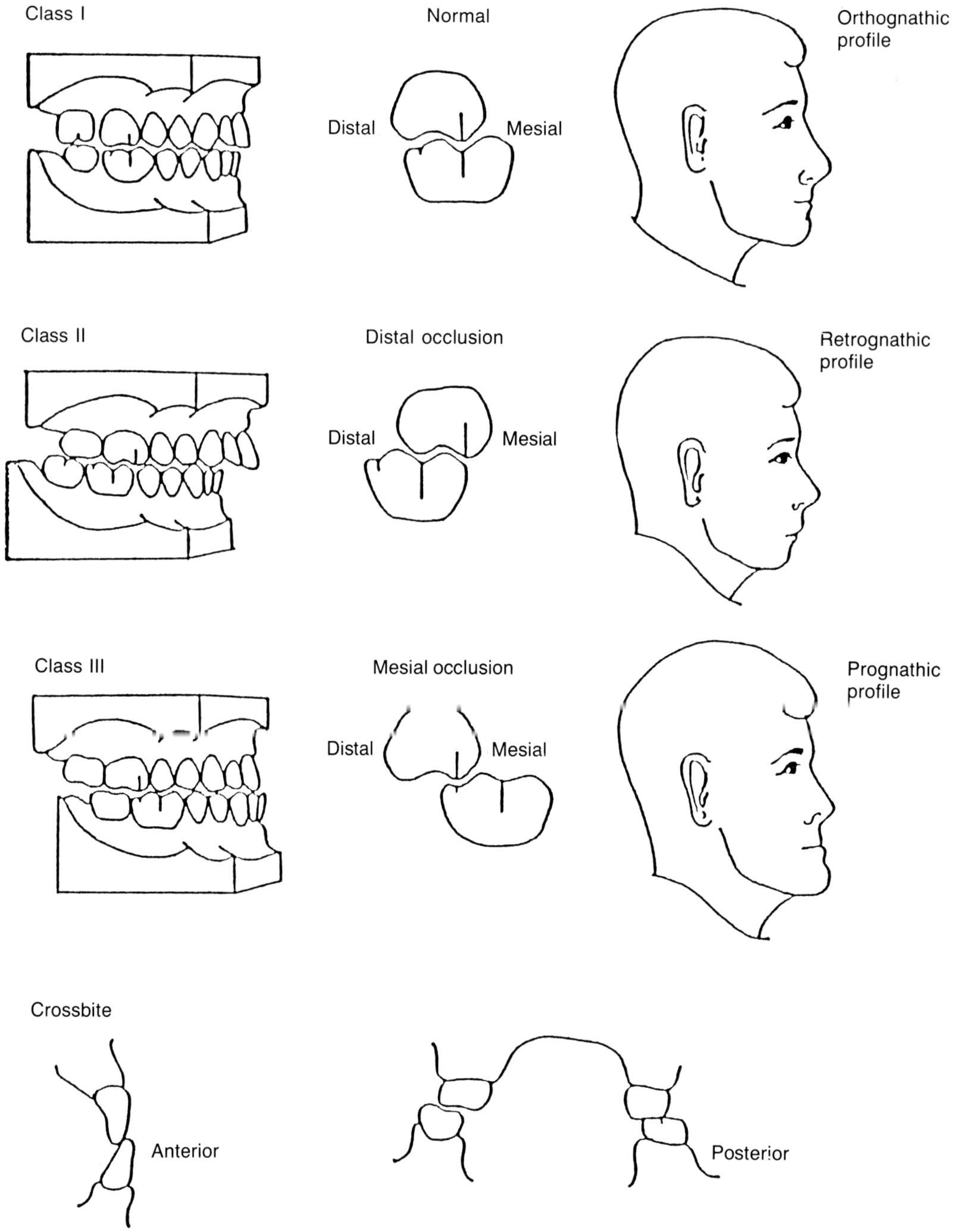

Figure 17–7 Classification of occlusal relationships showing casts in centric occlusion (left), facial view of maxillary and mandibular first molars (center), and the face profile that accompanies each of the three occlusal relationships (right). Anterior and posterior crossbites occur most frequently with a Class III malocclusion (below). Notice the typically large horizontal overlap of the maxillary incisors that typically accompanies Class II malocclusions.

Reviewing x-ray films from the child's dentist prior to treatment of maxillofacial injuries could be very helpful in achieving alignment of tooth-bearing bony fragments. It is advisable to consult with a pedodontist who can help provide proper treatment and care to children with maxillofacial injuries.

MANDIBULAR FRACTURES

The signs and symptoms of a fractured mandible are usually associated with the area of fracture, the displacement of the mandibular segment produced by unopposed muscle action on the fractured fragments, and localized swelling with ecchymosis and hematoma both in the soft tissues of the overlying skin and neck areas and in the mucosa and floor of the mouth. In addition, the patients all demonstrate some degree of malocclusion with deviation and displacement of the fractured segments.

Fractures involving the temporomandibular joint are accompanied by severe pain in the region of a condylar neck fracture when there is movement of the mandible. Tenderness is usually present and can be severe over the actual site of fracture and bony displacement. There is facial deformity due to swelling and distortion created by displacement of the fractured mandibular segments. Deviation toward the side of injury may be demonstrated when the patient attempts to open and close his mouth. It may be more apparent with the mouth open. Bilateral condylar neck fractures usually will appear with an anterior open-bite deformity due to the bilateral upward and posterior positioning of the ascending ramus (Fig. 17–8). This occurs because of the upward pull from the temporalis muscle as well as loss of vertical height due to medial forward displacement of the condylar segments out of the glenoid fossa by contraction of the external pterygoid muscles. There may also be signs of injury or laceration in the submental area or directly under the chin.

There is always a degree of malocclusion following fractures of the mandible where there is obvious or subtle displacement of the mandibular fragments. One need only have the patient open and close his mouth and hear the patient say that his "teeth do not feel like they are biting in a normal position." The area of swelling can appear early or may appear much later, especially in minimally displaced condylar fractures without other signs or symptoms. Opening and closing motions of the mandible can increase swelling overlying the fractured condylar neck segments. The child may also note a "cracking sound" whenever he tries to open and close his jaw, or there may be some grating of the bony fragments in the course of moving the jaw from side to side. Deviation from the midline may occur with a fracture through the mandibular angle on one side and without a contrecoup fracture on the other. These signs and symptoms of

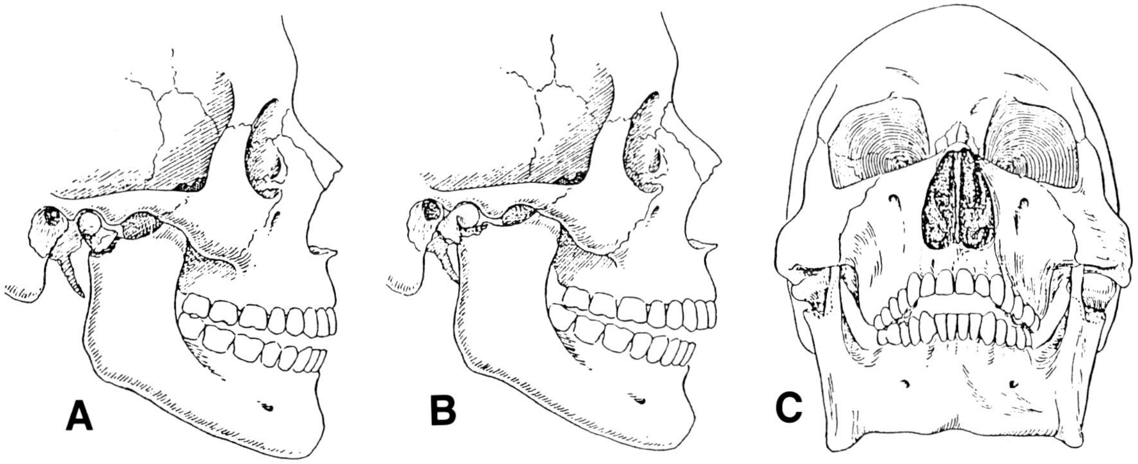

Figure 17–8 *A, B, C,* Displacement in unilateral and bilateral fractures of the neck of the mandibular condyles. Backward and upward displacement of the mandible is due to the powerful upward pull of the masseter, internal pterygoid, and temporalis muscles on the ascending rami. The bilateral ascending rami override the fractured and displaced condyles to produce an anterior open-bite deformity with only the maxillary and mandibular posterior molars in contact.

mandibular fractures can present clues to the diagnosis of the site of fracture and the muscles involved in the displaced segments. It is important to become familiar with the functions of the muscles of mastication to diagnose the fracture sites by clinical examination, especially if the child is uncooperative and frightened. Careful overall examination and evaluation can yield the correct diagnoses and allow for more rapid treatment planning.

Treatment

The precautions for maintaining airway and for débridement and careful examination of the endotracheal area following injury have already been noted. The airway must be open and clear before any type of maxillofacial surgical procedure is attempted. As noted previously, the use of a tracheostomy should be avoided, but if it is absolutely necessary, a low tracheostomy is usually preferred. During the first 5 years of life, however, because of the more superior location of the innominate vein, a low tracheostomy poses a danger to vascular structures. Likewise, the complications of tracheostenosis have to be considered when the higher approach is used for tracheostomy, especially if the first tracheal ring is incised. Because of these dangers, it is best to avoid the use of a tracheostomy. The airway can be maintained for several hours after surgery with an endotracheal tube left in place until the child is able to maintain his own airway and swallow his secretions.

Excluding nasal bone fractures, the most common facial bone fracture in young children is that of the mandible. Most fractures of the mandible occur in boys beyond 7 years of age; the incidence of injury to the mandible is virtually nil in children younger than 6. The anatomic growth differences between the facial skeleton in the child and adult explain the lower incidence of facial bone fractures in children (Fig. 17–9). As previously noted, the younger child is usually surrounded by a protected type of environment. Though the child may fall numerous times while learning to walk in contrast to the older, taller child, there is less force applied to the facial skeleton on impact. Since the distance traveled by the facial skeleton is less in the smaller and younger child than in the older and taller child, fewer facial bone fractures occur.[9a] The child's soft and resilient facial skeleton can withstand a considerable amount of trauma without fracture or complete separation of the bony segments. The cortical plates in the young child are thin, and the bone contains a greater proportion of cancellous substance, thus creating the high degree of elasticity present in a child's bones. It is for these reasons that fractures occur rarely and the green-stick nondisplaced fracture is more common in the younger child.[13,14]

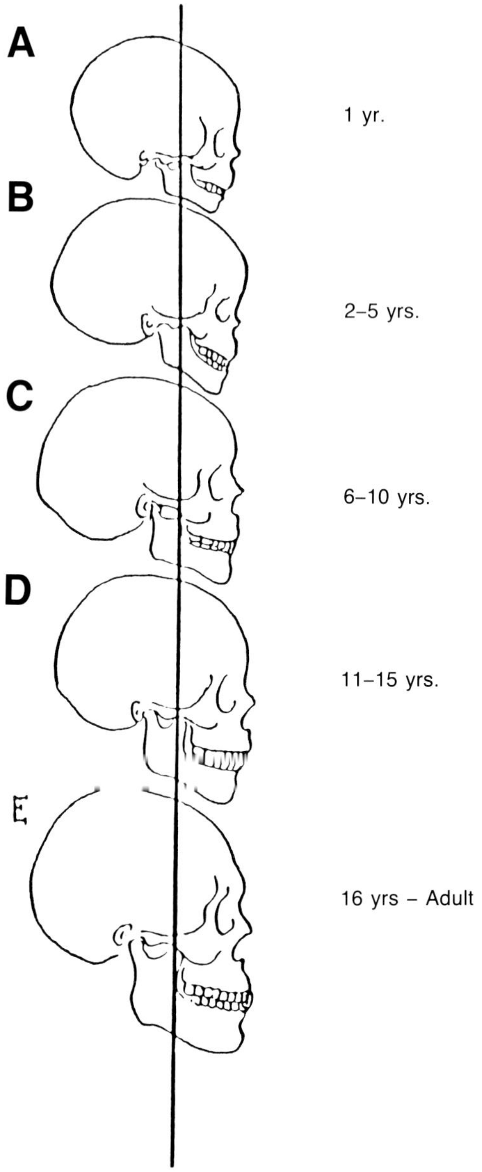

Figure 17–9 Tracings of a series of skulls showing changes in the size of the face and also of the position of the face in relation to the cranium. The growth of the face is associated with the growth of the jaws and the eruption of the teeth. From *C* through *E* the development of the sinuses along with growth of the maxilla and mandible increases the chance of maxillofacial injury.

The basal bone of the maxillary dentoalveolar segments is elastic and contains a number of deciduous and permanent teeth, thus creating a high tooth-to-bone ratio. The mandible as well as the alveolar segments of the maxilla contain a large amount of space occupied by the developing dental follicles separated by septae of delicate basal bone (Fig. 17–10). There is also a thicker inferior border of the mandible, along with the basal bony septae and dental follicles, which accounts for the nondisplaced green-stick fracture following a forceful blow through the follicular crypts and bony septae.

Along with a fractured mandible, most children appear with associated soft-tissue injuries in the form of facial lacerations and abrasions.[3] Skull fractures occurring concomitantly with closed head trauma and extremity and cervical spine injuries have been reported by McCoy and colleagues.[5]

The child seen immediately after injury is not a trustworthy historian and in many cases is quite uncooperative. A detailed account of the patient's injury is best obtained from a parent or an adult observer who might have been present at the scene of the accident. It is important to document the cause of injury and the force or direction of the blow to the injured site. The condition of the child's dentition as determined by radiographic views from the child's pedodontist or family dentist should be carefully reviewed and compared with the patient's existing dentition and occlusion at the time of examination. It is best, of course, to withhold sedation until the patient's sensorium and neurologic status have been cleared. When this is done, and the airway assured, it may be necessary to sedate the patient to examine the injured area and assess the severity of the fractures involved.

The site of mandibular fractures differs with age (Fig. 17–11) according to MacLennan.[4,15] Mandibular fractures in children under the age of 6 years most frequently occur as a *unilateral fracture of the body of the mandible*. The next most frequent is the *unilateral fracture of the body of the mandible* on one side with a contrecoup fracture of the mandibular condylar process on the opposite side. The third most frequent fracture is the *unilateral fracture of the mandibular condylar process only*. The fourth most frequent involves *both mandibular condylar processes* with or without a fracture in the incisor region of the body of the mandible. The fifth in frequency is *bilateral fractures of the body of the mandible in the region of the mental foramina*. Another interesting statistic is noted by Lehman and Saddawi[16] who reported a 66 percent incidence of condylar fractures in children under 10 years of age and a 44 percent incidence of condylar fractures in children 11 to 15 years of age. Children over 15 years old presented with 76 percent of the mandibular fractures occurring in the body and angle region of the mandible.

In reviewing the literature, growth and development of the midface, the bony orbits, and the max-

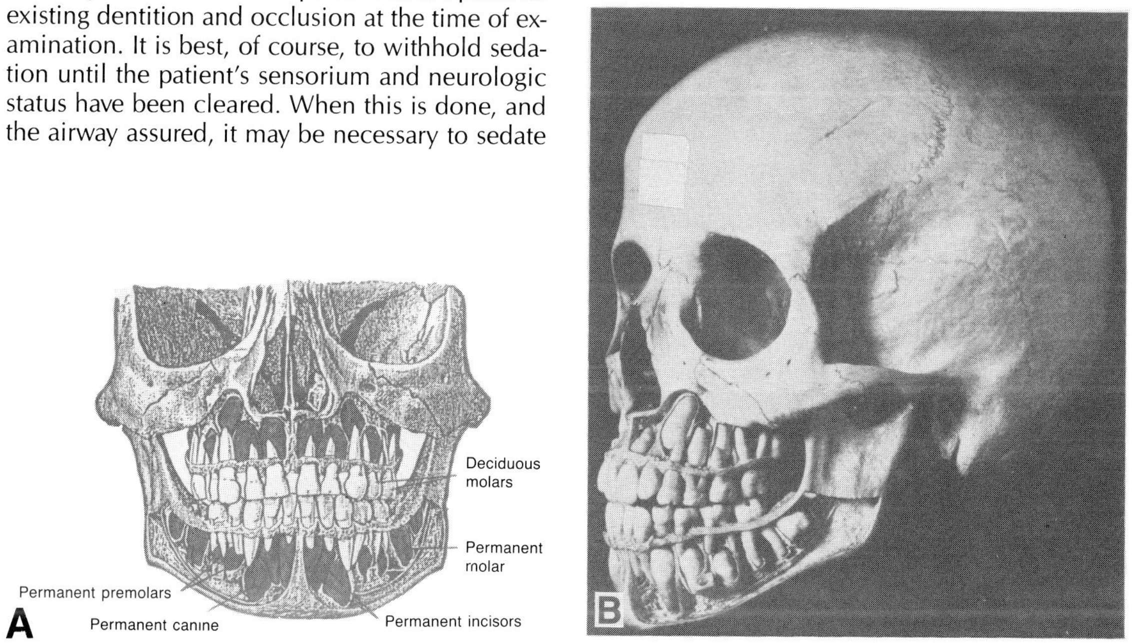

Figure 17–10 *A*, Mandible and maxilla with fully erupted deciduous dentition and developing follicles of the permanent dentition. The age of this child was 5 years. *B*, Skull of a 7-year-old child showing the position of the developing permanent dental follicles in relation to the temporary (deciduous) dentition.

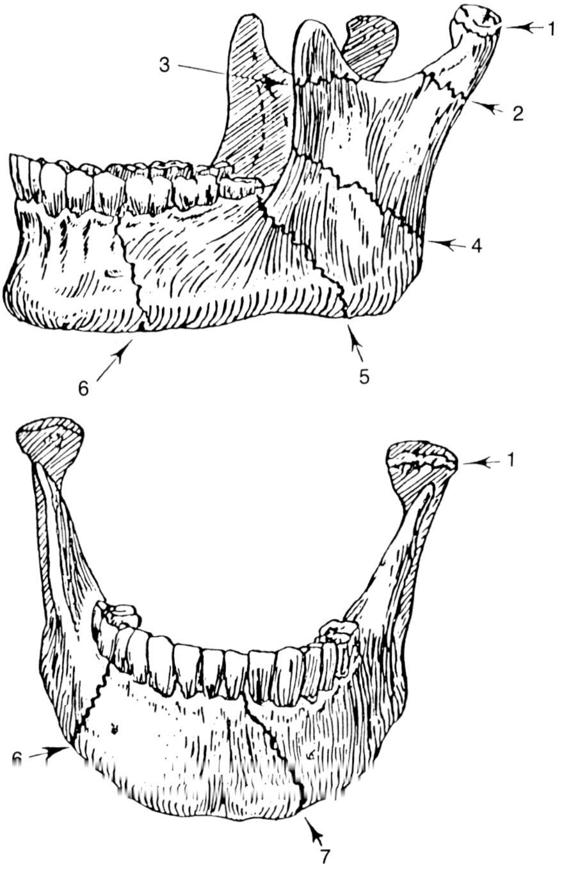

Figure 17–11 Sites of mandibular fractures. Most frequent mandibular fractures in children under 6 years of age: (1) unilateral fracture of body of mandible—6; (2) body fracture with contrecoup condylar fracture—6 and 1; (3) unilateral condylar fracture—1; (4) bilateral condylar fracture (with or without parasymphyseal or symphyseal fracture)— 1 and 1 or 1 and 7; (5) bilateral mental foramen body fractures—6 and 6.

illary and frontal sinuses account for the older child presenting with a higher incidence of multiple facial bone fractures. At 7 years of age, the bony orbits have reached adult dimensions, and at 6 to 10 years of age, the midfacial skeleton is made more vulnerable to fracture by simultaneous growth of the nasal aperture and development of the paranasal sinuses. Coupled with this fact is the increase in sports activity beyond the age of 7 years. From 7 to 16 years there is much more physical contact in sports and therefore a higher incidence of multiple facial bone fractures.

As I have noted, treatment of mandibular fractures in children essentially follows the same principles as in treating mandibular fractures in the adult. There are, however, definite anatomic dental features in the child that differ markedly from those of the adult patient. These anatomic differences are not only in the teeth but also in their bony and soft-tissue supporting structures. Understanding the growth potential in the developing permanent dentition, which occupies a large amount of the maxillary and mandibular alveolar bony areas of the child, should demonstrate the need to avoid surgical injury to these areas. Consequently, methods of immobilization; interdental wiring; application of arch bars, Ivy loops, and dental splints; and the use of the miniplate and screw techniques will all markedly differ from methods used in the adult, where there is a fully erupted permanent dentition and more solid bone in the alveolar segments of the mandible and maxilla.

Fractures in the young child most commonly occur in the developing body of the mandible which is packed with partially erupted and unerupted permanent dental follicles (Fig. 17–12). The fractures usually do not interfere with the tooth buds to any significant degree, and it is seldom necessary to remove these follicles to gain reduction of fractured segments. The bony fragments, when manipulated and reduced into good position, are usually aided in their reduction by the presence of these developing dental follicles and their bony septi which allow for more accuracy in fitting the pieces of the bony fracture "puzzle" together. Teeth or developing follicles in or near the line of fracture may demonstrate malformations or fail to develop fully and erupt. There has been no evidence in our series, however, that neoplastic transformation occurs in these follicles along the path of the fracture.

The child from 6 to 12 years of age has a mixed dentition. This means that there are erupted deciduous teeth with permanent developing follicles within the same bony body of the mandible so that both deciduous and permanent dentitions are present (Fig. 17–13). Since the roots of the primary teeth in this age group demonstrate various stages of absorption, they are not always suitable for interdental wiring of arch bars or intermaxillary fixation. Unlike the tapered shape of the permanent anterior dental crown, which is constricted at its lower cervical third, a comparable deciduous tooth is widest at its lower cervical third. Between the ages of 4 and 8 years, it is possible to apply arch bars around the deciduous teeth (Fig. 17–14). Careful placement of the interdental wires around the deciduous molars and canine teeth below their contact points may provide stable intermaxillary fixation for reduction and immobilization of a fracture (Fig. 17–15). Beyond 9 years of age, however,

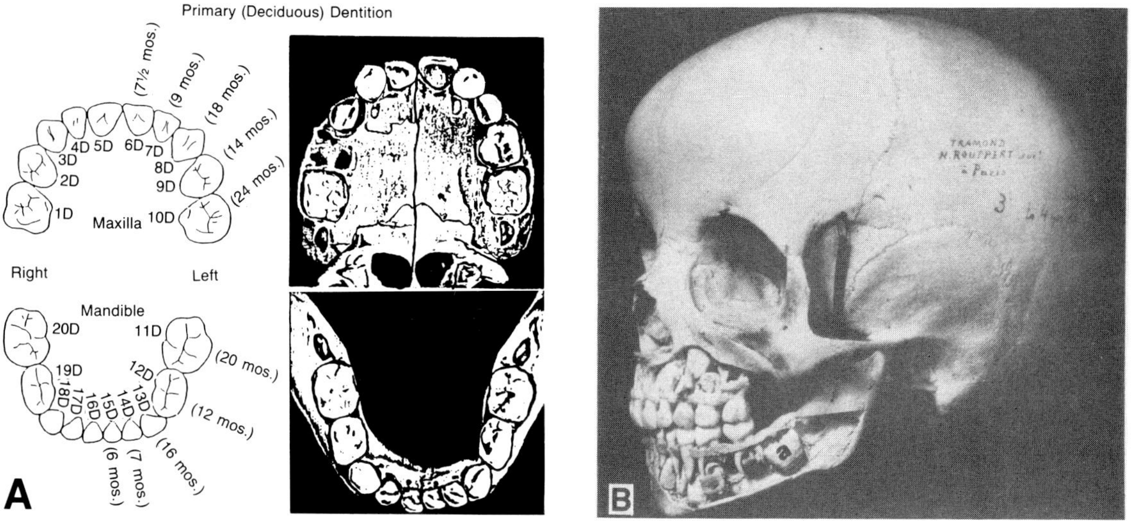

Figure 17–12 *A*, Fully erupted deciduous dentition of a 2-year-old child. *B*, A full deciduous dentition (20 teeth) and a developing first permanent molar (**a**) as well as incisors, canines, and premolar teeth.

fixation and immobilization in this manner could be unstable and unreliable due to erosion of the deciduous roots by the erupting permanent teeth and spreading of the interdental contact points. It is therefore necessary to use some other means of fixation.

A Jelenko or Winter type arch bar can be fixed to the deciduous dentition with interdental wires. In addition, circum-mandibular wires can be passed carefully around the mandible and the arch bar to stabilize the arch bar in position and support intermaxillary fixation in occlusion (Fig. 17–16B). In this case, one must be careful not to pass the wire through the bony mandible but rather around the mandible to avoid too much force, which can promote resorption of the malar bone. In applying an arch bar to the maxillary dentition with interdental wires, one can achieve stability by passing suspension wires from the arch bar through the pyriform rims and through the malar-maxillary buttresses (Fig. 17–16A). Subzygomatic circum-mandibular suspension wires can also be attached to a head cap to maintain the maxillary and mandibular dentition in intermaxillary fixation and the teeth in occlusion.

Another means of immobilizing or providing for interdental fixation and intermaxillary fixation is to fabricate an acrylic splint on a stone model made from an impression of the patient's teeth and alveolar structures. The splint can be cemented to the dentition or can be circum-mandibularly wired to the mandible or to the maxillary dentition with wires suspended from the pyriform rims as well as from the malar buttresses in the older child. It is also possible to bring out supporting subzygomatic circum-mandibular wires for suspension on a head cap.

A splint can be fabricated after an impression is taken of the fractured upper and lower jaws. The plaster model taken from the impression is then broken along the lines of fracture so that the fractured mandibular or maxillary segments can be put into proper occlusion on an articulator and thus create a means for fabricating an accurate acrylic splint. The mandibular splint can be wired to the mandible and fixed in place as can the maxillary splint. Segments of arch bars can be fixed to the acrylic splint so that intermaxillary elastic fixation can be applied (Fig. 17–17).

In the event that open reduction of a mandibular or maxillary fracture is necessary, one must be very careful to have good Panorex films or good anteroposterior and lateral open-bite films. The x-ray films of the mandible and maxilla are necessary to visualize the fracture and to determine the position of the developing permanent dentition and the unerupted follicles. It is prudent to place the interosseous wires along the thicker and more dense inferior border of the mandible through an appropriate incision so that the interosseous wire fixation will not impinge on any developing dental follicles.

There is a high degree of danger in the use of the miniplate and screw techniques for immobilizing fractures in the child's developing facial bone structures, including the mandible and maxilla.

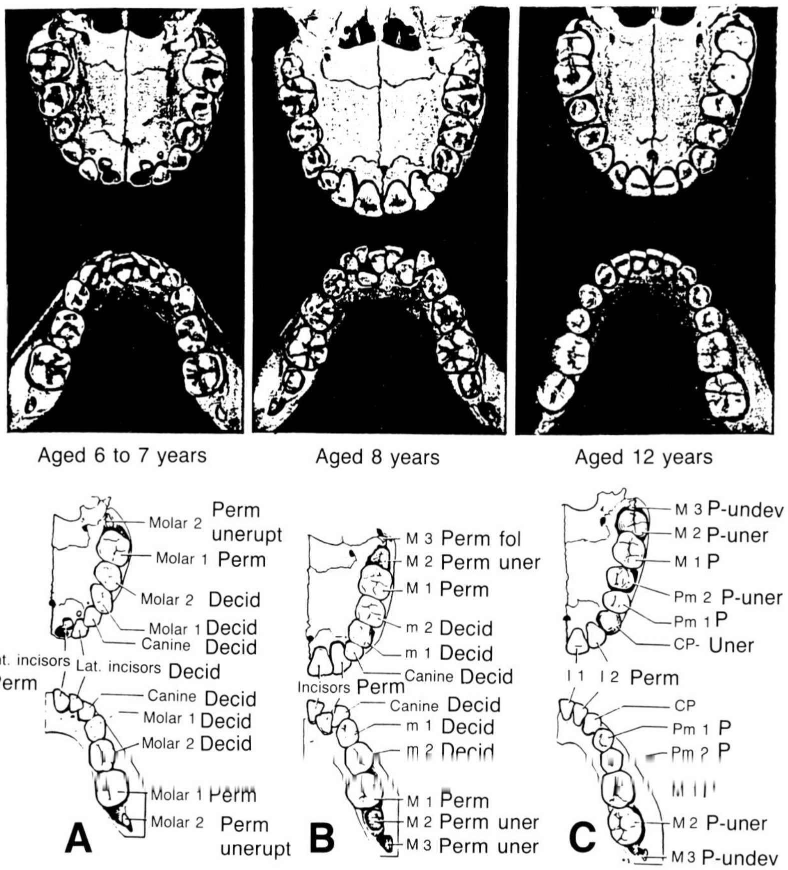

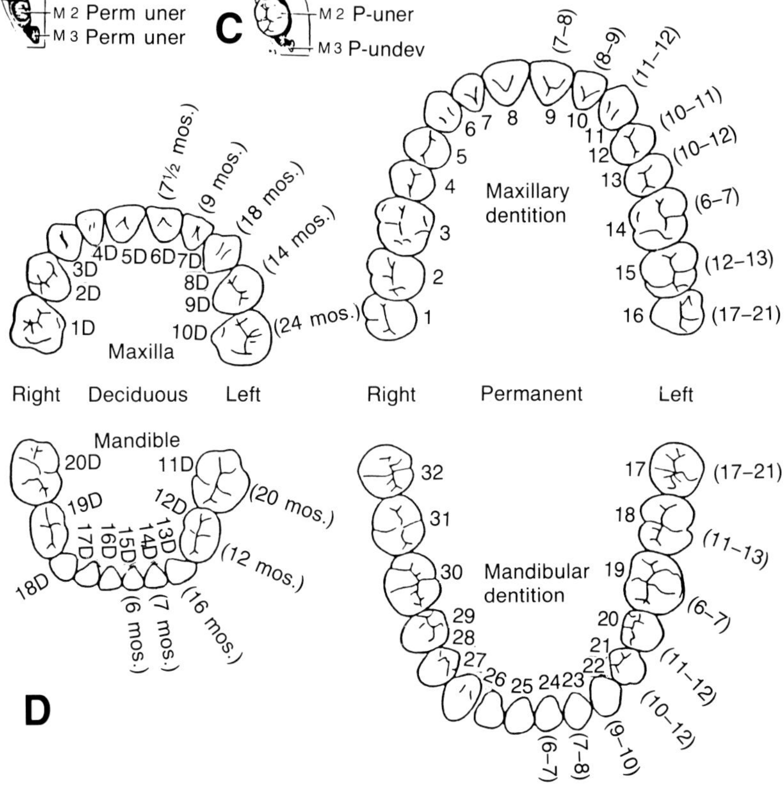

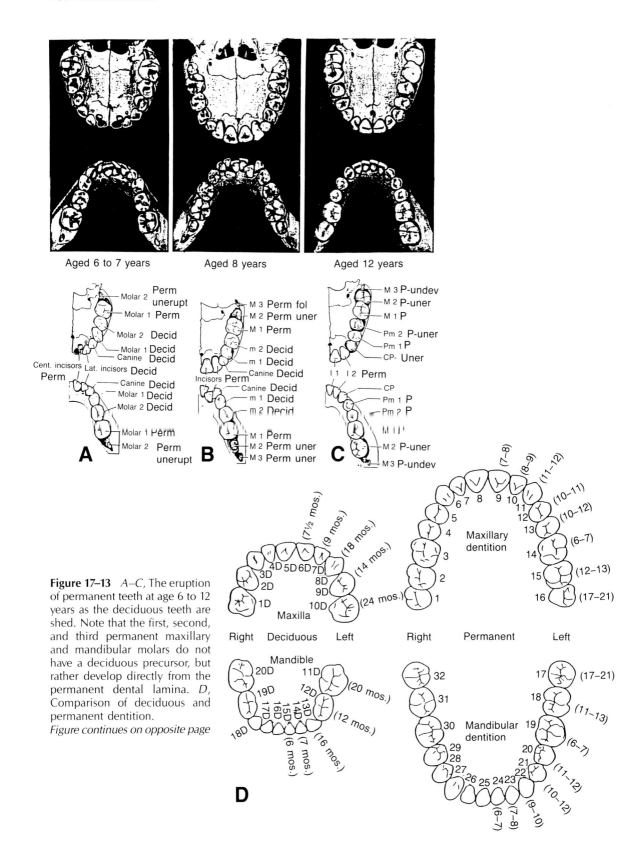

Figure 17–13 *A–C,* The eruption of permanent teeth at age 6 to 12 years as the deciduous teeth are shed. Note that the first, second, and third permanent maxillary and mandibular molars do not have a deciduous precursor, but rather develop directly from the permanent dental lamina. *D,* Comparison of deciduous and permanent dentition.

Figure continues on opposite page

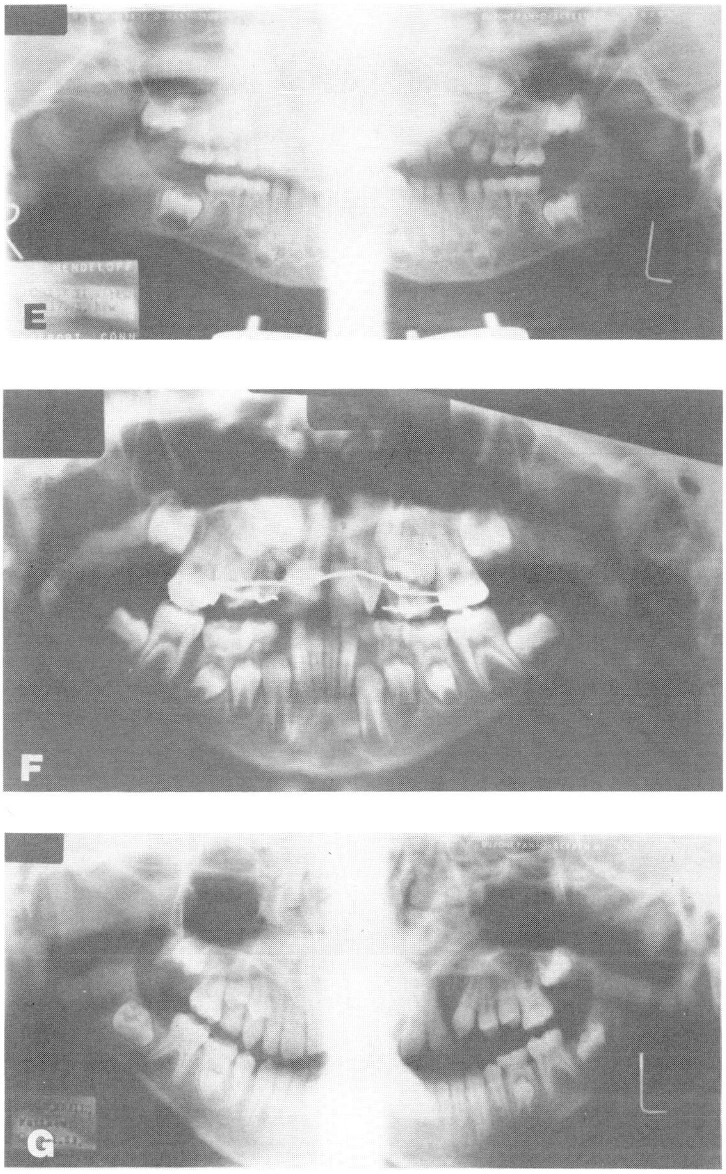

Figure 17–13 Continued. *E–G*, Examples of mixed dentition at various ages as seen on Panorex dental films. Ages 4–6 (*E*), 7–9 (*F*), and 10–13 years (*G*).

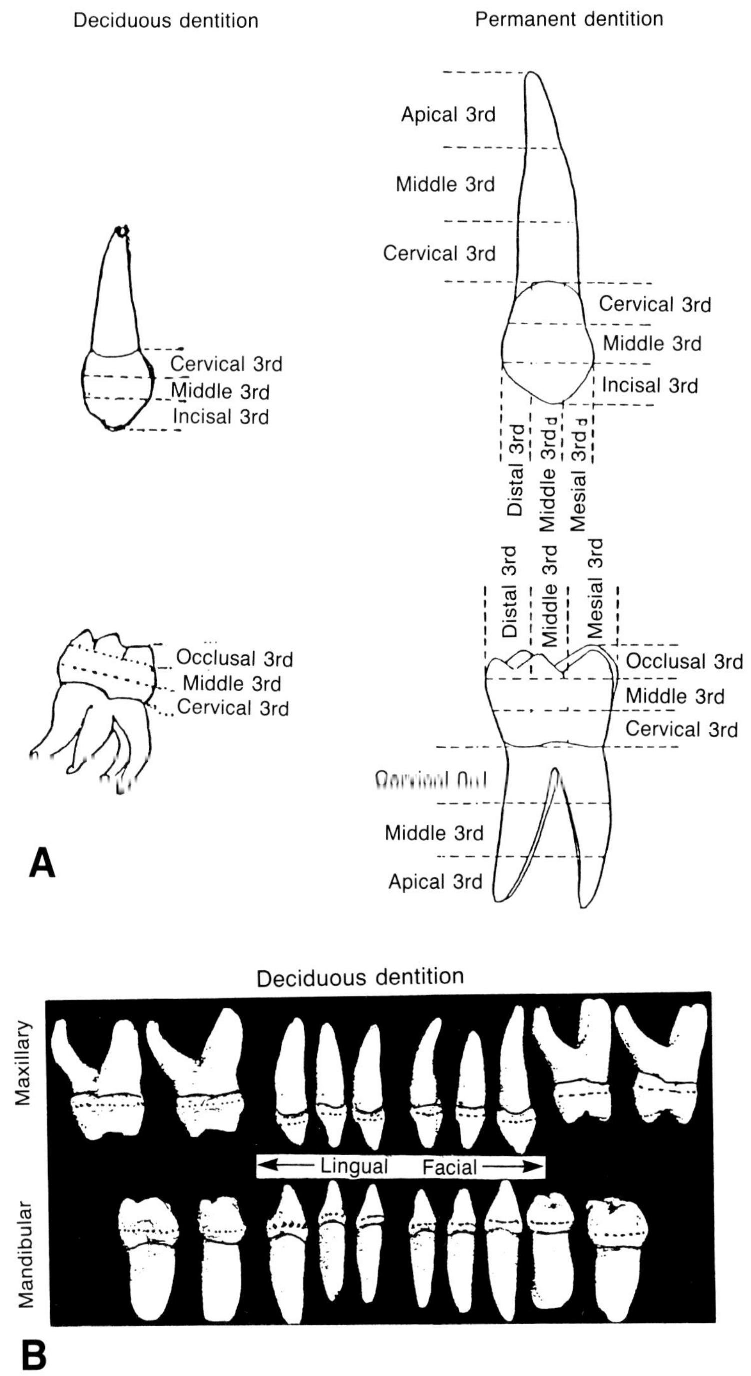

Figure 17–14 Permanent anterior and posterior dental crowns are widest at the junction of middle and incisal or middle and occlusal thirds. Thė anterior and posterior dental crowns of the deciduous teeth are widest at the junction of middle and cervical thirds and taper toward the incisal and occlusal surfaces. It is therefore difficult to maintain stable arch bar fixation to the deciduous dentition by interdental wires alone. Note that the deciduous teeth are marked at their widest circumference.

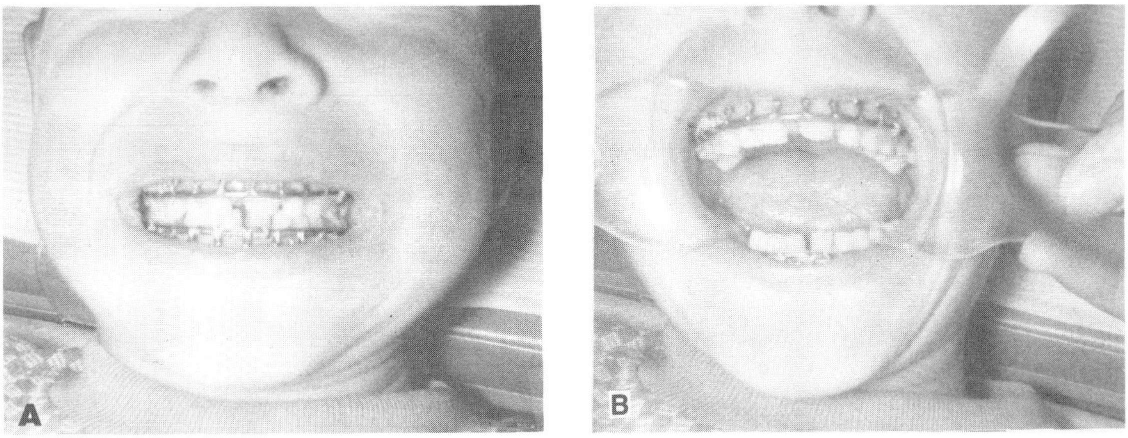

Figure 17–15 *A, B,* Jelenko dental arch bars adapted and secured to the deciduous dentition by carefully placed interdental wires around canine and molar teeth.

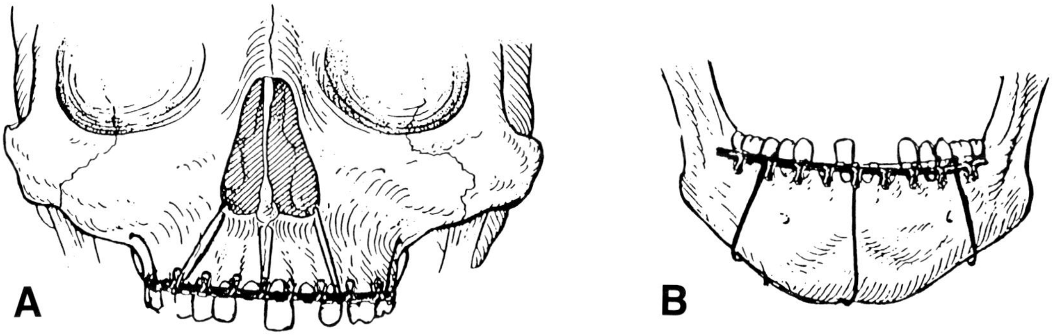

Figure 17–16 *A,* Circum-mandibular wires stabilizing mandibular arch bar on deciduous dentition. *B,* Maxillary arch bar stabilized by supplementary fixation wire through piriform margins, anterior nasal spine, and malar-maxillary buttress.

The screws and plates can injure the surrounding tissues as well as dental follicles and may impinge on potential growth centers. It is thus important that the surgeon treating injuries in children be familiar with the well-established "older" techniques for immobilization and interosseous fixation of facial bone fractures.

Young children have a high *osteogenic potential in the periosteum* of the facial skeleton for forming callus rapidly. This means that within 7 days of the injury, it may be very difficult to disrupt the callus bridging between the lines of fracture and to achieve a satisfactory reduction of the fractured segments.[9a] Once callus has formed and immobilization and fixation of the fractures are less than ideal in the young child, there is potential for alveolar bone growth and ability of the bone itself to remodel to some degree under the influence of mastication and occlusal forces.[4] There is also the "back-up" treatment through orthodontia[15] which can rectify many of the occlusal disharmonies that may result from the late treatment of fractures in children. Though this is a nice cushion to keep in mind, it must be emphasized that early reduction and immobilization of the fracture in good alignment is the treatment goal and should be carefully followed rather than leaving it for nature and the orthodontist to correct in the future.

If surgery and treatment of the facial bone fractures are contraindicated by the extent of acute injury, then the goal of early treatment has to be revised and the surgical treatment delayed until such time as it is safe to manipulate the fractured fragments. In that case, the growth potential and the expertise of the orthodontist should be considered. Even in the delayed treatment plan, however,

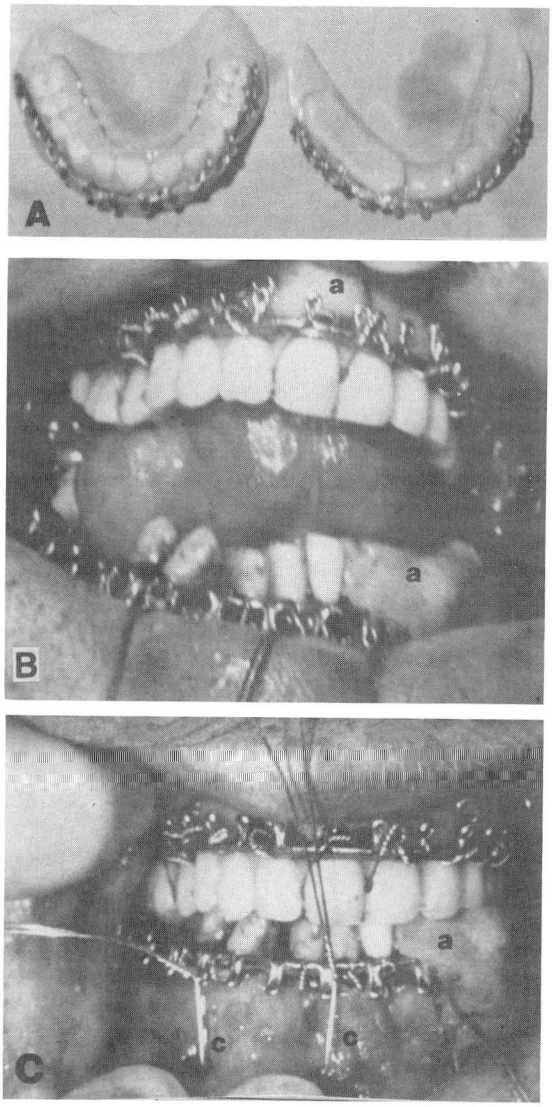

Figure 17–17 Acrylic dental splints with Jelenko arch bars (*A*) included and bonded to the splints so that the jaws can be immobilized in intermaxillary fixation. The maxillary and mandibular splints are attached to the mandible by circum-mandibular wires (*C*) and to the maxilla by interalveolar wires or by bilateral piriform interosseous and malar buttress wires. (**a**) indicates acrylic splints with attached Jelenko bar segments. (**c**) indicates circum-mandibular wires to secure splint to mandible.

there is a good possibility of correcting the malunited fracture if it does not jeopardize the integrity of the occlusion in the mandible or maxilla. Late repair and reconstruction is, of course, applicable in the form of orthognathic surgery and should be delayed until the growth potential has been fully realized. The major consideration in any fracture of the mandible or maxilla in a child is to protect the developing permanent follicles from injury. Therefore, techniques that involve interosseous wiring should be carefully and meticulously performed, and under no circumstances (where feasible) are any of the permanent follicles to be sacrificed.

The use of antibiotics pre- and postoperatively should be confined to compound fractures or to fractures communicating through lacerations where there has been contamination from foreign material. The definition of a compound fracture applies where fractures of the mandible pass through an area of dentition. The erupted tooth in the line of fracture is an open pathway to the fracture site and therefore is a compound fracture. Where the mandible is edentulous, the fracture, if not exposed intraorally or through the skin, is a well-contained fracture that has not been open to the "outside world" and therefore is not a compound fracture. The fracture in an area of dentition always communicates with the outside world through the periodontium.

Another consideration in the overall care of the patient with a fracture is to monitor fluid intake carefully as well as the child's hematocrit and hemoglobin. A moderate amount of bleeding can occur at the fracture site, and though transfusions are usually not required for the mandibular fractures, there may be other visceral injuries which can produce a significant blood loss that must be corrected. Proper healing of the wound and the fracture site is dependent on an adequate hematocrit and hemoglobin.

Caloric and fluid intake by means of a rubber tip syringe, straw, or cup should be carefully monitored. High-calorie, high-protein liquid diets that are tasty as well as nourishing are available in commercial form. The maintenance of good oral hygiene is most important for the healing process and can be facilitated by means of a Water Pik.

CONDYLAR FRACTURES

Condylar fractures in the child can be described as *intracapsular* or *extracapsular* (Fig. 17–18).

Intracapsular fractures are often comminuted crush (Fig. 17–18A) injuries involving the condylar head and its articular surface within an intact fibrous temporomandibular joint (TMJ) capsule. They also include high condylar neck fractures within the TMJ capsule and attachments of the external pterygoid muscle on the condylar neck above the sigmoid notch. This muscle attachment

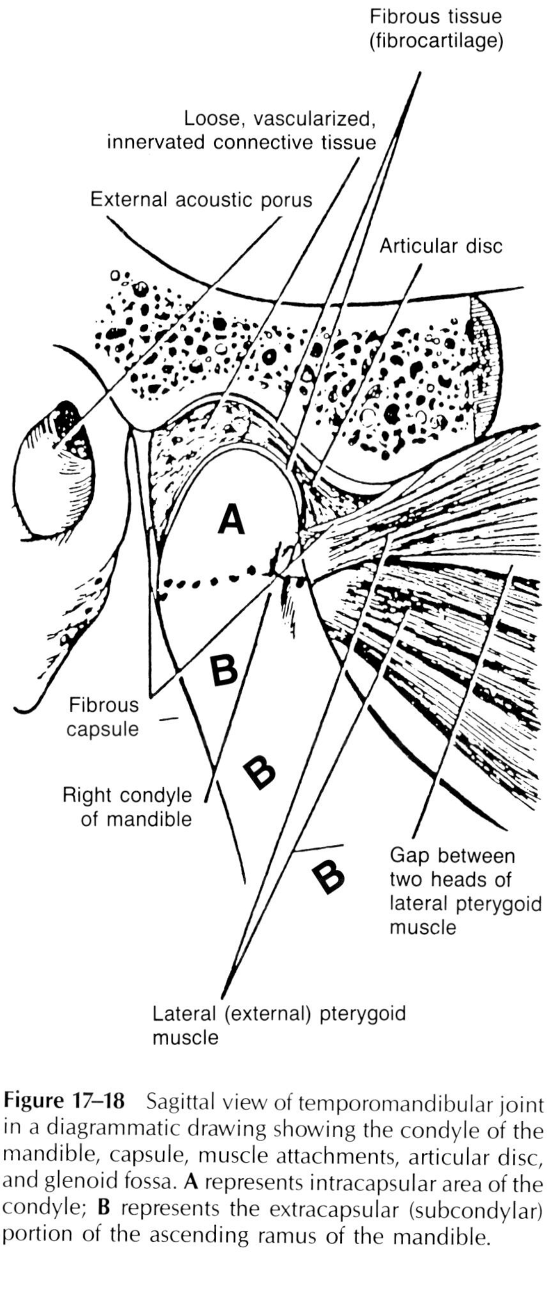

Figure 17–18 Sagittal view of temporomandibular joint in a diagrammatic drawing showing the condyle of the mandible, capsule, muscle attachments, articular disc, and glenoid fossa. **A** represents intracapsular area of the condyle; **B** represents the extracapsular (subcondylar) portion of the ascending ramus of the mandible.

produces medial and forward dislocation of the fractured condylar head and neck segment.

Extracapsular fractures are below the TMJ capsule and extend from the level of the sigmoid notch downward and backward below the neck of the condyle to the posterior aspect of the ascending ramus (Fig. 17–18B).

Open reduction and fixation is not indicated in the majority of condylar fractures. Where a deciduous or mixed dentition is present, adequate treatment involves immobilizing the jaws in occlusion to maintain vertical height of the ramus for a period of 2 weeks followed by gradual mobilization with opening and closing exercises of the mandible. The role of the mandibular condyle in facial growth is still controversial. For this reason, conservative treatment is recommended as injury to the growth center could result in an open-bite deformity. The conservative method of immobilization with intermaxillary fixation for 10 days to 2 weeks has stood the test of time and has produced good results with questionable interference in the growth potential and no open-bite deformities.

The TMJ is a ginglymodiarthrodial joint (Fig. 17–19) which differs from other bony joints in that the articulating segments are not separated by hyaline cartilage covering the articular surfaces, but rather by an articular fibrous disc with only a small number of cartilage cells scattered throughout the disc. The articulation is also unique in that the basic movements permitted by the TMJ complex are (1) a hinge movement between the condylar head of the mandible and the articular disc, and (2) an anteroposterior gliding movement of a condylar head combined with the articular disc in the glenoid fossa of the temporal bone. Both right and left condyles are coupled and move as a unit so that both TMJs pass through the same function at the same time unless the mandible is moving laterally.

Most surgeons recommend nonsurgical conservative treatment in pediatric patients regardless of the degree of condylar displacement. In his reviews of condylar fractures, MacLennan[4,17] stresses that complications arising from fractures of the mandibular condyle are "conspicuous by their absence." Many reports in the literature recommend that the typical unilateral subcondylar fracture presenting with minimal pain and without deviation be treated simply by a liquid diet and

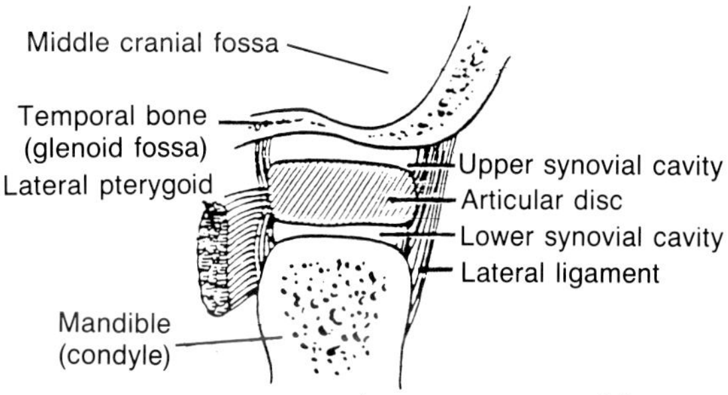

Figure 17–19 Diagrammatic representation of the temporomandibular joint. It is a ginglymoarthrodial joint with hinge and gliding movement.

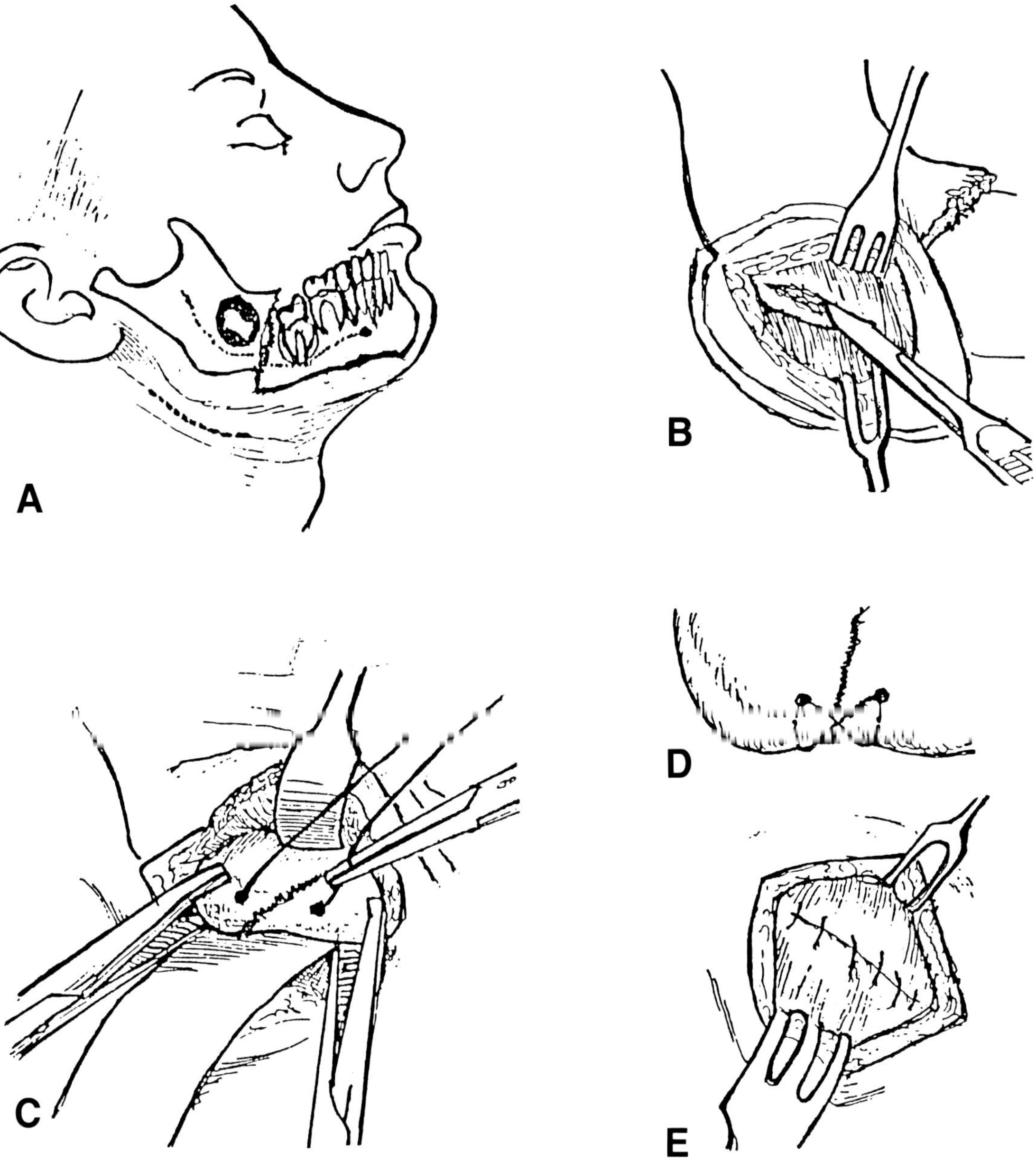

Figure 17–21 Open reduction of fracture at mandibular angle. *A*, Skin incision is marked in posterior neck crease approximately one finger's width below angle of mandible. *B*, Platysma muscle is incised with care taken not to injure mandibular branches of the facial nerve crossing over the posterior and common facial veins. *C*, The horizontal body and ascending ramus of the mandible are exposed at the mandibular angle by bluntly dissecting to the inferior border of the mandible and sharply incising the periosteum, which is then elevated from the mandible to expose the fracture along the inferior buccal and lingual surfaces. *D*, Drill holes are made along the inferior thick border of the fractured fragments. Care must be taken to avoid injury to the developing follicle of the third and erupting second molars. A figure-of-eight 25-gauge s.s. wire is placed to secure reduction as shown. *E*, Closure of platysma muscle and skin in layers.

an occlusal "stop" to prevent the mandible from riding upward. In general, though, fractures of the body of the mandible through the mental foramen area in children with noncarious teeth or even in children with minimal caries can be treated by fixing the Jelenko or Winter arch bar to the dentition of both the maxillary and mandibular segments with interdental wires and the fractured mandibular segments then reduced and brought into occlusion by elastic intermaxillary fixation. Intermaxillary fixation should be maintained for at least 3 to 4 weeks (Fig. 17–22).

PARASYMPHYSEAL AND SYMPHYSEAL FRACTURES

Fractures in the parasymphyseal and symphyseal areas are difficult to treat. Since there is a great deal of stress on the symphyseal line, it is most important that intermaxillary fixation be in accurate occlusion. Arch bar, Ivy loop, or acrylic splint fixation must be sufficiently rigid and stable to maintain the reduced position when intermaxillary fixation is applied. Surgical exposure of the inferior border of the mandible may be necessary to align the fracture fragments accurately and prevent tilting or distortion by pull from both the submandibular group of muscles and the external pterygoid, the masseter-pterygoid sling, and the temporalis muscles. With this in mind, an intraoral approach can be accomplished through a buccal or labial mucosal sulcus incision to expose the inferior border at the symphyseal area and place interosseous wire fixation through drill holes. Miniplates and screws are not to be used in the child's developing mandible, especially with the presence of a large number of developing permanent follicles in addition to the deciduous teeth.

The decision whether to use arch bars or individual Ivy loops is one of judgment. In most cases, simple Ivy loops between deciduous molars and between canine and deciduous molars can effectively immobilize the mandible and maxilla in correct occlusion. However, where there are parasymphyseal fractures, it is best to use an arch bar to distribute the forces of intermaxillary fixation evenly around the entire dental arch. With the child normally straining against fixation, elastic traction is preferred over wire for intermaxillary fixation. In the intractable child who attempts removal of these elastics, it may be necessary to augment the elastics with intermaxillary thin 28- or 30-gauge wire to discourage finger manipulation by the patient. Conservative treatment, careful technique and recognition of what structures lie within the child's mandible and maxillary alveolus are required of all surgeons treating maxillofacial injuries in children.

ALVEOLAR FRACTURES OF THE MANDIBLE AND MAXILLA

Alveolar fractures of the maxilla and anterior mandible are fairly common impact type injuries resulting from vehicular as well as occasional sports injuries. Maxillary alveolar fractures are more common than mandibular alveolar fractures. Most often the fracture consists of a buccal plate or labial plate with teeth attached to the bone and partially avulsed from the maxillary or mandibular alveolus. In this situation, the treatment of choice is to replace the teeth attached to the alveolar plate in the alveolar sockets. In many cases, vascularity is still intact and apical vessels are maintained in the alveolar segment so that the tooth need not be extracted or sacrificed. In addition, any follicles that appear to have been elevated or dislodged should be replaced in their crypts. The alveolar plates themselves, i.e., the labial or buccal plates, can be replaced in the alveolar segment from which they were partially avulsed or fractured provided the overlying gingival tissues are intact and attached by periosteum to the bone. These segments will survive and heal very well if they are fixed in position. There is a chance that the injured teeth within the alveolar sockets may lose their viability. To this end, the consultant pedodontist or the child's dentist should carefully follow the course of healing with pulp testing of involved teeth for viability. If root canal therapy is indicated, it should be done to salvage a permanent tooth. In general, placing the partially avulsed alveolus with the attached teeth back into their correct position and suturing the torn gingiva and alveolar mucosa should be performed as early as possible. A stent or a continuous interdental wire should be used to maintain the segment in correct position and occlusion with intermaxillary fixation applied between the uninvolved *posterior* teeth until the bony fragments are thoroughly healed and stable, at 3 to 4 weeks (Fig. 17–23).

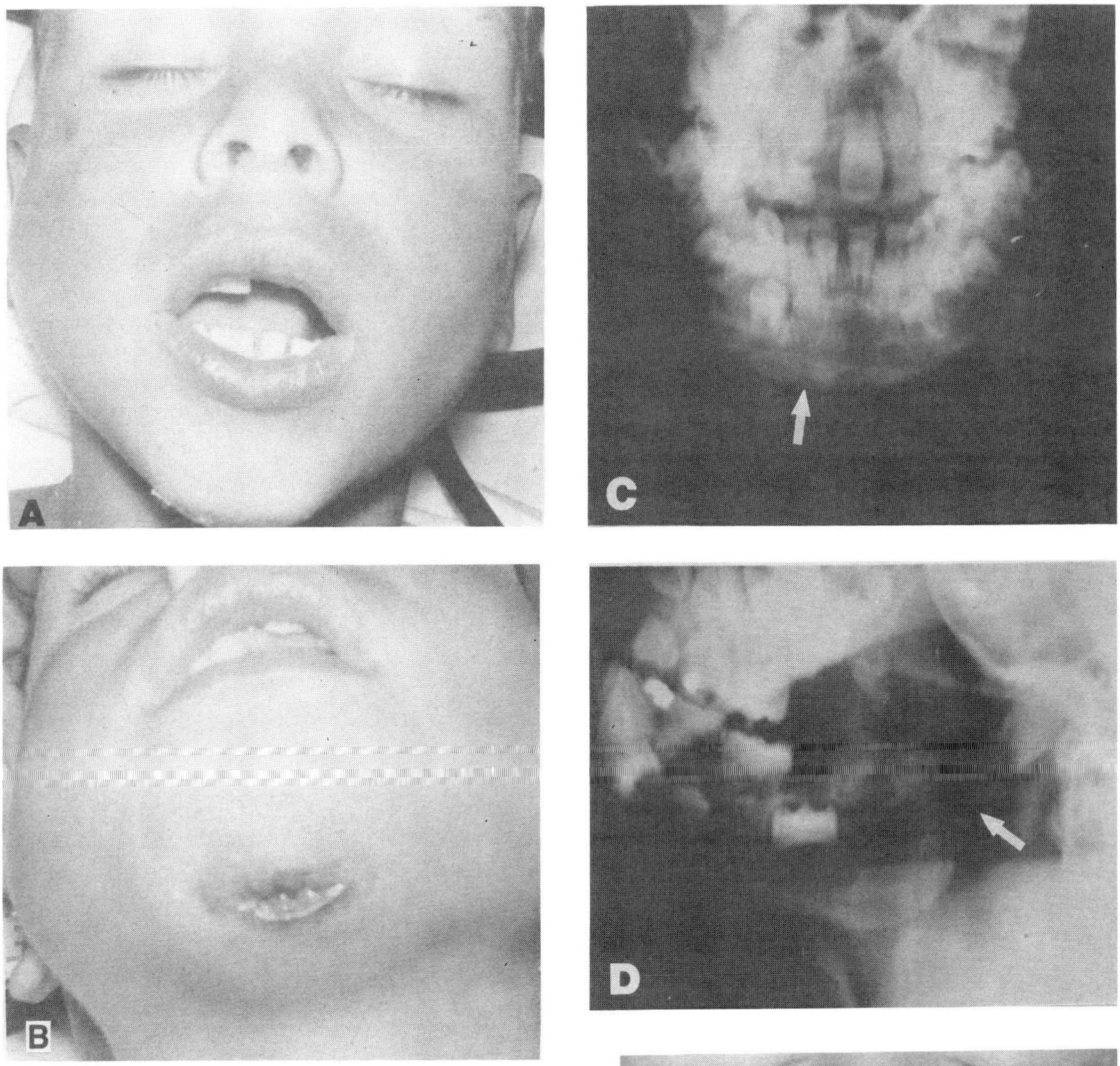

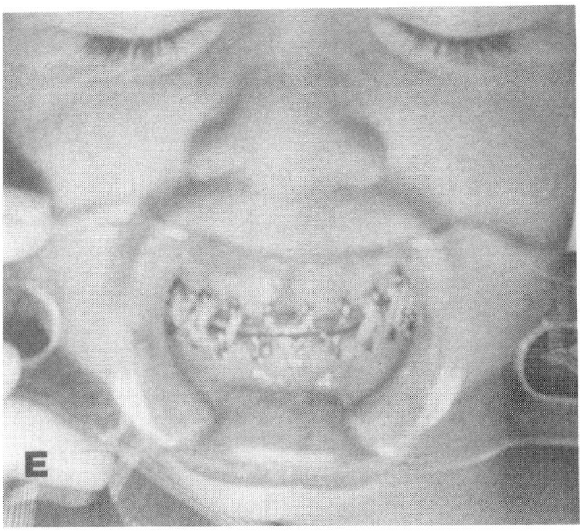

Figure 17–22 A 6-year-old boy was walking behind his horse and was kicked in the chin by its hind hoof. *A*, Swelling of right cheek, unable to close jaws in occlusion, and swelling in left cheek overlying left ramus. *B*, Laceration and contusion of chin at point of impact. *C*, X-ray film showing mandibular parasymphyseal fracture in a mixed dentition. Note the majority of the mandibular bony structure is occupied by the deciduous teeth and the permanent developing teeth within their follicles (arrow). *D*, Lateral oblique x-ray film showing fracture of ascending ramus (arrow). *E*, Arch bars in place and secured by interdental wires. Intermaxillary fixation elastic bands are in place. Note that no elastics are overlying the incisors.

Figure continues on opposite page

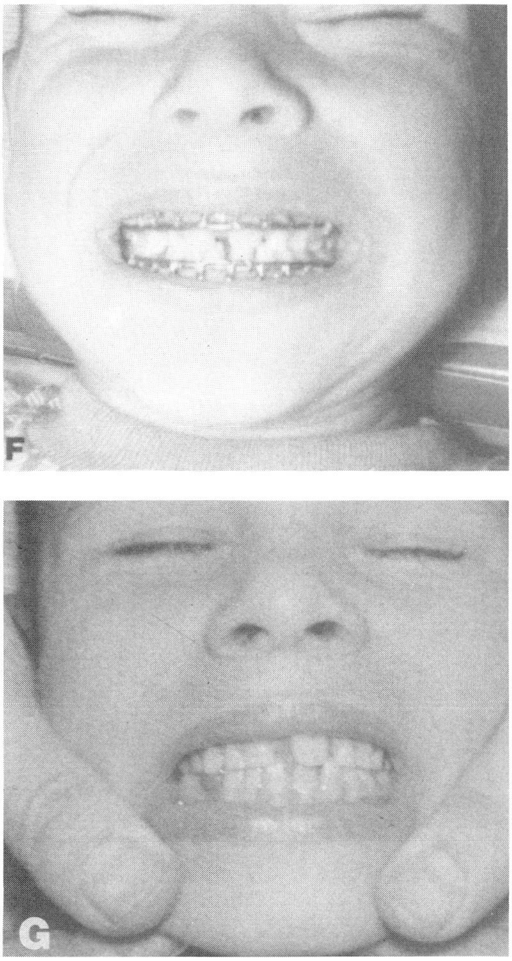

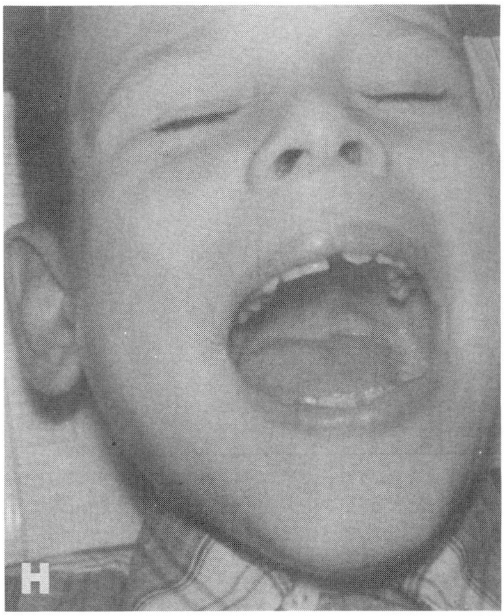

Figure 17–22 Continued. *F*, Intermaxillary fixation discontinued after 4 weeks. At the end of 3 weeks several of the elastic bands were removed to allow some early motion. The arch bars were left in place for a total of 5 weeks. Note good occlusal relationship. *G*, *H*, Patient 2 months after arch bars were removed. Patient in Class I occlusion and opens jaws fully.

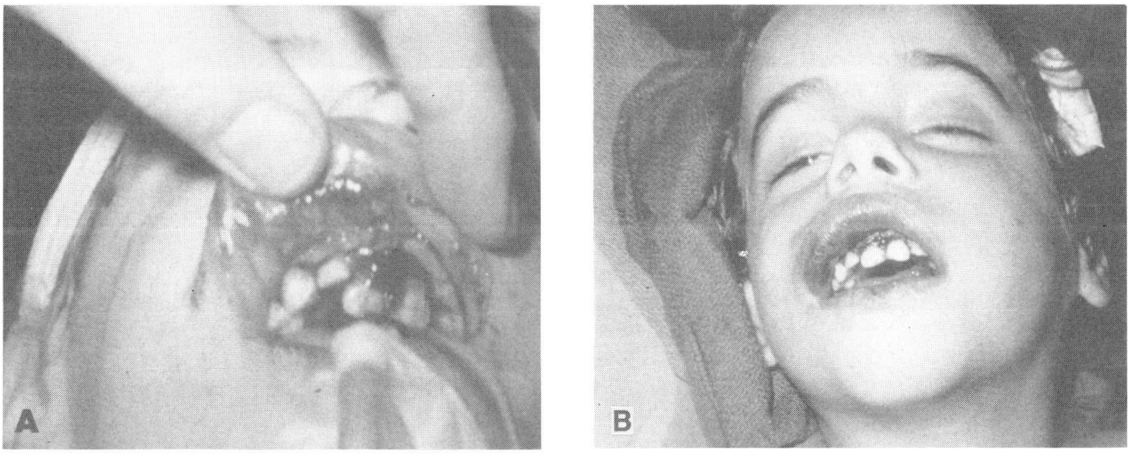

Figure 17–23 Alveolar fracture of anterior maxilla with partial avulsion of alveolar mucosa and gingiva but with teeth attached to alveolar fragment (*A*). Fractured alveolar segment was replaced in correct position along with the avulsed teeth which still demonstrated periodental attachment, and was stabilized by a continuous interdental wire along with an acrylic stent on the palate surface (*B*). Intermaxillary fixation was applied between the posterior teeth for 3 weeks.

FRACTURES OF THE MAXILLA

Fractures involving the midface and maxilla are less common than fractures of the mandible and nose. In early childhood, fractures of the maxilla are seldom seen until the age of 10 years but with pneumatization of the maxillary sinuses and growth of the maxilla itself these structures become more susceptible to injury. Alveolar fractures of the anterior maxilla are more common as a segmental fracture which has been noted in the preceding section of this chapter. The Le Fort II and Le Fort III fractures are for the most part nonexistent in early childhood, and in the child beyond 10 years of age, only the Le Fort II fracture is occasionally encountered (Figs. 17–24 to 17–26).

Segmental fractures of the maxilla, which can occur from a direct blow, should be reduced as soon as possible once pneumatization of the sinus has been initiated. A dental arch bar is applied with interdental wire fixation and suspended to the pyriform margin, as previously described, as well as around the anterior nasal spine or through the malar buttress to provide adequate stabilization of the arch bar on the mixed dentition. The maxillary arch is then placed in occlusion with the mandible and immobilized by elastic intermaxillary fixation. Again, where an arch bar is to be applied to unstable teeth in the mandible, stabilization can be secured by placement of circum-mandibular wires around the arch bar.

A very rare high Le Fort II or Le Fort III fracture of the midface can occur where the blow has been severe and where the impact force involves the maxillary-malar junction and malar-frontal junction. The problems of applying arch bars to a mixed dentition have been noted earlier in this chapter and apply in this case also. In addition to the application of arch bars, however, the stabilization of the fractured segment superiorly is also indicated. In these cases, the use of a headcap is questionable, since the child does not tolerate this type of suspension. The frontomalar area is moderately unstable as a supporting buttress; however, one can use a more superior portion of the frontal zygomatic process on the frontal bone and place suspension wires from there down to the maxillary arch bar. The arch bar should be carefully wired to the deciduous dentition and fixed to the piriform area of the maxilla anteriorly and to the malar buttress posteriorly. This whole segment can then be moved or pulled upward and suspended on the zygomatic process of the frontal bone bilaterally. In addition, an arch bar placed on the mixed dentition of the mandible and secured with circum-mandibular wires in the bicuspid area bilaterally can also be used in applying intermaxillary fixation and immobilizing the upper maxillary fragments. Immediate reduction and immobilization as well as intermaxillary fixation are of great importance in achieving a good anatomic result and accurate occlusion.

Open reduction of maxillary fragments can be achieved through a buccal and labial sulcus incision. However, one must be careful not to denude

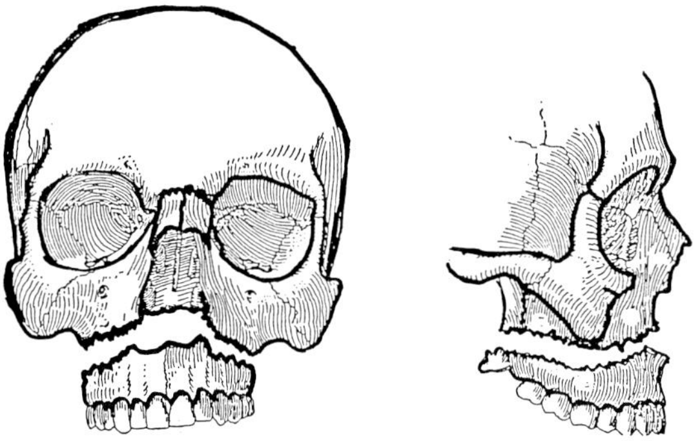

Figure 17–24 Le Fort I maxillary fracture.

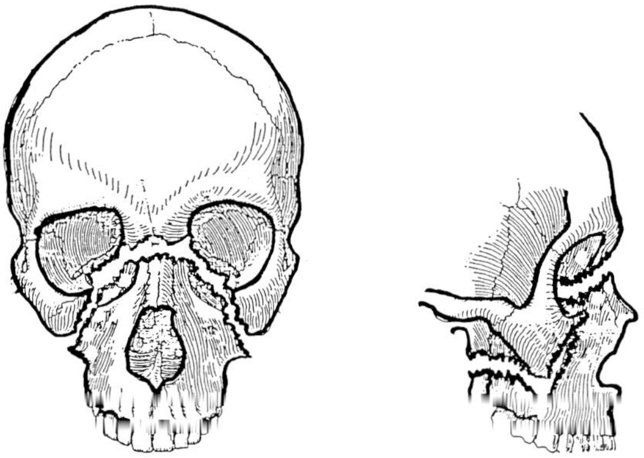

Figure 17–25 Le Fort II maxillary fracture.

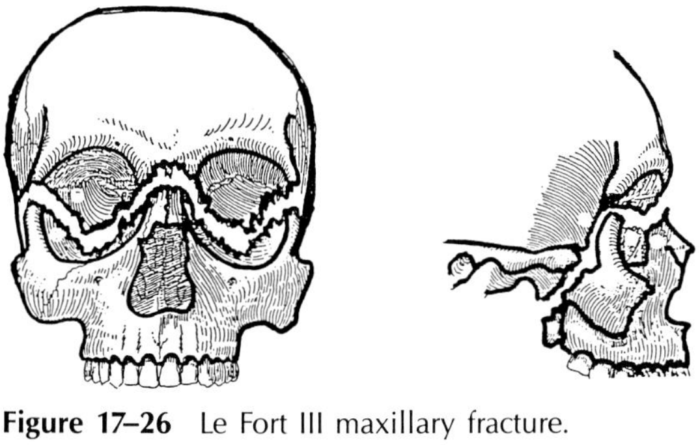

Figure 17–26 Le Fort III maxillary fracture.

wide areas of the bone with elevation of periosteum which can affect the vascularity of that area of bone. Again, use of miniplates and screws is not applicable in this type of fracture involving children under 14 years of age. Interosseous wiring of fragments can be achieved in the malar buttress area through appropriate drill holes using 26- or 28-gauge wire. Anatomic reduction and fixation of fragments using a combination of interosseous wires as well as intermaxillary fixation of correctly applied and stable dental arch bars will ensure good alignment of the bony fragments and restoration of the dental arch to provide for the normal eruption of permanent teeth. Injury to the dental follicle in the line of fracture may destroy the follicle and prevent the normal development of the permanent tooth. The tooth may never erupt and may remain partially formed and unerupted in situ.

In the case of a Le Fort type of maxillary fracture, intermaxillary fixation and stabilization of fracture fragments with suspension correctly applied should be maintained for 3 to 4 weeks. Elastic intermaxillary fixation is preferred over wire, and after 4 weeks mobilization should be initiated gradually and diet progress from liquid to soft food.

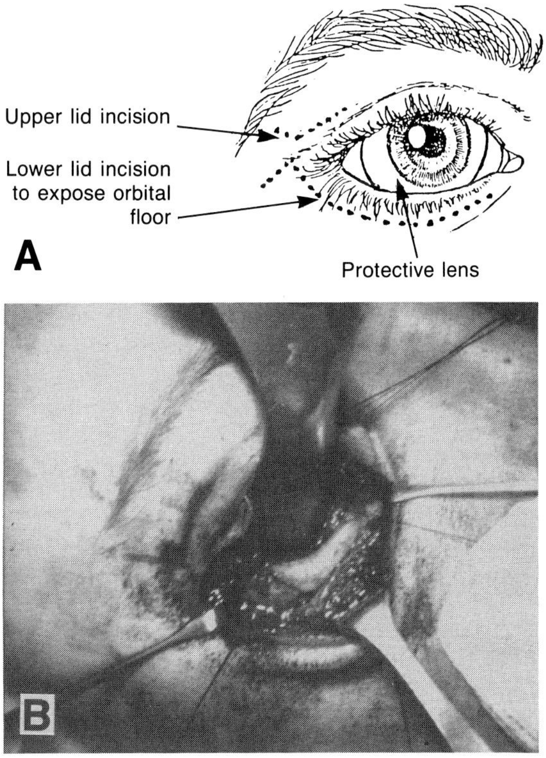

Figure 17–27 *A*, Lower eyelid blepharoplasty type incision to expose orbital floor. An upper lateral eyelid incision may also be used to expose the frontozygomatic suture. *B*, Intraoperative view of exposed orbital floor and rim fractures with wire fixation and orbital retractor in place. Note marking on lateral upper eyelid for an incision to expose the frontozygomatic suture.

ZYGOMATICOMAXILLARY ORBITAL FRACTURES

The malar bone forms the lateral wall of the maxillary antrum, the lateral wall of the orbit, and, at its junction with the malar processes of the temporal, frontal, and maxillary bones it forms an arch complex that is subject to injury, especially from the age of 10 years and up. Because this arch complex is readily struck by blows to the side of the face, fractures can involve the floor of the orbit, the malar bone, and the connections of malar bone to frontal, maxillary, temporal, and sphenoid bones. A crush injury can produce severe facial deformity as well as impair function of the globe and motion of the mandible. This deformity should be treated by open reduction and exploration of the orbital floor. A direct approach for visualization of the floor of the orbit is made through a lower lid blepharoplasty type incision which can be extended upward to visualize the frontozygomatic junction. Where the vertical height of the lateral orbital wall is such that a lower lid incision would not suffice to visualize fully the frontozygomatic suture, a lateral portion of an upper eyelid incision can also be made with an oblique upward extension that will provide excellent visibility of the frontozygomatic suture (Fig. 17–27).

It is important to visualize the floor of the orbit in these cases. Visualization under the orbital septum allows for examination of the infraorbital rim and the orbital floor as far back as the superior orbital fissure. Only by this means can a possible depressed posterior floor fracture be identified and corrected at the time of exploration. The lateral orbital rim should be stabilized at the frontozygomatic suture by interosseous 28-gauge wire through drill holes placed posteriorly behind the frontozygomatic junction and the malar-maxillary junction. The fractured orbital rim should likewise be elevated, reduced, and joined by interosseous wires in correct alignment with preservation of the infraorbital nerve, to re-establish a stable infraorbital malar, maxillary, and medial nasal rim.

The opinion of some surgeons that in the child two-point fixation is all that is needed in this type of malar-orbital fracture is not shared by all. It is my opinion that the fracture of the malar bone at the maxillary buttress must be reduced and held by the same type of interosseous wiring so as to provide a third point of stability. There are a number of instances in which only two-point fixation was used and subsequent herniation in the more posterior floor of the orbit resulted in enophthalmos. By stabilizing the malar-maxillary buttress area, the malar-orbital fracture fragment is invariably torqued back into position to elevate the posterior floor of the orbit and provide support for the globe.

Where there has been comminution of the floor of the orbit, it is preferable to use an autogenous bone graft rather than Silastic. Silastic support can be used as a temporary measure in the young child until there has been sufficient growth and development to replace the Silastic with an autogenous bone graft. In the older child (12 to 15 years of age) one can use rib or iliac bone without violating the iliac crest. The outer table of iliac bone can be harvested and presents a concavity that nicely accommodates the convexity of the globe. The bone graft can be inserted over the comminuted orbital floor to provide support for the globe. Onlay bone grafts in this area should be thin so that the globe is not distorted or excessively elevated. This requires harvesting a thinner graft with a small amount of cancellous material as well as contouring the graft before placing it on the orbital floor. A rib graft can be used but requires splitting the rib and inserting more than one fragment to maintain support of the globe. The bone graft is inserted beneath the orbital septum and periosteum directly onto the bony surface.

Attempts to manipulate and reduce the fractured fragments of the orbital floor are usually not rewarding. However, in some instances where there has been a fracture through the maxillary antrum, one can use that opening to manipulate fragments under direct vision into continuity with the remaining bone that is present in the floor. Even then, a thin bone graft is indicated for support of the globe.

Entrapment may occur in severe fracture deformity involving the malar orbital complex. In that case, release of entrapment is carried out in the same way one would for an adult (Fig. 17–28). Fixation of the bone graft placed on the orbital floor is often unnecessary. Where the bone is covering a large defect, however, it is best to drill a small hole at the orbital rim and through the graft to stabilize the graft anteriorly and prevent anterior movement of the bone graft. A 4–0 PDS suture works nicely in this area and is absorbed over a period of time.

The malar arch complex is subject to fracture and ordinarily the sharpness of the fracture fragments is such that, when reduced, they often stay in place. However, there are situations in which the fragments do not stay in place and in these cases open reduction is indicated. The malar arch complex fracture usually involves injury of the frontozygomatic area and the zygomaticotemporal area. A superior incision can be made for open reduction of the zygomaticotemporal segment, and an upper lateral eyelid incision can be used to approach the frontozygomatic segment. By wiring in these two areas, the fragment can be immobilized and secured in position.

The malar arch complex fracture is usually a simple fracture even though it may involve breaks at three points. A Gilles approach beneath the temporalis fascial envelope makes it possible to elevate and reduce the fracture, and in most cases the fracture will remain reduced.

The malar arch is rarely fractured in the child under 8 years of age. Between 8 and 14 years, fractures become much more severe from a direct blow to the malar arch complex and they often involve the floor of the orbit. The orbital floor must also be explored in older children with these complex malar injuries.

NASAL AND NASOFRONTAL FRACTURES

Nasal fractures occur more frequently than any other fracture involving the facial skeleton. Though mandibular fractures are the most common fractures in the child associated with the maxillofacial skeleton, nasal fractures, apart from fractures of the maxillary segments, occur in greater numbers. Many of the nasal fractures in children occur as simple fractures of the green-stick variety with no displacement or malposition of the nasal bones. These go on to heal without incident and often are not detectable 2 to 3 months after the injury. However, a lateral blow to a child's nose will displace the nasal bones medially or produce comminution and splaying out of the nasal bones, often creating a wider nasal pyramid.

A *septal hematoma* may develop which prevents the nasal bones from being brought into good apposition by manual manipulation. This hematoma must be evacuated if good anatomic reduction and healing are to take place following surgical treatment. The hematoma may result in a saddle-nose deformity which can be prevented if the hematoma is immediately evacuated or at least drained 2 to 3 days after the injury. The septal

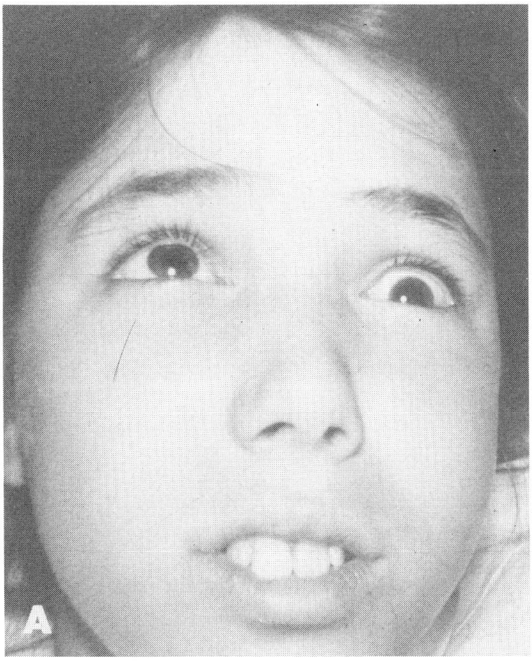

Figure 17–28 *A*, Entrapment of left globe in "blow-out" fracture floor of left orbit. Thirteen-year-old girl seen 5 weeks after injury. Note dilated left pupil and inability to raise globe superiorly on left. Compare position of left pupil with the right pupil on upward gaze. Diplopia is demonstrated on upward gaze. *B*, X-ray tomograms in anteroposterior (left) and lateral (right) views showing defect in orbital floor on the left. *C*, Cranial outer table bone graft for use in floor of left orbit after globe is freed from entrapment. *D*, Postoperative result 7 weeks after surgery.

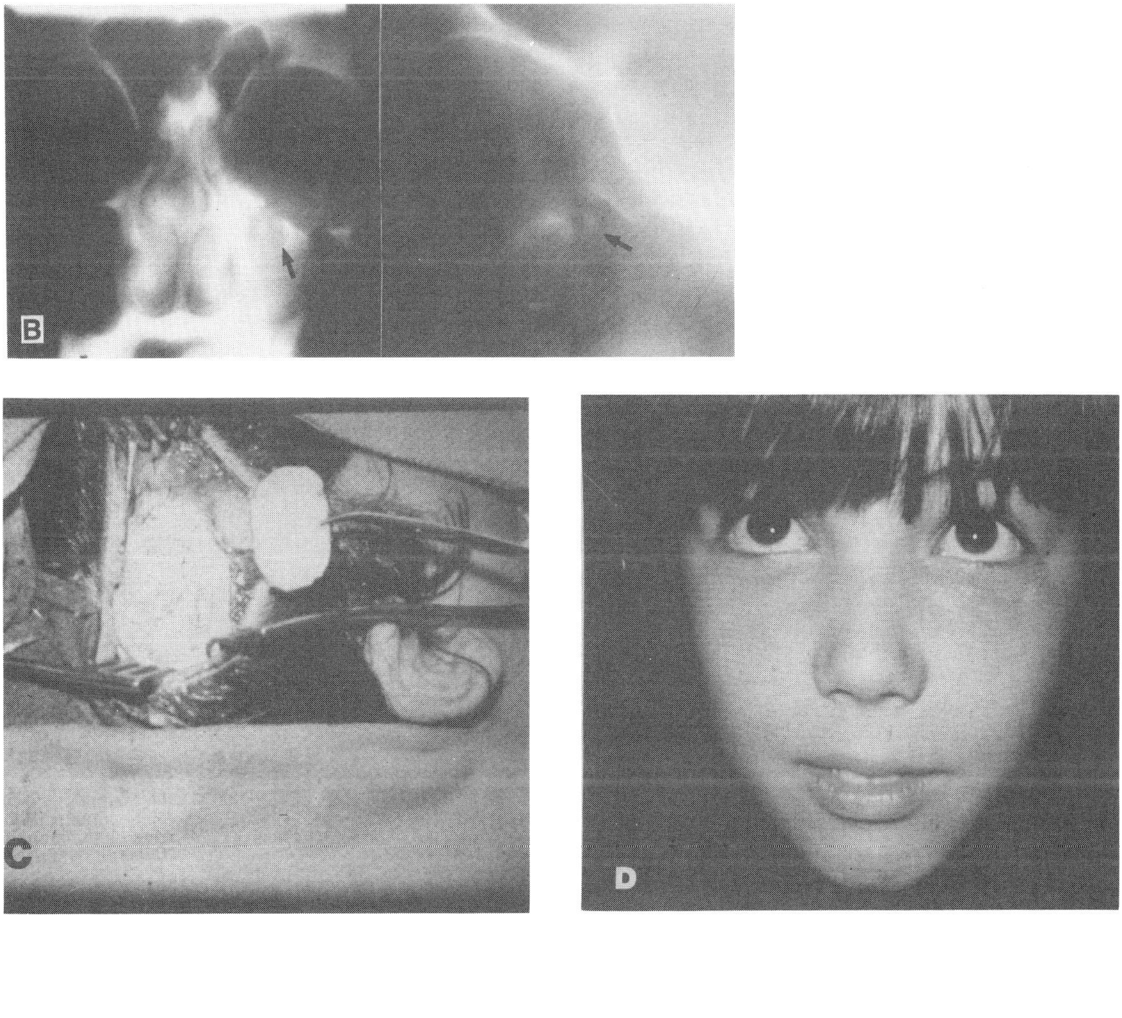

cartilage mainly serves as a mechanical support for the nasal bone and in this regard does not truly appear to be the growth center. However, injury to the septal cartilage or failure to evacuate a septal hematoma can definitely lead to a saddle-nose deformity and lack of normal nasal development. Since the fractured nasal bones heal quite rapidly, it behooves the surgeon to perform reduction within a week to 10 days after the injury. Otherwise there will be malunion of these nasal bones with a resulting nasal deformity.

Following the reduction of a nasal fracture, a nasal splint should be taped in position using transverse adhesive strips and a simple aluminum or plaster splint maintained in position. A septal hematoma is drained through mucosal incisions in a dependent portion of the septum. Where the hematoma is bilateral, a small window of cartilage can be removed from the septum or separate bilateral drainage incisions can be made through the mucoperichondrium.

With an injury occurring on the dorsum of the nose or side to side, the nasal septum can be dislocated and telescoped on itself through fractures in the vomer or in the vertical plate of the ethmoid. The fractured segments should be reduced and realigned with a through-and-through PDS suture which holds the mucoperichondrium or periosteum to help stabilize the fragments. Once the reduction has been completed, the usual nasal gauze packing is placed in each nostril to help maintain the nasal bones in position as well as to maintain the septum as a support for the nasal bones in the midline.

In many instances, not only are the nasal bones comminuted and fractured but the nasofrontal junction may be comminuted and fractured. Where the frontal portions of bone overlie the frontal sinus, a direct surgical approach to the area through an existing laceration can be extended if necessary. Where there is a closed type of injury, a transverse incision at the nasofrontal junction curving upward into the brow can be used to elevate the flap and expose the underlying multiple fractures that are present. Each of the fragments should be carefully preserved and left attached to periosteum. Small wires or PDS suture can be used to suture the bones together through tiny drill holes, which is indeed a tedious task but well worth the time. If these bones are still attached to periosteum and have not penetrated the inner table, simple reapproximation of the bony fragments will result in a well-healed restoration and reconstitution of the normal frontal contour.

Care must be taken to reposition the medial canthal bony attachment, which may be splayed out and in most cases is still attached to the medial canthal ligament. The lateral nasal bone or the nasal process of the maxilla where the medial canthus is attached usually remains attached to the ligament though it may be displaced. It is most important to bring these bones together and to maintain the normal distance between the right and left medial canthal attachments so as not to permit a traumatic telecanthus with widespread nasofrontal areas. To this end, the bones are brought together by through-and-through wires with the use of an external stent (which may be a Silastic button) to maintain compression against the right and left medial canthal attachments and the attached bony portion of the nasofrontal segment.

Nasoethmoidal as well as nasofrontal and maxillary fractures (Fig. 17–29) must be meticulously reduced and fragments realigned so that the medial canthal attachments on both sides can effectively bring the nasal pyramid together at the nasofrontal junction and narrow it to its preinjury state. Reduction and fixation should be maintained for at least 4 weeks from the time of injury. In many cases, the usual incision for exposure of this area does not permit satisfactory access to reduce these fragments. It is necessary to gain experience with a *coronal approach* (or bitemporal-frontal approach) to the site of injury because with this type of exposure the task of restoring the outer frontal table as well as the contour of the nasal frontal area and the entire bony pyramid can be more easily accomplished with access to the entire zone of injury.

COMPLICATIONS

Complications following treatment of facial fractures in children are reported in the series by Kaban and colleagues[3] as being in the neighborhood of 9.8 percent, and in most series the incidence of complications is low. Pulmonary complications may occur at the time of injury or shortly thereafter, or at any time during the period of healing. Airway obstruction postoperatively as well as hemorrhage, shock, and permanent central nervous system damage, including peripheral nerve damage or spinal damage, can occur, but fortunately the incidence is very low. Nonunion of fracture fragments is unusual though it can occur where reduction of the fragments has not been satisfactory and stabilization has been less than acceptable. Osteomyelitis as a result of delayed union or infection is rare but can occur, since all fractures

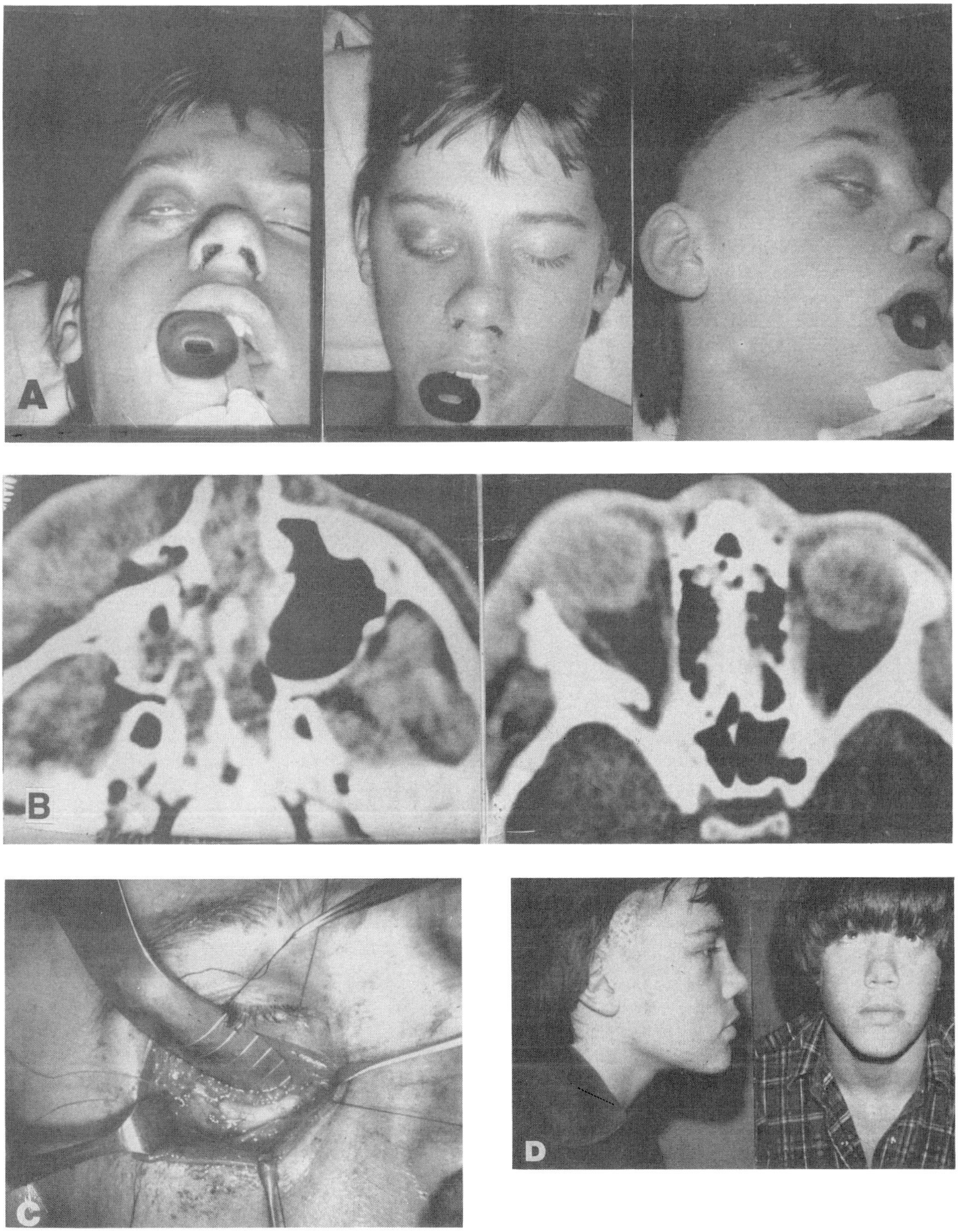

Figure 17–29 Nasoethmoidal, nasomaxillary, nasofrontal, and orbital fractures in a 14-year-old boy. *A*, At time of injury. *B*, Selected computed tomographic scan views. *C*, Intraoperative view of orbitomaxillary segment. *D*, 4 (left) and 10 (right) weeks postoperatively.

involving erupted teeth in the dental fragments are compound fractures. Meticulous care to maintain good oral hygiene postoperatively as well as at the time of the surgical treatment is necessary to avoid complications of infection, which fortunately are also rare.

The possibility of malocclusion, delayed eruption of teeth, and loss of permanent teeth as well as malformed dental follicles should be described to the child's parents prior to any surgical procedure. The complications can occur several years after injury when the permanent dentition erupts.

Interference with growth of the mandible and especially condylar development and development of the nasofrontal segment may also occur in rare instances. This should be considered part of the hazards of any procedure treating fractures in the maxillofacial and craniofacial areas. Ocular injury, permanent diplopia, blindness, injury to the lacrimal drainage apparatus, traumatic telecanthus—all of these are possible complications of injuries involving the maxillofacial and especially the nasofrontal segments.

Open-bite deformity, saddle-nose deformity, infraorbital nerve anesthesia, and anesthesia involving any of the branches of the trigeminal nerve in the areas of the mandible and maxilla can be complications, especially where there is marked comminution and surgical intervention is necessary. In general, the complications resulting from maxillofacial injuries that have been treated in a satisfactory manner are rare.

REFERENCES

1. Bales CR, Randall P, Lehr HB. Fractures of the facial bones in children. J Trauma 1972; 12:56–66.
2. Bernstein L. Maxillofacial injuries in children. Otolaryngol Clin North Am 1969; 2:397–401.
3. Kaban LB, Mulliken JB, Murray JE. Facial fractures in children: an analysis of 122 fractures in 109 patients. Plast Reconstr Surg 1977; 59:15–20.
4. MacLennan WD. Fractures of the mandible in children under the age of six years. Br J Plast Surg 1956; 9:125–128.
5. McCoy FJ, Chandler RA, Crow ML. Facial fractures in children. Plast Reconstr Surg 1966; 37:209–215.
6. Panagopoulos AP. Management of fractures of the jaws in children. J Int Coll Surg 1957; 28:806–815.
7. Rowe NL, Killey HC. Fractures of the facial skeleton. Ed. 1. Baltimore: Williams & Wilkins, 1955.
8. Rowe NL, Killey HC. Fractures of the facial skeleton. Ed. 2. Edinburgh: Churchill Livingstone, 1968.
9. Schultz RC. Pediatric facial fractures. In: Kernahan DA, Thomson HG, Bauer BS, eds. Symposium on pediatric plastic surgery. St. Louis: CV Mosby, 1982:249.

9a. Martin BC, Trabue JC, Leech TR. An analysis of the etiology, treatment and complications of fractures of the malar compound and zygomatic arch. Am J Surg 1956; 92:920–924.

10. Dingman RO. Symposium: malunited fractures of the zygoma: repair of the deformity. Trans Am Acad Ophthalmol Otolaryngol 1953; 57:889–896.
11. Freif MG, Baden E. Management of fractures in children. J Oral Surg 1954; 12:129–139.
12. Rowe NL. Fractures of the facial skeleton in children. J Oral Surg 1968; 26:505–515.
13. Rowe NL, Winter GB. Traumatic lesions of the jaws and teeth. In: Mustardé JC, ed. Plastic surgery in infancy and childhood. Philadelphia: WB Saunders, 1971:154.
14. Schultz RC. Facial injuries. Ed. 2. Chicago: Year Book Medical Publishers, 1977.
15. MacLennan WD. Injuries involving the teeth and jaws in young children. Arch Dis Child 1957; 32:492–494.
16. Lehman JA Jr, Saddawi ND. Fractures of the mandible in children. J Trauma 1976; 16:773–777.
17. MacLennan WD. Consideration of 180 cases of typical fractures of the mandibular condylar process. Br J Plast Surg 1953; 5:122–128.

18

PEDIATRIC TRAUMA: RESULTANT GROWTH CHANGES

DOUGLAS K. OUSTERHOUT, D.D.S., M.D., F.A.C.S.
KARIN VARGERVIK, D.D.S.

Normal growth and development of the craniofacial skeleton is a complex process, beginning with conception. While growth is most active in the early months and years, skeletal and soft tissue changes continue throughout life.[1,2] The interplay between genetic control mechanisms and function in the development of normal skeletal and soft tissue components can also be influenced by numerous pathological conditions, e.g., abnormal metabolism, tumors, and trauma.

While the human body is extremely resilient and usually can recover after trauma without significant long-term adverse effects, there are certain injuries, occurring within specific time frames, that can cause such effects in craniofacial growth and development. Injury to sutural tissue and growth cartilage would seem to be capable of effecting such growth disturbances. Post-traumatic growth disturbances usually involve deficiencies, but excessive growth may also occur.

In this chapter only growth disturbances as a consequence of childhood trauma are discussed. We do not discuss the residual deformities that result from the trauma itself or inadequate treatment following an injury. Also, we do not consider the sequelae of tumorous growth such as fibrous dysplasia, osteoid osteoma, and bone cysts, which in some cases may be the result of trauma and may cause significant deformity.

CHILDHOOD MIDFACIAL FRACTURES

Midfacial trauma is in general quite rare in children. McCoy and colleagues[3] reporting in 1966, stated that only 6 percent of all facial fractures were in children. Of 122 facial fractures reported by Kaban and associates[4] in 1977, none were midfacial except for nasal fractures, which accounted for 55 percent of the total. Only 0.5 percent of childhood facial fractures involved the midface according to a report by Rowe.[5] McCoy and colleagues[3] stated that in their series, of all the facial fractures that occurred in children, approximately 55 percent involved the midfacial area, which did not include nasal fractures treated on an outpatient basis. Based on Kaban and associates'[4] article, one would assume that this represents a significant portion of all facial fractures in children.

Maxillary Hypoplasia Secondary to Midfacial Trauma in Childhood

Converse and Dingman,[6] discussing facial fractures in children, stated that midfacial fractures may explain nasal deviation and nasal-maxillary hypoplasia which would otherwise have no apparent cause. They stated that "underdevelopment, maldevelopment, malocclusion .... are all potential complications of facial bone fractures in children." Unfortunately they do not make any specific statement as to how this opinion regarding hypoplasia following maxillary fractures was derived. McCoy et al, in the article mentioned above,[3] stated that "on the basis of this series, a properly reduced and stabilized facial fracture had no adverse effect on the growth of facial bones." They did not discuss whether cephalometrics were used in their long-term follow-up.

We have previously described three seemingly normal children who had midfacial fractures when they were younger and subsequently developed significant midfacial hypoplasia.[7] There were no preinjury cephalograms that would absolutely confirm that these children had totally normal faces prior to injury, and therefore conclusions reached in this regard were based on the pretrauma history of their normal facial appearance, the family history of normal facial appearances, and the fact that following the original treatment of their facial fractures their facial appearance reportedly was normal. It was only during subsequent craniofacial growth that their midfacial development fell behind.

The three patients reported had different types of fractures, but the common denominator was a fracture involving the midline structures of the midface including the ethmoidal area. We believe that this is a significant factor.

Clinical Example

The patient was 4½ years old when he was hit by a car and suffered multiple facial fractures. He apparently was unconscious for approximately 2 hours. He suffered fractures of both the maxilla and mandible, a nasal fracture, and right orbital fractures. These fractures were treated by open reduction and internal fixation. At that time the treating physician, a plastic surgeon and dentist, felt that the fractures were adequately reduced, the postoperative result was satisfactory, and the occlusion was normal. However, the midface did not develop normally, and significant maxillary hypoplasia with a severe class III malocclusion resulted. At age 14 the mandible was of normal size but the midface was in a markedly retruded position (Fig. 18–1). It was necessary to complete a Le Fort III maxillary advancement to establish a normal facial profile and occlusion. The postsurgical result was satisfactory (Fig. 18–2).

The other two patients in our series have a similar history of trauma in childhood. While their facial fractures were somewhat different, they did have in common fractures of the nasal septal and ethmoidal structures. The second patient, a girl, has had her midfacial advancement (Le Fort III) with an excellent result. The third patient is not old enough at this time, according to our treatment protocol, to have his midfacial Le Fort III advancement surgery. There is no question, however, that it will be necessary.

Diagnosis

Clues to the diagnosis of maxillary hypoplasia secondary to trauma lie in the pretrauma history of normal development, the midfacial trauma in childhood, and the subsequent demonstration of a midfacial growth disturbance. A class III malocclusion with a normal mandible, cheek hypoplasia, and decreased vertical height of the midface and nose are all indicators of a poorly developing maxilla. Cephalometric analysis employing accepted standards[8] should confirm the diagnosis of midfacial hypoplasia.

Treatment

Treatment will depend on the degree of hypoplasia but usually will include orthodontics and midfacial osteotomies, Le Fort III, with or without a Le Fort I procedure. For the optimal result, the surgical procedures should be performed after most of the craniofacial growth has been completed, usually after age 14. The pre- and postoperative care is similar to that recommended for congenital midfacial hypoplasia.[9]

Complications

There have been no complications as a result of this surgical procedure, and the position obtained at operation has been maintained with good aesthetic results, consistent with our Le Fort III advancements in syndrome patients, e.g., Crouzon and Apert.[9,10]

Discussion

Experimental studies in animal models demonstrate many effects of surgical trauma upon midfacial growth and the data are conflicting. Some studies have documented that growth is impaired while other studies have found no growth inhibition.[11,12,13] Munro[14] completed Le Fort I procedures on developing pigs and did not find any evidence of interference of growth. In contrast, recent surgical procedures on monkeys would indicate that surgery does cause growth interference. [illegible] and colleagues[15] have recently shown that midfacial growth was retarded by surgery in adolescent monkeys. The work of Shapiro and associates[12] and Wada and associates[13] is in agreement.

Rock and Brain,[16] in 1983, reported that, in a retrospective study of 29 adults being seen for nasal reconstruction for deformity secondary to childhood nasal injuries, these individuals showed a deficiency in forward growth of the midface when compared with random controls. In none of these 29 individuals was there evidence at the time of injury that damage to tissues outside of the nose had occurred.

Surgery itself must be considered to be a traumatic event. The tissue injuries in midfacial osteotomies are probably little different from those caused by a blunt object. Mullikan and coworkers[17] recently reported on midfacial hypoplasia resulting from the correction of hypertelorbitism in childhood. In all of these cases the upper portion of the septum and the adjacent medial tissues were involved to some degree in the hypertelorbitism repair (Kaban: Personal communication, 1986). This interference in midfacial growth was greater than what would be anticipated in these individuals with already deficient midfacial growth. In children undergoing Le Fort III osteotomies for midfacial hypoplasia secondary to craniosynosto-

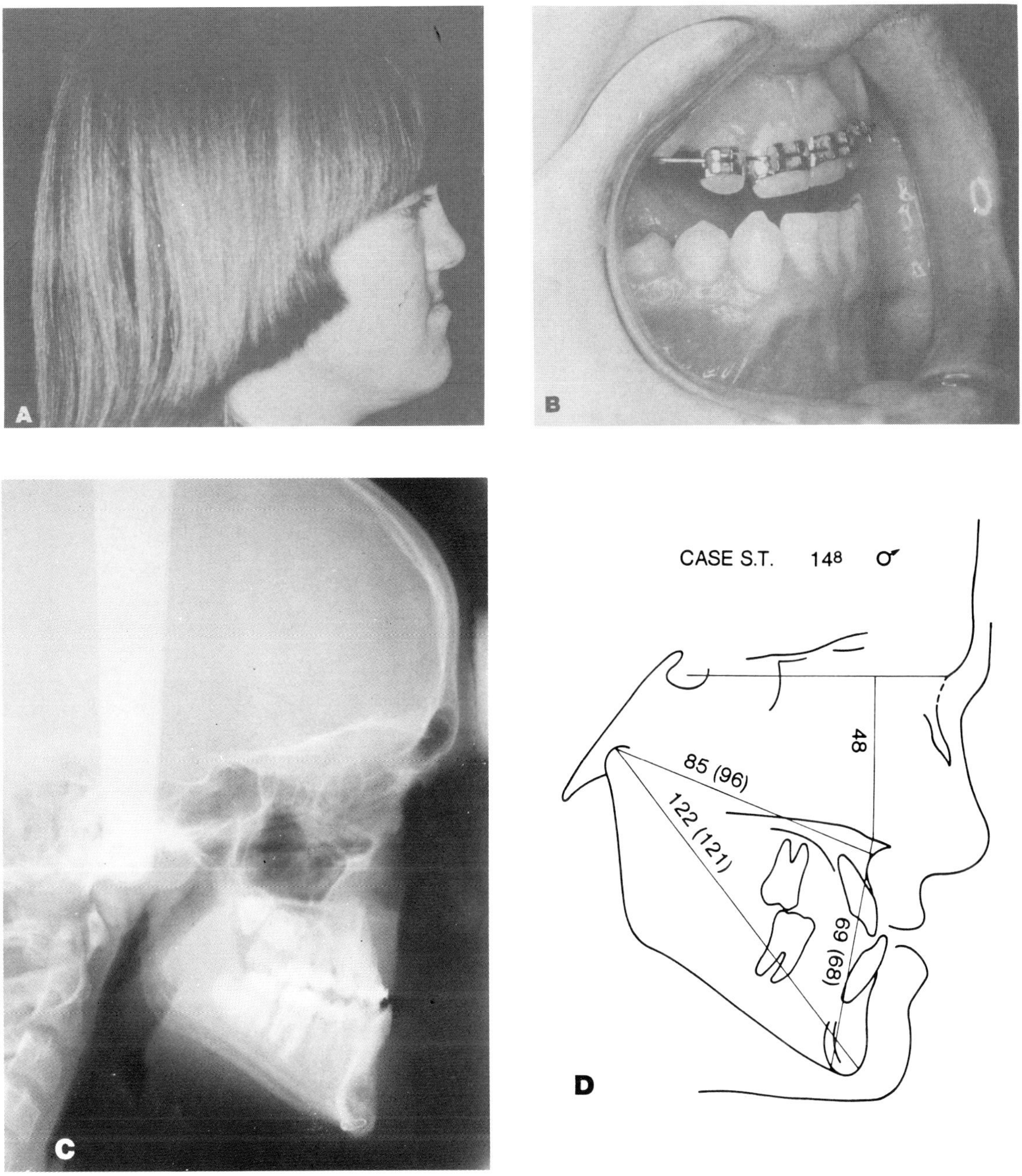

Figure 18–1 Patient at age 14. *A*, Prior to Le Fort III midfacial advancement; note moderate midfacial retrusion. *B*, Preoperative occlusion. *C*, Preoperative lateral cephalogram. *D*, Preoperative lateral cephalogram tracing.

sis syndromes, e.g., Crouzon syndrome, Bachmayer and Ross[18] have shown that the postsurgical midfacial growth will be less than expected were they not operated on, and in actuality they will show very little, if any, additional forward growth.

None of the post-traumatic midfacial hypoplasias we saw were nearly as severe as those seen in the average patient with Crouzon, Pfeiffer, or Apert syndrome. In these congenital conditions the growth disturbance started in utero, while in the

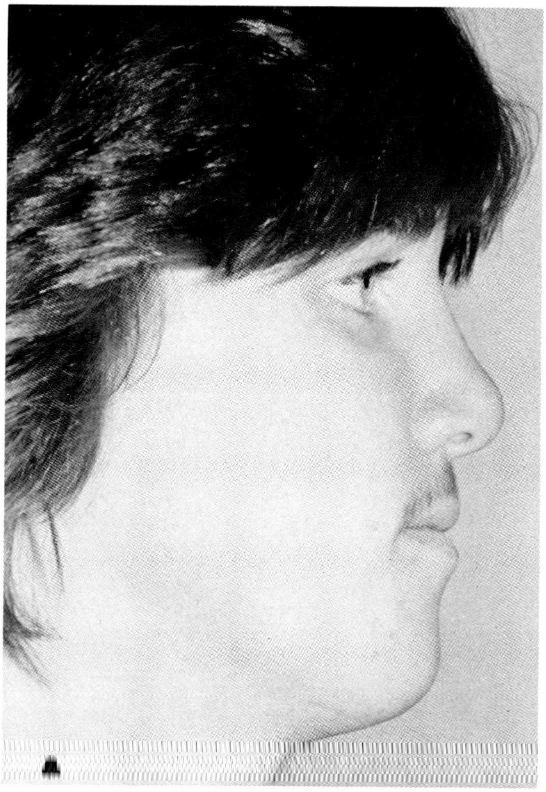

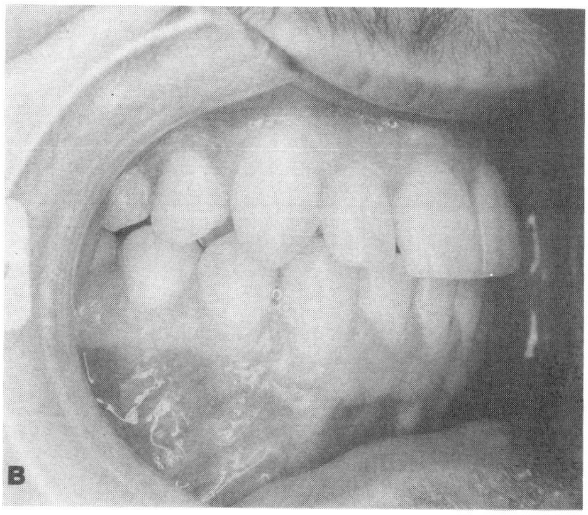

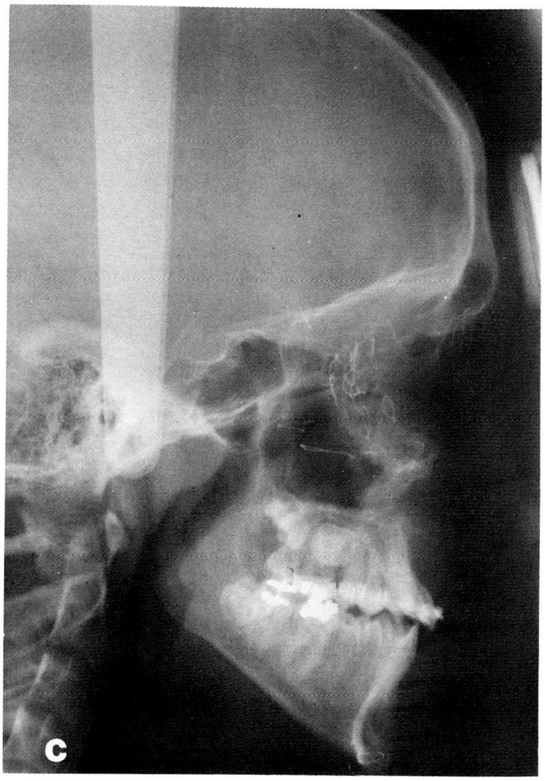

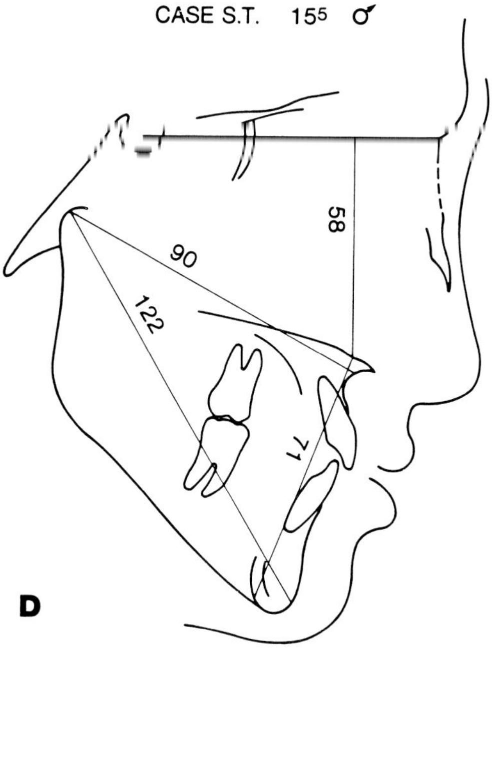

Figure 18–2 Same patient as in Figure 18–1. *A*, Post-operative appearance. *B*, Postoperative occlusion. *C*, Postoperative lateral cephalogram *D*, Postoperative lateral cephalogram tracing.

children with post-traumatic midfacial hypoplasia the injury occurred much later in childhood, well after the majority of normal growth was completed.

Trauma, whether by accident or by surgery, may cause bony bridging across sutures and damage to cartilaginous growth sites, but the exact nature of the traumatic injury is usually not clear. In our cases it cannot be documented that the trauma in childhood was the cause of the deformity (no preinjury cephalograms are available), but this certainly would seem likely.

It is important to recognize that such maldevelopment may occur in spite of the best of treatment. At the present time we do not know that there is anything that a practitioner can do to determine if a post-traumatic deformity will occur and what can be done during the initial treatment to prevent growth aberrations from occurring. It is possible that orthodontic procedures along with midfacial orthopedic maneuvers may be helpful in the early treatment of certain cases. If early diagnosis is made, such techniques could be attempted. Recognition of the possible occurrence of midfacial hypoplasia would seem to be the most important factor to be obtained from a history of such an injury in childhood.

CHILDHOOD NASAL FRACTURES

Nasal fractures are the most common facial fracture in children. Their frequency is not known because probably a considerable number of nasal injuries go undiagnosed and untreated. Kaban and associates[4] reported that 55 percent of the fractures in children were of the nose. The previous section of this chapter described the midfacial deformity occurring as a result of midfacial injury. Rock and Brain[16] studied in particular the midfacial deformity resulting from nasal fracture in childhood. An unresolved question is whether it is possible that nasal fractures can cause developmental deformities within the nose itself. McCoy and colleagues[3] suggested such a complication in their article.

Nasal Hyperplastic Growth Following Trauma in Childhood

Grymer and associates[19] reported on 57 patients who were treated between birth and 16 years of age for nasal fractures by closed reduction techniques. This group was compared with a control group of 50 individuals without a history of nasal trauma. Functional complaints were no different between the two groups, but a considerable number of developmental abnormalities were found in the post-trauma group, including (1) deviations of the osseous and cartilaginous pyramid, (2) dorsal humps, (3) spine formations, and (4) deviations of the septum.

While not discussed in their paper, each of these deformities could have resulted from various causes such as incompletely reduced deformity, but they also could have resulted from hyperplastic growth of bone and/or cartilage. Grymer and coworkers stated that 70 percent of those identified with deviations (bony pyramid or cartilaginous septum) at follow-up reported a satisfactory appearance following fracture reduction. A long nose was the most common late deformity. This deformity appeared at puberty, during the usual rapid adolescent growth spurt. These findings suggest an overactive growth disturbance rather than a postinjury surgical reduction problem.

We have seen numerous adolescents who have had nasal trauma some years before. The history would indicate that at the time of the initial injury, the treatment seemed to reduce the deformity adequately. When they were seen some years later the profile size of the nose was consistent with the hereditary expectations, yet the nose was deviated to one side and internally there was a marked septal deviation. There has been little question that in these individuals the septum had markedly overgrown. With the possible constraints of a post-trauma bony wedge (vomer and perpendicular plate of the ethmoid above and behind and the maxilla below), the quadrilateral cartilage may have had little choice but to buckle and deviate with the overgrowth.

The nose continues to grow throughout life and the amount of growth varies among ethnic groups. The potential for certain cartilages to grow is apparently present throughout life. It is reasonable to consider the possibility of excessive growth following trauma.

Nasal Hypoplastic Growth Following Trauma in Childhood

Grymer and colleagues,[19] mentioned in the section on nasal hyperplasia following trauma, also described saddle deformities resulting from injury. The most likely cause is inadequate surgical reduction, but the possibility of hypoplastic cartilaginous growth must be considered.

The work of Sarnat[20] on nasal and maxillary growth following trauma, while not totally consistent with other studies, is very interesting and of marked importance. The experimental model is obviously a very difficult one. Sarnat has not only shown maxillary hypoplasia secondary to septal experimental surgery but cartilage hypoplasia as a result of injury as well.

Discussion

It would appear that the nasal septal area may be very vulnerable to trauma. It is certainly conceivable that growth could be either retarded or stimulated as a result of injuries to the cartilages. It is not possible to determine from published clinical studies[19,21] whether the deformities described are the result of a growth disturbance or not. Considerably more needs to be studied in this regard. Long-term prospective studies of a large patient population may be more fruitful than laboratory studies.

CHILDHOOD MANDIBULAR FRACTURES

Like the nose, the mandible is a much more common site of injury in children than the midfacial area. McCoy and colleagues[3] found that of all facial fractures in that area, only 6 percent were in children. Kaban and associates[4] described a 32 percent incidence of mandibular fractures among all facial fractures in children 15 years of age and younger. The sex distribution was equal.

The most commonly recognized long-term complication of mandibular trauma in childhood is unilateral or bilateral ankylosis with resulting mandibular hypoplasia. Much less commonly recognized is the condition of condylar hyperplasia following trauma. Sections on both of these conditions follow.

Mandibular Hypoplasia Secondary to Trauma in Childhood

According to published long-term follow-up records of children who suffer condylar fractures, approximately 25 percent demonstrate deficient mandibular growth, while the majority will have regeneration of the condylar process and re-establishment of adequate function.[22] If function is impaired with restriction of mandibular movements, reduced growth of that side of the mandible must be anticipated. In the majority of mandibular trauma cases the fracture is unilateral and at the neck of the condyle. If the fracture site is below the attachment area of the lateral pterygoid muscle, the condylar fragment will usually be dislocated medially and anteriorly by the lateral pterygoid muscle pull as the muscle shortens. The dislocated fragment generally resorbs and a new condylar process may regenerate toward the glenoid fossa. It is likely that many condylar fractures go undiagnosed because the symptoms often are mild.

Restoration of a new condyle and normal function does not always occur, and mandibular growth deficiency and concomitant unfavorable maxillary adaptations may result. A comprehensive overview of the growth effects and treatment of early condylar fractures has been presented by Proffit and colleagues.[23]

The damage to the mandibular condyle and joint structures may be more extensive than just a condylar fracture, and the subsequent healing of damaged tissues may result in fibrous or bony ankylosis. A combination of these two types of interfaces may even develop, as seen in Figure 18–3.

Clinical Examples

The records of the 9-year-old boy shown in Figure 18–3 were obtained 3 years after a car accident that caused a left condylar fracture and presumably additional damage to temporomandibular joint tissues. No treatment was instituted after the accident. The condylar fragment became ankylosed to the glenoid fossa, most likely following the development of a hematoma that organized into fibrous tissue and bone. The mandible, which was not stabilized after the accident, continued to function and the movements resulted in the development of a pseudoarticulation in the fracture site (see Fig. 18–3A). This tight fibrous union allowed only minimal rotational movement and no forward translation. Untreated, this condition did not allow any further growth of the mandible on that side and mandibular and maxillary asymmetry developed as the normal side continued to grow (see Fig. 18–3B, D).

At the time of the first visit to our clinic, 3 years after the trauma, jaw opening was severely restricted. The left (fractured) side of the mandible was approximately 10 mm shorter than the right, the chin was positioned to the left of the face midline, and the maxillary occlusal plane was canted. The recommendation was to surgically remove the ankylosed condyle and to start treatment with a functional appliance. The condyle was not removed, however, and it was then decided to start treatment with a spring-loaded appliance that forced the jaws apart and was adjusted to hold the affected side forward. This appliance was worn evenings and nights for 2½ years with the result

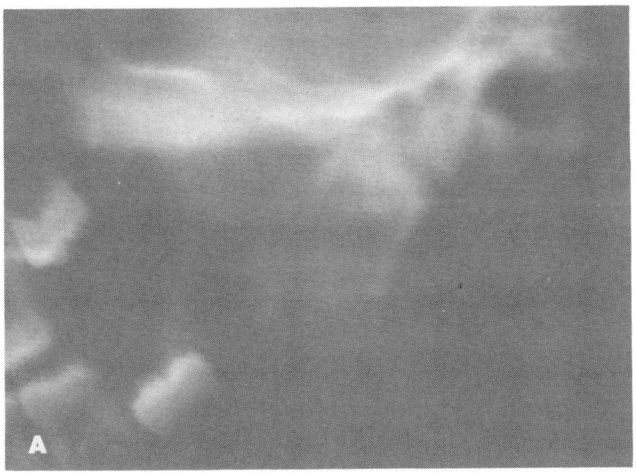

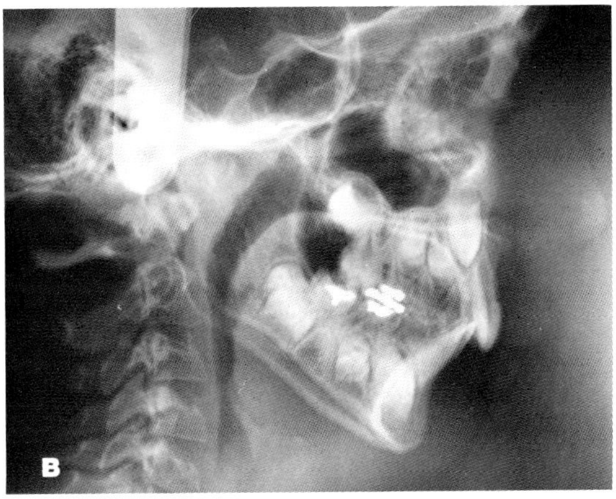

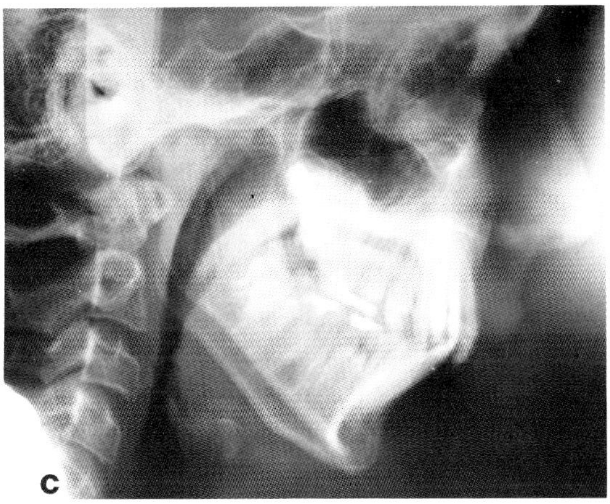

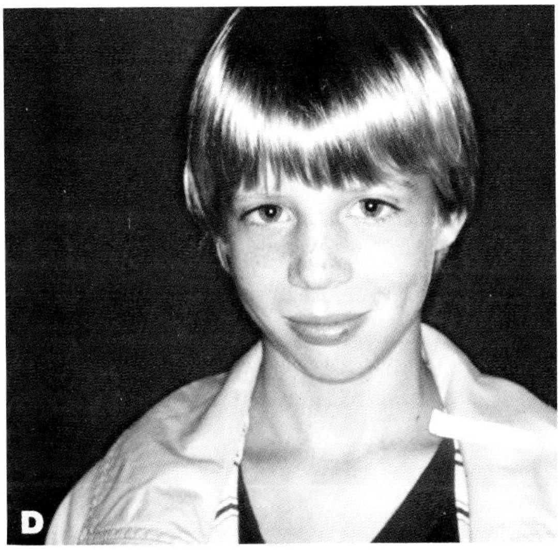

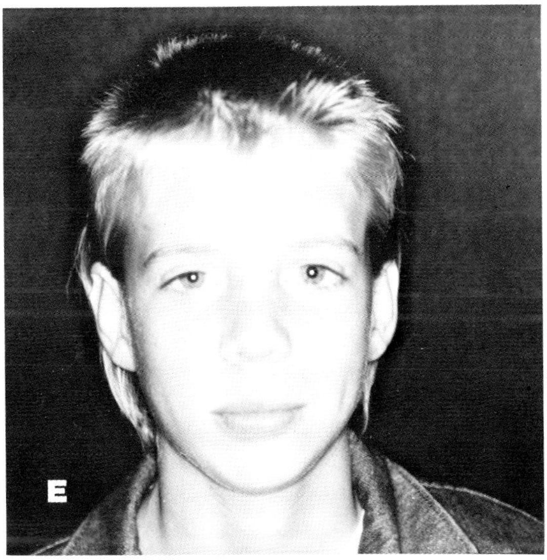

Figure 18–3 *A*, Tomogram of fractured and ankylosed mandibular condyle three years after the injury, which occurred when this boy was 6 years old. A pseudoarticulation has developed between the distal and proximal segments. During jaw opening a slight movement takes place between the two segments, allowing slight opening but no forward translation. *B*, Lateral head film obtained three years after trauma demonstrates reduced ramus height on the damaged side and class II jaw relationship. *C*, Lateral head film obtained 2½ years later, following the use of a functional appliance, shows improvement in jaw relationship but persistence of ramus height deficiency. *D*, Three years after mandibular injury, before any treatment had been instituted. *E*, Following 2½ years of functional appliance treatment the position of the mandible has improved and the mandibular asymmetry is less apparent.

that the ankylosed side did increase 12 mm in length, the same amount of growth as the normal side, and the asymmetry did not increase. The treatment resulted in improved jaw relationship and clinically the chin became positioned closer to the face midline (see Fig. 18–3C, E). Jaw movements are still restricted, however, and surgery to create a better functioning temporomandibular joint is still indicated.

Trauma to the mandible may cause similar injury to both temporomandibular joints, and the effects on the growth of the mandible and maxilla may be bilateral and symmetric, as seen in the child shown in Fig. 18–4. This child suffered major craniofacial injuries at age 4. The hospital records describe a fracture of the mandible in the area of the right cuspid, but condylar fractures were not noted. Radiographs of the skull and temporomandibular joints were obtained during his first visit to our clinic, 1½ years after the accident (see Fig. 18–4A, B). It can be seen on the tomograms that the jaw could rotate open, but forward movements of the condyles did not occur during jaw opening. The lack of anterior translation could be due to tight fibrous scar tissue that developed subsequent to the trauma combined with reduced lateral pterygoid muscle function. The fibrous ankylosis resulted in lack of growth of the mandible (see Fig. 18–4C). A severe overjet developed and it became difficult to achieve lip closure over the maxillary teeth. The lower lip started to function behind the maxillary incisors, causing them to become more protrusive and allowing them to overextrude (see Fig. 18–4D). Treatment for this child required extraction of maxillary bicuspids, orthodontic coordination of the dental arches, and surgical advancement of the mandible with reconstruction of temporomandibular joints using cartilage. The use of a functional appliance under these circumstances is not effective in increasing mandibular length because the mandible cannot be held in a forward position by the appliance. An optimal treatment approach for this child would have been a surgical release and advancement of the mandible at an earlier stage, preventing some of the unfavorable maxillary adaptations. A disadvantage with early mandibular advancement is the uncertainty that still exists with regard to subsequent mandibular growth of the lengthened rami through the rest of the growth period.

General Treatment Considerations

To minimize growth disturbances, function of the mandible should be restored as soon as possible following an injury. If the occlusion is intact and function, including translatory movements, is restored, it can be expected that the injured condyle will remodel and continue to grow. Under such circumstances continued growth can be enhanced by the use of a functional appliance.[24] If, after the initial healing, mandibular movements are restricted and the joint structures do not allow forward movement of the mandible, it must be anticipated that further mandibular growth will be minimal. Undesirable dentoalveolar adaptations will occur in response to the diminished and asymmetric growth of the mandible. Under those circumstances, surgical release of the restrictions with or without reconstruction of the jaw and placement of a bone graft must be considered. If mandibular deficiency exists when growth is completed, a surgical lengthening may be indicated at that time.

Mandibular Hyperplasia Secondary to Trauma in Childhood

Jacobsen and Lund[25] reported two carefully analyzed cases of children who had unilateral fractures of the condylar neck. In both of these cases there was a resulting ipsilateral overgrowth of the mandible with gross asymmetry. Their findings were clearly illustrated using cephalometric data. Lund, in a more extensive study,[26] followed the mandibular development into adolescence in 38 children who suffered condylar fractures at a younger age. Interestingly, in 78 percent of these patients there was accelerated mandibular growth on the side of the fracture that can best be termed compensatory growth. This compensatory growth was most dramatic during adolescence. Thirty percent of these patients developed an overgrowth with resulting asymmetric mandibular hypertrophy on the side of the fracture. Lund's study showed that in a majority of cases of condylar fractures in children there is a period of accelerated mandibular growth on the side of the injury. This active phase could go on to overgrowth and asymmetry. Unfortunately the article did not state the incidence of clinically significant malformation as a result of condylar trauma in children with mandibular injuries.

Proffit and associates in 1980 presented a discussion of Lund's findings but used only those cases of hypoplastic mandibular growth following condylar fracture, a pattern that Lund identified as occurring in 2 percent of the group. We could find no other papers documenting condylar trauma as a cause for condylar hyperplasia and resulting mandibular asymmetry.

In each of our three patients previously

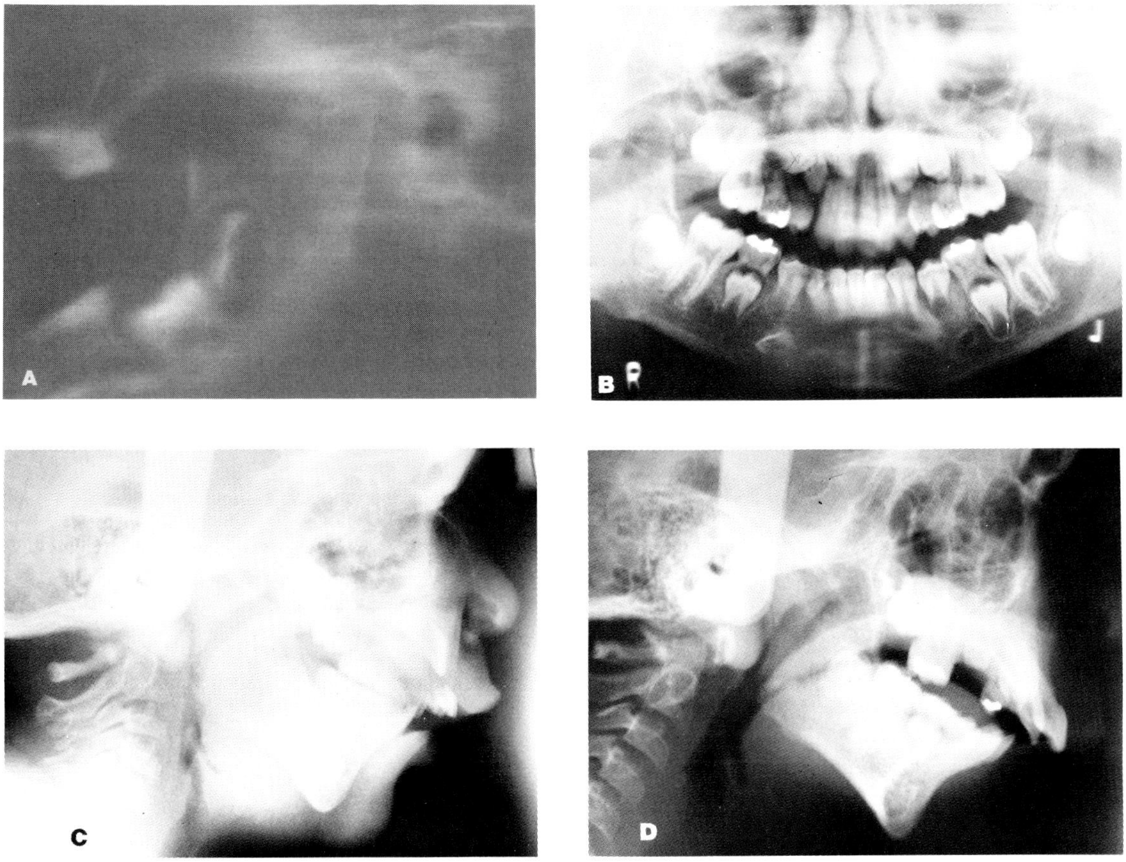

Figure 18–4 *A*, Tomogram of the right side obtained 1½ years after trauma to the mandible at age 4. During jaw opening the malformed condylar process rotates but does not translate forward. *B*, Panoramic radiograph demonstrates condylar hypoplasia bilaterally. *C*, Lateral head film obtained 1½ years after the accident demonstrates severely underdeveloped mandible with developing maxillary excess. *D*, Five years later the mandible has grown only minimally while the maxilla has continued to overdevelop.

reported[27] there is a history of significant mandibular injury but there is no documentation of condylar fractures. If fractures occurred they were missed, not recorded, or were not evident in the initial radiographic evaluation. The condylar hyperplasia and the resulting mandibular asymmetry that resulted could possibly be the result of compressive or rotational trauma and may even occur as a contrecoup injury. As described in the section on mandibular hypoplasia, the injury to tissues may be less where a fracture occurred than in nonfracture cases. The incidence of mandibular asymmetry secondary to a condylar injury may be as high as 30 percent.

The deformity resulting from condylar hyperplasia affects the mandibular condyle itself, the ramus and body, and also the maxilla where secondary adaptations occur. The condyle becomes enlarged and may become displaced out of the glenoid fossa, resulting in partial subluxation. With the increased size there will be a vertical change which will lower the body of the mandible on that side, causing the occlusal plane to be asymmetrically lowered also. In addition there may be bone apposition on the inferior border of the mandible, lowering it even farther. The chin becomes deviated to the opposite side (Figs. 18–5, 18–6).

The maxillary adaptations consist mainly of increased alveolar bone height on the ipsilateral side. As the mandibular occlusal level becomes lower with the developing condylar hyperplasia, the maxillary alveolar process follows the development in order to maintain occlusion. The result is an increase in alveolar bone height. In addition, the

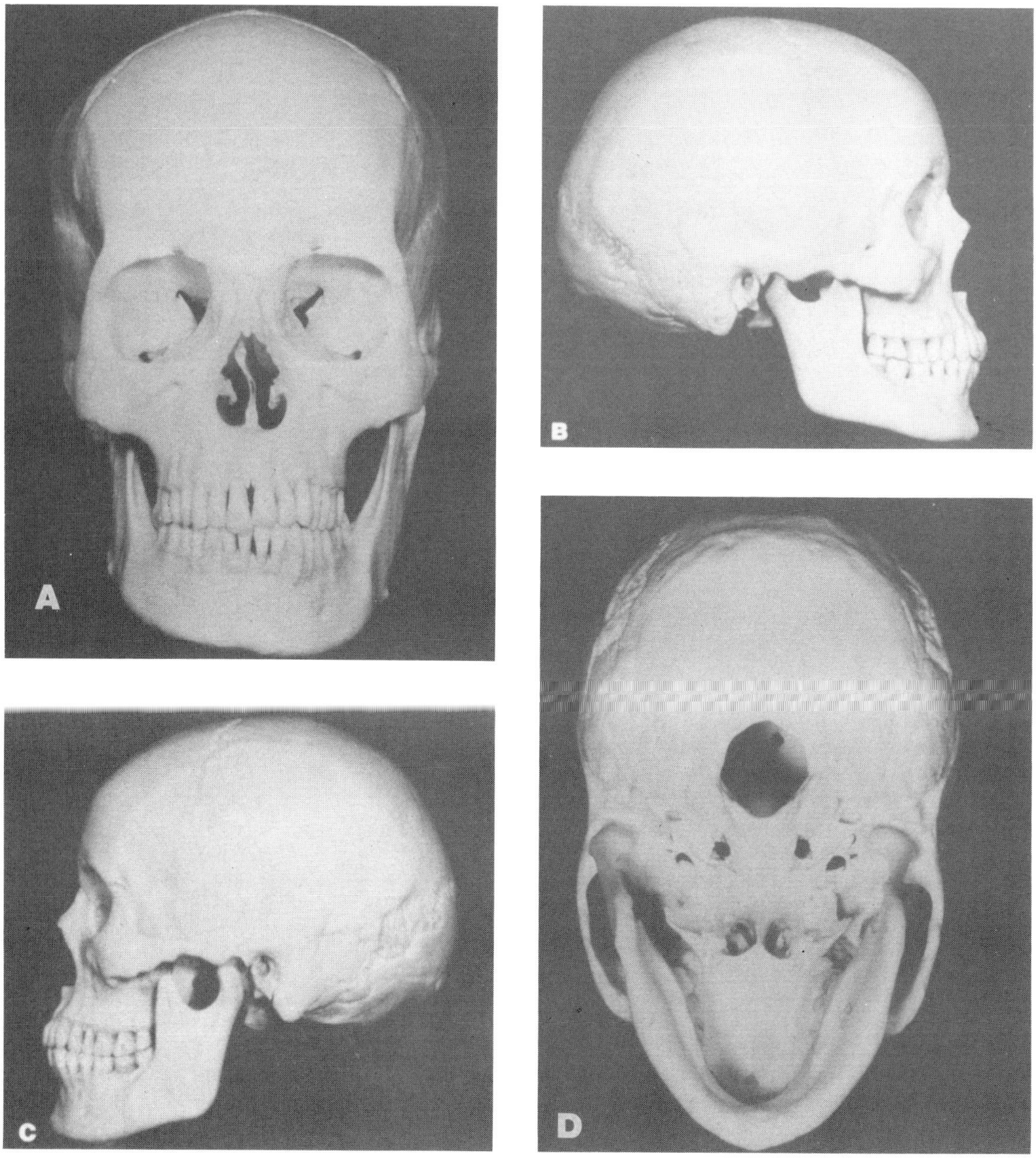

Figure 18–5 *A–D*, This series of four views of the same skeleton shows exactly the same deformities seen in condylar hyperplasia. This skeleton is in the Arne Bjork skull collection, Royal Dental College, Copenhagen, Denmark.

nasal floor on the ipsilateral side may become somewhat lower if the mandibular overgrowth starts early in the growing child. If the condylar hyperplasia occurs very rapidly, the dental adaptations cannot maintain the occlusal relationship and an open bite or cross bite may develop.

We have seen condylar hyperplasia without a history of trauma which has very similar morphologic characteristics. In these cases there is usually a generalized hemifacial hyperplasia involving all tissue elements. For example, the eye on the ipsilateral side may be elevated compared with the contralateral side and the adjacent ear may have a longer vertical measurement. There may be a familial hisory of hyperplasia in some portion of the body, not just the face.

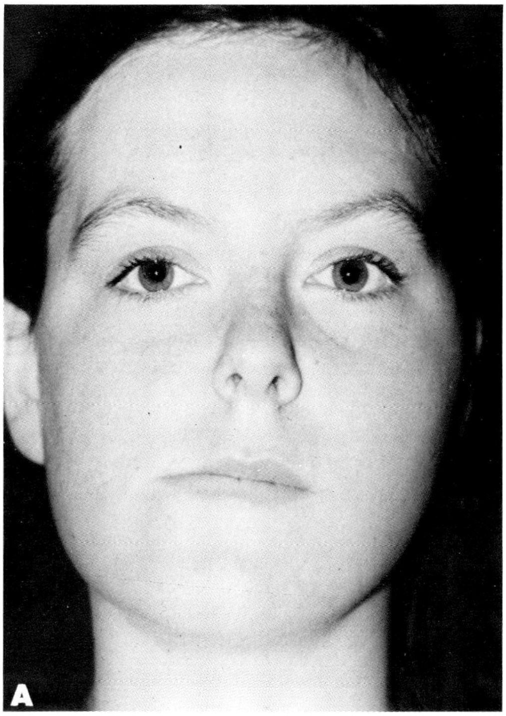

Clinical Example

In 1978, a 14-year-old girl was involved in a motor vehicle accident in which she sustained blunt facial trauma. No fractures were identified at that time. Within a year she demonstrated gross mandibular asymmetry. None of her routine dental examinations prior to the accident showed mandibular bony deformities. By 1979, radiographs demonstrated left condylar hyperplasia and relative enlargement of the left side of the mandible, and the chin deviated to the right of the midline (see Fig. 18–6A, B). By 1980 the condylar hypertrophy had caused a displacement of the condylar head from the glenoid fossa.

Following orthodontic treatment, the patient underwent first a Dautrey arthroplasty to stabilize the condylar head in the glenoid fossa, and six months later a bilateral sagittal split of the mandible to correct the skeletal asymmetry. A symmetric appearance and satisfactory occlusion resulted (see Fig. 18–6C).

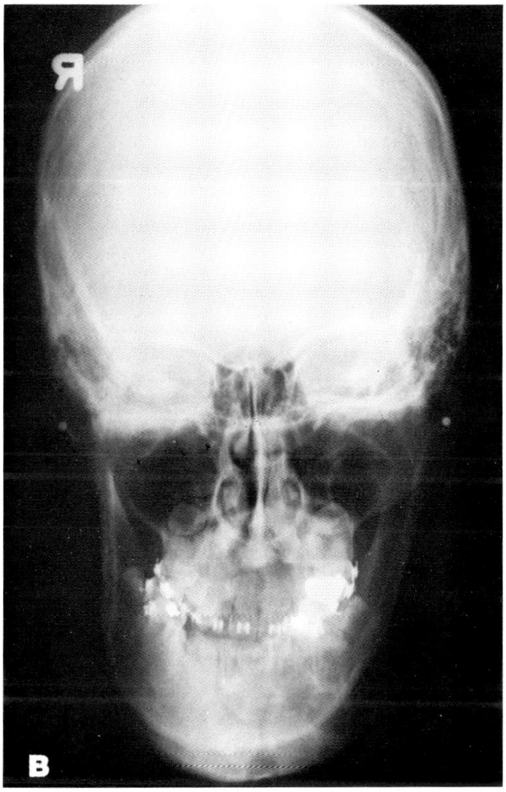

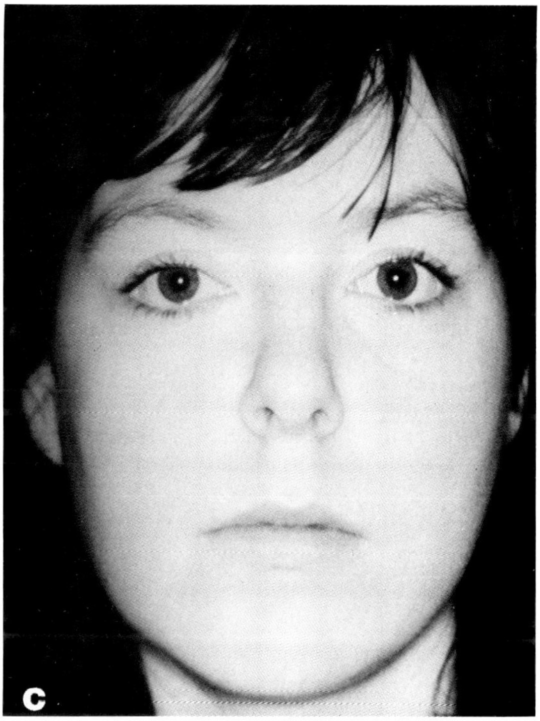

Figure 18–6 *A*, Patient at age 16; note the lower facial asymmetry. *B*, Posteroranterior cephalogram showing skeletal asymmetry. *C*, Postoperative view demonstrating improved appearance.

Treatment

Treatment of these deformities has primarily consisted of a unilateral or, if necessary, bilateral mandibular sagittal split to allow elevation and rotation of the mandible to a more normal position. If necessary, a simultaneous Le Fort I procedure elevating the ipsilateral side is also completed.

The inferior border of the mandible on the ipsilateral side can be reduced, but as the inferior alveolar nerve seems to run close to the inferior cortical bone, the reduction is limited unless the nerve is carefully dissected free from the bone. We have not completed this maneuver. A reduction of the inferior border of the mandible is usually not very successful, as the soft tissue does not come up following the bone reduction as one would like. A sliding, asymmetric genioplasty may be very helpful in these individuals for final adjustment of the facial profile and symmetry.[28]

It is not known what might be done to prevent progression of the deformity if the diagnosis is made early in the development of the condition. Surgery on the condylar head growth cartilage might be considered.

Complications

There have not been any complications as a result of these surgeries. The position of the mandible has been nicely maintained with the techniques we use in our hemifacial microsomia patients for establishing bony union.[29]

REFERENCES

1. Behrents RG. An atlas of growth in the aging craniofacial skeleton. Monograph 18, Craniofacial Growth Series. Ann Arbor: Center for Human Growth and Development, 1985:160.
2. Enlow DH. Handbook of facial growth. Control process in facial growth. Philadelphia: WB Saunders, 1982:486.
3. McCoy FJ, Chandler RA, Crow ML. Facial fractures in children. Plast Reconstr Surg 1966; 37:209–215.
4. Kaban LB, Mulliken JB, Murray JE. Facial fractures in children, an analysis of 122 fractures in 109 patients. Plast Reconstr Surg 1977; 59:15–20.
5. Rowe NL. Fractures of the jaws in children. J Oral Surg 1969; 27:497–506.
6. Converse JM, Dingman RO. Facial injuries in children. In: Converse JM, ed. Reconstructive plastic surgery. Philadelphia: WB Saunders, 1977:794.
7. Ousterhout DK, Vargervik K. Maxillary hypoplasia secondary to midfacial trauma in childhood. Plast Reconstr Surg 1987; 80:491–497.
8. Harvold EP, Vargervik K. Morphogenetic response to activator treatment. Am J Orthod 1971; 60:478–490.
9. Ousterhout DK, Vargervik K, Clark S. Stability of the maxilla after Le Fort III advancement in craniosynostosis syndromes. Cleft Palate J (Suppl) 1986; 23:91–101.
10. Ousterhout DK, Vargervik K. Aesthetic improvement resulting from craniofacial surgery in craniosynostosis syndromes. J Craniomaxillofac Surg 1987; 15:189–197.
11. Freihofer HPM. The timing of facial osteotomies in children and adolescents. Clin Plast Surg 1982; 9:445–456.
12. Shapiro PA, Kokich VG, Hohl TH, Low C. The effects of early Le Fort I osteotomies on craniofacial growth of juvenile Macaca nemestrea monkeys. Am J Orthod 1981; 79:492–499.
13. Wada T, Kremenak CR, Miyazaki T. Midfacial growth effects of surgical trauma to the area of the vomer in beagles. J Osaka University Dental School 1980; 20:241–276.
14. Munro IR. The effect of total maxillary advancement on facial growth. Plast Reconstr Surg 1986; 62:751–762.
15. Nanda R, Bouayad O, Topozian RG. Facial growth subsequent to Le Fort I osteotomies in adolescent monkeys. J Oral Maxillofac Surg 1987; 45:123–136.
16. Rock WP, Brain DJ. The effects of nasal trauma during childhood upon growth of the nose and midface. Br J Orthod 1983; 10:38–41.
17. Mulliken JB, Kaban LB, Evans CA, et al. Facial skeleton changes following hypertelorbitism correction. Plast Reconstr Surg 1986; 77:7–16.
18. Bachmayer D, Ross RB. Stability of Le Fort III advancement surgery in children with Crouzon's, Apert's and Pfeiffer's syndromes. Cleft Palate J (Suppl) 1986; 23:69–74.
19. Grymer LF, Gutierrez C, Stoksted P. Nasal fractures in childhood: influence on development of the nose. J Laryngol Otol 1985; 99:735–739.
20. Sarnat BG. The postnatal maxillary-nasal-orbital complex: some considerations in experimental surgery. In: McNamara JA Jr. Factors affecting the growth of the midface. Monograph 6, Craniofacial Growth Series. Ann Arbor: Center for Human Growth and Development, 1976:399.
21. Mann W, Jonas I, Schlenter WW, Meltzer-Splitt B. The development of the nose following trauma in the growing stage. Laryngol Rhinol Otol (Stuttg) 1983; 62:266–269.
22. Gilhuus-Moe O. Fractures of the mandibular condyle in the growth period. Stockholm: Scand Univ Books Universitetsforlaget, 1969.
23. Proffit WR, Vig KWL, Turvey TA. Early fractures of the mandibular condyles: frequently an unsuspected cause of growth disturbances. Am J Orthod 1980; 78:1–24.
24. Vargervik K. Appliances utilized in the treatment of hemifacial microsomia. In: Harvold EP, Vargervik K,

Chierici G, eds. Treatment of hemifacial microsomia New York: Alan R Liss, 1983:139.

25. Jacobsen PV, Lund K. Unilateral overgrowth and remodeling processes after fracture of the mandibular condyle. Scand J Dent Res 1972; 80:68–74.
26. Lund K. Mandibular growth and remodelling processes after mandibular fractures. Acta Odontol Scand 1974; 32:(Suppl 64) 117.
27. Lineaweaver W, Vargervik K, Tomer BS, Ousterhout DK. Post traumatic condylar hyperplasia. Plast Reconstr Surg (in press).
28. Thompson ERE. Sagittal genioplasty: a new technique of genioplasty. Br J Plast Surg 1985; 38:70–74.
29. Vargervik K, Ousterhout DK, Farias M. Factors affecting long-term resulting in hemifacial microsomia. Cleft Palate J (Suppl) 1986; 23:53–68.

INDEX